Working with Children and Adolescents

A Guide for the Occupational Therapy Assistant

Janet V. DeLany, DEd, OTR/L, FAOTA

Associate Professor
Department of Occupational Therapy and Occupational Science
Towson University
Towson, Maryland

Margaret J. Pendzick, MOT, OTR/L, BCP

Senior Instructor
Occupational Therapy Assistant Program
The Pennsylvania State University, DuBois Campus
DuBois, Pennsylvania

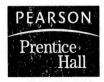
PEARSON
Prentice
Hall

Upper Saddle River, New Jersey 07458

Library of Congress Cataloging-in-Publication Data

DeLany, Janet V.
  Working with children and adolescents : a guide for the occupational therapy assistant / Janet V. DeLany, Margaret J. Pendzick.
    p. ; cm.
  Includes bibliographical references and index.
  ISBN-13: 978-0-13-171917-0
  ISBN-10: 0-13-171917-3
  1. Occupational therapy for children.   2. Occupational therapy for teenagers. [DNLM: 1. Occupational Therapy—methods. 2. Adolescent Development. 3. Adolescent. 4. Child Development. 5. Child. 6. Disabled Children—rehabilitation. WS 368 D337w 2008] I. Pendzick, Margaret J. II. Title.
  RJ53.O25D45 2008
  615.8`2'083—dc22

                      2007035117

Notice: The authors and publisher of this volume have taken care that the information and technical recommendations contained herein are based on research and expert consultation, and are accurate and compatible with the standards generally accepted at the time of publication. Nevertheless, as new information becomes available, changes in clinical and technical practices become necessary. The reader is advised to carefully consult manufacturers' instructions and information material for all supplies and equipment before use, and to consult with a healthcare professional as necessary. This advice is especially important when using new supplies or equipment for clinical purposes. The authors and publisher disclaim all responsibility for any liability, loss, injury, or damage incurred as a consequence, directly or indirectly, of the use and application of any of the contents of this volume.

Publisher: Julie Levin Alexander
Executive Editor: Mark Cohen
Associate Editor: Melissa Kerian
Editorial Assistant: Nicole Ragonese
Managing Editor for Production: Patrick Walsh
Production Liaison: Christina Zingone
Production Editor: Karen Berry, Pine Tree Composition
Manufacturing Manager: Ilene Sanford
Manufacturing Buyer: Pat Brown

Design Director: Jayne Conte
Cover Designer: Bruce Kenselaar
Director of Marketing: Karen Allman
Senior Marketing Manager: Harper Coles
Marketing Specialist: Michael Sirinides
Marketing Assistant: Wayne Celia
Composition: Pine Tree Composition, Inc.
Printer/Binder: Hamilton Printing
Cover Printer: Coral Graphics

Cover Photos: Young girl arranges blue and white tiles, David Mager/Pearson Learning Photo Studio; Two girls making cakes, Vanessa Davies © Dorling Kindersley; Boy in wheelchair, Richard Haynes/Prentice Hall School Division; Girl standing by plant, Susanna Price © Dorling Kindersley.

Pearson Education Ltd., *London*
Pearson Education Australia Pty. Limited, *Sydney*
Pearson Education Singapore, Pte. Ltd.
Pearson Education North Asia Ltd., *Hong Kong*
Pearson Education Canada, Ltd., *Toronto*
Pearson Educación de Mexico, S.A. de C.V.
Pearson Education—Japan, *Tokyo*
Pearson Education Malaysia, Pte. Ltd.
Pearson Education, Upper Saddle River, New Jersey

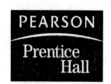

PEARSON
Prentice
Hall

10 9 8 7 6 5 4 3 2 1

ISBN-13: 978-0-13-171917-0
ISBN-10: 0-13-171917-3

Contents

Section II   Occupations of Children and Adolescents

Section IV   Implementing Occupational Therapy Interventions for Children and Adolescents

Contents

Appendices

Preface

The idea for this text emerged from many years of teaching occupational therapy assistant students about occupational therapy practice for children and adolescents. As have many other educators teaching in occupational therapy assistant programs, we struggled during those years to find texts and learning resources for our students that concurrently examined the occupations of children and adolescents, the interface between growth and development of the children and adolescents and their occupational capacities, and the use of occupation-based conceptual models to work with children and adolescents. Appreciating that more than 25 percent of occupational therapy assistants work with children and adolescents, we endeavored to write a text that occupational therapy assistants could use to think about and provide services to children and adolescents in a manner consistent with best practice models.

We assume that students using this text will have taken courses about the history and philosophy of occupational therapy, and about human growth and development. Rather than reiterating what occupational therapy assistant students already learned, we have tried to expand upon this by providing multiple examples of application for children and adolescents. This text is divided into four sections. Each section serves as a building block for the next section. Section I provides an overview of occupational therapy for children and adolescents. Chapter 1 examines the domain and process of occupational therapy practice and the value of occupations for the health and well-being of children and adolescents. It emphasizes the importance of family and culture in the therapeutic process. Chapter 2 addresses the importance of using occupation-based conceptual models to guide occupational therapy practice decisions, and illustrates how to use four different occupation-based conceptual models to work with children and adolescents. Chapter 3 reviews several non–occupation-based frames of reference frequently used with children and adolescents, and how to incorporate them into occupational therapy practice to foster best practice methods. Chapter 4 provides an overview of various practice settings that focus on children and adolescents, and the roles of the occupational therapists and occupational therapy assistants working in these practice settings. The chapter concludes with a discussion about the elements and importance of the supervisory relationship between the occupational therapy and the occupational therapy assistant.

Section II focuses on the occupations of children and adolescents within the context of their developmental capacities. This section is divided into four chapters; each of these contains vignettes about children and adolescents engaging in multiple occupations throughout various developmental stages. The vignettes provide a backdrop for exploring how cognitive, physical, social, emotional, and contextual factors interact to influence the occupational performance of children and adolescents. Developmental charts highlight the major milestones of development. Chapter 5 focuses on how development influences the occupations of infants and toddlers. Chapters 6 and 7 examine the interplay between development and occupations of young children and school age children. Chapter 8 explores the relationship between development and the occupations of adolescents.

Section III focuses on the delivery of occupational therapy services that is grounded in knowledge about occupations, occupation-based and non–occupation-based conceptual models, and the occupational development of children and adolescents. Chapter 9 describes the evaluation process. It outlines areas within the domain of occupational therapy practice to evaluate, and delineates systematic steps to follow to gather and organize the evaluation data. It takes into account how the children's and adolescents' stages of development, their performance skills, the tasks they need to perform, and the context in which they perform their occupations influence the evaluation process. Chapter 10 outlines the general principles for providing occupation-based interventions for children and adolescents. This chapter addresses the general goals for occupational therapy intervention, and the role of occupational therapy assistants in the intervention planning and implementation. It considers the appropriateness of directing interventions toward the person, the occupations, and the environment; it also examines the use of preparatory activities, occupations, and therapeutic use of self when providing these interventions. Chapter 11 provides a review of the various types of documentation procedures used in occupational therapy and the importance of these procedures for quality assurance, communication, reimbursement, and outcome research. The responsibilities of occupational therapy assistants in the documentation process are clarified. Strategies for writing documentation that is relevant to the occupational needs of the children and adolescents, reflects observable and measurable behaviors, and serves as benchmarks for judging the effectiveness of the intervention processes are discussed.

Chapters 12, 13, 14, and 15 focus on specific interventions that address the various areas of occupations in which children and adolescents engage. Each of these chapters explores the developmental and contextual relevance of the interventions and the role of the occupational therapy assistant in the planning and delivery of these interventions. Chapter 12 discusses intervention approaches for activities of daily living including dressing, feeding, eating, bathing, showering, functional mobility, hygiene, grooming, and toileting. Chapter 13 examines interventions that focus on selected instrumental activities of daily living. These include care of pets, community mobility, communication device use, financial management, meal preparation and cleanup, safety procedures and emergency responses, and shopping. Chapter 14 explores formal and informal education opportunities and paid and volunteer work activities for children and adolescents, and explains legislation that influences occupational therapy services in educational and work settings. Chapter 15 describes interventions that address the play, leisure, and social participation occupations of children and adolescents.

Section IV, the final section of the text, contains seven chapters. These chapters focus on how to implement occupational therapy interventions for children and adolescents who are experiencing specific health and learning challenges. Each chapter probes various health and learning challenges, and provides stories to examine how children and adolescents with these health and learning challenges participate in their daily occupations. The stories illustrate the underlying conditions and diagnoses and how they impact the daily lives of the children and adolescents within the context of the family and their environment. These stories help the occupational therapy assistant students to visualize the need for occupational therapy services and how they are delivered. From these readings the students learn how to use the knowledge from sections I, II, and III of the text to provide client-centered occupational therapy services to children and adolescents. Chapter 16 focuses on children and adolescents with cognitive challenges. Chapter 17 examines the daily life needs of children and adolescents with psychosocial, emotional, and behavioral challenges. The occupational needs of children and adolescents with orthopedic and muscular conditions, and with neural tube defects are addressed in Chapter 18 and Chapter 19, respectively. Chapter 20 considers the occupational challenges of children with neuromuscular challenges. Chapter 21 addresses autism spectrum disorder. Chapter 22, the last chapter of the book, provides information about the range of learning disabilities and attention deficit disorders. The appendixes support the content in the chapters. They include developmental charts, assessment tool resources, legislative summaries, and web site sources.

From reading this book, we hope that occupational therapy students gain an understanding of the theoretical underpinnings of occupational therapy practice for children and adolescents. We also hope that they have a broad overview of the occupations in which children and adolescents engage at various stages of development. Studying the core of the text will enable occupational therapy assistant students to become knowledgeable about the occupational therapy evaluation, intervention, and outcome processes to address occupational challenges of children and adolescents. They also will be able to describe various educational and medical diagnoses impacting children and adolescents. Integrating this knowledge, occupational therapy assistant students will be able to apply it to provide client-centered, best practices approaches to address the various occupational challenges of children and adolescents. The learning activities posed in Applying Key Concepts at the end of each chapter provide opportunities to combine their knowledge with the practice of occupational therapy.

We hope that this text achieves these objectives. Most important, we hope this book provides a rich resource of information that prepares occupational therapy students to deliver occupational therapy practices in a manner conducive to client-centered best practice approaches.

Janet V. DeLany and Margaret J. Pendzick

Acknowledgments

During the past two years, many people have supported our effort and contributed to the writing process. With sincere gratitude, we would like to acknowledge a few of those special individuals.

The Penn State DuBois Occupational Therapy Assistant Program Class of 2006—Terri Barrett, Ashley Fryer, Theresa Hayward, Tristen Kelly, Roxanne Pearce, Martha Poague, Matthew Reasinger, Sally Round, Lyndsey Rowles, and Tiffany Nero, who provided critical feedback on chapter content and writing style—you were a wonderful class and we appreciate all the effort you put into this project!

The Towson University research assistants Amy Mateer and Cristina Torres, who cheerfully found needed resources, created tables and charts, and assisted with the multiple rewrites of the chapters and appendices. We are deeply appreciative of your many hours of dedication. Perhaps you will write a text book in the future!

Our professional colleagues, Lisa Crabtree, Shannan Dixon, LuAnn Demi, David Kresse, and Doadi Rockwell, who squeezed precious hours out of their heavy schedules to read critically and offer insights about the philosophical lenses and content of the book. We are grateful for your collective wisdom and expertise.

Our husbands, Pat and Robert, who provided computer support, and patiently listened to our ideas and frustrations while quietly giving up couple time so we could complete this project—you are two special fellows who are loved dearly!

Our children, Shannan, Keith, Kolin, John, and Sara, who allowed us to integrate our knowledge of occupation and development as we viewed childhood and adolescent experiences through their eyes—it's sometimes tough having a mom who is an occupational therapist, and we are very proud of you!

Contributing Authors

Janet V. DeLany, EdD, OTR/L, FAOTA
Associate Professor
Department of Occupational Therapy
  and Occupational Science
Towson University
Towson, Maryland
Chapters 1, 2, 3, 4, 7, 8, 9, 12, 15, 17, 21

Barbara B. Demchick, MS, OTR/L, BCP
Lecturer
Department of Occupational Therapy
  and Occupational Science
Towson University
Towson, Maryland
Chapter 20

LuAnn Demi, MS, OTR/L
Instructor
Occupational Therapy Assistant Program
The Pennsylvania State University, DuBois
  Campus
DuBois, Pennsylvania
Chapters 16, 18

David Kresse, MS, OTR/L
Instructor
Occupational Therapy Assistant Program
The Pennsylvania State University, Berks Campus
Berks, Pennsylvania
Chapter 21

Margaret J. Pendzick, MOT, OTR/L, BCP
Senior Instructor
Occupational Therapy Assistant Program
The Pennsylvania State University, DuBois
  Campus
DuBois, Pennsylvania
Chapters 5, 6, 10, 11, 13, 14, 16, 18, 20, 22

Dorothy L. Rockwell, MS, OT/L
Senior Instructor
Occupational Therapy Assistant Program
The Pennsylvania State University, Mont Alto
  Campus
Mont Alto, Pennsylvania
Chapters 14, 19

Reviewers

Deena Baenen, MA, BA, AAS
Preceptor, Fieldwork Coordinator
Cuyahoga Community College
Cleveland, Ohio

Judy Blum, MS, OTR/L
Associate Professor
Community College of Baltimore County
Baltimore Maryland

Carolyn O. Cantu, MS, OTR
Associate Professor, Department Chair
Austin Community College
Austin, Texas

Lisa Carruth, OTR/L
Program Director
Northwestern Technical College
Rock Spring, Georgia

Carla Douglas, OTR/L
Adjunct Professor
St. Charles Community College
St. Peters, Missouri

Eve Fischberg, OTR/L
Clinical Coordinator, Assistant Professor
Lincoln Land Community College
Springfield, Illinois

Judith S. Gonyea, OTD
State University of New York at Canton
Canton, New York

Helen Grothem
Program Coordinator
Madisonville Community College
Madisonville, Kentucky

Tia Hughes, MBA, OTR/L
Department Chair, Associate Professor
Florida Hospital College of Health Sciences
Orlando, Florida

Anita Lane, M.Ed., OTR
OTA Program Chair
Navarro College
Corsicana, Texas

Kathleen Larson, MS, OTR
Faculty
Fox Valley Technical College
Appleton, Wisconsin

Nichelle Miedema, ORT/L
Program Director, Associate Professor
Kirkwood Community College
Cedar Rapids, Iowa

Barbara J. Natell, MSed, ORT/L
Director, Associate Professor
Penn College of Technology
Williamsport, Pennsylvania

Michelle Parolise, MBA, OTR/L
Program Director
Santa Ana College
Santa Ana, California

Joyce Wandel
Director, OTA Program
Wright College
Chicago, Illinois

Understanding the Domain and Process of Occupational Therapy

Janet V. DeLany

Key Terms

Activities of daily living (ADL)
Activity
Activity demands
Adaptation
Areas of occupation
Client
Client factors
Concept
Construct
Context
Education
Environmental factors
Evaluation
Habits
Instrumental activities of daily living (IADL)

Intervention
Leisure
Occupation
Occupational form
Occupational profile
Outcome
Participation
Performance patterns
Performance skills
Play
Ritual
Roles
Routines
Social participation
Work

Objectives

- Define and understand the value of occupation.
- Identify and explain the domain of occupational therapy as related to working with children and adults.
- Identify and explain the process of occupational therapy as related to working with children and adolescents.
- Articulate the importance of client-centered practice in the therapeutic process.

UNDERSTANDING OCCUPATIONS

Since its founding, the importance of **occupation** for the health and well-being of individuals has been at the cornerstone of occupational therapy. It is central to the services that occupational therapists and occupational therapy assistants provide. The term occupation is a complex **construct** (Kramer, Hinojosa, & Royeen, 2003). A construct is built from interconnected **concepts**; a concept is an abstract or intangible idea built from a number of concrete or tangible examples (Merriam-Webster, 2007). Intelligence is an example of a construct built on interconnected concepts such as memory, thought, perception, and types of intelligence. Because the concrete examples used to build a concept can change as a result of people's diverse experiences and temporal influences, the precise meaning of a concept also may change. As the precise meaning of the concept changes, so does the meaning of the construct. The precise meaning of the word occupation continues to evolve in response to changing societal experiences and temporal influences.

Early founders of the profession of occupational therapy talk about the healing powers of work, leisure, daily living, and rest occupations (Meyer, 1922). Letters between Barton and Dunton explain that they and other founders of the profession chose the title *occupational therapy* because they wanted a name that was sufficiently broad to reflect the therapeutic nature of active engagement in occupations to address any mental or physical condition (Christensen, 1991; Kramer et al., 2003; Quiroga, 1995).

Recent scholars continue to clarify the construct of occupation within the profession of occupational therapy and the discipline of occupational science. Such clarification helps occupational therapists and occupational therapy assistants who work with children and adolescents to maintain a focus on, as well as appreciate, the complexity of their occupations. Kielhofner (2007) defines human occupation as:

> the doing of work, play, or activities of daily living within a temporal, physical, and sociocultural context that characterizes much of human life. . . . Time, space, society, and culture intersect with each other to create conditions that affect what people do, and how and why they think and feel about what they do (pp. 1–2).

Applying Kielhofner's definition, occupational therapists and occupational therapy assistants who work with children and adolescents in a hospital setting consider how the physical space and location of the medical facility, the uncertainty and intensity of the hospital stay, the blend of family and hospital cultures, and the health conditions of the children and adolescents affect the daily living, educational, and play occupations of the children and adolescents. Similarly, occupational therapists and occupational therapy assistants who work with children and adolescents in an emergency shelter consider how the physical layout and geographic location of the shelter, the temporality of the living arrangements, the heterogeneous mixture of family cultures, and the survival needs of the family members affect the daily living, educational, and play occupations of the children and adolescents. In both settings, the occupational therapists and occupational therapy assistants concern themselves with what and how the children think and feel about themselves, their health and safety, and their occupational capacities.

Nelson and Jepson-Thomas (2003) offer another definition of occupation that provides important distinction between occupation and **occupational form**. They define occupation as a person doing something at a particular time. According to Nelson and Jepson-Thomas, people have unique developmental structures that reflect the capacities of their bodies to perform. These physical, sensory, cognitive, and psychosocial structures influence what people choose to do and how they do it. The occupational form involves all of the physical and sociocultural factors that surround the person, but are not part of the person. The occupational form influences or bounds how people perform their occupations. Occupations involve a dynamic relationship among the person, the occupational form, the meaning and purpose the person attaches to the occupational form, and the resulting occupational performance. For example, the type of clothing, the dressing area, other people in the dressing area, the language, the time of day or year, and the country in which the children live are part of the occupational form, and influence the occupation of dressing. The children attach meaning and purpose to the dressing occupation, based upon the culture in which they live. Thus, the occupation of dressing by a five-year-old boy in his bedroom who is to attend a Korean holiday festival, as seen in Figure 1.1■, differs in skills, form, purpose, and meaning from the occupation of dressing by adolescent boys on an outdoor field in preparation for lacrosse practice. (See Figure 1.2■.)

Pierce (2001) provides helpful clues for distinguishing between **activities** and occupations. Though occupational therapists and occupational therapy assistants often use these words interchangeably, Pierce suggests that they differ in an important way. Pierce views activities as actions people do to achieve a goal, and occupations as the activities people do that hold a central meaning and purpose and contribute to a sense of identity and competency. What is considered an activity for one person may be considered an occupation for another depending on the meaning, purpose, and sense of identity and competency associated with it. For example, in the above scenario, the five-year-old boy or the adolescent boys may consider dressing as an activity, a

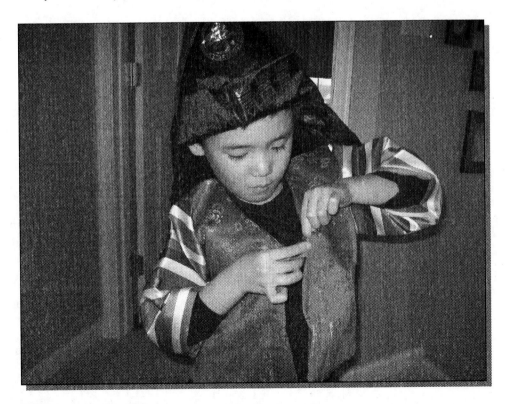

■ Figure 1.1
A young boy dressing for a Korean festival.

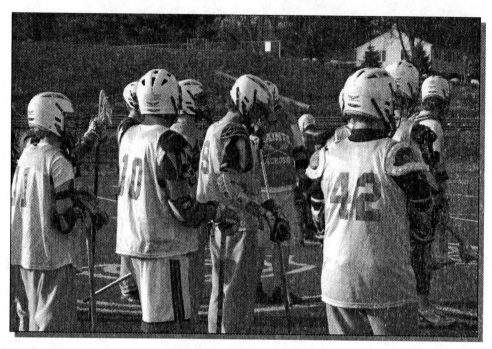

■ Figure 1.2
Lacrosse players putting on gear for practice.

goal-directed chore necessary to attend the holiday activity or to participate in the sport. Likewise, the five-year-old boy or the adolescent boys may consider dressing an occupation that reflects their sense of competency and their self-image as a member of a community or a sports team. They may have developed a ritual for dressing and ascribed symbolism to items they wear that reflect the rituals and symbols of the larger community.

Zemke and Clark (1996), who were instrumental in developing the discipline of occupational science, offer another way to define occupation. They define occupations "as chunks of daily activity that can be named in the lexicon of the culture" (p. vii). They further explain that people's daily occupations expand or shift over time, and reflect varying amounts of self-choice and cultural expectations. For example whether or not adolescents work, and where they work, are influenced by their sense of self-choice and the expectations of the family and communities to work. Geographic location, gender, age, ability status, and socioeconomic needs also influence engagement in work. It is more likely that children who live in rural communities begin to help with farm work and drive tractors as young as 10 years of age, whereas adolescents who live in the city may not begin to work in a retail shop or drive until the age of 16. Occupational therapists and occupational therapy assistants need to examine the environments in which children and adolescents live to understand the occupations in which they engage and the way they perform those occupations.

Law, Polatajko, Baptiste, and Townsend (1997) offer yet another definition of occupation. They explain that:

> Occupations are activities . . . of everyday life, named, organized, and given value and meaning by individuals and a culture. Occupation is everything peo-

ple do to occupy themselves, including looking after themselves . . . enjoying life . . . and contributing to the social and economic fabric of their communities (p. 32).

As indicated in this definition, occupations involve both a process of doing as well as the activity that is done. As applied to children and adolescents, both the process and the activity are identifiable. They are valuable and meaningful to the children and adolescents, and the broader cultures in which they live. Children and adolescents most clearly benefit from an occupation when the challenge of performing it matches their neurological, biological, and psychological capacities and needs (Velde & Fidler, 2002).

Though it is easy to become confused by the differences among these definitions, it is more important to consider the similarities. Doing so provides a way to explain occupation to children, adolescents, and their caregivers. The word occupation implies that the children and adolescents are "doing" or performing everyday life activities that are recognized and named by the culture in which they live. Occupations are broader than simple acts or activities (Christiansen & Baum, 1997; Christiansen, Baum, and Bass-Haugen, 2005; West, 1984). Occupations include a series of acts or activities that, when combined, become meaningful and purposeful to the children and adolescents and their larger communities. The temporal and physical environments in which the children and adolescents live affect how and why they perform these occupations. The physical, cognitive, and social-emotional capacities of the children and adolescents also affect how and why they perform these occupations. Occupations contribute to their health, well-being, and sense of self.

OCCUPATION AND THE LANGUAGE OF *ICF*

Members of the World Health Organization (WHO) spent a number of years collaborating with health professionals in many countries and in many areas of health practice to create standardized terminology that was culturally acceptable, and could be used worldwide to describe health and health-related states. The result of their work was a document called the *International Classification of Functioning, Disability, and Health (ICF)* (WHO, 2001). Its purpose was to provide a structure for discussing, researching, and documenting the health and health-related states of all individuals, not just those with disabilities. The ICF uses the words **activity**, **participation**, and **environmental factors** to discuss the concepts embedded in the definition of occupation described above, without using the word occupation. This combination of words conveys some but not all of the same rich notions embedded in the word occupation, as used by occupational therapists and occupational therapy assistants. In ICF, activity is defined as "the execution of a task or action by an individual" (WHO, p. 123). Participation is defined as "the involvement in a life situation" (WHO, p. 123). Environmental factors "make up the physical, social, and attitudinal environments in which people live and conduct their lives" (WHO, p. 171). In addition, the ICF provides a comprehensive list of tasks individuals perform as part of their lived experiences. There is overlap in the language found in the ICF and the language used in occupational therapy to describe human activities and restrictions to those activities. Such overlap allows for congruity of the language used in occupational therapy with that used in other health professions. Depending upon where occupational therapists and occupational therapy assistants work, they may find themselves using language that is more consistent with that found in the occupational therapy literature, or that outlined in ICF. Additionally, practice setting and funding agencies may influence the language used to share ideas and record services.

DOMAIN OF OCCUPATIONAL THERAPY PRACTICE

In 2002, the American Occupational Therapy Association (AOTA) first published the *Occupational Therapy Practice Framework: Domain and Process*. It was particularly important because it was the first official AOTA document that outlined the domain and process of occupational therapy, and stated that the focus of occupational therapy intervention was to facilitate "engagement [of individuals] in occupation to support participation in context or contexts" (AOTA, 2002, p. 611). A domain of a profession is the area of human concern that it addresses. For lawyers, this might be the legal concerns. For dieticians, this might be nutritional concerns. For occupational therapists and occupational therapy assistants, this is the occupations of people. As part of its responsibility to ensure currency and accuracy of all AOTA official documents, the Commission on Practice initiated a revision of the Occupational Therapy Practice Framework in 2006. Both the original Practice Framework (AOTA, 2002) and the revised Practice Framework (AOTA, nd) clarify that the domain of occupational therapy includes consideration of **areas of occupation, performance skills**, and **performance patterns** needed to accomplish those occupations, the context and environments in which those occupations are performed, the **activity demands** inherent with the occupations, and **client factors** that influence the occupational engagement. Occupational therapists and occupational therapy assistants use their knowledge of occupations and the therapeutic power of occupations to help children and adolescents participate in meaningful lives.

Areas of Occupation

In the Practice Framework, activities of daily living, instrumental activities of daily living, education, work, play, leisure, and social participation are considered the areas of occupation. These categories are an expansion of the daily living, work, and play areas found in older occupational therapy literature (AOTA, 1994).

ADL occupations are activities that people perform to take care of their bodies (Rogers & Holm, 1994). These include bathing, bowel and bladder management, dressing, eating, feeding, functional mobility, personal device care, sexual activity, sleep and rest, toilet hygiene, and grooming and hygiene (AOTA, 2002). When working with children and adolescents, it is important to remember that their chronological and developmental ages, as well as their experiences, influence their capacity to perform activities of daily living. To perform her ADL occupations, an infant girl may nurse, cry when her diaper is soiled, splash in a sink, and sleep in a sling attached to her parent for three-hour intervals throughout most of the day. A baby may feed himself with his fingers (see Figure 1.3■), intermittently control his bowel and bladder functions throughout the day, play in a tub, and sleep for 12 hours through the night in the family bed. An older child may feed himself independently with chopsticks (see Figure 1.4■), locate and use a variety of toilet and bathing facilities, and determine the time to go to bed.

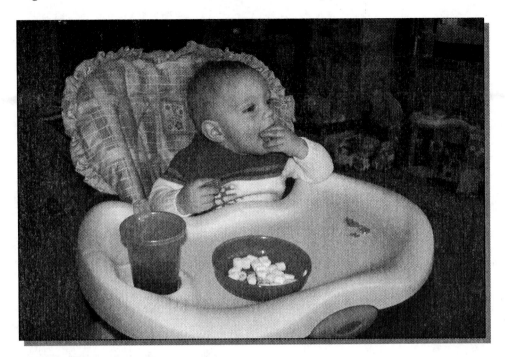

■ **Figure 1.3**
A young child finger feeding.

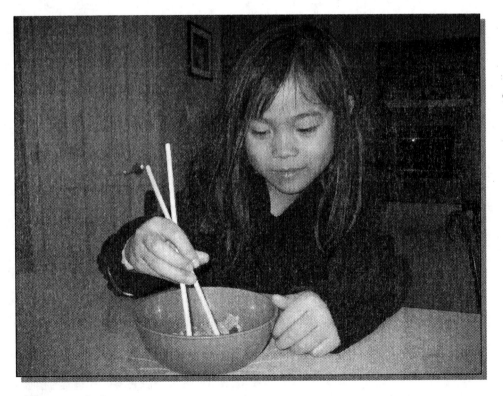

■ **Figure 1.4**
A girl eating with chopsticks.

Beyond their apparent self-caring features, activities of daily living also serve a social function (Christiansen & Baum, 1997). Societies place expectations on the manner in which children are to perform activities of daily living and the age at which children are expected to perform them independently. Children who do not meet these expectations may be judged negatively or isolated from their peers. Occupational therapists and occupational therapy assistants work with children and adolescents to develop or restore their capacities so that they can participate more fully in their daily living occupations in the contexts where they live, learn, and play. Intervention approaches used to accomplish this goal are discussed in Section III.

Instrumental activities of daily living are more complex than activities of daily living and involve additional interaction with the environment (Rogers & Holm, 1994). They may involve a sequence of tasks that require decision making and responsibility to and for other people or objects. Care of other people or pets, child rearing, communication device use, community mobility, financial management, health management and maintenance, home establishment and management, meal preparation, safety procedures and emergency response, and shopping are examples of activities of daily living (AOTA, 2002). As part of the instrumental activities of daily living a young child may help to feed family goats, collect the mail, wash the fruit and vegetables, and save coins in a bottle. An older child may be responsible for caring for siblings after school, preparing supper, taking the family dog to the vet, and maintaining a savings account. Unlike activities of daily living, children and adolescents may be expected to accomplish some but not all instrumental activities of daily living. Responsibility for accomplishing instrumental activities of daily living may be determined by the gender of the child or adolescent. For example, in some families, meal preparation and child care may be assigned to the female children (see Figure 1.5■). Safety and activities requiring community mobility may be assigned to the male children. Occupational therapists and occupational therapy assistants must be sensitive to the cultural and family expectations when helping children and adolescents acquire the skills to participate in instrumental activities of daily living.

Education occupations include formal, informal, and exploration learning activities (AOTA, 2002). Formal learning activities are those associated with an educational institution or program. For children and adolescents these often include academic, extracurricular, and vocational programs. Informal learning activities allow children and adolescents to gain knowledge and skills about areas of personal interest beyond the scope of educational institutions in such places as their homes, local community settings, craft and art stores, museums, and parks. Exploration learning activities allow children and adolescents to discover areas of personal interest or areas for potential skill development, and can occur within or outside structured learning settings. Children and adolescents can participate in educational occupations alone or with others. Computers have created opportunities for virtual formal, informal, and exploratory learning activities. As part of their education occupations, infants and toddlers may participate in swimming and tumbling programs at a community wellness center. Young children may enroll in preschool programs, visit zoos, and watch education based television programs. Elementary age children may enroll in a formal school, home school, and religious education classes. Summer camps have gained increased popularity as a method to help school age children to explore sports, science, and creative arts. Adolescents may attend driver education, college test preparation, and military preparation classes, form music groups, and join career exploration groups.

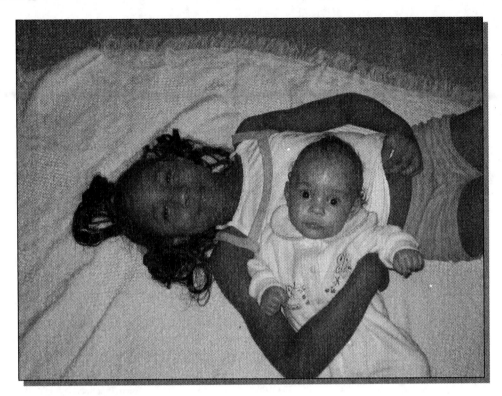

■ **Figure 1.5**
A girl caring for her baby sister.

Occupational therapists and occupational therapy assistants serve an important role in adapting the educational environments and modifying the learning tools so that children and adolescents, regardless of their ability levels, can participate in the variety of educational occupations.

Work occupations involve paid and volunteer activities. Identifying paid and volunteer interests, seeking and acquiring paid or volunteer employment, and performing paid and volunteer activities are part of work (AOTA, 2002). Families and the larger societies in which they live establish norms and laws regarding the appropriate age for children and adolescents to participate in work occupations. Families and societies also may regulate the tools, tasks, places of employment, pay scales, and hours associated with the work occupations of children and adolescents. There may be different norms and regulations for paid and volunteer work, and different expectations of work based on the socioeconomic status of the family. Occupations associated with instrumental activities of daily living, such as pet care, child care, and home management may be considered work if the children and adolescents are remunerated for their efforts. Some young children may work by collecting firewood and watering the plants. School age children may work by selling produce at their family's roadside stand, walking the neighbors' pets, or volunteering as a reading buddy at a senior citizen center. Adolescents may work by washing dishes in a restaurant, modeling or acting, and volunteering in youth service corps. Some of these work experiences may lead to future career opportunities and academic pursuits; others will not. As children and adolescents approach the end of their formal schooling, the expectation for them to work increases. The type of work and the ability to work contribute to their self-concept and independence. Occupational therapists and occupational therapy assistants may contribute to the ability for children and adolescents to engage in their work occupations in many ways, including training them how to perform specific skills, exploring areas of potential interest, and modifying and adapting work environments, procedures, and tools.

Play occupations involve exploratory and participatory activities that provide pleasure or amusement, stimulate curiosity and creativity, or offer diversion and entertainment (Parham & Fazio, 1997). The pleasure of play stimulates a desire to repeat and master the motor, sensory, social, language, and cognitive skills associated with it (see Figure 1.6■). With this repetition comes a sense of mastery motivation and self-efficacy, that is, a desire to find solutions and a belief in the capacity to master new skills (Cronin & Mandich, 2005).

Children and adolescents participate in both spontaneous and organized play activities. They can play alone or with others. For example, one child walking along the beach might spontaneously begin a game of finding and chasing sand crabs, while a group of children on that same beach organize themselves to play a game of beach volleyball. Rules for how to play may not be part of the spontaneous activity or may be few and fluid, as the play evolves. Rules for the organized play may be more formally established; changes in the rules may need to be negotiated among the players. Materials for play may be very few or very elaborate. A child might use only his body and natural items found in the environment to engage in play such as when rolling or dancing in a pile of leaves. Children playing on-line video simulation games with one another require computers, adapters, joysticks, adapted motherboards, voice synthesizers, and software programs. Adolescents playing ice hockey require specialized

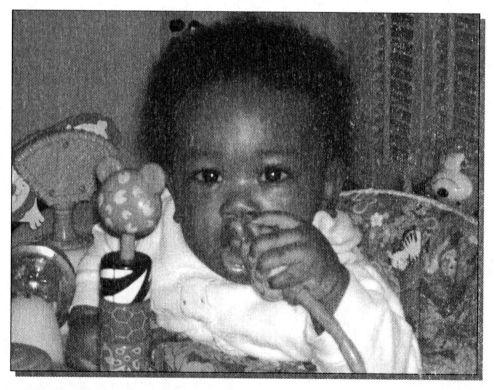

■ **Figure 1.6**
A baby at play.

equipment and skating surfaces. Families and societies have expectations as to the kind of materials that are appropriate for play. As well, the socioeconomic level of the family and the community place bounds on money allocated for play materials. In one community, children may play with dolls made from cornhusks, while in another community children play with dolls and doll accessories manufactured by multimillion dollar corporations. In the Amish community, toys are to be made from natural materials, and are not to be powered by electricity or battery.

Occupational therapists and occupational therapy assistants frequently use play as an intervention method when working with children and adolescents. Play can be a powerful medium for facilitating development and occupational performance, fostering self-esteem and empowerment, and improving the quality of life and health. For play to have these therapeutic benefits, the occupational therapist and occupational therapy assistant carefully select play activities that match the capacities, interests, and needs of the children and adolescents, and respect the values, beliefs, and socioeconomic conditions of their families and cultures.

Leisure occupations involve exploratory and participatory activities. They are nonobligatory and are done during discretionary time (Parham & Fazio, 1997). They may satisfy an area of curiosity or interest, may be done alone or with others, and may provide pleasure or opportunities to learn and create. Attempts have been made to classify leisure occupations, though no one universal system exists (Christiansen & Baum, 1997). Kite flying, model building, hip hop dancing, painting, singing, sewing, orienteering, fishing, biking, and boating are examples of leisure occupations in which children and adolescents engage. By participating in leisure pursuits with their older siblings, parents, and grandparents, children may begin to develop interest in similar leisure occupations such as gardening, hunting, and coin collecting. Membership in youth groups and community centers also may provide a venue for developing interest in such leisure occupations as drama, magic, metalwork, camping, and astronomy.

Families, societies, and living environments influence what are considered appropriate leisure occupations for children and adolescents. Ice fishing may be considered an appropriate leisure occupation in Newfoundland; flamenco dancing may be considered an appropriate leisure occupation in Spain. As well, the socioeconomics of the families and societies in which they live place bounds on the leisure occupations in which children and adolescents can engage.

Because of their knowledge of activities and occupations, and their ability to modify activities and adapt environments to match the performance capacities, occupational therapy assistants can work with occupational therapists to design programs that support participation of children and adolescents in healthy occupations. This is an important service not only to the children and adolescents but also the communities in which they live, because those who participate in healthy leisure activities are less likely to experiment with risky behaviors, substance abuse, sex, and illegal activities (Farnworth, 1999).

Social participation occupations involve interactions with family, friends, peers, and community members in organized patterns that are recognized by society (Mosey, 1996). Attending birthday parties, celebrating community holidays, and visiting family members are examples of social participation. Language, social, emotional, cognitive, and moral development occurs through participation in social occupations. Bandura and his colleagues conducted numerous studies that examined how children learn through participation in social situations, and the affects of that participation on emotional development, self-perception, and motivation. He also studied how children learn social norms by observing others in social situations (McDevitt & Ormrod, 2004). Vygotsky pioneered research on how social participation in everyday activities affects

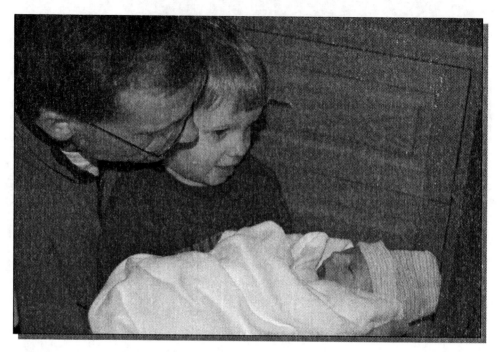

■ **Figure 1.7**
Social participation of father, son, and baby sister.

the cognitive development of children. He offered insights into how cultures and the tools used in those cultures to participate in everyday activities affect cognitive development of children and adolescents (McDevitt & Ormrod, 2004).

Through smiling and cooing in response to their parents' vocalizations, infants participate in early social exchanges. Opportunities for social participation quickly expand as extended family members and friends involve the infant in their daily activities and rituals. (See Figure 1.7■.)

Young children may participate in playgroups in one another's homes, day care, or early education activities. As children enter elementary school, opportunities for social participation expand beyond family connections to include the larger community. Children may divide their time among family social activities, peer related social activities, and community and school structured social activities. By adolescence, social participation with peers may occupy more time than social participation with family members. Similar to the other areas of occupation, families and cultures may have established norms regarding the appropriateness of social participation activities, and the age at which children and adolescents can participate in those activities. Occupational therapy assistants, working with occupational therapists, may develop programs to assist children and adolescents develop necessary skills to engage in a variety of social participation occupations. They also may design environments, and modify tools and materials to maximize access for children and adolescents to social situations.

Performance Skills and Performance Patterns

To engage in occupations requires children and adolescents to develop and master many skills. Texts on human growth and development often discuss physical, sensory, cognitive, and social-emotional skills needed to engage in daily life tasks (Feldman, 2007; McDevitt & Ormrod, 2004; Vander Zanden, Crandell, & Crandell, 2003). They are considered performance skills when individuals actually perform or demonstrate the skills, not just potentially possesses the capacity for the skills (Fisher, 2006; Fisher & Kielhofner, 1995; Kielhofner, 2007). For example, though a child appears to have the ability to communicate verbally, it is not until he talks that he demonstrates the ability to perform the skill of talking. Fisher categorizes performance skills into three areas: motor, processing, and communication and interaction. Motor skills are those skills necessary to move, to perform the task, and to interact with objects and the environment (Fisher, 2006; Kielhofner, 2007). Motor skills that children demonstrate when playing baseball include *bending* their trunks backward then forward to throw the ball, *calibrating* the force of the throw, *reaching* with their arms to catch the ball, and *gripping* the thrown ball with a mitt. Processing skills are those skills necessary to think about, sequence, and modify actions to complete the task (Kielhofner, 2007). Some processing skills that children demonstrate when playing baseball include *choosing* and *using* the appropriate bat, *judging* when to *initiate* swinging the bat, and *attending* to the trajectory of the ball as it travels through the air. Communication and interaction skills are those skills necessary to share thoughts and to engage in social interactions with others (Fisher, 2006; Kielhofner, 2007). Some communication skills that children might demonstrate when playing baseball include *asking* about and *conforming* to the rules of the game, *gesturing* to other players about where to throw the ball, and *speaking* with the coach about game strategies.

Genetic inheritance and opportunities to learn, or nature and nurture, influence the development of skills in children and adolescents. Thus, children of the same chronological age will display a range of physical, sensory, cognitive, and social-emotional capacities (Feldman, 2007; McDevitt & Ormrod, 2004; Vander Zanden, et al., 2003). One child might develop communication skills very quickly, but motor skills more slowly. In contrast, another child the same age might develop motor skills very quickly, but communication skills more slowly. Skills develop over time as children mature, enabling them to engage in more complex and more diverse occupations. For example, the motor, processing, and communication skills that five-year-old children use to play T-ball emerge over time to the skills that adolescents use to play on the high school baseball team. Likewise, participating in occupations influences the development of increasingly more complex and integrated skills. Those children who play ball games more frequently are more likely to develop complex and integrated skills necessary to participate in highly competitive sports programs. Those children who play ball games less frequently are more likely to participate in noncompetitive or mildly competitive recreational baseball games.

Because performance skills require an act of doing, occupational therapists and occupational therapy assistants can observe, measure, and record how children and adolescents perform their daily life occupations. Based on this information, as well as information about occupations and the environments in which they are performed, occupational therapists and occupational therapy assistants design intervention plans to develop, strengthen, or restore the performance skills of those children and adolescents who struggle to perform their daily life occupations.

Performance patterns include habits, routines, rituals, and roles that individuals use when engaging in daily life activities. **Habits** are automatic behaviors that allow a person to respond in a consistent way in familiar environments (Kielhofner, 2007). A toddler may suck her thumb to calm herself at bedtime; an adolescent may bite his lip to focus his thoughts before beginning to write. **Routines** are sequences of behaviors that individuals cluster together to accomplish a task and organize time.

Routines allow children and adolescents to perform familiar parts of the task efficiently and without careful attention to each step (Kielhofner, 2007).

Habits and routines can be *useful, impoverished,* or *dominating* (AOTA, 2002). Useful habits and routines provide enough structure to enable children and adolescents to perform their daily life tasks efficiently, yet allow enough flexibility to enable them to adapt to various situations. As part of her nightly routine, the toddler may get a book and blanket, sit on the bed, and suck her thumb while her grandparent reads to her. As part of his writing routine, the adolescent may get a drink and a snack, gather textbooks, turn on the radio and the computer, and bite his lip. Impoverished habits and routines do not provide enough structure to enable children and adolescents to effectively organize time and activities. An adolescent who cannot organize himself to gather his drink, snacks, and books, and then sit down to write may demonstrate impoverished habits and routines. As a result of impoverished habits and routines, he loses valuable study time. In contrast, dominating habits and routines restrict adaptation by requiring rigid adherence to a specific way to perform the behavior. An adolescent who can only drink one type of liquid from one particular glass, eat the snack only if placed on the plate in a particular direction, use the text only if stacked on the desk in a particular manner, and bite his lip until it bleeds when preparing to write may be demonstrating dominating habits and routines.

A **ritual** is a type of action that holds special meaning and purpose to the person. These rituals can be socially, culturally, and spiritually influenced. A young child may participate in a family holiday ritual that involves food preparation, gift exchanges, and storytelling. An adolescent may participate in a high school sports ritual that includes a pep rally, dressing in school colors, and attending a post game dance.

Roles are scripts of expected behaviors placed on people within the social systems that they belong to (Christiansen & Baum, 1997; Kielhofner, 2007). The habits, routines, and rituals in which children and adolescents engage contribute to the roles they assume. Conversely, the roles that children and adolescents perform contribute to the habits and routines that they learn. For example, the habit of tapping out rhythms on tabletops, the routine of practicing on her drums every night, and the ritual of dressing in a particular costume contribute to the adolescent's role as a drummer in a band. Likewise, her role as drummer contributes to the development of hand and foot tapping habits, the routine of writing down percussion patterns she hears in songs and nature, and the candle lighting ritual she uses to connect with her spiritual self prior to a performance.

Perhaps the first roles infants assume are those of child and sibling. As young children, their roles might expand to include those of playmate, house hold helper, and preschooler. By adolescence, these roles can become quite varied based upon societal expectations, experiences, and learned performance skills. The various roles that children and adolescents assume help to organize their days. For example, in a given day, a 12-year-old girl may assume the role of a student from 8 A.M. to 3 P.M., a jazz pianist from 4 P.M. to 5 P.M., and a cast member of a community theatre production from 7 P.M. to 10 P.M. In between those scheduled activities, she may assume the role of daughter, friend, sibling, or peer mentor. For each of these roles, she may perform different tasks, wear different clothes, and use different language styles. Roles become internalized and contribute self-concept and self-esteem. Children and adolescents who possess useful habits and routines, and healthy role repertoires tend to have a stronger sense of their self-efficacy and worth. Occupational therapy assistants, working with occupational therapists, may help children and adolescents to develop or strengthen healthy habits and routines, and expand their roles so that they can participate more fully and more successfully in daily life activities.

Context

Context is that which is part of and external to the person, and influences what tasks a person performs and how the person performs those tasks. The cultural, physical, social, personal, temporal, and virtual contexts influence how children and adolescents perform their daily life tasks (AOTA, 2002). These contexts often are interconnected with and influence one another.

The *cultural* **context** is comprised of the beliefs, attitudes, values, and expectations of a society. The culture of a society may be depicted in its politics, laws, and customs. The more diverse a community, the more likely that children and adolescents negotiate among several cultures to engage in their occupations. This cultural negotiation occurs when children from various Asian, South American, and European backgrounds attend school together.

The *physical context* incorporates the nonhuman objects, terrains, buildings, plants, and animal aspects. Because of these physical features, the occupations of a child growing up in an apartment complex in New York City differ substantively from those of a child growing up on a Native American reservation in Arizona.

Social context refers to the relationships of people with one another in groups, organizations, and societal systems. The norms associated with the social context affect how children and adolescents assume their roles and behave within them. An adolescent may be very reserved and respectful in the social context of a school board meeting, but very boisterous and assertive when in the social context of a party with peers.

Personal contexts are the nonhealth features of a person such as age, gender, education level, and economic status. The occupations of a 3-year-old girl who attends a Head Start preschool program differ substantively from the occupations of a 15-year-old male who attends a private, exclusive high school.

Temporal context refers to the point in time in the day, year, activity cycle, or life stage in which the individual engages in the occupation. Measurement of time is personally and culturally determined. The age of a child also affects the perception of time passage. When children and adolescents enjoy the activities in which they engage, time may move quickly. When they do not, time moves slowly.

Virtual context refers to those electronic and other nonphysical interactions with occupations across a distance. As computer access increases, so do opportunities for children and adolescents to participate in long distance, virtual based occupations. Concurrently, demands for face-to-face social skills may decrease.

By examining the environment that affects development, Bronfenbrenner provides important perspectives about these various contexts. Bronfenbrenner (1979, 1997), in his ecological theory, proposes that development is a reflection of the interaction between the person with the environment. This interaction is dynamic, and remains fluid over time. Bronfenbrenner designed a schema of five concentric circles to represent the interaction of the person with the environment. In the innermost circle is the individual as described by *personal* characteristics. The next circle is the *microsystem*, which reflects the social system, that is, those social systems such as church, school, and family with which a person interacts each day. The next circle is the *mesosystem*. It represents the interrelationship among the systems that impact the person's development. The next system is the *exosystem*, which consists of systems external to the person. The exosystem directly and indirectly affects the individual. Extended family members, school systems, government agencies, and mass media are part of the exosystem. The outermost circle is the *macrosystem*, which represents the cultural beliefs and ideologies of the society at large. To understand the occupations of children and adolescents, occupational therapists and occupational therapy assistants must consider and respect these contexts and environments.

Activity Demands

When engaging in occupations, individuals may perform various activities. These activities require the use of specific objects and tools, space, body actions, and body parts, and involve sequence and timing demands, and adherence to social rules. In the *Occupational Therapy Practice Framework*, these are labeled activity demands. They are an inherent part of the activity, independent of a person's ability to do it. Activity demands inherent within the occupation of meal preparation on a camping trip may include the use of: kettles, bowls made from shells, and cooking utensils made from sticks; an open pit fire; body parts such as arms, trunk, and legs to lift and manipulate the pots and carry firewood; sequence and timing to prepare and completely cook the food; and social rules regarding food preparation and cleanliness. Some adolescents may possess the ability to meet all of the demands of the activity independently. Younger children may need assistance because the activity demands inherent within the cooking occupation are beyond their developmental and experiential capacities. Occupational therapy assistants possess the knowledge and skills necessary to modify and grade the activity demands so that children and adolescents, who may not otherwise be able to do so, can complete the activities. This process of modifying and grading activity demands is referred to as **adaptation**.

Client Factors

Client factors include the beliefs, values, spirituality, body functions, and body structures an individual uses to engage in the occupations (AOTA, nd). Beliefs are the constructs, principles and assumptions that individuals hold as true. These beliefs may arise from personal experiences, from community practices, and from historical perspectives passed down through the generations. Values are the importance a person attributes to beliefs and behaviors. Spirituality refers to the sense, purpose, and meaning that individuals associate with their lives. It may incorporate religious beliefs. An adolescent who believes that the meaning and purpose of his life rests in the quality of life of all humanity might volunteer at a homeless shelter.

Body structures are the anatomical parts of the human body; body functions are the actions associated with each of those body structures that reside within the person. Body structures include the nervous system; eyes and ears; voice and speech, cardiovascular, immunological, and respiratory systems; digestive system; genitourinary and reproductive systems; neuromuscular system; and skin. The World Health Organization (2001) classifies body functions according to: affective, cognitive, and perceptual mental functions; sensory functions and pain; neuromuscular and movement related functions; and cardiovascular, immunological and respiratory functions. Body functions also may be classified according to other groupings such as neuromusculoskeletal, cognitive, and psychosocial. Though often used interchangeably, body function abilities differ from performance skills. Performance skills, as previously discussed, are the observable actions associated with each of these body functions. In the cooking activity described above, the campers complete the cooking activity through blending of body structures and body functions. Specifically, the campers use the body structures of their nervous system to be able to think about, have feelings about, and interpret cues related to the food preparation process; use the structure of their eyes and ears to be able to see and smell the fire; use their voice structures to be able to communicate about the cooking with one another; use their cardiovascular and respiratory systems to be able to pump blood and oxygen to their body parts; use their musculoskeletal systems to move their bodies and to lift and carry the wood, and use their skin to feel the fire heat.

Occupational therapists and occupational therapy assistants have general knowledge about all of the body functions and body structures. Depending upon their area of specialty, they may have more in-depth knowledge about specific body functions, particularly those associated with the nervous, musculoskeletal, sensory, cardiovascular, and respiratory systems. This knowledge enables occupational therapists and occupational therapy assistants to work with children and adolescents to develop, strengthen, or restore performance skills they need to engage in their daily life occupations.

PROCESS OF OCCUPATIONAL THERAPY

The process of delivering occupational therapy services involves **evaluation**, **intervention**, and **outcome** processes. Though perhaps using different terminology, other professionals use these same overarching processes to deliver the services of their profession. Evaluation involves the identification of problems, needs, and capacities. Intervention requires the design and implementation of services or solutions. Outcomes measure the degree to which the interventions addressed the issues identified during the evaluation. Occupational therapists and occupational therapy assistants use these processes to deliver services within the bounds of the domain of occupational therapy. The occupational therapy process is grounded in occupation-based and related theories and frames of reference that guide clinical reasoning and decision making. These theories and frames of reference are discussed in Chapters 2 and 3. The occupational therapy process requires knowledge about occupations, occupational performance challenges, and various diagnostic conditions that limit the ability of children and adolescents to participate in their daily life activities.

During the evaluation, the occupational therapist and the occupational therapy assistant develop **occupational profiles** of the children and adolescents to assess their capacities and occupational performance challenges. As part of the occupational profile, the occupational therapist and the occupational therapy assistant gather information about what the children or adolescents could do previously, currently have difficulty doing, and need and want to be able to do (AOTA, 2002). They then develop intervention plans based on an analysis of the collected data related to occupational performance. When developing intervention plans, the occupational therapist and the occupational therapy assistant must be knowledge about the priorities, values, and culture of the children and adolescents, and about methods for modifying the occupations, tasks, and environments, that respect these priorities, cultures, and values. The intervention is developed in collaboration with the children and adolescents, and their family or caregivers. Based on identified goals, the intervention plan is implemented and reviewed periodically to determine whether it should be continued, modified, or discontinued. Outcome studies are conducted to determine the benefits of the intervention plan and the intervention.

The occupational therapist is responsible for initiating and directing each stage of the occupational therapy process, for interpreting the data obtained, and for making judgments about the outcomes of occupational therapy services. The occupational therapy assistant contributes to the process by carrying out designated assessments and

■ **Table 1.1**
Occupational Therapy Domain–Process Grid

	EVALUATION		INTERVENTION			OUTCOMES— ENGAGEMENT IN OCCUPATIONS TO SUPPORT PARTICIPATION
	OCCUPATIONAL PROFILE CAPACITIES AND NEEDS	ANALYSIS OF OCCUPATIONAL PERFORMANCE CAPACITIES AND NEEDS	INTERVENTION PLAN	INTERVENTION IMPLEMENTATION	INTERVENTION REVIEW	
Performance in Areas of Occupation						
Performance Skills						
Performance Patterns						
Context						
Activity Demands						
Client Factors						

interventions, and by providing written and verbal reports to the occupational therapist about the observations made related to the capacity of the children and adolescents to engage in their daily life occupations (AOTA, 2004a). Chapter 4 of this text goes into further detail about the roles and responsibilities of occupational therapists and occupational therapy assistants when providing occupational therapy services (AOTA, 2004a; 2004b).

To provide safe, competent, and effective services requires the occupational therapist and the occupational therapy assistant to understand the domain and process of occupational therapy. Table 1.1■ is a grid depicting the relationship between the domain and the process of occupational therapy. It highlights each aspect of the domain considered during each step of the process. By filling in each of the cells during every step of the occupational therapy process, occupational therapists and occupational therapy assistants can routinely consider all aspects of the domain. Thus, it can be used to organize observations about the abilities and needs of the children and adolescents related to each part of the occupational therapy domain. It also can provide a structure for designing interventions based on those capacities and needs, and evaluating the effectiveness of the interventions.

CLIENT-CENTERED PRACTICE

A basic tenet of occupational therapy is that occupations gain their therapeutic value from the meaning and purpose attributed to them by the individuals engaged in them. Consistent with this tenet is the belief that the occupational therapy process must be client centered. In client centered practice, children, adolescents, and their family members or caregivers are actively involved in the decision about the need for services, the goal of those services, and the types of services received. The children, adolescents, and their families or caregivers are the experts about their shared life experiences. The occupational therapist and the occupational therapy assistant are experts about occupations and occupational performance challenges. They advise the children, the adolescents, and their families or caregivers about factors contributing to occupational performance challenges, intervention strategies to address those challenges, evidence-based studies regarding the effectiveness of those strategies, and the consequence of available choices (Dunn, 2000). The occupational therapist and the occupational therapy assistant use developmentally appropriate language when conveying such information to children, adolescents, and their caregivers and family members. In collaboration with these individuals, the occupational therapist and occupational therapy assistant outline a course of action. Client-centered practice requires the occupational therapist and the occupational therapy assistant to understand and respect the values, beliefs, priorities, goals, and performance context of the children and adolescents and their family or caregivers. Because client centered practice is culturally sensitive, occupational therapists and occupational therapy assistants participate in continuing education initiatives to learn about the customs, practices, and language of various cultures.

SUMMARY

Occupations involve the doing of activities that are meaningful, purposeful, and recognizable for the individuals, and the societies in which they live. The domain, or area of human concern, of occupational therapy is the occupations of people. The domain of occupational therapy includes consideration of areas of occupation, performance skills, and performance patterns needed to accomplish those occupations, the context in which those occupations are performed, the activity demands inherent in the occupations, and client factors that influence the occupational engagement. Consistent with this domain is the belief that participation in occupations can contribute to the health and well-being of children and adolescents. Occupational therapists and occupational therapy assistants can use occupations and purposeful activities therapeutically to facilitate the ability of children and adolescents to participate in meaningful lives.

When providing occupational therapy services to children and adolescents, occupational therapists and occupational therapy assistants conduct an evaluation, design and implement an intervention, review the intervention, and measure the outcomes of the provided services. The occupational therapist assumes full responsibility for each stage of the occupational therapy process. The occupational therapy assistant, supervised by the occupational therapist, contributes to and collaborates in each stage of this process.

Consistent with the core tenet of the profession, the occupational therapy process is client centered. In client centered practice the children, adolescents, and their family members or caregiver are actively involved in the decision about the need for services, the goal of those services, and the types of services received. The children, adolescents, and their families or caregivers are the expert about their shared life experiences. The occupational therapist and the occupational therapy assistant are experts on occupations and occupational performance challenges. In client centered practice, the occupational therapist and the occupational therapy assistant respect the values, beliefs, priorities, goals, culture and other performance context of the children and adolescents and their family or caregivers.

REVIEWING KEY POINTS

1. Define the following terms:

Activity	Activity demands
Activities of daily living	Adaptation
Areas of occupation	Client
Client factors	Concept
Construct	Context
Education	Environmental factor
Evaluation	Habits
Instrumental activities of daily living	Interventions
	Occupation
Leisure	Occupational profile
Occupational form	Participation
Outcome	Performance skills
Performance patterns	Preparatory methods
Play	Rituals
Purposeful activity	Roles
Routines	Social participation
Work	

2. Paraphrase two explanations of occupation and explain how they are similar and different from one another.
3. Explain how the language in *ICF* relates to the definition of occupation used in occupational therapy.
4. Explain what is meant by the domain of occupational therapy.
5. Explain each aspect of the domain of occupational therapy.
6. Explain what is meant by the process of occupational therapy.
7. Explain each aspect of the process of occupational therapy
8. Outline the steps of the occupational therapy process.
9. Explain what is meant by client centered care.

APPLYING KEY CONCEPTS

1. Using language that is consistent with their roles and experiences, audiotape an explanation of occupation and occupational therapy for the following people: family members of a preschooler with a developmental disability; an educator deciding the scope of occupational therapy services in the school system; an adolescent coping with depression; a community based nurse working with medically fragile children in their homes.
2. Using the language of the *Occupational Therapy Practice Framework*, give three examples of activities children or adolescents might do for each of the following areas of occupations: activities of daily living, instrumental activities of daily living, education, work, play, leisure, and social participation.
3. Observe two children or adolescents from different cultures engaging in several occupations. Give examples of when opportunities for self-choice and the cul-

tural expectations influenced how the children or adolescents engaged in their occupations.

4. Watch a video of a child or adolescent who is having some difficulty performing a daily life activity. Use Table 1.1 to record the observations and the potential intervention plans. Outline what you think might be possible outcomes of the intervention.

REFERENCES

American Occupational Therapy Association (1994). Uniform terminology for occupational therapy (3rd ed.). *American Journal of Occupational Therapy, 48,* 1047–1054.

American Occupational Therapy Association (2002). Occupational therapy practice framework: Domain and process. *American Journal of Occupational Therapy, 56,* 609–639.

American Occupational Therapy Association (2004a). Guidelines for supervision, roles, and responsibilities during the delivery of occupational therapy. *American Journal of Occupational Therapy, 58,* 663–667.

American Occupational Therapy Association (2004b). Scope of practice. *American Journal of Occupational Therapy, 58,* 673–677.

American Occupational Therapy Association (nd). Occupational therapy practice framework: Domain and process (2nd ed.). Draft.

Christiansen, E. (1991). *A proud heritage: The American Occupational Therapy Association at seventy-five.* Rockville, MD: AOTA.

Christiansen, C., & Baum, C. (Eds.). (1997). *Occupational therapy: Enabling function and well-being* (2nd ed.). Thorofare, NJ: SLACK.

Christiansen, C., Baum, C., & Bass-Haugen, J. (Ed.). (2005). *Occupational therapy: Performance, participation, and well-being.* Thorofare, NJ: SLACK.

Cronin, A., & Mandich, M. (2005). *Human development and performance throughout the lifespan.* Clifton Park, NY: Thomson Delmar Learning.

Bronfenbrenner, U. (1979). *The ecology of human development: Experiments by nature and design.* Cambridge, MA: Harvard University Press.

Bronfenbrenner, U. (1997). Systems vs. associations: It's not either/or. *Families in Society, 78,* 124.

Dunn, W. (2000). Best practice occupational therapy: In community service with children and families. Thorofare, NJ: SLACK.

Farnworth, L. (1999). Time use and leisure occupations of young offenders. *American Journal of Occupational Therapy, 54,* 315–324.

Feldman, R. (2007). *Child development* (4th ed.). Upper Saddle River, NJ: Prentice Hall.

Fisher, A. (2006). Overview of performance skills and client factors. In H. McHugh Pendelton and W. Schultz-Krohn (Eds.), *Pedrettti's occupational therapy: Practice skills for physical dysfunction* (6th ed.). St. Louis: Mosby Elsevier.

Fisher, G., & Kielhofner, G. (1995). Skill in occupational performance. In G. Kielhofner (Ed.), *A model of human occupation: Theory and application* (2nd ed.) Philadelphia: Lippincott & Wilkins.

Kielhofner, G. (2007). *Model of human occupation: Theory and application* (4th ed.). Baltimore: Lippincott Williams & Wilkins.

Kramer, P., Hinojosa, J., & Royeen, C. (2003). *Perspectives in human occupation: Participation in life.* Philadelphia: Lippincott, Williams, & Wilkins.

Law, M., Polatajko, H., Baptiste, W., & Townsend, E. (1997). Concepts of occupational therapy. In E. Townsend (Ed.), *Enabling occupation: An occupational therapy perspective* (pp. 29–56). Ottawa, ON: Canadian Association of Occupational Therapists.

McDevitt, T. M., & Ormrod, J. E. (2004). *Child development: Educating and working with children and adolescents* (2nd ed.). Upper Saddle River, NJ: Prentice Hall.

Merriam-Webster Collegiate Dictionary (11th ed.) (2007). Retrieved October 2, 2007 from http://www.Merriam-WebsterCollegiate.com.

Meyer, A. (1922). The philosophy of occupational therapy. *Archives of Occupational Therapy, 1,* 1–10.

Mosey, A. (1996). *Applied scientific inquiry in the health professions. An epistemological orientation* (2nd ed.). Bethesda, MD: American Occupational Therapy Association.

Nelson, D. L., & Jepson-Thomas, J. (2003). Occupational form, occupational performance, and a conceptual framework for therapeutic occupation. In P. Kramer, J. Hinojosa, & C. Royeen (Eds.), *Perspectives in human occupation: Participation in life,* pp. 87–155. Philadelphia: Lippincott Williams & Wilkins.

Parham, L. D., & Fazio, L. S. (Eds.) (1997). *Play in occupational therapy for children.* St. Louis: Mosby.

Pierce, D. (2001). Untangling occupation and activity. *American Journal of Occupational Therapy, 55,* 138–146.

Quiroga, V. (1995). *Occupational therapy: The first 30 years.* AOTA: Bethesda, MD.

Rogers, J., & Holm, M. (1994). Assessment in self-care. In B. R. Bonder & M.B. Bonder (Eds.), *Functional performance in older adults,* pp. 181–202. Philadelphia: F.A. Davis.

Vander Zanden, J., Crandell, T., & Crandell, C. (2003). *Human development* (7th ed. rev). Boston: McGraw-Hill.

Velde, B., & Fidler, G. (2002). *Lifestyle performance: A model for engaging the power of occupation.* Thorofare, NJ: SLACK.

West, W. (1984). A reaffirmed philosophy and practice of occupational therapy for the 1980's. *American Journal of Occupational Therapy, 38,* 15–23.

World Health Organization (2001). *International classification of functioning, disability, and health.* Geneva, Switzerland: Author.

Zemke, R., & Clark, F. (Eds.) (1996). *Occupational science: The evolving discipline.* Philadelphia: Davis.

Chapter

Occupation-Based Conceptual Models for Guiding Practice

Janet V. DeLany

Key Terms

Affordance
Conceptual models
Environmental factors
Frame of reference
Habituation
Human agency
Interests
Occupational competence
Occupational form
Participation
Performance capacity

Performance range
Person factors
Person variables
Personal causation
Physical environment
Press
Social environment
Tasks
Temporal factors
Values
Volition

Objectives

- Articulate the importance of occupation-based conceptual models for making practice decisions.
- Explain basic constructs and assumptions of selected occupation-based conceptual models: the Ecology of Human Performance Model, the Model of Human Occupation, the Person-Environment-Occupational Performance Model, and the Person-Environment-Occupation Model.

INTRODUCTION

A **conceptual model** is set of constructs and assumptions organized in a systematic manner to represent their interrelatedness. A conceptual model defines these constructs, clarifies these assumptions, and explains the linkages among them (Burke, 2003). It helps to define the focus of a profession and its relationship to other professions (Mosey, 1981). It also guides the therapeutic practices and research questions of the profession. Sometimes, a conceptual model is called a conceptual framework (Dunn, 2000) or a professional model (Mosey, 1981). A conceptual model differs from a **frame of reference** in that it applies to the entire profession. In contrast, a frame of reference applies to a specific area of practice to guide evaluation, intervention, and outcome procedures (Burke, 2003; Mosey, 1981). Occupation-based conceptual models are discussed in this chapter. Frames of reference used in occupational therapy practice are discussed in Chapter 3.

Initially, as did other professions, occupational therapy relied on conceptual models developed by other disciplines, particularly education, psychology, sociology, anthropology, and biology, to understand human development and to frame therapeutic practice. As the profession of occupational therapy became more established, a number of occupational therapists and occupational scientists developed occupation-based conceptual models to guide the thinking about and delivery of occupational therapy. Some of the conceptual models currently used in occupational therapy practice are the Ecological Model of Human Performance (Dunn, Brown, & McGuigan, 1994), the Model of Human Occupation (Kielhofner, 2002), the Person-Environment-Occupational Performance Model (Christiansen & Baum, 1997; Baum & Christiansen, 2005), and the Person-Environment-Occupation Model (Law, Cooper, Strong, Steward, Rigby, & Letts, 1996). Each of these models is discussed in the following sections. Other occupation-based conceptual models, such as the Canadian Model of Occupational Therapy (CAOT, 1997), the Lifestyle Performance Model (Velde & Fidler, 2002), the Conceptual Model for Therapeutic Occupation (Nelson & Jepson-Thomas, 2003), and the Occupational Adaptation Model (Schkade & Schultz, 1992; Schultz & Schkade, 1992.), are worth reviewing but are beyond the scope of this text.

Though each of these conceptual models has distinct features, common to all is an appreciation of the person, the occupations and the activities that the person performs, and the contexts or environments in which the person performs these activities and occupations. Each model acknowledges that individuals are complex beings, influenced by and reflecting intersecting biological, social, cognitive, and psychological processes. Each model also acknowledges that the individuals' stages of development influence the tasks and roles they can and are expected to accomplish. Finally, each model supports the assumption that participation in occupations promotes health and wellness when there is a match among the person, the tasks, and the environments in which the occupational performance occurs (Baum & Christiansen, 2005).

More commonly, occupational therapists assume the responsibility for determining the conceptual model most applicable for the needs of the particular children and adolescents with whom they and occupational therapy assistants work. However, it is important for occupational therapy assistants to understand the conceptual models so that they can work effectively with the occupational therapists to consider systematically the occupations, the performance skills and patterns, the performance contexts, and the body functions of children and adolescents, and the demands of the activities they are trying to accomplish. The ability to articulate the occupation-based conceptual model guiding clinical reasoning clarifies the distinction of professional roles and responsibilities between occupational therapy and other professional disciplines, and justifies the appropriateness of occupational therapy services. Occupational therapists and occupational therapy assistants use the supervisory, professional, and continuing education processes within their practice settings, and within the state and national occupational therapy associations to learn about and use occupation-based conceptual models.

OCCUPATION-BASED CONCEPTUAL MODELS

Ecological Model of Human Performance

The Ecological Model of Human Performance was developed by the occupational faculty at the University of Kansas (Dunn, Brown, & McGuigan, 1994). They incorporated the work of Bronfrenbrenner (1979; 1997), who emphasized the significance of environmental influences on how children learn, develop, and perform. The Ecological Model of Human Performance underscores the dynamic relationship among the context, the person, and the task on the scope and quality of human performance. When using this model to work with children and adolescents, the occupational therapist and the occupational therapy assistant consider the relative importance of directing interventions toward the person, and toward modifying and adapting tasks and contexts (Dunn, 2000). This model contrasts with other models that direct focus primarily on the person, giving only limited focus to the task or context. For example, when using the Ecological Model of Human Performance to guide the intervention for a preschool child with spastic cerebral palsy, the occupational therapist and the occupational therapy assistant consider strategies to address the task and the context in addition to those that address the neuromuscular abilities of the child. They consider how to adapt the toys and classroom materials to maximize the ability of the child to use his existing skills to play with them. They also consider the layout of the classroom, the placement of the toys and materials, the temporal sequence of the classroom activities, the culture of the child and the preschool, and the capacities of the other preschoolers to partner with and include the child in the play and learning activities. Below is the schema that depicts the Ecological Model of Human Performance (see Figure 2.1■).

Constructs of the Ecological Model of Human Performance

Person, task, context, and performance are the four central constructs of the model. Because the Ecological Model of Human Performance was designed as an interdisciplinary model, the construct **occupation** is not stated explicitly in the schema. Rather, it is implied as part of the dynamic relationship between the person and the context that defines and gives meaning to a series of integrated tasks (Dunn, Brown, & Youngstrom, 2003).

Within this model, the **person** is considered a unique individual who brings a set of **personal variables**, that is, personal values, interests, experiences, and skills, to the task. Similar to the language often found in educational setting, skills in this model include sensorimotor, cognitive, and psychosocial skills. The personal variables, in conjunction with the surrounding context, influence the tasks that the person can and chooses to perform. They affect the performance level of and meaning that the person attaches to the task. Thus, two children or adolescents working on a similar task such as counting money may perform the task differently because of how they value money,

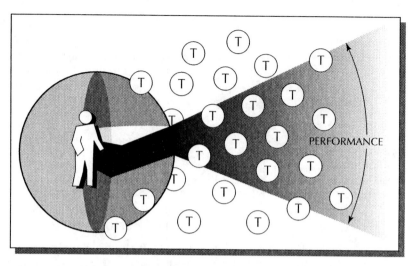

■ Figure 2.1
Schemata of a typical person within the Ecology of Human Performance framework.
Copyright Dunn, W., Brown, C., & McGuigan, A. (1994). The ecology of human performance: A
framework for considering the effect of context. *American Journal of Occupational Therapy, 48.*
Used by permission.

their interest in the specific counting activity they are performing, their current skills
for thinking about and executing the counting task, and the context which supports
or creates barriers for their performance. The personal variables change in response
to new experiences the person has, to shifts in the context, and to the passage of time.
Changes in these person variables may increase or limit the person's ability to perform
various tasks.

Tasks are the series of objective behaviors sequenced to achieve a specific goal
(Dunn et al., 2003). Counting money includes the tasks of picking up the money, sorting the money by denominations, placing the money in specified containers, recording the money, and exchanging money for goods or services. When clustered together
and given meaning, these tasks can define the roles and occupations of the person. One
adolescent may incorporate the money counting tasks in her role and occupation as a
store clerk. Another adolescent may incorporate them into her role and occupation as
a shopper (see Figure 2.2■). The children and adolescents are surrounded by a potentially unlimited number of tasks. Their person and context variables influence the
tasks they can access and accomplish.

According the Ecological Model of Human Performance, **context** is the temporal
and environmental factors that continually surround and provide support to and barriers for the person. This definition of context differs in some respects from the definition of context in the *Occupational Therapy Practice Framework* (AOTA, 2002). In the
Ecological Model of Human Performance, **temporal factors** are made up of the temporal features of the person and temporal features of the task. The person's chronological age, developmental stage, life cycle, and health status, are the temporal features of
that person. The number of task steps, the duration and recurrence rate of the task, and
the time when the task occurs are the temporal factors of the task. The physical, social,
and cultural dimensions external to the person are the environmental factors (Dunn et
al. 1994; 2003). For example, an eighteen-year-old adolescent male with Down Syndrome, employed as a part-time clerk at the school book store, may count money by first
using one tray to sort bills and coins according to denominations, and then by using a
second tray to count and bag a specified number of identical bills or coins. In contrast,

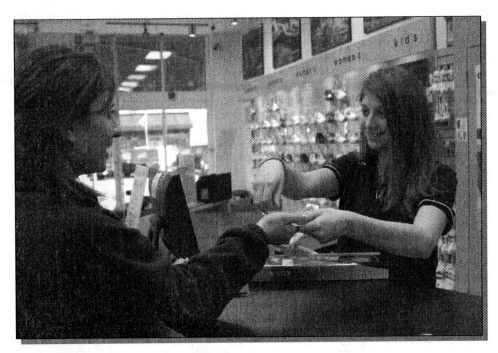

■ **Figure 2.2**
The store clerk and the shopper exchanging money.

a fifteen-year-old teen parent who lives in an emergency shelter may keep careful count of her weekly expenditure of food stamps to stretch limited resources for the month.

Performance involves the selecting and doing of tasks. The Ecological Model of Human Performance highlights that individuals have performance ranges available to them. Inside this range are those tasks the person can and wants to accomplish. Outside the range are those tasks that exist, but are not meaningful, available, or within the skill capacity of the person. Some individuals have a narrow range of performance, while others have a wide range of performance (Dunn et al., 2003). In the above scenarios, the cognitive skills of the adolescent male and the economic factors of the adolescent female limit their range of performance. In contrast, the money counting adaptations provided to the adolescent male, and the food stamps provided to the adolescent mother broaden their performance range.

Assumptions of the Ecological Model of Human Performance

Key assumptions embedded within the model tie together the person, task, context, and performance constructs. To use the Ecological Model of Human Performance effectively, it is important to appreciate that children and adolescents are understood only within the context that surrounds them. This context influences their performance and their performance range; children and adolescents also affect the context where they perform. It is through their performance of tasks that the children and adolescents sustain or change their personal variables and the context that surrounds them. According the Ecological Model of Human Performance, it is best to assess the performance of the children and adolescents and provide interventions to them in their natural environments. Contrived contexts affect their performance and performance range. When they provide additional supports, contrived environments make it easier for the children and adolescents to perform; when they introduce unfamiliar objects and procedures, contrived environments make it more difficult for the children and adolescents to perform. Occupational therapy interventions provided to the children and adolescents should be directed at the wants and needs they and their family identify as important (Dunn et al., 2003).

Interventions

Within the Ecological Model of Human Performance, interventions can be directed at the person, the task, the context, or a combination of all three. Similar to those identified in the *Occupational Therapy Practice Framework* (AOTA), these interventions include establishing or restoring the ability of the person to accomplish the task, altering the context for performing the task, adapting or modify the task or context, preventing the development of a performance problem, and creating circumstances that support the performance capacities of all individuals (Dunn et al., 1994, 2003). Thus, an occupational therapy assistant may establish the ability of the male adolescent in the above scenario to put piles of 30 dimes into three separate $1 wrappers by using clear plastic tubes to modify the sorting and counting tasks. The occupational therapy assistant may prevent additional financial problems for the teen mother by helping her to transition to a foster home and by teaching her money management strategies. In some situations, it may be more efficient and effective to improve the performance of children and adolescents by directing the intervention strategies at the tasks they need to perform or context surrounding them rather than at their personal variables.

Model of Human Occupation

Similar to the Ecological Model of Human Performance, the **Model of Human Occupation** also considers the person, the occupation or activities, the performance, and the context. However, whereas the Ecological Model of Human Performance directs particular attention to the context, the **Model of Human Occupation** directs particular attention to the person. Building upon the concepts of occupational behavior formulated by Mary Reilly (1962, 1969), Kielhofner, Burke, and Heard published the first version of the Model of Human Occupation in 1980. Since that time, the model has evolved into its current, dynamic form (Kielhofner, 2002). The goal of the authors was to create a model that fostered understanding of occupations in the daily lives of people and the role occupations played in health and illness. They wanted a model that expanded the conceptual understanding of the nature of occupation, applied to practice, and guided research. To achieve these goals, the authors and other colleagues published extensive literature about the theoretical underpinnings of human occupation, conducted studies to evaluate the efficacy of using the Model of Human Occupation with various populations, generated case examples, and developed and field tested assessment tools. Much of the information related to the Model of Human Occupation can be found at the Model of Human Occupation Clearinghouse at the University of Illinois at Chicago or at its website at http://www.uic.edu/hsc/acad/cahp/OT/ (Forsyth & Kielhofner, 2003).

The Model of Human Occupation provides a structure to consider the:

- Motivational aspects of occupations **(volition)**
- Routines and patterns imbedded within the behaviors used to perform the occupations **(habituation)**
- Level and types of skill needed to perform the occupations **(performance capacities)**
- Influence of the environment on the performance

The model helps occupational therapists and occupational therapy assistants to look at what occupations children and adolescents choose to perform, what motivates them to engage in various daily life occupations, and how these occupations contribute to their sense of who they are. The model also directs occupational therapists and occupational therapy assistants to take into consideration the children's and adolescents' existing and needed routines and roles, their existing and needed skill levels, and the environmental influence on what they do. The constructs and assumptions of the Model of Human Occupation are depicted in a drawing that helps to clarify how the pieces of the model fit together to convey the dynamic nature of human occupation (see Figure 2.3■) (Forsyth & Kielhofner, 2003; Kielhofner, 2002).

Constructs of the Model of Human Occupation

The three main constructs of the Model of Human Occupation are **person, environment**, and **occupational performance**. Of these, the person construct is the most fully detailed.

Person.   In the Model of Human Occupation, the person is described in terms of **volition, habituation**, and **performance capacities**. In the model, each of these terms is further divided.

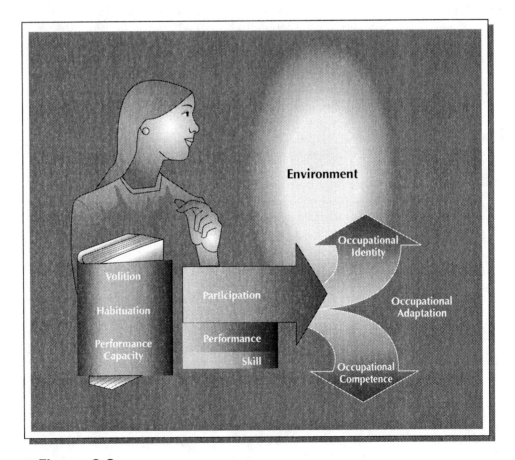

■ Figure 2.3
The process of occupational adaptation.
Copyright Kielhofner, G. (2002). *Model of human occupation. Theory and application* (3rd ed.). Baltimore, MD: Lippincott Williams & Wilkins. Used by permission.

As related to children and adolescents, **volition** is the patterns of feelings and thoughts they have about what is important to them (**values**), what they believe they are capable of doing (**personal causation**), and what they find pleasurable and satisfying to do (**interests**). Volition motivates children and adolescents to participate in various activities and occupations. As part of the volitional process they

- **Anticipate** what activities and occupations to do
- **Choose** and **experience** those activities and occupations
- **Interpret** their choices and experiences

This process allows them to reflect on their actions over time and develop a sense of their current and potential abilities (Forsyth & Kielhofner, 2003; Kielhofner, 2002).

The patterns of feelings and thoughts associated with volition can alter over time for children and adolescents based on their biological propensities, developmental stages, life experiences, changing capacities, awareness of these capacities, and environmental influences (Kielhofner, 2002). As children and adolescents succeed, their **sense of their personal capacity** and **self-efficacy** strengthen and motivate them to engage in more complex and healthy occupations. When children and adolescents confront challenges and barriers that prohibit their success, they experience a diminished sense of personal capacity and self-efficacy, resulting in more limited and unhealthy occupations. For example, two seven-year-old boys may value the opinions of their teachers over those of his peers, believe they are capable learners, and find pleasure in school activities. By the time they become thirteen, one of these boys successfully blends together the values of his teachers and peers, believes he can assume leadership roles within his school, and enjoys a number of athletic and creative arts activities. In contrast, the other boy may devalue the opinions of his teachers, feel that he is failure as a student, and become involved in risky, gang behaviors. Children and adolescents with disabilities confront additional difficulties that challenge their volition. The disability itself, in conjunction with negative societal attitudes toward disabilities and nonsupportive environments, can limit options for testing values, developing a sense of personal capacity, and forging interests.

Within the Model of Human Occupation, **habituation** refers to the repeated patterns and behaviors that provide routine and familiarity to people's daily lives. As applied children and adolescents, these patterns and behaviors create a rhythm and structure within the physical, social, and temporal dimensions of their lives. The **habits** and **roles** that are part of these patterns help the children and adolescents accomplish portions of their tasks efficiently and semi-automatically. Habits refer to how the children and adolescents repeatedly perform an activity, allocate time, and demonstrate particular styles of behavior. Roles provide a way for them to identify who they are and what they do within a social system. Various social systems identify children and adolescents by these roles, placing expectations on how they should behave and perform. Once internalized, roles shape how they look and think about themselves and the world (Forsyth & Kielhofner, 2003; Kielhofner, 2002). Occupational therapists and occupational therapy assistants help children and adolescents develop healthy habits and roles so that they can participate actively in their daily life occupations. For example, an occupational therapy assistant might help a young child with attention deficits to develop her roles as a student. This may include helping the student to organize her morning school routine by developing the habit of hanging her coat on the locker hook, placing her homework assignments on the teacher's desk, and then putting her books inside her desk, within the first five minutes of arrival. The occupational therapy assistant also might help a child who has autism to expand his narrow range of morning habits so that he develops the ability to respond to novel classroom situations.

According to the Model of Human Occupation, **performance capacity** involves not only the objective physical and mental components necessary to do the activity but also the subjective experience. Both occur at the moment of doing the activity within a given environment. By acknowledging the subjective and the objective aspects of performance, the model attempts to unify the mind and body in the act of doing. This acknowledgement helps to clarify that the feeling of the experience is central to and occurs simultaneously with the doing of the activity. Feeling of the experience can help guide and modify the doing. In contrast to research associated with other models that focus primarily on understanding the objective aspects of performance capacity, research associated with the Model of Human Occupations focuses primarily on understanding the subjective aspects (Forsyth & Kielhofner, 2003; Kielhofner, Tham, Baz, & Hutson, 2002). Using this model to work on the morning routines in the above scenarios, the occupational therapy assistant would be concerned with understanding how the children feel when they practice their new habits, and how these feelings reinforce or alter new performance behaviors.

Environment.   According to the Model of Human Occupations, environments include **physical** and **social environments**. As applied to children and adolescents, these physical and social environments influence what is accessible for them to do and what they are allowed to do. Physical environments can be natural, such as rivers, forests, and oceans. They can be man made, such as schools, hospitals, and community centers. Objects within these environments can be natural, such as plants and rock, or fabricated, such as desks, beds, and chairs. Social environments are the **social groups** and the **occupational form**. Social groups set norms about what children and adolescents can do and where they can do the activities. Families, neighbors, church groups, and classmates are some of the social groups that set norms about what children and adolescents can do. Occupational forms are the activities that are available for children and adolescents to do within a particular social and physical environment. Occupational form involves a sequence of rule-bound actions that are recognized, named, and understood by the members of the society. Occupational forms available to children and adolescents in the natural environment of a river might be fishing, swimming, and canoeing. Occupational forms available at a community center might be cooking, painting, or dancing.

Occupational performance.   As outlined in the Model of Human Occupation, **occupational performance** is the actual doing of the occupational forms. It is the doing of the fishing, swimming, and canoeing on the river, and the cooking, painting, and dancing at the community center. To perform these occupations requires **skills**. These skills include the motor skills, process skills, and communication and interaction skills described in Chapter 1 (Fisher, 2006). Skills are discernable, goal-directed actions. Through combining and sequencing these skills, children and adolescents perform their activities and occupation. This performance allows the children and adolescents to **participate in their occupations**. Consistent with the philosophy of occupational therapy, the ability of children and adolescents to participate in occupations leads to their self-identity, their sense of competency, and their capacity to adapt to life changes (Forsyth & Kielhofner, 2003; Kielhofner, 2002).

Assumptions of the Model of Human Occupation

To use the Model of Human Occupation effectively, it is important to understand the foundational assumptions that underlie these constructs. Within the Model of Human Occupation it is assumed that motivational factors, daily life patterns and routines, performance capabilities, and the environment influence the occupations that the children and adolescents can and choose to do. Each of these influences acts in concert with one another to influence occupational choices and behaviors of the children and adolescents. As well, it is through the performing of their occupations that the children and adolescents maintain and change their daily life patterns and routines, their performance capabilities, the environments, and internal and external motivational factors. The children's and adolescents' repertoire of occupational behavior changes over time. How and why the occupational behaviors change is dependent on the inner characteristics of the children and adolescents, and the context in which the occupations occur. It is through the doing of occupations that children and adolescents shape and define who they are. Thus, occupations are self-organizing. By using occupations, occupational therapists and occupational therapy assistants help children and adolescents to organize themselves and shape their identities (Forsyth & Kielhofner, 2003; Kielhofner, 2002).

Interventions

Within the Model of Human Occupation, intervention is directed at the person, the environment, and the occupational performance with the intent of fostering occupational competency and adaptation. When using the Model of Human Occupation to work with children and adolescents, careful attention is paid to their sense of personal causation, values, interests, habits, roles, and the subjective experience of their performance capacities. In addition, particular consideration is given to how the disabilities of the children and adolescents, and society's view of their disabilities contribute to the health or dysfunction of their occupational choices and behaviors (Forsyth & Kielhofner, 2003).

Person-Environment-Occupational Performance Model

Participation of people in occupations that are important and meaningful to them is the central focus of the Person-Environment-Occupational Performance Model. Developed by Christiansen and Baum (1991,1997; Baum and Christiansen, 2005), the model highlights that the person, the environment, and what people need and want to do intersect at the point of **occupational performance** and **participation**. The model is client centered; the client may be the individual, the organization, or the community. As applied to children and adolescents, the model emphasizes that the interaction between their person factors and environmental factors either can support or create barriers to the performance of and participation in occupations. These occupations include roles, tasks, and activities that the children and adolescents value.

The model uses a top-down approach. This means that the model directs occupational therapists and occupational therapy assistants to learn first what the children and adolescents perceive as their primary occupational performance and occupational participation challenges. Based on this knowledge, the model then directs occupational therapists and the occupational therapy assistants to collect information about the personal factors and environmental factors contributing to these performance and participation challenges (Baum & Christiansen, 2005).

When using this model, occupational therapists and occupational therapy assistants first consider what occupations are necessary and of value for the children and adolescents to perform, then the personal and environmental factors that contribute to and impede their performance and participation.

The following scenario illustrates how to use the top-down approach of the Person-Environment-Occupational Performance Model to conduct social skills groups for children and adolescents. First, the occupational therapist and occupational therapy assistant might talk with the children and adolescents to ascertain what social situations such as in-class, recreational, and performing arts activities are important to and challenging for them. Then, using additional interviews, observations, and measurement tools, the occupational therapist and occupational therapy assistant gather needed information about the children's and adolescents' personal capacity to participate in those social situations, and environmental factors that influence where and how they participate. The schema below depicts the Person-Environment-Occupational Performance Model (see Figure 2.4■).

Constructs of the Person-Environment-Occupational Performance Model

As implied by its title, person, environment, occupation, and occupational performance are the four main constructs of the model. Its core emphasis is on competent occupational performance so that people can lead productive and meaningful lives.

Person factors include genetically predisposed capacities and those that are nurtured and developed in response to experiences. Engagement in occupations, such as social participation occupations, strengthens person factors. Conversely, the more developed their person factors, the more successfully children and adolescents can perform their occupations. **Person factors** include the neurobiological, physiological, cognitive, psychological, emotional, and spiritual factors intrinsic to the child or adolescent.

- **Neurobehavioral** factors include the sensory and motor systems working in concert to produce behaviors necessary to perform.
- **Physiological** factors involve the physical health and level of fitness necessary to perform.
- **Cognitive factors** include the language, attention, reasoning, memory, and organizational capacities to participate in the occupation.

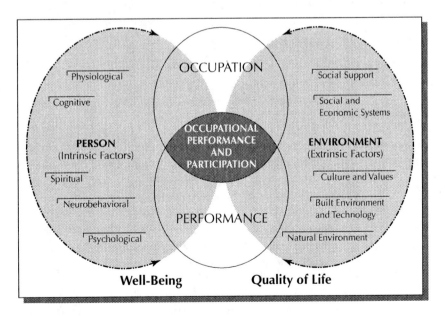

■ Figure 2.4
The Person-Environment-Occupation-Performance (PEOP) model.
Copyright Christiansen, C., Baum, C. M., & Bass-Haugen, J. (Eds). (2005). *Occupational therapy: Performance, participation, and well-being* (3rd ed). Thorofare, NJ: SLACK. Used by permission.

- **Psychological and emotional factors** include personality traits, motivational factors, and internal processes that affect self-concept, self- identity, and sense of well-being.
- **Spiritual factors** focus on the meanings attributed to the nature of the situation and the experiences, the symbols attached to objects and actions within those situations and experiences, and the contributions these meanings and symbols make to individuals' sense of self and place within the world. It is important to note that the Person-Environment-Occupational Performance Model is one of the few occupation-based conceptual models that explicitly identify spirituality as a person factor (Baum & Christiansen, 2005).

Environmental factors include societal factors, social interactions, social and economic systems, culture environment, built environments and technology, and natural environment. They are extrinsic to the child or adolescent.

- **Societal factors** are the values and attitudes of a society that affect the standing of the children and adolescents within the group and influence policies and laws regarding access to and availability of resources.
- **Social interactions** are the networks children and adolescents have with other people that foster social interactions and provide practical, informational, and emotional support.
- **Social and economic systems** create the social and fiscal policies and practices to generate and allocate resources.
- The **cultural environment** includes the customs, values, beliefs, and norms that the children and adolescents share intergenerationally with other people within a particular society.
- **Physical environments and technology** are the buildings, spaces, objects, tools, and technologies that the children and adolescents use to in their daily living.
- **Natural environments** include the geographic terrain, weather, temperature, amount of sunlight, and noise level and air quality within nature.

The degree of compatibility between the person factors and the environmental factors influence the inclination children and adolescents have to explore and interact in their worlds (Baum and Christiansen, 2005). Thus, for the above social skills group scenario, the occupational therapist and occupational therapy assistant would gather information about how these environmental factors affect the ability of the children and adolescents to participate in social situations. Children and adolescents are more likely to explore and interact with those environments that they perceive are safe and offer the right amount of challenge for their particular set of person factors. Children and adolescents are more likely to avoid environments that they perceive as threatening or offering too much or too little challenge for their particular set of person factors.

Environments create **press** or expectations to perform in particular manner and offer **affordance** to support performance (Christiansen & Baum, 2005). For example, social situations in school environments create press and offer affordance to sit and speak quietly, and to use paper, pencils, and computers. In contrast, social situations in playground environments create press and offer affordance to run, to jump, and to experiment with and learn through movement activities. Occupational therapists and occupational therapy assistants work with children, adolescents, and their families to identify and design environments that provide the amount of press and affordance to support their participation in the daily occupations.

Occupations, according the Person-Environment-Occupational Performance Model, involve the doing of everyday life pursuits. They are goal directed, extend over a period of time, hold particular meaning for the children and adolescents, and involve sequencing and integrating multiple tasks. **Tasks** are a combination of observable actions that have shared purpose. Occupations have structure and defined expectations. Their structure and expectations come from their purpose, temporal properties, and social dimensions (Baum & Christiansen, 2005). Occupations that children and adolescents perform shape their roles; likewise, the roles children and adolescents have shape the occupations they perform.

Occupational performance joins together the occupation with the act of doing. It involves doing or performing a sequence of integrated tasks that form an occupation meaningful to the individual. To do or perform the occupations may require intrinsic capacities of the person, the extrinsic support from the environment, or blend of both. When working with children and adolescents, occupational therapists and occupational therapy assistants need to carefully assess their intrinsic capacities, and the environmental affordance and press to design interventions that support their existing and developing occupations and roles.

Assumptions of the Person-Environment-Occupational Performance Model
Several assumptions underscore the constructs of the Person-Environment-Occupational Performance Model. As applied to children and adolescents, it is assumed that they are naturally motivated to explore and master their environments. Labeled **human agency,** this motivation enables the children and adolescents to effectively use the social, material, and personal resources available within their environments to learn, problem solve, and achieve goals that contribute to life satisfaction. A second assumption is that when children and adolescents experience success, they feel good about themselves and thus confront new challenges with a greater sense of competency. They derive a sense of fulfillment and mastery when they accomplish occupational goals that have personal meaning. Over time these experiences help the children and adolescents to define who they are and their place in the world (Baum & Christiansen, 2005). As applied to the social skills group, occupational therapists and occupational therapy assistants would design interventions that allow the children and adolescents to derive a sense of fulfillment and mastery from effectively using resources to explore and master their environments. This may involve providing practice sessions, adapting activities and tools, modifying environments, and providing buddy systems.

Interventions
In this model it is assumed that children and adolescents benefit from support from others to overcome the personal, societal, and disability–related barriers that limit participation. Occupational therapy is viewed as a process for enabling the children and adolescents to engage or re-engage in occupations that are important and meaningful to them when such engagement is limited or threatened by their health conditions, societal factors, or disabilities (Baum & Christiansen, 2005). Occupational therapy focuses on developing **occupational competence,** that is, competent occupational performance so that the children and adolescents can lead satisfying and meaningful lives.

Occupational therapists and occupational therapy assistants can use a wide range of client-centered strategies to help the children and adolescents develop skills or use resources so that they can participate in their occupations. Guided by this model, occupational therapists and occupational therapy assistants sometimes direct interventions at the person factors; other times, at the environmental factors. Interventions directed at the person factors strengthen, restore, or develop needed capacities. Those directed at the environment expand it and thus make it more accessible. Sometimes occupational therapists and occupational therapy assistants engage the children and the adolescents in performing occupations; at other times they work with them to develop goals and strategies for removing environmental barriers that limit their roles and activities (Baum & Christiansen, 2005). For example, when providing interventions for a group of elementary age children who live in a homeless shelter, occupational therapists and occupational therapy assistants may use building and construction activities to develop social skills and coping mechanisms. They might work with the administrators of the homeless shelter to create indoor and outdoor play areas for the children. They may introduce the children to a variety of low and no cost games and crafts to practice their social skills and expand their occupational choices. The occupational therapist and occupational therapy assistant also may work with the children and their parents to learn about fee waivers and scholarships for joining the local community center. The combination of these activities may lead to increased capacity for the children to participate in successfully and perform a variety of play and leisure occupations that promote their health and well-being.

Person-Environment-Occupation Model

Law, Cooper, Strong, Stewart, Letts, and Rigby developed the Person-Environment-Occupation Model as part of the Environmental Research Group at McMaster University (Law et al., 1996). They incorporated environmental theories of Lawton and Nahemow (1973), flow theories of Csikszentmihalyi (1988), and the Canadian Guidelines for Occupational Therapy (CAOT, 1997) into the model (Law et al., 1997). It is similar in a number of ways to the Person-Environment-Occupational Performance model and the Ecological Model of Human Performance previously discussed. The Person-Environment-Occupation model supports occupation-based practice and views human development as a life long process. According to the model, occupational performance results from the dynamic relationship among the person, the environment, and the occupation. Maximal occupational performance occurs when there is congruence among the person, the occupation, and the environment (Law et al., 1996). The model has provided a framework to direct education, research, practice, and professional papers in such countries as Canada, the United States, India, and Russia. Because of the clarity of its language, the model also has proven useful when communicating with legislators about health care policy (Crist et al., 2000). The model guides occupational therapists and occupational therapy assistants to consider the child's and adolescent's sense of themselves and their physical and psychosocial capacities, the occupations they need and want to perform, and the environments that surround them and affect their occupational performance. For example, as a coordinator of a Special Olympics program, the occupational therapist and occupational therapy assistant would consider the children's and adolescents' perceptions of themselves as athletes, the athletic related occupations they need and want to perform, their capacities to perform athletic related activities, and the environments affecting their performance. Figure 2.5■ depicts the Person-Environment-Occupation Model (Law et al., 1996).

Constructs of Person-Environment-Occupation Model

As indicated by its name, three constructs of the model are person, environment, and occupation. The construct of occupational performance emerges from the first three constructs.

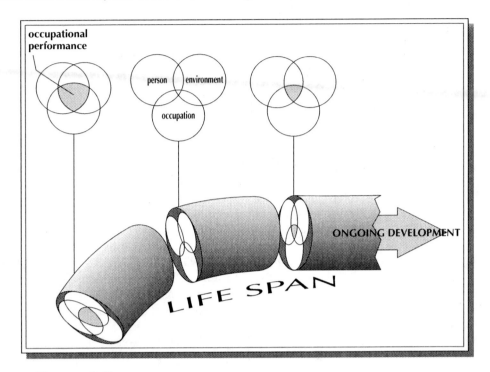

■ Figure 2.5
Person-environment-occupation model.
Copyright Law, M., Cooper, B., Strong, S., Stewart, D., Rigby, P., & Letts, L. (1996). The person-environment-occupation model: A transactive approach to occupational performance. *Canadian Journal of Occupational Therapy, 63*, 1. Used by permission.

Within the model, the **person** can apply to an individual, a group, or a community. The term person incorporates the body, mind, and spiritual aspects of individuals. Persons are viewed as dynamic, motivated, and developing beings who interact with and affect their environments. When working with children and adolescents in the Special Olympics program, the model directs the occupational therapist and occupational therapy assistant to consider the various skills and attributes they possess, their capacity to develop, and the roles they assume within the environment where they prepare for and participate in the Special Olympics program. The model also encourages the occupational therapist and occupational therapy assistant to consider the children and adolescents' previous and emerging sense of themselves as athletes, and their view of their abilities and disabilities (Law, 2000).

Environment includes the physical, social, cultural, and institutional dimensions that influence how and what occupations people perform (Law et al., 1996). Similar to the layers of environment described by Bronfenbrenner (1979, 1997), layers of the environment include the "person, . . . family, neighborhood, community, province or state, country, and world" (Crist et al., p. 113). Such environments can provide supports and barriers to occupational performance (Law, 2000; Law et al., 1996). As Special Olympics coordinators, the occupational therapist and occupational therapy assistant would consider how the environments support or discourage participation in Special Olympics programs, and celebrate or negate the children and adolescents as athletes.

As defined by the model, **occupations** are clusters of self-directed tasks or activities in which people participate throughout their life. They contain psychosocial and physical components. People establish occupational routines that create patterns of time for them during their days, and throughout their weeks and years (Law, 1997). As Special Olympics coordinators, the occupational therapist and occupational therapy assistant would focus on the immediate and long term athletic occupations of the children and adolescents. They also may concern themselves with the self-care occupations of the children and adolescents so that they can prepare themselves to participate in the competitions. In addition, they may concern themselves with the play and social occupations of the children and adolescents that are part of the Special Olympic competitions, buddy programs, and ceremonies.

Occupational performance results when the children and adolescents actively engage in purposeful activities and tasks in a particular environmental setting. Attention is paid to the subjective experience of the performance and to the observable performance. Maximal occupational performance occurs when there is congruency among the person, the environment, and the occupation (Law, 2000). Guided by the Person-Environment-Occupation Model in the role of Special Olympics coordinators, the occupational therapist and occupational therapy assistant focus on the (1) the personal characteristics of children and adolescents; (2) the physical, social, cultural, and institutional environments influencing the Special Olympics program; and (3) the occupations wanted by and expected of the children and adolescents. They endeavor to achieve a goodness of fit among these factors to maximize the occupational performance of the children and adolescents and their subjective experience of that performance.

Assumptions of the Person-Environment-Occupation Model

Underscoring these constructs are central assumptions. The model assumes that the person, the environment, and the occupations change across time and space. The interactions among these factors are fluid, shaping and changing occupational performance throughout the person's life span. When working with children and adolescents, it is important to remember that their behaviors are inseparable from their physical and psychological characteristics, their environments, and their temporal and spatial contexts (Law et al., 1996). While it is healthy for them to have a balance among the areas of occupational performance, this balance is individualized (Crist et al., 2000). The Person-Environment-Occupation model serves as a tool for examining the fit of the children and the adolescents with their environments and their occupation factors, and for analyzing their resultant occupational performance (Crist et al., 2000; Law et al., 1996).

Intervention

Rather than immediately focusing on skills necessary to perform a task, this model guides occupational therapists and occupational therapy assistants to work with the children and adolescents first to consider what they can, need, and want to do, and to examine occupational performance issues. Based on this understanding, evaluation and interventions are directed at the performance challenges and the environmental conditions. When using this model, occupational therapists and occupational therapy assistant work in conjunction with the children, the adolescents, and their families to eliminate barriers and find supports for occupational performance. Intervention is directed toward occupational performance of those activities and tasks the children, the adolescents, and their families identified as important (Crist et al., 2000; Law et al., 1996). In certain circumstances, it may be more effective and efficient for the occupational therapist and the occupational therapy assistant to direct interventions toward changes in the environment that affect the occupational performance than toward changes in the person characteristics of the children and adolescents (Crist, Royeen & Schkade, 2000). The ultimate goal is to establish a fit among the person, the environment, and the occupations.

CONNECTING TO THE OCCUPATIONAL THERAPY PRACTICE FRAMEWORK

Chapter 1 of this text reviewed the purpose and structure of the domain and process of occupational therapy. Specifically, it clarified those areas of human concern that occupational therapy addresses, and delineated the general evaluation, intervention, and outcome procedures occupational therapists and occupational therapy assistants follow to deliver occupational therapy services. This chapter reviewed four occupation-based conceptual models: the Ecological Model of Performance, the Model of Human Occupation, the Person-Environment-Occupation-Performance Model, and the Person-Environment-Occupation Model. Each of the models organizes constructs and assumptions about the nature of human beings, occupations, and environments that influence human beings and occupations, and the performance of those occupations. Their purpose is to provide a particular structure to guide the clinical reasoning occupational therapists and occupational therapy assistants use to direct their knowledge and skills to work with children and adolescents. There are similarities and differences as to how each of the conceptual models organizes these constructs and assumptions, and guides clinical reasoning. It is useful for occupational therapists and occupational therapy assistants to consider how the Occupational Therapy Practice Framework and the conceptual models relate to one another. Doing so strengthens their ability to deliver occupational therapy services to children and adolescents. Table 2.1■ offers one approach for organizing the key constructs and language of the Practice Framework and parts of the occupation-based conceptual models. It demonstrates a method for linking the language of the Practice Framework with some of the concepts and constructs of the four occupation-based practice models reviewed in this chapter. Remember that the language and structure of the Occupational Therapy Practice Framework and these conceptual models will evolve over time in response to research findings and current and emerging occupational therapy practice issues. This makes it necessary for occupational therapists and occupational therapy assistants to revisit the Occupational Therapy Practice Framework and the conceptual models periodically as they practice occupational therapy. Doing so helps keep clear the domain and process of occupational therapy and clinical reasoning processes to follow to provide effective, best occupational therapy practice to the children and adolescents.

■ Table 2.1
Connecting the Language of the Practice Framework with Conceptual Models

Conceptual Models	Occupational Therapy Practice Framework—Domains							Occupational Therapy Practice Framework Process		
	Areas of Occupation	Performance Skills	Performance Patterns	Context	Activity Demand	Body Function	Body Structure	Evaluation	Intervention	Outcome
Ecological Model of Human Performance Person—personal values, interests, experiences, and skills	Cluster of meaningful tasks	Performance—selecting and doing tasks	Person—roles	Context	Temporal and environmental features of the task	Person—skills, values		Directed at performance within context	Intervention approaches	Performance, range of performance
Model of Human Occupation Person—volition, habituation Performance capacity	Nature of occupation	Occupational performance	Habituation—roles and routines	Environment—physical and social		Performance capacity—subjective experience and objective component		Eight assessment tools to use with children or adolescents	Directed at person factors, environmental factors, and occupational performance	Occupational adaptation and occupational competency
Person-Environment-Occupational Performance Person—neurobiological, physiological, cognitive, psychological, emotional, spiritual factors	Participation in Actions and performance of occupations	Participation in Actions and tasks		Environment factors		Person factors		Directed at personal factors, environmental factors, activities, tasks, and roles	Directed at personal factors and environmental factors, activities, tasks, and roles	Health and well-being
Person-Environment-Occupation Person—mind, body spirit	Occupation—cluster of self-directed activities and tasks	Observable aspects of occupational performance		Environment		Physical and psychosocial capacities		Directed at the person, environment, and occupation	Directed at the person, environment, and occupation	Occupational performance

SUMMARY

A conceptual model is a set of constructs and assumptions, organized in a particular manner to clarify their interrelatedness. Within a profession, conceptual models help to define the focus of a profession and its relationship to other professions. Members of the profession use these conceptual models to guide their clinical reasoning, frame their research questions, and advance the efficacy and effectiveness of their therapeutic practices. Conceptual models evolve over time. As well as affecting change in practice, research, and policy decisions, they are affected by changes in practice, research, and policy.

A number of occupation-based conceptual models have developed within the field of occupational therapy during the last several decades. That a profession has a number of overlapping conceptual models capable of evolving over time is a sign of its strength and maturation. Four of the occupation-based conceptual models directing current occupational therapy practice are the Ecological Model of Human Performance, the Model of Human Occupation, the Person-Environment-Occupational Performance Model, and the Person-Environment-Occupation Model. Underscoring each of these models is the assumption that individuals are complex beings, influenced by and reflecting their intersecting biological, social, and psychological processes and life stages. Each of these models addresses the constructs of person, environment, occupation, and performance. Each supports the philosophical belief that participation in meaningful, developmentally relevant occupations promotes health and well-being.

However, the models differ in the particular way they organize, define, and emphasize these assumptions, constructs, and philosophical beliefs. Designed as an interdisciplinary conceptual model, the Ecological Model of Human Performance emphasizes the dynamic relationship among the context, the person, and the task on the scope and quality of human performance. It considers the range of performance available to and achievable by the person in a given context. The model places particular emphasis on contextual factors, and guides occupational therapists and occupational therapy assistant to consider modifying and adapting tasks and contexts, in addition to focusing on the person when providing interventions. The Model of Human Occupations has its roots in occupational behavior, anthropology, psychology, and philosophy. While also addressing the environment and occupational performance, the model places particular emphasis on understanding the person and the nature of occupation. Consistent with the initiatives of the World Health Organization, the Person-Environment-Occupational Performance Model focuses on occupational performance and participation. The model directs occupational therapists and occupational therapy assistants to consider how the innate and acquired capacities of the person, and supports and barriers within the environment, influence people's performance of and their participation in occupations that promote health and well-being. The Person-Environment-Occupation model has its roots in environmental and occupation-based theories. The model acknowledges both the subjective experiences and observable behaviors associated with occupational performance. It supports the belief that maximal occupational performance results from goodness of fit among the person, the environment in which the occupational performance occurs, and the occupation performed.

The particular occupation-based conceptual model that occupational therapists and occupational therapy assistants use to guide their clinical reasoning, when working with children and adolescents, is influenced by the capacities and needs of the children and adolescents. It also is influenced by the knowledge and comfort level of the occupational therapist and occupational therapy assistant in using that model, and the philosophy and mission of the practice setting. What is essential is for the occupational therapist and the occupational therapy assistant to use an occupation-based conceptual model to guide their clinical reasoning and to focus their therapeutic interventions. Using the occupation-based conceptual model helps them to maintain their professional identity, provide services that are within the scope of occupational therapy practice, and justify the rationale of their interventions approaches to the funders, administrators, and recipients of their services.

REVIEWING KEY POINTS

1. Explain why it is important to use an occupation-based conceptual model when providing occupational therapy services to children and adolescents.
2. List and define the key terms associated with the Ecological Model of Human Performance.
3. Outline four assumptions of the Ecological Model of Human Performance.
4. Describe the focus of occupational therapy intervention when using the Model of Human Occupation.
5. List and define the key terms associated with the Model of Human Occupation.
6. Outline four assumptions of the Model of Human Occupation.
7. Describe the focus of occupational therapy intervention when using the Model of Human Occupation.
8. List and define the key terms associated with the Person-Environment-Occupational Performance Model.
9. Outline four assumptions of the Person-Environment-Occupational Performance Model.
10. Describe the focus of occupational therapy intervention when using the Person-Environment-Occupational Performance Model.
11. List and define the key terms associated with the Person-Environment-Occupation Model.
12. Outline four assumptions of the Person-Environment-Occupation Model.
13. Describe the focus of occupational therapy intervention when using the Person-Environment-Occupation Model.

APPLYING KEY CONCEPTS

1. With a partner, select one of the conceptual models described in this chapter. Using the constructs, assumptions, and language of the model, draft a series of questions that can be used to interview a child, an adolescent, or the caregiver of a child. The child or adolescent does not need to have special needs. Focus the interview questions to learn about the unique personal aspects of the child or adolescent, the occupations and activities the child or adolescent performs, and the environments in which the child or adolescent performs these activities and occupations. Conduct and audio tape a 30 to 45 minute interview. Afterward, listen to the audiotape and review the information gathered. Consider how the model structures and directs the interview process. Consider what additional information would have been helpful to gather.
2. With a partner, select a second conceptual model described in this chapter. Using the constructs, assumptions, and language of this second model, draft a series of questions that can be used to interview a child, an adolescent, or the caregiver of a child. The child or adolescent does not need to have special

needs. Focus the interview questions to learn about the unique personal aspects of the child or adolescent, the occupations and activities the child or adolescent performs, and the environments in which the child or adolescent performs these activities and occupations. Conduct and audio tape a 30 to 45 minute interview. Afterward, listen to the audiotape and review the information gathered. Consider using the model to structure and direct the interview process. Consider what additional information would have been helpful to gather.

3. Compare the types of questions asked and the types of information gathered from the above two learning activities. Consider the benefits and limitations of each model for guiding the interview and for gathering information needed to provide occupational therapy services. Consider what additional knowledge and skills are needed to use the conceptual models effectively to guide interviewing techniques.

REFERENCES

Baum, C. M., & Christiansen, C. (2005). Person-environment-occupational performance: An occupation-based framework for practice. In C. Christiansen, C. Baum, & J. Bass-Haugen (Eds.), *Occupational therapy: Performance, participation, and well-being*. Thorofare, NJ: SLACK.

Bronfenbrenner, U. (1979). *The ecology of human development: Experiments by nature and design*. Cambridge, MA: Harvard University Press.

Bronfenbrenner, U. (1997). Systems vs. associations: It's not either/or. *Families in Society, 78*, 124.

Burke, J. P. (2003). Philosophical base of human occupation. In P. Kramer, J. Hinojosa, & C. B. Royeen (Eds.), *Perspectives in human occupation*. Philadelphia: Lippincott Williams & Wilkins.

Canadian Occupational Therapy Association (1997). *Enabling occupation: An occupational therapy perspective*. Ottawa: Author.

Christiansen, C., & Baum, C.M. (Eds.). (1991). *Occupational therapy: Overcoming human performance deficits*. Thorofare, NJ: SLACK.

Christiansen, C., & Baum, C. M. (Eds.). (1997). *Occupational therapy: Enabling function and well-being* (2nd ed). Thorofare, NJ: SLACK.

Christiansen, C., Baum, C. M., & Bass-Haugen, J. (Eds.). (2005). *Occupational therapy: Performance, participation, and well-being* (3rd ed). Thorofare, NJ: SLACK.

Crist, P., Royeen, C. B., & Schkade, J. (Eds.). (2000). *Infusing occupation into practice* (2nd ed.). Bethesda, MD: AOTA.

Csikszentmihalyi, M., & Csikszentmihalyi, I. S. (1988). *Optimal experience: Psychological studies in flow in consciousness*. Cambridge: Cambridge University Press.

Dunn, W. (2000). *Best practice occupational therapy: In community service with children and families*. Thorofare, NJ: SLACK.

Dunn, W., Brown, C., & McGuigan, A. (1994). The ecology of human performance: A framework for considering the effect of context. *American Journal of Occupational Therapy, 48*, 595–607.

Dunn, W., Brown, C., & Youngstrom, M. (2003). Ecological model of occupation. In P. Kramer, J. Hinojosa, & C. B. Royeen (Eds.), *Perspectives in human occupation*. Philadelphia: Lippincott Williams & Wilkins.

Fisher, A. (2006). Overview of performance skills and client factors. In H. McHugh Pendelton and W. Schultz-Krohn (Eds.), *Pedrettti's occupational therapy: Practice skills for physical dysfunction* (6th ed.). St. Louis: Mosby Elsevier.

Forsyth, K, & Kielhofner, G. (2003). Model of human occupation. In P. Kramer, J. Hinojosa, & C. B. Royeen (Eds.), *Perspectives in human occupation*. Philadelphia: Lippincott Williams & Wilkins.

Kielhofner, G. (2002). *Model of human occupation. Theory and application* (3rd ed.). Baltimore, MD: Lippincott Williams & Wilkins.

Kielhofner, G., Burke, J., & Heard, I. C. (1980). A model of human occupation. Part four: Assessment and intervention. *American Journal of Occupational Therapy, 34*, 777–788.

Kielhofner, G., Tham, K., Baz, T., & Hutson, J. (2002). Performance capacity and the lived body. In G. Kielhofner (Ed), *Model of human occupation: Theory and application* (3rd ed.). Baltimore, MD: Lippincott Williams & Wilkins

Kramer, P., Hinojosa, J., & Royeen, C. B. (Eds.). (2003). *Perspectives in human occupation*. Philadelphia: Lippincott Williams & Wilkins.

Law, M. (1997). Theoretical context for the practice of occupational therapy. In C. Christiansen, & C. Baum (Eds.), *Occupational therapy: Enabling function and well-being* (2nd ed.). Thorofare, NJ: SLACK.

Law, M., Cooper, B., Strong, S., Steward, D., Rigby, R., & Letts, L. (1996). The person-environment-occupational model: A transactive approach to occupational performance. *Canadian Journal of Occupational Therapy, 63*, 9–23.

Law, M. (2000). Person-environment-occupation model. In P. A. Crist, C. H. Royeen, & J. K. Schkade (Eds.), *Infusing occupation into practice* (pp. 111–114). Bethesda, MD: American Occupational Therapy Association.

Lawton, M. P., & Nahemow, L. (1973). Towards an ecological theory of adaptation and aging. In W. Preiser (Ed.), *Environmental design research*. Stroudsburg, PA: Dowden, Hutchinson & Ross.

Mosey, A. (1981). *Occupational therapy: Configuration of a profession*. NY: Raven Press.

Nelson, D., & Jepson-Thomas, J. (2003). Occupational form, occupational performance, and a conceptual framework for therapeutic occupation. In P. Kramer, J. Hinojosa, & C. B. Royeen (Eds.), *Perspectives in human occupation*. Philadelphia: Lippincott Williams & Wilkins.

Reilly, M. (1962). Occupational therapy can be one of the great ideas of 20th century medicine. *American Journal of Occupational Therapy, 16,* 1–9.

Reilly, M. (1969). The educational process. *American Journal of Occupational Therapy, 23,* 299–307.

Schkade, J. K., & Schultz, S. (1992). Occupational adaptation: Toward a holistic approach to contemporary practice, part 1. *American Journal of Occupational Therapy, 46,* 829–837.

Schultz, S. & Schkade, J. K. (1992). Occupational adaptation: Toward a holistic approach to contemporary practice, part 2. *American Journal of Occupational Therapy, 46,* 917–926.

Velde, B., & Fidler, G. (2002). *Lifestyle performance: A model for engaging the power of occupation*. Thorofare, NJ: SLACK.

Chapter 3

Other Theories and Frames of Reference to Support Occupation-Based Conceptual Models

Janet V. DeLany

Key Terms

Accommodation
Acquisitional frame of reference
Adaptation
Assimilation
Autonomy
Behavioral theory
Biomechanical model
Centration
Cognitive theory
Concrete operations
Conservation
Dissociative movements
Dyspraxia
Egocentric
Epigenetic principle
Equilibrium
Extinction
Frame of reference
Formal operations
Identity
Imaginary audience
Industry
Initiative
Intrinsic reinforcement

Metacognition
Mobility
Negative reinforcement
Neurodevelopmental model
Object permanence
Person permanence
Personal fable
Positive reinforcement
Praxis
Preoperational
Psychosocial theory
Punishment
Reinforcement
Reversibility
Role confusion
Role experimentation
Role fixation
Schema
Sensory integration
Sensory modulation
Shaping
Stability
Transformation
Trust

Objectives

- Understand the relationship of non–occupation-based theories and frames of reference to occupation-based conceptual models.
- Explain basic principles of selected theories of development related to occupational therapy practice with children and adolescents.
- Explain basic concepts of other selected theories and frames of reference used in occupational therapy practice with children and adolescents: social learning, behavioral, acquisitional, sensory integrative, biomechanical, and neurodevelopmental model.
- Articulate the importance of theories and frames of reference to direct the delivery of occupational therapy services.

RELATIONSHIP OF OTHER THEORIES AND FRAMES OF REFERENCE TO OCCUPATION-BASED CONCEPTUAL MODELS

Chapter 2 examined various occupation-based conceptual models. These conceptual models focused on the capacities and needs of children and adolescents, the nature of their occupations, and the influence of the environment and occupational tasks on their ability to participate in daily life occupations. However, to more fully understand how children and adolescents engage in their daily life occupations, it is necessary to examine non–occupation-based theories and frames of reference. Specifically, it is important to review theories and frames of reference that provide clues as to how children and adolescents develop the performance skills and patterns they need to perform their occupations and how their body structures and body functions influence the way they perform their occupations.

A theory is a set of constructs organized in a particular manner to provide a systematic understanding of and predictions about the relationship between events or phenomena. A frame of reference is a method for organizing information and knowledge to serve as a guide for evaluation and intervention. Frames of reference link together and apply theory to the practice of the profession (Kramer & Hinojosa, 1999; Mosey, 1981). Though occupational therapists have developed a few theories and frames of reference, occupational therapists and occupational therapy assistants also rely heavily on those crafted by theorists in other disciplines such as psychology, neurophysiology, sociology, and anthropology. These theories and frames of reference provide more detailed schemata than do the occupation-based conceptual models regarding specific aspects of how children and adolescents grow, develop, process information, move their bodies, think, behave, feel, and act socially with others.

This chapter provides an overview of several non–occupation-based theories and frames of reference applicable to children and adolescents. The theories and frames of reference can guide clinical reasoning skills used during the occupational therapy evaluation and intervention processes regarding how to promote or restore person factors, and to modify or adapt task and environmental factors. Though it is the responsibility of the occupational therapist to determine which theory or frame of reference to use, it also is important for occupational therapy assistants to know these theories and frames of reference. Doing so enables the occupational therapist and the occupational therapy assistant to provide collaboratively effective occupational therapy services to children and adolescents. By combining overarching conceptual models that focus on occupation, with specifically focused theories and frames of reference that focus on body functions and structures, occupational therapists and occupational therapy assistants can design and deliver best-practice occupational therapy services.

THEORIES OF DEVELOPMENT

An Overview

Theories of human development are explanations of how individuals grow, mature, and learn. These theories assume that development occurs in physical, cognitive, social, emotional, and spiritual areas, and in an orderly and sequential manner throughout the lives of individuals. These theories also assume that changes in growth, maturation, and learning occur within and are affected by physical, cultural, social, and temporal environments.

There are a number of notable theories about development. Because human development is so complex, each of the theories tends to focus on a particular area rather than all areas of development. Because they are used frequently in occupational therapy practice, this chapter focuses on Erikson's **psychosocial theory** of development and Piaget's **cognitive theory** of development. Other developmental theories include Bronfenbrenner's ecological theory of development, Freud's psychoanalytic theory, Maslow's humanistic model, and Vygotsky's sociocultural theory. Texts on human growth and development are a good source to obtain an overview of these latter theories.

Erikson's Psychosocial Theory of Development

As suggested by its name, Eric Erikson expanded upon psychological explanations of development to also consider the social influences on human development. In contrast to the prevailing psychoanalytic theories of his time that emphasized psychosexual issues, Erikson concentrated on the influence of history, culture, and society on healthy development. His theory encapsulated the **epigenetic principle**, that is, each of the part of the personality has a particular time for development to occur until all the parts develop to form the whole of the individual. Though he believed that unfavorable development of one stage negatively affected the development of later stages of personality, he did allow for second opportunities to develop areas that may have been missed (Vander Zanden, Crandell, & Crandell, 2003). Erikson outlined nine stages of development. The first five of these apply to the psychosocial growth and development of children and adolescents.

- Trust versus mistrust
- Autonomy versus doubt and shame
- Initiative versus guilt
- Industry versus inferiority

- Identity versus role confusion
- Intimacy versus isolation
- Generativity versus stagnation
- Integrity versus despair
- Despair versus hope and faith (Erikson & Erikson, 1997)

The words Erikson used to label each of the stages reflect the central issue or crisis of emotional and social development that he believed individuals addressed during that time period. Rather than indicators of bipolar dichotomies, Erikson saw the words as indicators, along a continuum, of those stage-specific central issues. Each of the stages built upon one another; mastery of one stage allowed for development to emerge in a following stage.

According to Erikson, the stage of **trust versus mistrust** occurs during infancy. During this stage, infants learned to form basic trusting relationships as a result of positive and secure interactions with their caregivers (McDevitt & Ormrod, 2004; Vander Zanden et al., 2003). Consider the children and adolescents who receive occupational therapy services. Those who were fed when they were hungry, were soothed when they were distressed, were held and stimulated when they needed social interactions, and who lived in secure, predictable surroundings most likely developed a sense of trust in their caregivers and environments. In contrast, those who were abused and neglected physically, emotionally, and socially, or experienced significant trauma in their living situations may have developed mistrust in their caregivers and environments. Having a sense of basic trust of others and environments, tempered by a sense of mistrust of potentially harmful situations contributes to healthy development. Though the foundation for trust and mistrust emerges during infancy, children and adolescents continue to refine their sense of trust and mistrust as they develop and participate in their daily life occupations. Occupational therapists and occupational therapy assistants can foster the development of trust through therapeutic interactions that occur within safe and predictable environments. For example, when working with children who are **tactually defensive**, occupational therapists and occupational therapy assistants introduce tactile input in a slow and predictable manner, thus allowing the children to accommodate to, feel safe about, and positively respond to the sensations. When working with young adolescents living in homeless shelters, occupational therapists and occupational therapy assistants work to ensure that food is readily available, that the sleeping arrangements are safe and private, and that daily routines are established.

Erikson's second stage, **autonomy versus shame and doubt**, typically occurs during toddlerhood when children become more mobile and are able physically to explore their environments. According to Erikson, during this stage of psychosocial development, young children address issues of self-certainty versus self-consciousness. They decide when and how to assert their will. They endeavor to develop self-control while maintaining a sense of self-esteem. As with other stages of development, a sense of autonomy balanced by sense of doubt reflects healthy development (Erikson & Erikson, 1997; McDevitt & Ormrod, 2002). Children who receive encouragement to voice their opinions and to act on their choices within flexible, safe boundaries are more likely to develop a sense of autonomy. Children who are criticized routinely for their opinions and choices are at greater risk for developing feelings of shame and doubt. To help young children with chronic medical conditions develop a healthy sense of autonomy, occupational therapists and occupational therapy assistants might design developmentally appropriate play stations in the hospital that promote making independent, healthy choices regarding the toys they wish to try. Similarly, they might foster a positive sense of autonomy in older children by allowing for and respecting their right to choose from among several appropriate preparatory or occupation-based therapeutic activities.

Erikson's third stage of psychosocial development, **initiative versus guilt**, expands upon his second stage. Children between the ages of 4 and 5 years confront the central issue of this stage, **role experimentation** versus **role fixation** (Erikson & Erikson, 1997). Role experimentation implies that children risk new roles and stretch the boundaries of the roles they currently have. Consider commonly spoken phrases such as "Let me do it" and "See what I made." Role fixation implies that children do not take such risks. A healthy balance between a desire to initiate actions and a sense of guilt allows children to pause and reflect on their actions. Children who are safe and secure to explore their environment and manipulate objects within it, develop a sense of initiative. As a result, they develop a sense of purpose for and direction to their actions (Vander Zanden et al., 2003). Children who are restricted from or criticized for such exploratory and manipulative activities may develop a sense of guilt when attempting these actions. To support young children with physical challenges to develop a healthy sense of initiative, occupational therapists and occupational therapy assistants create safe, secure environments for them to explore various developmentally appropriate occupational roles. For preschool children, these roles might include pet caretaker, parent helper, and book buddy.

According to Erikson's fourth stage, children ages 6 through 12 years of age address issues of **industry versus inferiority**. They are interested in how things work and are constructed. Through their explorations they develop a sense of mastery and competency (Erikson & Erikson, 1997). Similar to the above stages, children who are afforded opportunities to experiment with materials in a safe environment that allows for mistakes and fosters success develop a sense of mastery. Those children who routinely are criticized for their efforts or who are restricted from participating in such endeavors may develop a sense of inferiority. Occupational therapists and occupational therapy assistants can encourage this stage of psychosocial development by designing activities that allow children to experiment with alternative methods for manipulating and combining materials and that result in a final product. Cooking, construction, craft, and science projects are examples of such activities.

During the fifth stage of psychosocial development, Erikson believed adolescents worked through issues of **identity versus role confusion**. During this stage, adolescents attempt to develop a coherent sense of who they are. They also attempt to find tasks and roles that are meaningful to them, desire to be themselves, and seek mutual recognition of self and others (Erikson & Erikson, 1997). According to Erikson, those adolescents who struggle with role confusion have a sense of task futility, role inhibition, self-doubt, and isolation. Successful resolution of the issues at all of the former stages of psychosocial development, coupled with opportunities to experiment with and successfully participate in various roles and tasks, contributes to the adolescents' sense of their identity. To promote the development of self-identity, occupational therapists and occupational therapy assistants design multiple opportunities for adolescents to plan, carry out, and reflect upon occupation-based activities and their feelings associated with doing them. For example, occupational therapists and occupational therapy assistants might organize an after-school youth group that allows adolescents to investigate various career and leisure pursuits and to reflect about their various group membership roles while performing the occupations.

Piaget's Cognitive Theory of Development

In contrast to Erikson, who focused on psychosocial development across the lifespan, Piaget examined cognitive development of children. He studied how children think, gain knowledge, become self-aware, and understand their environments. Piaget viewed development as a process of **adaptation**. Through the process of adaptation, he believed children modify their behaviors to meet the demands of the environment. As part of this, children use **schemas**, or mental frameworks, to cope with and respond to this environmental information. Adaptation requires the children to assimilate and accommodate to new information. **Assimilation** means that children take in new information and interpret it in a manner that conforms to their existing view or schema of the world. When they cannot assimilate the information into their existing schema, they experience a sense of **disequilibrium**. Through a process called **accommodation**, the children then modify their existing schema to incorporate and make sense of the new information and achieve a new state of equilibrium (Vander Zanden et al., 2003). The children again experience a sense of equilibrium as long as they can use the newly acquired schema to assimilate and make sense of environmental information. When they cannot, the above cycle of disequilibrium, then accommodation repeats itself.

It is helpful to use the concepts of assimilation, accommodation, equilibrium, and disequilibrium to consider how children and adolescents engage in their existing occupations and learn new occupations. Periods of equilibrium allow children time for practice and mastery. During this time, they observe and acquire new information but do not change the fundamental way they think about how to perform their occupations. Periods of disequilibrium require the children and adolescents to grow by modifying their existing schema to accommodate new ways of engaging in their daily occupations.

Piaget outlined four major stages of cognitive development. He believed that children went through these stages of development sequentially, as a result of their biological growth and interactions with the environment. The stages are:

- Sensorimotor
- Preoperational
- Concrete operational
- Formal operational (Piaget, 1965, 1970)

According to Piaget, the sensorimotor stage lasts from birth to approximately 2 years of age. During this period, children learn about their world through integrating sensory and motor experiences. They learn about sounds, textures, and sights and objects from hearing, touching, seeing, smelling, and moving themselves and objects. They develop a sense of **cause and effect** related to their own body movements. Specifically, they learn that an action they cause has an effect on an object. For example, they learn first accidentally, then intentionally, that bumping the mobile with their arm makes it move, and that crying makes their caregiver attend to them. Around 7 months of age, they develop a sense of **person permanence** and about 8 months of age, they develop a sense of **object permanence.** Person permanence means that the children realize that people exist independent of their ability to see and hear those people; object permanence means that the children realize that objects exist independent of their ability to see and hear those objects. Occupational therapists and occupational therapy assistants who work with young children frequently design sensory and motor activities to help them develop their ability to process sensory input and to move their bodies. When consistent with the children's level of ability to assimilate and accommodate, these activities enable the children to interact effectively with their environments and objects in it. Examples of activities might include playing with water, sand, and nontoxic paints, and climbing through mazes and jungle gyms.

Piaget's second stage of cognitive development, the **preoperational stage**, occurs between 2 through 7 years of age. During this period, children learn to use symbols such as pictures, language, and pretend objects to represent real objects and events in the world. As their ability to use symbols expands, they engage in increasingly more complex storytelling, and fantasy or imaginary play. They have an **egocentric** understanding of events, seeing and interpreting situations from their own vantage point, rather than also from that of another person. They can categorize objects but focus on one detail at a time and ignore other details. This process is called **centration**. For example, when playing with dishes, they can stack them by a single feature such as shape, but not by two features simultaneously, such as shape and color. Thus, they are likely to separate red and green bowls and plates into two stacks: one of plates and one of bowls. They are not likely to have four stacks, one of red plates, one of green plates, one of red bowls, and one of green bowls. They think that a tall 8-ounce glass holds more liquid than a short 8-ounce glass because they focus on the height rather than also the width dimension.

Likewise, children at this age of development focus on the existing state or condition of an object. That is, they focus on what the object looks like at the present moment. They do not attend to the **transformation** of an object, that is, how an object can change in size, shape, consistency, and color. For example, young children may have difficulty understanding that cookie dough transforms into a cookie when it is baked, or that cut hair grows again into longer hair over a period of time. A family member who has changed hair color may upset them.

They also have difficulty with the concept of **reversibility**, that objects such as melted ice cream or water can be reversed to their original state of frozen ice cream or snow. When they become sick they may struggle to understand that their state of health will reverse, and that they will become well again. Board games that involve forward and backward movement and chances for winning and losing also are difficult for them because they see states as nonreversible. Occupational therapists and occupational therapy assistants can help children grow and develop through this stage of development by integrating frequent opportunities for them to engage in storytelling, story acting, and pretend play occupations during therapy sessions. Simple props such as sticks, balls, and old sheets that can be used in multiple ways to stimulate the imagination. Allowing the children to experiment with, create, and change the characteristics of objects rather than providing finished products helps them to decenter their perspectives and begin to understand concepts of transformation and reversibility.

Concrete operations, the third stage of development occurs between the ages of 7 and 11 years. During this period, children develop their ability to use inductive logic. They can use arithmetic to manipulate numbers and complete measurements. They use classification to establish set and class relationships and identify hierarchical structures. For example, they can differentiate between classes and types of motorized vehicles and establish a hierarchical relationship among them based on their purpose, power, and durability. Because they can use the concepts of transformation and reversibility, they attend to how objects change from one state to another and how they can return to their original state (Vander Zanden et al., 2003). Thus, at this age, they are ready for games that involve chances for winning and losing. Similarly, they now understand the concept of **conservation,** that is, the quantity of an object remains unchanged even when it is reshaped or rearranged (McDevitt & Ormrod, 2002). For example, they understand that a piece of fruit is the same amount whether it is divided into several pieces or kept whole, that a piece of clay is the same amount whether it is molded into a ball or a square, and that a stack of coins is the same amount whether it is divided into two or five piles. Occupational therapists and occupational therapy assistants can help children advance through this stage of cognitive development by providing occupations that allow them to master concepts of classification, conservation, hierarchical order, and inductive logic. Examples include cooking, building, crafts, science projects, magic tricks, and math and visual-perceptual games.

The fourth stage examined by Piaget, **formal operations,** develops from age 12 through 16 years of age. During this time period, some but not all adolescents develop the ability to use formal logic. Those who do are able to use abstraction and deductive reasoning and to systematically solve problems by sequentially testing single factors at a time to find the final solution. Called **metacognition,** they think about their own thinking capacities. As part of this process, they consider how they look for and attend to information, and how they organize and memorize details (McDevitt & Ormrod, 2002). Because they can imagine multiple possibilities inherent in situations, and multiple solutions to problems, they are not fixed to present time and real objects. Rather than needing physical objects, they can mentally restructure information to form a new understanding of it and the categories of events (Bee & Boyd, 2002). Though egocentrism continues, its form changes to take on the notions of **personal fable** and **imaginary audience.** Personal fable implies that adolescents create romantic and heroic images and stories about themselves, believing that no one can understand what they are experiencing. Imaginary audience refers to the adolescents' belief that everyone in the environment is attending to and making judgments about their behavior and appearance (Elkind, 1970). Thus, they are simultaneously undersensitive to the experiences of others and overly sensitive to the scrutiny of others. When providing occupational therapy services to adolescents, it is useful to use scenario-building activities, brainstorming sessions, and role-playing scripts. Using such strategies to help adolescents think about their occupational performance capacities and behaviors before, during, and after completing the occupational tasks fosters the development of their formal logic capacities and enables them to assume responsibility and control over their choices and actions.

It is important to note that studies conducted in recent years have challenged some of Erikson's and Piaget's work. Erikson is criticized for focusing primarily on male development without also attending to the importance of relationships associated with female development (Bee & Boyd, 2002). Piaget is criticized for his fixed notions of development. For example, Ciancio et al. (1999) found that children as young as 2 and 3 years of age demonstrate conservation principles for simple projects. Brownell (1990) and Dunn (1994) observed that young children are not completely egocentric in their view of the world but do adapt their language patterns and emotions to adjust to the needs of their siblings and peers. Flavell (1986) found that by age 4, children can identify what features of an object will cause another person to distinguish between its real and false appearance. Given the finding of such studies, it is important for occupational therapists and occupational therapy assistants to attend to the clues that the children and adolescents provide regarding their level of cognitive development rather than strictly adhering to Erikson's or Piaget's stages.

LEARNING THEORIES AND FRAMES OF REFERENCE

An Overview

Learning frames of reference provide clues as to how children and adolescents acquire knowledge to interact with their environments. The field of cognitive psychology focuses on trying to understand the complexities of this phenomenon. Within occupational therapy practice, behavioral and social learning theories, and the acquisitional frame of reference are commonly used.

Behavioral Theory

Skinner (1953, 1980) has provided substantive insight into the use of operant conditioning, a learning technique that influences a person to continue or to cease a behavior because of the consequence of that behavior. These consequences occur after the initial behavior and include **punishment, extinction**, and **reinforcement**. According to Skinner, punishment and extinction cause a behavior to cease; positive and negative reinforcement cause a behavior to continue. Forms of punishment commonly used with children and adolescents include scolding, curtailment of privileges, time outs, and removal of wanted objects. Though being banned increasingly as violations of human rights, some cultures continue to sanction corporal forms of punishment such as spankings and beatings. Extinction involves the systematic reduction and elimination of a behavior. When used with children and adolescents, this often occurs through ignoring or not reinforcing that behavior. **Positive reinforcement** increases the likelihood that the initial behavior will occur again. Positive reinforcers usually are pleasant consequences. Positive reinforcers for children and adolescents may include increased attention, time with a special person, verbal praise, food, privileges and token gifts. **Negative reinforcement** increases the likelihood that a behavior will increase so that something unpleasant will stop (Bee & Boyd, 2002). Like punishment, negative reinforcers can include scolding, removal of privileges and favorite objects, and time outs. The critical distinction is that, when used as punishment, the intent of these consequences is to stop an unwanted behavior; when used as negative reinforcement, the intent is to increase a desired behavior.

To make this clearer, consider the following scenarios. Suppose at an inclusionary preschool program, a young child routinely scratches other children when he wants to play with their toys. The occupational therapy assistant working with the child says, "Do not scratch" and puts the child in time-out for a two-minute interval. In this scenario, the occupational therapy assistant uses time out as a form of punishment to stop the unwanted behavior of scratching. However, suppose the occupational therapy assistant puts the child in time-out and says, "Say please when you want the toy." After two minutes of time out, the occupational therapy assistant allows the child to return to the other children. In this scenario, the occupational therapy assistant uses time out as a negative reinforcer to increase the desired behavior of asking for the toy. The intent is for the child to demonstrate the asking behavior and thus decrease the unpleasant experience of being removed from the other children. In reality, time out may be used concurrently as a punishment to stop the scratching behavior, and as a negative reinforcer to increase the asking behavior. In addition, once the child returns to the group of other children, the occupational therapy assistant may use positive reinforcement such as praise or hug when the child asks for the toy. To complicate the scenario, assume that the child begins to whine before he asks for the toy. Because the whining does not pose a physical threat to the other children, the occupational therapy assistant may choose to ignore the whining, but respond with praise immediately when the child asks for the toys. Thus, the occupational therapy assistant is trying to extinguish the whining behavior and positively reinforce the asking behavior.

Skinner and his colleagues introduced other concepts as part of their behavioral theory that are used in occupational therapy practice. Three of these concepts include **shaping**, **continuous reinforcement**, and **intermittent reinforcement**. Shaping involves reinforcement of progressively closer approximations of the desired behavior. In the above scenario, this might mean first praising the child for standing near other children without scratching them, then praising him for saying the name of the toy, then finally praising him for asking for the toys. Continuous reinforcement requires providing positive or negative reinforcement every time the child demonstrates the desired behavior. Intermittent or partial reinforcement requires providing positive or negative reinforcement occasionally at either random or predetermined intervals when the child demonstrates the desired behavior. Desired behaviors increase more quickly with continuous reinforcement; however, it is difficult to sustain that level of reinforcement. Once continuous reinforcement stops, the extinction of the behavior can occur. It takes longer to increase a positive behavior with intermittent reinforcement; however, such behaviors are resistant to extinction once they are established (Bee & Boyd, 2002). To change the scratching behavior to the asking behavior in the above scenario, an effective strategy might be for the occupational therapy assistant to put the child in time out every time he scratches, inform him that he is to use language to ask for the toy, return him to the group, and model the desired behaviors. Initially, every time the child approximates asking for the toy, the occupational therapy assistant praises or hugs him. As the consistency and accuracy of the desired behavior increases, the occupational therapy assistant switches to intermittent use of praise and hugs.

Social Learning Theory

Through his development of social learning theory, Bandura (1977, 1989) made important contributions to and modifications of traditional behavioral theory. He highlighted the importance of **intrinsic reinforcement** that occurs within the person and vicarious reinforcement that occurs through observational learning within a social context (Bee & Boyd, 2002; Royeen & Duncan, 1999). Thus, external reinforcement is not always necessary for learning to occur. Intrinsic reinforcement occurs when the children experience a sense of internal satisfaction from their accomplishments, independent of any external feedback. Vicarious reinforcement through observational learning occurs as children learn, make generalizations, and modify their behaviors based on watching the reinforcement or punishment others receive for their behaviors. As a result, modeling becomes an important avenue for learning. Attention and memory are central to observing and apply the modeled behaviors. The age and capacities of the children influence the behaviors that they observe, and their emotional reaction to and memory of those behaviors (Bee & Boyd).

Consider how Bandura's concepts apply to the scenario of the child who scratches others to get a toy. It may be that the act of scratching provides intrinsic satisfaction to the child because it affords the pleasure of physical contact or the release of frustration. Sitting in the time out chair may provide intrinsic reinforcement because it feels soft, comfortable, and secure. Equally plausible, playing in the presence of other children may provide intrinsic reinforcement. It may be possible that the child learned to scratch to get what he wants by observing others perform the same behavior, and the increased attention they received for that behavior. The child may have learned to ask for what he wanted solely by observing his peers ask for toys or by feeling happy when he got the toys.

It can be confusing as to what is the most effective approach to modify a child's behavior. There is not one correct answer. It is only through careful observation of the child's complex and intertwined behaviors, and the antecedents to and consequences of those behaviors, that such a decision can be made.

Acquistional Frame of Reference

The acquisitional frame of reference uses principles and assumptions from a combination of learning theories, including Skinner's behavioral theory and Bandura's social learning theory. According the acquistional frame of reference, behavior occurs in response to environmental cues (Royeen & Duncan, 1999). Thus, when applying this frame of reference in their work with children and adolescents, occupational therapists and occupational therapy assistants use the environment to facilitate skill acquisition and adaptive responses. For example, when teaching driving skills to an adolescent with spina bifida, the occupational therapy assistant might set up on-the-road sessions using an automobile that has hand controls, rather than clinic based sessions with computer simulations.

Emphasis is placed on those functional behaviors children and adolescents need to acquire to develop the broader skills needed to participate in their specific environments. Intervention is directed toward shaping and reinforcing those behaviors that contribute to the acquisition of the needed skills. For example, when working with an adolescent on computer skills needed for communication in the school environment, the occupational therapy assistant might work to increase functional behaviors such as activating switches and keys, controlling a mouse, and scanning visual displays.

The acquisitional frame of reference incorporates reinforcement techniques and reinforcement schedules consistent with Skinner's operant conditioning principles. It also incorporates the concept of shaping and generalization, that is, applying the specifically learned behavior to other tasks (Royeen & Duncan, 1999). In this way, a specific behavior does not need to be relearned for another task. Four basic assumptions underlie the acquisitional frame of reference. The first assumption is that the past and present environment shapes behavior. Thus, behaviors occur in response to interactions with the physical, social, and cultural environment external to the person. Second, the occupational therapist and occupational therapy assistant accept the child unconditionally and believe that the child is capable of learning functional skills. Third, through the acquisition of skills, a child becomes competent. Fourth, acquisition of skills does not always follow a developmental sequence. Rather, skills needed to succeed in a particular environment are what is essential (Royeen & Duncan).

When using the acquisitional frame of reference, the occupational therapist and the occupational therapy assistant first observe how the child or adolescent demonstrates the necessary behaviors and performs the tasks within a specific environment. In the computer scenario above, the occupational therapy assistant would observe how the adolescent accesses and controls the keys, mouse, and other switches, organizes the workstation, and attends to and reads the display monitor. The occupational therapy assistant also would consider the physical and sociocultural aspects of the environment, such as the classroom and library, where the adolescent needs to perform the task. Next, the occupational therapy assistant and the occupational therapist would decide what other skills the adolescent needs to perform the task. These might include the use of alternative key commands and switches, work organization strategies, and visual processing skills. The occupational therapy assistant would begin the process of teaching those skills through shaping and reinforcing. Initially, the focus would not be on the quality of the performance, but on the attempts to perform the task. So that the adolescent meets with success, the occupational therapy assistant might modify it or make it simpler (downgrade it). As the adolescent gains computer competency skills, the occupational therapy assistant would make the task more complex (upgrade it) until it is at a level consistent with the expectation of the student's school environment. The occupational therapy assistant would decrease the amount of reinforcement directly provided to the adolescent as he receives increasing reinforcement from progressive mastery of the computer skills. This progressive mastery reinforces the adolescent to learn more demanding skills and to generalize what he has learned, such as organizational and visual perceptual skills to other tasks.

SENSORY INTEGRATION FRAME OF REFERENCE

Sensory integration, a frame of reference widely used in occupational therapy practice for children, is complex, and requires an in-depth understanding of the central nervous system. First postulated by Ayres (1972, 1979), it addresses how the brain receives, processes, interprets, and responds physically and emotionally to sensory information. The sensory systems include the auditory, visual, tactile, proprioceptive, visual, and olfactory systems. Six basic assumptions underlie the sensory integration frame of reference:

- The central nervous system (CNS) is hierarchical; cortical structures rely on lower brain centers for accurate input.
- The CNS first must register meaningful sensory information before it can respond to it.
- The CNS has plasticity, or flexibility and adaptability.
- The brain functions in such a way that people innately seek beneficial and self-organizing stimulation.
- Input from each sensory system can inhibit or stimulate every other sensory system.
- Normal human develop occurs sequentially (Bundy, Lane, & Murray, 2002).

Children and adolescents whose sensory systems are functioning normally demonstrate a moderate level of arousal to sensory input. They are able to seek an optimum level of sensation, called sensory diet, to organize and integrate their central nervous system. Their functional support capabilities help to integrate and modulate sensory input. For example, they demonstrate synchronized suck-swallow-breathe patterns, normal muscle tone, and developmentally appropriate level of reflexes. They can discriminate sensory input in each of the sensory systems, maintain their balance and equilibrium, and cocontract agonist and antagonistic muscles, that is, simultaneously contract opposing sets of muscles to work against force and gravity. They receive accurate input from their joints, muscles, and skin receptors, that is, accurate proprioceptive feedback, to understand their body position in space. They are able to lateralize hand, foot, and eye movements, and to integrate movements of both sides of the body, called bilateral integration (Bundy et al., 2002; Kimball, 1999).

In contrast, children and adolescents with sensory processing and **sensory modulation** difficulties may demonstrate under or over responsiveness to tactile, auditory, visual, oral, gravitational, rotary, or other movements. They also may demonstrate under or over emotional reactions and attention levels. When these children or adolescents are over aroused, they can become disorganized and display anxiety, chronic stress, and other negative emotions. Their sympathetic nervous systems become activated, resulting in fight-flight-freeze responses, the body's response to perceived danger. They may continue to remain physiologically over aroused, the fight response, or may become physiologically under aroused, the flight-freeze response. Those children and adolescents who demonstrate emotional under reactivity may look as if they are depressed. In addition to sensory modulation, they may demonstrate difficulties with other functional support capacities. That is, they may have difficulty with functional suck-swallow-breathe patterns and tactile and sensory discrimination. They may have difficulty initiating and sustaining muscle cocontraction and maintaining their balance and equilibrium against gravity or force. They may exhibit low muscle tone and delayed reflex integration, and have difficulty with lateralization or bilateral integration. They may not receive clear proprioceptive feedback regarding the position of their bodies (Ayres, 1979; Bundy et al., 2002; Kimball, 1999).

Children and adolescents with over reactive sensory systems may demonstrate tactile defensiveness, oral defensiveness, gravitational insecurity, auditory defensiveness, olfactory defensiveness, or visual defensiveness. Children and adolescents who are tactually defensive are hypersensitive to touch. They react aversively to human touch, the texture of clothing, and to grooming and bathing activities. Children and adolescents who are orally defensive have difficulty tolerating oral hygiene activities, and the textures and taste of food, thus potentially compromising their oral health and nutritional intake. Those with gravitational insecurity are fearful of actions that require them to move their heads beyond the upright position such as climbing, tumbling, or moving quickly. In contrast, children and adolescents who are under aroused by gravity may seek out strong, frequent, and dangerous movements to get the sensory input they need. Children who demonstrate auditory defensiveness have difficulty tolerating and habituating to environmental sounds, and those with olfactory defensiveness may become emotionally agitated or physically nauseated by typical smells. Those who are visually defensive have difficulty tolerating bright lights, too many visual materials, or too many people (Kimball, 1999; Wilbarger & Wilbarger, 2002).

As a result, children and adolescents with sensory integration problems may demonstrate difficulty with end-product abilities. These include praxis, form and space perception, behavioral control, language and articulation, academics, activity levels, and emotional response. **Praxis** is the ability to plan and execute nonhabitual motor acts and to consider how to and adapt body movements to complete coordinated, complex movements. Children and adolescents with **dyspraxia** may have difficulty developing the idea of how to move their bodies, planning and sequencing the course of actions to move the body, and using feedforward and feedback input to fluidly execute and modify their movements in response to environmental clues. Children and adolescents with form and space perception problems may have difficulty with writing, reading, building activities, and physically moving through their environments without bumping objects. Those with behavioral control problems may explode or act aggressively toward others. Those who have difficulty regulating their activity level may be restless, fidgety, and nonfocused during school, social, and sports activities. Those who have difficulty modulating their emotional tone may demonstrate increased levels of stress or compulsive levels of organization to keep their environments under control. It is important to remember that when working with other professionals not all may view these behavioral, activity level, and emotional difficulties from a sensory integrative perspective. Others may view them from psychosocial or educational perspectives. Thus, knowledge about and respect for each other's professional expertise is essential for providing coordinated interventions.

Academics, language, and articulation also may be an area of struggle for these children and adolescents because of difficulty with attending, planning their motor actions, perceiving form and space, and modulating their emotional tone. Lastly, these children and adolescents may struggle with mastering tasks and objects in their environment (Bundy et al., 2002; Kimball, 1999). Clustered together, these difficulties manifest themselves in four main areas of sensory integrative dysfunction: dysfunction in sensory modulation, dysfunction in praxis, dysfunction with visual perception and visual motor skills, and auditory-language dysfunction (Bundy et al.).

When occupational therapists and occupational therapy assistants use a sensory integration as a frame of reference, they first direct intervention toward modulating the sensory systems. Under the direction of the occupational therapist, occupational therapy assistants might provide a sensory diet either to excite or inhibit the children's sensory systems. They might provide excitatory activities such as fast dancing, rapid swinging, loud music, and fast-moving sports activities. They might provide inhibitory activities including soft music, heavy deep pressure, cuddling, heavy lifting, and quiet rooms. To help the children and adolescents modulate their sensory responses within the classroom environment, the occupational therapy assistant might propose chewing gum, sucking on sour candies, rocking in a chair, or squeezing fidget toys. The occupational therapy assistant also might encourage the children to sit in a bean bag chair or on a bouncing ball since the proprioceptive and vestibular input they provide sometimes has a calming effect.

Once the sensory system is modulated, occupational therapy intervention focuses on developing the functional support capacities and the end-product abilities described above (Kimball, 1999). Under the guidance of the occupational therapist, occupational therapy assistants might use candy chewing, bubble blowing, and whistling activities to work on suck-swallow-breathe patterns. They might use jungle gym, swinging, scooter board, trampoline, and push-pull games and activities to work on proprioception, balance and equilibrium, muscle tone and cocontraction, lateralization, and bilateral integration. They might use activities such as skating, biking, karate, and swimming to work on motor planning, self-initiation, organization, equilibrium, and bilateral integration. For the particular activity to facilitate sensory integration, it must be at the appropriate level of challenge for the children and adolescents, allow initiation and control by them, and generate the production of quality movement patterns, an adaptive response by them. As implied by the above overview, to accurately and effectively use the sensory integrative framework requires education beyond that included within the occupational therapy assistant curriculum. It is important for occupational therapy assistants to acquire supervision by an occupational therapist with advanced training in sensory integration to effectively incorporate some of the approaches during intervention. When using sensory integration approaches, remember that:

- Each of the sensory systems influences another, and that overload of one system may result in overload in other systems.
- The state and function of the underlying sensory systems affects the quality and adaptability of the children's and adolescents' functional support capabilities and end-product habilitations.

- Appropriate registration of and adaptive responses to sensory input from several systems contributes to sensory integration.
- Activities at the upper range of the children's and adolescents' abilities facilitate the greatest adaptation and integration (Kimball, 1999).

MOVEMENT RELATED FRAMES OF REFERENCE

Movement related frames of reference provide structure for evaluating and providing interventions to address **neuromuscular** and **musculoskeletal** difficulties. Neuromuscular focuses on the relationship between the nervous and the muscular systems of the body; musculoskeletal focuses on the relationship between the muscular and skeletal systems of the body. Though not exclusively designed for children and adolescents, two of the movement related frames of reference used when working with them are the **biomechanical** and **neurodevelopmental frames of reference**. The following section examines each of these and considers their application within occupational therapy practice.

Biomechanical Frame of Reference

The biomechanical frame of reference has its foundation in biological and mechanical principles of how nerves, muscles, and bones work. It draws on theories of physics and physiology to explain how gravity affects the body physically, mechanically, and physiologically as it moves. Occupational therapists and occupational therapy assistants use the biomechanical frame of reference to address the postural control, body alignment, and head, trunk, and limb movements of children and adolescents with central nervous system (CNS) trauma and physical disabilities.

Biomechanical Frame of Reference and the Central Nervous System

During infancy, reflexes contribute to early postural control, body alignment, and body mobility. Reflexes are stereotypical motor reactions stimulated by gravity, tactile, proprioceptive, and vestibular input. Examples of primitive reflexes that infants display within the first month include the asymmetrical tonic neck reflex, the symmetrical tonic neck reflex, and tonic labyrinthine reflex; these are described in Appendix B. In infants with intact central nervous systems, reflexes contribute to the early development of muscle tone and muscle movements needed for motor control. Typically, these primitive reflexes fade as the infant develops more control in the muscles of the neck and trunk, and as righting, protective extension, and **equilibrium** reactions emerge. A description of these also can be found in Appendix B. Righting reactions enable the infant to align or right the head in space and maintain head and neck alignment. Protective extension and equilibrium reactions emerge after righting reactions. Protection extension reactions stimulate young children to extend their arm and leg in the direction they are falling to protect themselves from harm. Equilibrium reactions enable young children to maintain their balance against gravity and against external forces. Young children with intact CNS demonstrate well developed righting, protective extension, and equilibrium reactions shortly after one year of age (Bly, 1994; Colangelo, 1999).

Children and adolescents who have experienced CNS trauma, such as cerebral palsy, brain attack, or closed head injury, demonstrate primitive reflexes beyond the age when they should have faded, and do not demonstrate righting, protective, and equilibrium reactions by the age they should occur. In addition, they may exhibit too low muscle tone, called hypotonicity, or too high muscle tone, called hypertonicity. Both hypertonicity and hypertonicity can lead to abnormal posture and shortening of muscles because of mechanical misalignment of the joints (Bly, 1994; Colangelo, 1999).

Guided by the occupational therapist, occupational therapy assistants might use biomechanical principles to address muscle tone, muscle movement, and bone alignment concerns. For example, the occupational therapy assistant might show parents of a young child with cerebral palsy how to roll him and range the muscles to prevent muscle contractures. The occupational therapy assistant also might show the parents how to modify the furniture at home to help the child maintain balance when sitting. When working with an adolescent with a brain injury from an automobile accident, the occupational therapy assistant might demonstrate where to place the food and how to use adaptive equipment to reteach self-feeding skills. The occupational therapy assistant might demonstrate to the caregiver how to stabilize or hold the adolescent's jaw so that she can chew her food. The occupational therapy assistant also might teach the adolescent how to use the movement patterns she has to activate assistive technologies, her wheelchair, computer, and other electronic equipment.

The following key principles are important to remember when using biomechanical principles with children and adolescents who experienced trauma to their CNS.

- Postural control depends on the body's ability to use to vestibular, tactile, and proprioceptive input to respond to gravity.
- The development of posture follows a sequential and developmental pattern; impairments to the bones, muscles, or CNS may interfere with this development.
- The body uses substitute movements to compensate for postural reactions that do not develop normally.
- These substitute movements can lead to additional difficulties with body alignment and movement control.
- Biomechanical approaches provide external support to compensate for abnormal posture; these external supports reduce the effects of gravity (Colangelo, 1999).

Intervention approaches for children and adolescents who have experienced trauma to their CNS are discussed in more detail in Chapter 19.

Biomechanical Frame of Reference and Joint Mobility

In addition to those with trauma to their CNS, occupational therapists and occupational therapy assistants use biomechanical approaches to work with children and adolescents with joint mobility problems such as juvenile arthritis, hip fractures, and arthrogyroposis. The principles they use with children and adolescents are similar to those used with individuals of any age who have joint mobility problems. Depending on the joint mobility impairment, occupational therapists and occupational therapy assistants might encourage these children and adolescents to:

- Use the largest joints possible to complete the motor task.
- Keep the joints warm and the muscles stretched to maintain flexible movement.
- Use low weight, low resistant activities with frequent repetitions to keep muscles strong.

- Divide heavy loads into several smaller, light loads, or use wheels to push rather than carry heavy loads.
- Keep shoulders aligned over hips, and hips aligned over feet when standing, bending, and sitting.
- Bend at the knees rather than at the waist.
- Carry objects near the midline of the body.

Rather than teaching discrete biomechanical principles, it may be best to incorporate them within the daily occupations of the children and adolescents. For example, occupational therapy assistants might encourage children with arthritis to use wheeled school bags rather than backpacks for their books or to petition the school to have a set of books at home and at school. They also may encourage the children and adolescents to participate in swimming and water play activities to keep joints mobile and muscles strong. They might teach children with arthrogryposis how to turn resistive lids by also using hip movements if they do not have full range of movement in their elbows or shoulders. As with all other intervention approaches, it is important to select activities appropriate for the developmental age and cultural context of the children and adolescents when applying biomechanical principles.

Neurodevelopmental Frame of Reference

The neurodevelopmental frame of reference applies sensorimotor techniques to address movement related difficulties and developmental delays. Developed originally by Bobath and Bobath in the 1940s, the approach is used with children and adolescents with neuromuscular disorders, immature CNS, and developmental disabilities. The approach now incorporates current information about the organization of the CNS, motor development, and motor control theory (Shumway-Cook & Woollacott, 2001). Rather than viewing motor development as sequential only, it considers the importance of genetics, environment, and experience on that development. It views cephalo to caudal, proximal to distal, and gross to fine motor development as interactional rather than hierarchical, a belief formerly held. This means that (1) head and trunk control develop in relationship with one another to produce head and body alignment, (2) control of muscles near the midline and peripheral parts of the body develop in relationship to one another to produce limb control, and (3) gross and fine motor development occur separately and in relationship to one another to produce controlled movement. The neurodevelopmental frame of reference also recognizes the importance of feedforward as well as feedback information throughout the execution of a movement. As part of feedforward, muscles ready themselves to cocontract in preparation for a goal directed movement. Sensory feedback provides input on the accuracy of the goal directed movement once it is executed. Goal directed movements, that is, those movements associated with accomplishing a task, provide more accurate feedforward and feedback information to stimulate motor development than do non–goal directed movements (Schoen & Anderson, 1999; Shumway-Cook & Woollacott, 2006).

Three components of normal development are central to neurodevelopmental treatment (NDT). NDT focuses on the relationship between **stability** and **mobility** for controlled movement, postural tone and postural alignment, and **dissociate** or differentiated **movements** of various body parts. Children and adolescents who demonstrate normal development are able to execute progressively more advancing levels of dynamic movement, that is, fluid, coordinated, controlled movement. Dynamic movement involves stabilizing a portion of the body to allow for controlled mobility of other parts of the body. The size of the base of support decreases as children and adolescents advance in their skills. Children demonstrate these principles when they are learning to sit. Initially, they lean forward at the waist, position their legs in front of them on the ground, and prop themselves on their arms. This position provides for a wide base of support. As children gain more pelvic girdle and trunk stability, they begin to be able to free their arms to pick up and play with objects and to free their legs to kick (see Figure 3.1■). As the children advance in their skills, they learn to stabilize themselves on their buttocks while lifting and turning their legs to pivot and reach for toys beyond their immediate grasp. As two-year-olds, they can stand on narrow stools to reach higher objects (see Figure 3.2■). By the time they become preschoolers, young children can maintain dynamic sitting on bouncing balls and T-stools.

Children and adolescents who demonstrate normal motor development also exhibit progressively more advancing quality of postural tone and postural alignment to hold a position (stability) and to move against gravity (mobility). As young children learn to sit, they first develop postural control in the sagittal plane through extension and flexion movement to shift weight forward and backward. Next, they refine postural control in the frontal plane to shift their weight laterally. Then they exhibit control in the transverse plane to rotate their bodies and prepare to crawl.

Children and adolescents who demonstrate normal motor development also exhibit an increasingly progressive ability to separate (dissociate) and combine movements of various parts of their bodies. As children progress in their ability to draw and write, they demonstrate this principle. Initially, children use their entire arm to draw and write. They also may stick out and move their tongues as they draw and write. This is called an associative movement. Shoulders, fingers, and tongues display similar rotary movements. As the children gain more control concurrently over their scapular, elbow, wrist, and finger movements, they make progressively smaller

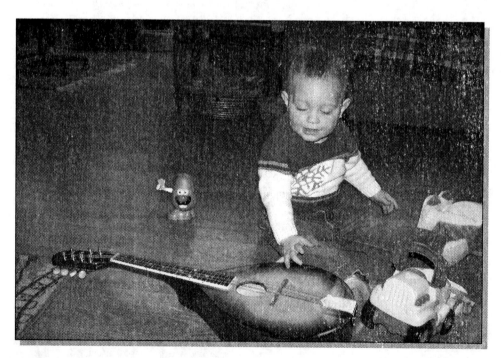

■ Figure 3.1
Child reaching for a toy.

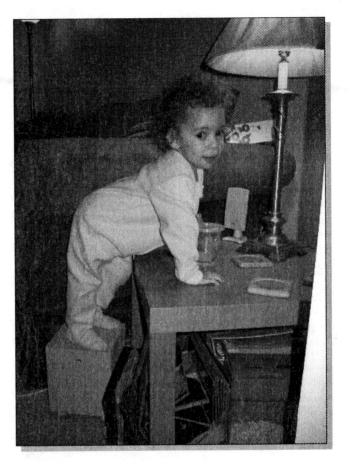

■ **Figure 3.2**
Child standing on a narrow stool.

movements with the shoulder, elbow, and wrist, and progressively more complex and rapid movements with their fingers.

In contrast to children and adolescents who demonstrate normal development, those who demonstrate atypical motor development may have problems with stability and mobility, postural tone and alignment, and dissociative movements. Children with atypical postural tone have difficulty mastering a number of automatic movement patterns, including automatic righting, protective extension, and equilibrium reactions. Difficulty with the feedforward and feedback mechanisms interferes with the development of postural control and movement skills. Excessive postural tone restricts joint movements and can lead to shortening and intrinsic changes in the surrounding muscle fibers (Keshner, 1990; Schoen & Anderson, 1999; Shumway-Cook & Woollacott, 2006). This restriction of movement interferes with the ability to dissociate movements. Children with severe developmental disabilities may have this difficulty. Rather than separately moving their head, shoulders, trunk, and legs to roll, they roll their body as a unit, called log rolling. When trying to activate a switch on a toy or electronic device, they may need to swing their entire arm to make contact, rather than to isolate finger movements.

Children and adolescents with neurodevelopmental problems also may exhibit atypical posture, as manifested by increased or decreased postural tone throughout their bodies, and increased or decreased tension and mobility in their joints. They may use atypical or compensatory strategies to maintain their stability, such as walking with a wider gait, W-sitting, and using upper extremities for additional balance. They may display atypical postural alignment, such as excessive extension of trunk and head and excessive flexion when standing. When moving, they may exhibit synergistic movements such that flexion of the arms results in flexion of the hands, and extension of the hips results in extension of the hips and ankles. They also may develop contractures or deformities such as scoliosis. If intervention is not provided, the children continue to repeat and thus reinforce these abnormal and compensatory movements, compromising their ability to participate in their daily life activities (Schoen & Anderson, 1999).

As with the sensory integration frame of reference, the use of the neurodevelopmental framework requires education beyond that included within the occupational therapy assistant curriculum. It is important for occupational therapy assistants to receive supervision from an occupational therapist with advanced training in NDT, or to receive training in NDT to effectively incorporate some of the approaches during intervention. When using NDT approaches, occupational therapists and occupational therapy assistants might adjust the amount of sensory input associated with occupational tasks to elicit efficient rather than over or under reactive movement patterns. They also might use handling techniques, that is, placing hands in specified positions on the child, with specific degrees of pressure to facilitate desired movement patterns. Key points for handling typically include the shoulder girdle, trunk, and pelvis. To use these sensory and handling techniques, occupational therapists and occupational therapy assistants need to possess a firm knowledge of typical development and movement and carefully observe the child's shift in postural tone, level of stability and mobility, and dissociative movements as he performs the occupation. These techniques also require the occupational therapist and the occupational therapy assistant to judge when to reduce the amount of handling so that the child can initiate and execute the movements necessary to independently complete the desired occupation. When incorporating NDT principles interventions:

- Strive for good alignment of trunk, extremities and head during functional activities. When adjusting alignment, start with the pelvic area and monitor how gravity affects alignment and function.

- Observe changes in postural tone during movement and activity. Strive to facilitate fluid movement by feeling and adjusting to how the body is reacting to environmental stimulation.

- Provide a stable base of support during activities and occupations that require refined distal movement, since proximal stability enhances distal movement patterns.

- Position materials in relationship to the child's or adolescent's midline and below eye-level, to encourage good alignment.

- Apply deep pressure to the child's pelvic girdle to strengthen that base of support.

- Apply deep pressure to the child's pectoral muscles to elongate them and move the scapula in a downward rotating position.

- Cocontract weight-bearing joints to facilitate their ability to stabilize the shoulders and hips for movement of the arms and legs.

- Intermittently compress the muscle around the joint to facilitate the ability of the child to stabilize it.
- Provide graded sensory input based on the children's ability to integrate and generate motor responses.

When engaging the child in movement:

- Incorporate spontaneous play activities to encourage automatic movement.
- Encourage the reciprocal use of agonist and antagonist muscles as the child engages in meaningful occupations and within the natural environment.
- Allow for multiple repetitions to encourage integration and habituation of the movement patterns (Schoen & Anderson, 1999).

CONNECTING TO THE OCCUPATION-BASED CONCEPTUAL MODELS AND THE OCCUPATIONAL THERAPY PRACTICE FRAMEWORK

Chapter 2 concluded with a table that connected occupation-based models to the Occupational Therapy Practice Framework. Some of the occupation-based conceptual models provide guidance for thinking about occupations; others provide guidance for considering the context or activity demands. Still others focus more directly on performance patterns or performance skills.

This chapter reviewed some of the non–occupation-based theories and frames of reference. They offered perspectives for viewing the psychosocial development, cognitive development, learning processes, sensory integrative processes, and movement development and capacities of children and adolescents. Though not covered in this chapter, other non–occupation-based theories and frames of reference exist that provide perspectives on social skills, coping skills, play skills, environmental influences, physical context, and visual processing skills of children and adolescents, to name a few. Each of the non–occupation-based theories and frames of reference provides useful structures for considering what factors influence the way children and adolescents perform, and how to evaluate those specific factors. However, the non–occupation-based theories and frames of reference do not provide guidance for considering the actual occupations that children and adolescents perform or why they engage in those occupations. It is through combining the non–occupation-based theories and frames of reference with occupation-based conceptual models that occupational therapists and occupational therapy assistants obtain a fuller understanding of the interrelationship between performance and the occupational engagement. This knowledge leads to best practice services to children and adolescents.

Table 3.1■ offers one way to view the relationship among the occupation-based conceptual models, non–occupation-based frames of reference, and the Occupational Therapy Practice Framework. It expands upon Table 2.1. Remember that Table 3.1 is neither a complete list of all of the occupation-based conceptual models nor of the non–occupation-based frames of reference. Others can be added to it. The table will need to be modified as conceptual models, frames of reference, and the Practice Framework evolve.

■ Table 3.1
Connecting Practice Framework with Conceptual Models, Theories, and Frames of Reference

NON OCCUPATION-BASED THEORIES AND FRAMES OF REFERENCE

		OCCUPATIONAL THERAPY PRACTICE FRAMEWORK—DOMAINS							OCCUPATIONAL THERAPY PRACTICE FRAMEWORK-PROCESS		
(Non OT theories)		Cognitive Learning Neurodevelopmental	Behavioral Acquisitional	Social learning	Cognitive Learning, Social Learning, Acquisitional Neurodevelopmental, Psychosocial, Behavioral Biomechanical, Sensory Integrative			Biomechanical Sensory Integrative	Behavioral, Sensory Integrative, Neurodevelopmental, Acquisitional Biomechanical		
CONCEPTUAL MODELS		AREAS OF OCCUPATION	PERFORMANCE SKILLS	PERFORMANCE PATTERNS	CONTEXT	ACTIVITY DEMAND	BODY FUNCTION	BODY STRUCTURE	EVALUATION	INTERVENTION	OUTCOME
Ecological Model of Human Performance	Person—personal values, interests, experiences, and skills	Cluster of meaningful tasks	Performance—selecting and doing tasks	Person—roles	Context	Temporal and environmental features of the task	Person—skills, values		Directed at performance within context	Intervention approaches	Performance, range of performance
Model of Human Occupation	Person—volition, habituation Performance capacity	Nature of occupation	Occupational performance	Habituation—roles and routines	Environment—physical and social		Performance capacity—subjective experience and objective component		Eight assessment tools to use with children or adolescents	Directed at person factors, environment factors, and occupational performance	Occupational adaptation and occupational competency
Person-Environment-Occupational Performance	Person—neurobiological, physiological, cognitive, psychological, emotional, spiritual factors	Participation in and performance of occupations	Actions and tasks		Environment		Person factors		Directed at personal factors, environmental factors, activities, tasks, and roles	Directed at personal factors and environmental factors, activities, tasks, and roles	Health and well-being
Person-Environment Occupation	Person—mind, body spirit	Occupation—clusters of self-directed tasks or activities	Observable aspects of occupational performance		Environment		Physical and psychosocial capacities		Directed at the person, environment, and occupation	Directed at the person, environment, and occupation	Occupational performance

SUMMARY

A theory is a set of constructs organized in a particular manner to provide a systematic understanding of and predictions about the relationship between events. A frame of reference is a method for organizing information and knowledge to serve as a guide for evaluation and intervention. Frames of reference link together and apply theory to the practice of the profession (Mosey, 1981; Kramer & Hinojosa, 1999). Occupational therapists and occupational therapy assistants who work with children and adolescents need to understand theories and frames of reference related to growth and development, learning, sensory integration, and motor development and control.

Erikson, through his theory of psychosocial development, provides a structure for understanding the psychological and social crisis children and adolescents must resolve throughout various stages of development. Piaget, through his work on cognitive learning, offers a framework for examining how children develop their thinking capacities and their awareness of self. Skinner's work in behavioral theory highlights the role of reinforcement and punishment in learning. Bandura, through his work on social learning theory, considers the influence of the environment and connectedness with other people on how and what children and adolescents learn. The learning principles associated with acquisitional frame of reference offer a systematic approach to facilitate the skill acquisition and adaptive responses of the children and adolescents. A review of the sensory integrative framework offers insights about the sensory system and strategies for providing interventions to children and adolescents with sensory integrative and sensory modulating difficulties. The biomechanical frame of reference provides an approach for considering the principles underlying how gravity affects the nerves, bones, and muscles. Finally, the neurodevelopmental model offers a perspective about the CNS, motor development, and motor control theory, and strategies for applying sensorimotor techniques to address movement related difficulties and developmental delays.

These theories and frames of reference detail a more in depth schemata than do the occupation-based conceptual models regarding how children and adolescents grow, develop, process information, move their bodies, think, behave, feel, and act socially with others. Some also provide a rationale for how to evaluate and provide interventions for children and adolescents who have difficulty in these areas. The chapter concludes with a perspective on the importance of combining occupation-based conceptual model with non–occupation-based theories to guide occupational therapy practice.

REVIEWING KEY POINTS

1. Explain why it is important to use non–occupation-based theories and frames of reference when providing occupational therapy services to children and adolescents.
2. List the eight theories and frames of reference discussed in this chapter. For each:
   - Define the key terms.
   - Outline four assumptions.
   - Describe two examples of how to apply it to occupational therapy practice.

APPLYING KEY CONCEPTS

1. Observe four different children and adolescents for 30 minutes each. Observe children and adolescents who are approximately 3, 6, 10, and 14 years old. Use each of the eight theories and frames of reference presented in this chapter to explain the behaviors observed. Use the following chart to record the observations. Adjust the size of the chart to accommodate the amount of observations recorded.

   Age of child or adolescent _____

   Setting for observation _____

   Occupations in which the child or docent engaged _____

   Relationship of other people present to the child or adolescent _____

   THEORY OR FRAME OF REFERENCE   OBSERVATION OF RELATED BEHAVIORS
   Psychosocial development
   Cognitive development
   Social learning
   Behavioral
   Acquistional
   Sensory integrative
   Biomechanical
   Neurodevelopmental

2. Cut and paste the observations recorded about each child's and adolescent's psychosocial development onto one page. Using the psychosocial theory of development, describe how and why the behaviors changed or remain the same for each of the four ages. Use the following chart to organize the observations. Adjust its size to accommodate your observations.

   Theory or Frame of Reference _____

   AGE OF CHILD OR ADOLESCENT   OBSERVATIONS
   3-year-old
   6-year-old
   10-year-old
   14-year-old

   Description of how and why the behaviors changed _____

   _____

   _____

   _____

   _____

3. Follow the directions for activity 2 substituting cognitive theory for psychosocial learning theory. Do the same for each of the other six theories and frames of reference.

REFERENCES

Ayres, A. J. (1972). *Sensory integration and learning disorders.* Los Angeles: Western Psychological Services.

Ayres, A. J. (1979). *Sensory integration and the child.* Los Angeles: Western Psychological Services.

Bandura, A. (1977). *Social learning theory.* Englewood Cliffs, NJ: Prentice Hall.

Bandura, A. (1989). Social cognitive theory. *Annals of Child Development, 6,* 1–60.

Bee, H., & Boyd, D. (2002). *Lifespan development* (3rd ed.). Boston: Allyn & Bacon.

Bly, L. (1994). *Motor skill acquisition during the first year of development and abnormal motor development.* Birmingham, AL: Neuro-Developmental Treatment Association.

Brownwell, C. A. (1990). Peer social skills in toddlers. Competencies and constraints illustrated by same-age and mixed-age interaction. *Child Development, 61,* 836–848.

Bundy, A., Lane, S., & Murray, E. (Eds.). (2002). *Sensory integration: Theory and practice* (2nd ed.). Philadelphia: F. A. Davis.

Ciancio, D., Sadovsky, A., Malabonga, V., Trueblood, L. et al. (1999). Teaching classification and seriation to preschoolers. *Child Study Journal, 29,* 193–205.

Colangelo, C. (1999). Biomechanical frame of reference. In P. Kramer & J. Hinojosa (Eds.), *Frames of reference for pediatric occupational therapy* (2nd ed.). Philadelphia: Lippincott Williams & Wilkins.

Dunn, J. (1994). Experience and understanding of emotions, relationships, and membership in a particular culture. In P. Ekman & R. J. Davidson (Eds.), *The nature of emotion: Fundamental questions* (pp. 353–355). New York: Oxford University Press.

Elkind, D. (1970, April). Eric Erikson's eight stages of man. *New York Times Magazine,* 24.

Erikson, E. H., & Erikson, J. M. (1997). *The life cycle completed.* New York: Norton & Company.

Flavell, J. H. (1986). The development of children's knowledge about the appearance-reality distinction. *American Psychologist, 41,* 418–425.

Keshner, E. (1990). Coordinating stability of complex motor systems. *Physical Therapy, 70,* 844–854.

Kimball, J. (1999). Sensory integration frame of reference: Theoretical base, function/dysfunction continua, and guide to evaluation. In P. Kramer & J. Hinojosa (Eds.), *Frames of reference for pediatric occupational therapy* (2nd ed.). Philadelphia: Lippincott Williams & Wilkins.

Kramer, P., & Hinojosa, J. (Eds.). (1999). *Frames of reference for pediatric occupational therapy* (2nd ed.). Philadelphia: Lippincott Williams & Wilkins.

McDevitt, T., & Ormrod, J. (2002). *Child development: Educating and working with children and adolescents* (2nd ed.). Upper Saddle River, NJ: Prentice Hall.

Mosey, A. C. (1981). *Configuration of a profession.* New York: Raven Press.

Piaget, J. (1965). *The child's conception of the world.* New York: Littlefield Adams.

Piaget, J. (May, 1970). Conversations. *Psychology Today, 3,* 25–32.

Royeen, C. B., & Duncan, M. (1999). Acquisitioned frame of reference. In P. Kramer and J. Hinojosa (Eds.), *Frames of reference for pediatric occupational therapy* (2nd ed.). Philadelphia: Lippincott Williams & Wilkins.

Schoen, S., & Anderson, J. (1999). Neurodevelopmental treatment frame of reference. In P. Kramer and J. Hinojosa (Eds.), *Frames of reference for pediatric occupational therapy* (2nd ed.). Philadelphia: Lippincott Williams & Wilkins.

Shumway-Cook, A., & Woollacott, M. (2006). *Motor control: Translating research into clinical practice* (3rd ed.). Philadelphia: Lippincott Williams & Wilkins.

Skinner, B. F. (1953). *Science and human behavior.* New York: Macmillan.

Skinner, B. F. (1980). The experimental analysis of operant behavior. A history. In R. W. Reibes and K. Salzinger (Eds.), *Psychology: Theoretical-historical perspectives.* New York: Academic Press.

Vander Zanden, J., Crandell, T., and Crandell, C. (2003). *Human development* (revised 7th ed.). New York: McGraw Hill.

Wilbarger, P., & Wilbarger, L. (1991). *Sensory defensiveness in children 2–12: An intervention guide for parents and other caregivers.* Denver, CO: Avanti Education Program.

Wilbarger, P., & Wilbarger, J. (2002). The Wilbarger approach to treating sensory defensiveness. In A. Bundy, S. Lane, & E. Murray (Eds.), *Sensory integration: Theory and practice* (2nd ed.). Philadelphia: F. A. Davis.

Williams, M. S., & Shellenberger, S. (1994). *How fast does your engine run?* Albuquerque, NM: TherapyWorks.

Chapter 4

Role of the Occupational Therapist and Occupational Therapy Assistant in Various Practice Settings

Janet V. DeLany

Key Terms

Assessment

Client

Clinical reasoning

Code of Ethics

Evaluation

Interdisciplinary team

Intervention

Multidisciplinary team

Occupational profile

Outcomes

Re-evaluation

Screening

Supervision

Transdisciplinary team

Objectives

- Define the role of the occupational therapy assistant and the occupational therapist in the delivery of occupational therapy services.
- Explain the supervisory relationship between the occupational therapy assistant and the occupational therapist.
- Explain the influence of regulations on the roles and supervisory process.
- Identify various practice settings where occupational therapy assistants and occupational therapists provide services for children and adolescents.
- Explain the composition of teams and the role of occupational therapy assistants and occupational therapists in these practice settings.
- Apply the AOTA **Code of Ethics** to these practice settings.

ROLES WHEN PROVIDING OCCUPATIONAL THERAPY SERVICES

When working with children and adolescents, occupational therapists and the occupational therapy assistants perform complementary but distinct roles in each stage of the occupational therapy delivery process. As explained in Chapter 1, the occupational therapy delivery process involves three stages: evaluation, intervention, and outcomes. These stages do not necessarily follow a strict sequential progression, but can occur in tandem with one another (AOTA, 2002), based on the needs of the children and adolescents, practice setting guidelines, and the length of time services are provided. The entire occupational therapy process is grounded in occupation-based conceptual models and other theories and frames of reference. As discussed in Chapters 2 and 3, they guide clinical reasoning and decision making.

Evaluation

The words **screening**, **evaluation**, and **re-evaluation** are used in some practice settings to differentiate among the different types of evaluations that occur at various times during the occupational therapy process. Screening refers to the prestep of the overall evaluation process. During the screening, the occupational therapist and the occupational therapy assistant gather preliminary data about the child or adolescent to determine the need for a more comprehensive occupational evaluation or intervention plan. Evaluation is the initial, comprehensive step of the occupational therapy delivery process. It involves gathering and interpreting all of the relevant data to make judgments about the need for, scope of, and types of occupational therapy services. **Assessments** are the specific observations, chart reviews, interviews, and measurement tools that are used to gather the information. These are discussed in more detail in Chapter 9. The re-evaluation occurs after intervention has begun to determine the need to continue, modify, or discontinue occupational therapy services (AOTA, 2005b).

Regardless of the terminology used in the practice setting, the occupational therapy evaluation requires knowledge about occupations, occupational performance challenges, and various diagnostic conditions that limit the ability of children and adolescents to participate in daily life activities. As part of the evaluation, the occupational therapist and the occupational therapy assistant consider the:

- Activities and occupations that the children and adolescents can and want to do in their daily lives
- Motivations for the children and adolescents to do these activities and occupations
- Characteristics of the children and adolescents that influence how they perform these activities and occupations
- Environment where the occupations are performed (Law et al., 2005)

The occupational therapist is responsible for initiating and directing the occupational therapy evaluation, and for integrating and analyzing the data to develop an intervention. The occupational therapist may designate aspects of the evaluation to occupational therapy assistant. However, before doing so, the occupational therapist and the occupational therapy assistant first must review applicable practice setting guidelines, and state and federal regulations. This is necessary because the scope of practice for occupational therapy assistants differs among practice settings, and state and federal jurisdictions. What is reimbursed by the funding agency also must be considered (AOTA, 2004b, 2005a). Some practice settings, state and federal jurisdictions, and funding agencies permit occupational therapy assistants to complete designated aspects of the occupational therapy evaluation. Others do not.

When designating aspects of the evaluation to the occupational therapy assistant, the occupational therapist must provide appropriate **supervision**. The occupational therapist must ensure that the occupational therapy assistant has demonstrated service competency to carry out the designated aspects of the evaluation at a level appropriate to address the complexities of the children's and adolescents' occupational, health, and learning challenges. To demonstrate service competency, the occupational therapy assistant must conduct the assessment according to established procedures, and obtain results similar to those that the occupational therapist would have obtained. The occupational therapy assistant may contribute to the evaluation process by carrying out designated assessments and by providing written and verbal reports to the occupational therapist about the information collected related to the capacity of the children and adolescents to engage in their daily life occupations (AOTA, 2004b, 2005a).

The occupational therapy assistant may help with developing **occupational profiles** and with gathering data to analyze the performance capacities of the children and adolescents. The occupational profile includes information about the children's and adolescents' occupational histories or life experiences, daily living routines, interests, values, problems with performing their daily life tasks, and priorities. For example, the occupational profile of an adolescent female with arthritis who rides horses might include information about her horseback riding and school experiences, her daily routines to care for the horse and complete her school obligations, her interest in becoming a veterinarian, her current difficulties completing her riding activities and school obligations because of arthritis, and her priorities for continuing to participate in riding and school activities. The occupational therapy assistant may help to gather data about the adolescent's daily occupations, her performance skills and routines, the environments that influence how she performs her activities and occupations, the demands associated with those activities, and how her body moves (AOTA, 2002). Using an observation sheet, the occupational therapy assistant might record how and where the adolescent carries out her horse riding–related activities. The occupational therapy assistant also might use other assessments such as an ADA environmental accessibility checklist to identify physical barriers, and a time chart to record the other time demands. The occupational therapy assistant then provides verbal and written documentation to the occupational therapist and discusses possible intervention approaches. Table 1.1 (in Chapter 1) provides a grid for organizing the evaluation information.

Intervention

As with the evaluation, the occupational therapist assumes responsibility for all aspects of the **intervention**. The occupational therapy assistant works with the occupational therapist to develop the intervention in collaboration with the client. When working with children and adolescents, the term **client** includes not only the children and adolescents, but also their parents, caregivers, and extended family, when applicable. The intervention has three aspects: the intervention plan, the intervention implementation, and the intervention review. The intervention plan is directed by the:

- Client's beliefs, values, and goals for therapy
- Client's performance skills and performance patterns

- Client's physical, social, and cultural environments
- Demands of the activity
- Functioning capacity of the client's body structures
- Setting for or circumstances of intervention (AOTA, 2002)

When working with children and adolescents, overarching goals for intervention focus on:

- Establishing, restoring, and maintaining their capacity and skill to perform their occupations
- Modifying or adapting tasks and environments so that they can participate in their daily life tasks
- Preventing the development of barriers that limit their occupational participation
- Designing occupationally supportive environments (AOTA, 2002; Dunn, 2000).

Goals related to the above horse riding scenario might focus on: establishing the ability of the adolescent to develop coping strategies to manage her pain while performing daily routines; modifying the riding gear and grooming supplies to protect her joints; and eliminating accessibility barriers so that she can walk to the stable and mount the horse.

Occupational therapy assistants can assume responsibility for implementing those aspects of the intervention that the occupational therapist delegates to them. Given supervision from the occupational therapist, they can select, implement, and make modifications to therapeutic activities and interventions that are consistent with their demonstrated service competency, the intervention plan, the requirements of the practice setting, and state and federal regulations (AOTA, 2004a). For the adolescent in the above riding scenario, the occupational therapy assistant might recommend a padded saddle and shock absorbing stirrups, grooming equipment with straps and cushioned handles, a wheeled school bag, and scheduled rest period. The interventions need to be culturally sensitive, contextually relevant, and consistent with the goals, priorities, and values of the children and adolescents, and their families.

When implementing the interventions, occupational therapists and occupational therapy assistants use their professional selves, activities, and occupations in a therapeutic manner to help the children and adolescents achieve their occupational performance goals. Sometimes, they use preparatory methods to prepare the children and adolescents to participate in purposeful activities and occupations. Other times, they use purposeful activities to help the children and adolescents develop skills for engaging in their occupations. In the above scenario of the adolescent horseback rider, preparatory methods might include stretching, nonresistive exercises, and visual imaging. Purposeful activities might involve braiding hair, lifting, carrying, and role-playing activities. The ultimate goal is to use occupations to enable the children and adolescents to develop their capacity to participate fully in meaningful lives (AOTA, 2002).

Embedded within the intervention process is the need to systematically review the intervention plan to determine whether to continue, modify, or terminate occupational therapy services (AOTA, 2002). The occupational therapist is responsible for making that decision. Occupational therapy assistants contribute to the decision making process by providing information and documentation to the occupational therapist regarding any changes in the capacity of the children and adolescents to engage in their occupations, and their statements about their capacities, needs, and the occupational therapy intervention (AOTA, 2004a).

Outcomes

Recipients and payers of occupational therapy services seek evidence of the benefits of occupational therapy services. Measuring the **outcomes** of occupational therapy service at the individual and the program levels provides this evidence. Indicators of the benefits of occupational therapy services include positive changes in the ability of children and adolescents to:

- Engage in a variety of healthy occupations and occupational roles
- Master skills necessary to perform their occupations
- Adapt to varying environmental or contextual demands
- Feel satisfied with their occupational performance capacities and quality of life (AOTA, 2002)

For the adolescent in the riding scenario, data collected to measure the outcome of occupational therapy might include: the frequency and length of time she can participate in her riding and school activities free of pain, the amount of useful environmental and task modifications she can identify and implement to enable her to engage in her occupations, and her self-appraisal of her ability to continue her riding and school activities.

The occupational therapist is responsible for designing, implementing, and interpreting evidence-based outcome procedures that measure changes in the children's and adolescents' ability to engage in their occupations. Occupational therapy assistants participate in this process by implementing evidence-based procedures and systematically collecting data related to outcome measures (AOTA, 2004a).

SUPERVISORY PROCESS WHEN PROVIDING OCCUPATIONAL THERAPY SERVICES

Occupational therapy assistants provide occupational therapy services under the supervision of and in partnership with the occupational therapist. Within occupational therapy, supervision is viewed as a cooperative process. The occupational therapist, as the supervisor, and the occupational therapy assistant, as the supervisee, are mutually responsible for the content, format, quality, and frequency of the supervision (AOTA 2004b; 2005a).

The goal of supervision is twofold: (1) to ensure the safe and effective delivery of occupational therapy services; and (2) to foster professional development. As the supervisor, the occupational therapist needs to consider the occupational therapy assistant's current and advancing knowledge and skills, **clinical reasoning** abilities, and educational and career aspirations. Supervision includes discussions about the benefits and limits of various intervention methods (procedural reasoning), affective strategies to interact with children and adolescents (interactive reasoning), the past and present life experiences and future expectations of the children and adolescents (narrative reasoning), and resources available to provide occupational therapy services (pragmatic reasoning). Supervision also focuses on professional development such as continuing education initiatives to enrich clinical skills and to advance levels of competency (AOTA 2004b; 2005a).

As the supervisor, the occupational therapist is responsible for providing timely and appropriate information, guidance, and oversight to enable the occupational therapy assistant to provide occupational therapy services safely and effectively. As the supervisee, the occupational therapy assistant is responsible for seeking and procuring the supervision needed, and for providing accurate information to the occupational therapist about the children and adolescents, the occupational therapy services, and service competencies. Supervision can occur directly and indirectly. Direct supervision involves face to face or video conferencing contact between the occupational therapist and the occupational therapy assistant. Face to face discussions, modeling, cotreatment, teaching, and observations are examples of direct supervision. Indirect supervision involves telephone contact, electronic exchanges, and written correspondence. These methods do not provide opportunities for the occupational therapist and occupational therapy assistant to see what is occurring during the occupational therapy process. Since the occupational therapist is responsible for all aspects of the evaluation, intervention, and outcomes process, it is imperative that supervision includes some level of direct contact (AOTA 2004b; 2005a).

The American Occupational Therapy Association does not specify the frequency or amount of time the occupational therapy assistant is to receive direct or indirect supervision. Rather, as outlined in the *Guidelines for Supervision, Roles, and Responsibilities During the Delivery of Occupational Therapy Service* (AOTA 2004b), the frequency, amount and type of supervision depends on the:

- Occupational therapy assistant's demonstrated service competencies and skills
- Occupational therapist's supervisory and practice competencies and skills
- Needs and complexities of the children and adolescents receiving services from the occupational therapy assistant
- Number of children and adolescents receiving services from the occupational therapy assistant
- Guidelines of the practice setting, and regulatory requirements (AOTA 2004b; 2005a).

For example, the amount, type, and frequency of supervision appropriate for an occupational therapy assistant to safely and effectively conduct one on one dressing programs for elementary age children with moderate cognitive challenges may be different than what is appropriate to safely and effectively conduct a leisure pursuit group for adolescents with an eating disorder. State and federal agencies and practice settings may have established regulations that specify the minimum type, frequency, and amount of supervision occupational therapy assistants are to receive when providing occupational therapy services. Since these regulations supersede AOTA guidelines, occupational therapists and occupational therapy assistants are obligated to know and abide by them. If the occupational therapy assistant or the occupational therapist deems it necessary and appropriate for more supervision to occur than is outlined in these regulations to provide safe and effective services to the children and adolescents, then it is the right and responsibility of the occupational therapy assistant to obtain it (AOTA, 2005a).

Roles and Supervision When Providing Services Outside the Scope of Occupational Therapy

Occupational therapy assistant education also prepares occupational therapy assistants to work with children and adolescents in roles other than occupational therapy positions. For example, occupational therapy education might prepare occupational therapy assistants to work as play therapists at a rehabilitation hospital for children, as assistive technology specialists within a school setting, or as Special Olympics program coordinators in the community. Sometimes occupational therapy assistant education provides occupational therapy assistants with the necessary credentials to assume these work roles. Other times, occupational therapy assistants need to procure additional education and credentials to assume these work roles.

When assuming such roles, the occupational therapy assistants use the job title and credentials consistent with that position. This makes it clear to the recipient of the services what kinds of services they are receiving and the qualifications of the occupational therapy assistant to provide those services. The following questions help differentiate between when an occupational therapy assistant is providing occupational therapy services to children and adolescents, and when the occupational therapy assistant is using occupational therapy knowledge and skills to provide non–occupational therapy services. In the former situation, the occupational therapy assistant is to abide by occupational therapy supervision guidelines; in the latter situation, occupational therapy assistants abide by supervisory expectations outlined for that area of practice. The questions are as follows:

- What is the written or verbal understanding the agency, the payer, and the children, adolescents, and their families have about the types of services being provided?
- Are these services within the domain of occupational therapy practice?
- How do the state practice acts define the education, credentials, and supervision needed to offer the services?
- How do other relevant regulatory agencies define the education, credentials, and supervision needed to offer the services? (AOTA, 2004b).

If after answering these questions, it is determined that the occupational therapy assistant is providing occupational therapy services, then the assistant abides by the occupational therapy supervision and role requirements of the state practice acts, regulatory agencies, and the American Occupational Therapy Association. If after answering these questions, it is determined that the assistant is not providing occupational therapy services, though may be using occupational therapy knowledge and skills, then the occupational therapy assistant is to abide by the supervision and role requirements governing those services.

Practice Settings

Occupational therapy assistants work in a variety of practice setting with children and adolescents. One way to organize and think about the practice settings where occupational therapy assistants might work is to cluster them into institutional settings, outpatient settings, school based settings, and home and community settings.

Institutional settings include acute care, rehabilitation, and psychiatric hospitals, residential placements, and prisons. Occupational therapy assistants working in acute care or rehabilitation settings might help a child learn to feed himself with a prosthesis, or assist an adolescent who experienced a traumatic brain injury in relearning bathing skills. In a psychiatric hospital, occupational therapy assistants might work with an occupational therapist to conduct a playgroup for children coping with conduct disorders, or a leisure interest group for adolescents coping with eating disorders. At a residential setting for children and adolescents with severe developmental delays, occupational therapy assistants might provide adaptive seating devices, or direct a prevocational skills training program in preparation for sheltered workshop employment. Within a juvenile detention center, they might conduct a creative writing program with the occupational therapist to facilitate communication skills. In these same settings, they might use their occupational therapy knowledge and skills and other required credentials to assume the role of a recreation coordinator or behavioral health worker.

Outpatient settings include hospital clinics, medical offices, and therapy practices. In a hospital clinic, occupational therapy assistants might provide driver education to adolescents who have spina bifida or a learning disability. In a medical office, occupational therapy assistants might help with splint construction for children with neuromuscular complications. In a therapy practice, they might conduct a sensory exploration group for young children with autism. In these same settings, they might combine their occupational therapy assistant education with other education to work as a case manager, or sales consultant for therapeutic equipment and durable goods.

School based settings include preschools, elementary schools, middle schools, high schools, vocational education schools, and specially focused schools such as those for children and adolescents with vision or hearing challenges. School systems are one of the largest employers of occupational therapy services. In a preschool setting, occupational therapy assistants might work on pre-K readiness skills, or conduct an outdoor exploration group for children with and without mobility challenges. At the elementary and middle school levels, they might offer a keyboarding group for children who have difficulty with cursive writing, or assist with a social skills group for children with behavioral management difficulties. At the high school level, they might run a prevocational skills group for adolescents with cognitive limitations. In these same settings, they might use their occupational therapy assistant education, in combination with additional education and credentials, to assume a role as a preschool teacher, an assistive technology specialist, or a school-to-work counselor.

Community settings include health and wellness programs, day care programs, camps for children, homeless shelters, emergency shelters, and community social service programs. Given the funding sources and the social service model influencing these work settings, occupational therapy assistants may use their occupational therapy knowledge and skills to fill positions other than that of an occupational therapy assistant. They might work as a counselor or a director at a camp for children with chronic health conditions, as an instructor at a community gym for children with developmental delays, or as a home health care advocate for pregnant and parenting teens. They also might consider a position as a youth activities coordinator for a risk prevention community program, a group home supervisor, an employment coach, or as a respite program coordinator for families of children with special needs.

Professional Teams

In these institutional, outpatient, school based, and community settings, occupational therapy assistants serve as a member of a team of professionals. In client-centered practice, the client is the core member of the team. Physical therapists, speech and language therapists, audiologists, nurses, physicians, educators, social workers, case managers, and community agency professionals also may serve as team members.

There are three main types of teams: multidisciplinary, interdisciplinary, and transdisciplinary. In **multidisciplinary teams**, the members inform one another of their evaluation results and their interventions. However, there is not an effort to work collaboratively with one another or to keep the client as the central member of the team. Occupational therapists and occupational therapy assistants who work at a number of schools as part of their school based practice may function as part of a multidisciplinary team because there is little time for all members of the team to meet on a regular basis to coordinate services. Discussions among members may occur over the phone or through leaving notes in a central file. In **interdisciplinary teams**, members from different disciplines collaborate with one another to share and interpret their findings and design integrated interventions. When providing services, each member incorporates goals from other disciplines. The client is the central member of interdisciplinary teams. Clinic based practices that have regularly scheduled meetings with the family members and where the occupational therapist or the occupational therapy assistant provide interventions jointly with other professionals adhere to interdisciplinary team concepts. In **transdisciplinary teams**, the members work together throughout the evaluation, intervention, and outcome processes. Early intervention programs tend to use transdisciplinary teams. Rather than all members of the team providing direct services, they integrate and share their knowledge with one another. Some provide direct services while others act as consultants to provide additional support and expertise. For example, when the primary concerns for the child are related to feeding and play skills, the occupational therapist may provide the direct intervention; the speech and language therapist may provide consultation to the occupational therapist regarding strategies for incorporating language into the play activities; the social worker may offer recommendations to address family interaction patterns; and the psychologist may propose methods for managing disruptive behaviors. In this manner, the child and the family can establish a more in depth and trusting relationship with one professional, instead of trying to prioritize and integrate the recommendations of numerous professionals (Dunn, 2000). This approach minimizes the number of professionals coming into the home or classroom to provide direct interventions.

APPLYING THE CODE OF ETHICS WHEN WORKING WITH CHILDREN AND ADOLESCENTS

Regardless of the practice setting, occupational therapy assistants are to abide by the AOTA Code of Ethics (AOTA, 2005c). The Code of Ethics is a set of principles regarding adherence to a high standard of professional behaviors. Consistent with the Code of Ethics, occupational therapy assistants are committed to supporting the ability of children and adolescents to participate in their daily life activities in all of their environments regardless of their health status (AOTA, 2005c). There are seven principles.

Abiding by the principle of beneficence, occupational therapy assistants are to demonstrate concern for the well-being of the clients. They are to respect the clients' cultural, religious, social, and economic contexts; to advocate for needed service; and to charge fees that are fair and reasonable. For example, when working on feeding and dressing programs, they are to abide by religious sanctioned codes for food and clothing. If they are responsible for billing, they are to consider the family's ability to pay and alternative funding sources.

Consistent with the principle of nonmaleficence, occupational therapy assistants are not to exploit or impose harm on the clients. They are to avoid interactions with the clients that compromise their professional judgment and objectivity. Consistent with the principle of nonmaleficence, they are not to use punishment techniques, such as spankings and public embarrassment to discipline children and adolescents.

Adhering to the principle of autonomy, privacy, and confidentiality, occupational therapy assistants are to collaborate with the clients throughout the occupational therapy process. They are to inform the clients of the benefits and risks of interventions, protect their confidentiality, and respect their right to refuse occupational therapy services. Abiding by this principle, they are to respect the right of the clients to select and prioritize intervention goals. They are not to discuss the clients in public places, or with people not directly involved with providing services to them.

In accordance with the principle of duty, occupational therapy assistants are to maintain high level of competency. If they work with children and adolescents who speak a language other than English, they are to learn that language for effective communication. They are to seek appropriate levels of supervision, remain current in their professional knowledge and skills, and participate in continuing education and professional development initiatives related to their area of practice. Becoming a member of the AOTA Developmental Disabilities or School Based Special Interest Section is one way to do this. In addition, occupational therapy assistants are to procure and maintain state and national credentials consistent with the services they offer. The National Board for the Certification of Occupational Therapy (NBCOT), AOTA, and state practice acts have established criterion for continuing competency.

Consistent with the principle of procedural justice, occupational therapy assistants are to be knowledgeable about and to comply with all local, state, national, institutional, and AOTA policies. They are to understand laws and legislation related to American with Disabilities Act (ADA), Individuals with Disabilities Education Act (IDEA), Section 504 of the Rehabilitation Act, and No Child Left Behind. They are to inform their employer of the AOTA Code of Ethics, and record and report their professional activities in a timely manner to their state licensure boards, National Board for the Certification of Occupational Therapy, and their practice setting.

Respecting the principle of veracity, occupational therapy assistants are to be truthful about their credentials, education, qualifications, and competencies, and the services they provide. They are to disclose any potential conflict of interest in their professional and contractual work. For example, they are to disclose if they have a second job as a distributor of rehabilitation equipment for children, if they are responsible for purchasing such equipment at the pediatric hospital where they work.

In accordance with the principle of fidelity, occupational therapy assistants are to treat their colleagues and other professionals with integrity. They are to deal with them fairly, and respect their confidentiality. Finally, they are to discourage, correct, and report any violations of the Code of Ethics. They are not to talk disparagingly about other professionals who are providing services to the children and adolescents, nor are they to cover up for professional wrongdoing by their coworkers (AOTA, 2005c).

SUMMARY

Occupational therapists and occupational therapy assistants perform complementary, distinct roles when providing occupational therapy services to children and adolescents. The occupational therapist is responsible for all aspects of the occupational therapy process. Occupational therapy assistants work under the supervision of and in partnership with the occupational therapist to provide services to children and adolescents. Several documents published by the AOTA and state regulatory agencies provide detailed explanations of the roles, responsibilities, and supervision requirements for occupational therapy assistants. (AOTA, 2003, 2004a, 2004b, 2004c, 2005a, 2005b). It is important for occupational therapy assistants to read these documents to gain a full understanding of their roles and responsibilities. As a member of the American Occupational Therapy Association (AOTA), occupational therapy assistants can access the AOTA documents at www.aota.org. They also can access the state licensure laws at the state occupational therapy association web site.

Occupational therapy assistants work with children and adolescents in various practice settings. Working with other professionals and the family as a member of a team, they may provide occupational therapy services in institutional, outpatient, school based, and community settings. They also may use their occupational therapy assistant knowledge and skills, along with other required educational and credentialing requirements, to work with children and adolescents in a role other than that of an occupational therapy assistant. Funds available through private sources, insurance, local taxes, grants, and state and federal allocations, may be used to pay for occupational therapy services. Federal policy mandates eligibility criteria for children and adolescents to receive governmental funds for occupational therapy services within the various practice settings. When providing occupational therapy services, occupational therapy assistants must abide by the principles outlined in the AOTA Code of Ethics.

REVIEWING KEY POINTS

1. Describe the role of the occupational therapist and the occupational therapy assistant during the evaluation process.
2. Describe the role of the occupational therapist and the occupational therapy assistant when providing occupational therapy intervention.
3. Explain the role of the occupational therapist and the occupational therapist in the supervisory process.
4. Explain the influence of regulations on the roles and supervisory process.
5. Explain the difference between working as an occupational therapy assistant and using occupational therapy assistant knowledge and skills to provide non–occupational therapy services. Explain the supervisory requirements for each of these situations.
6. Provide 10 examples of practice settings where occupational therapy assistants and occupational therapists provide services for children and adolescents.
7. Give an example of the role of the occupational therapy assistant in these practice settings.
8. Apply the AOTA Code of Ethics to working with children and adolescents.

APPLYING KEY CONCEPTS

1. Role-play interviewing for a position as an occupational therapy assistant at a school setting, a medical facility, or a community agency. Explain to the interviewer, who is not an occupational therapist, the knowledge and skills an occupational therapy assistant brings to the work setting, the roles and responsibilities an occupational therapy assistant can assume, and the supervision needed. Use information from Chapters 1 and 2 and personal experience to answer this question.

2. Role-play interviewing for a non–occupational therapy assistant position at a school setting, a medical facility, or a community agency. Explain to the interviewer, who is not an occupational therapist, the knowledge and skills occupational therapy assistants bring to the work setting that make them qualified for the position, the roles and responsibilities they can assume, and the supervision they need. Use information from Chapters 1 and 2 and your own experience to answer this question.

3. Interview a group of occupational therapy assistants who work with children and adolescents. List the settings where they work. Describe the services they provide, and the funding sources used to pay for these services. Discuss ethical dilemmas they confront when advocating for or providing occupational therapy services.

REFERENCES

American Occupational Therapy Association (2002). Occupational therapy practice framework: Domain and process. *American Journal of Occupational Therapy, 56,* 609–639.

American Occupational Therapy Association (2003b). Policy 5.3: Licensure. *Policy Manual* (2003 ed.). Bethesda, MD: Author.

American Occupational Therapy Association (2004a). Definition of occupational therapy practice for the AOTA Model Practice Act. (Available from the State Affairs Group, American Occupational Therapy Association, 4720 Montgomery Lane, P.O. Box 31220, Bethesda, MD 20824-1220.)

American Occupational Therapy Association (2004b). Guidelines for supervision, roles, and responsibilities during the delivery of occupational therapy services. *American Journal of Occupational Therapy, 58* (November/December).

American Occupational Therapy Association (2004c). Occupational therapy services in early intervention and school-based programs. *American Journal of Occupational Therapy, 58* (November/December).

American Occupational Therapy Association (2005a). Model state regulation for supervision, roles, and responsibilities during the delivery of occupational therapy services. (Available from the State Affairs Group, American Occupational Therapy Association, 4720 Montgomery Lane, P.O. Box 31220, Bethesda, MD 20824-1220.)

American Occupational Therapy Association (2005b). Standards of Practice for Occupational Therapy. *American Journal of Occupational Therapy, 59* (November/December), 663–665.

American Occupational Therapy Association (2005c). Occupational therapy code of ethics. *American Journal of Occupational Therapy, 59,* 639–642.

Dunn, W. (2000). *Best practice occupational therapy: In community service with children and families.* Thorofare, NJ: SLACK.

Law, M., Baum, C., & Dunn, W. (2005). *Measuring occupational performance supporting best practice in occupational therapy* (2nd ed.). Thorofare, NJ: SLACK.

Developmental Influences on the Occupations of Infants and Toddlers

Margaret J. Pendzick

Key Terms

Expressive language
Hand-to-mouth movements
Inferior pincer grasp
Object permanence
Pincer grasp
Receptive language

Reflex
Secondary circular reactions
Superior pincer grasp
Symbolic representation
Temperaments
Voluntary release

Objectives

- Identify occupations and roles of infants and children.
- Identify factors that influence occupational performance.
- Understand the developmental and interrelated nature of factors that influence occupational performance.
- Explain how these factors influence the occupations of infants and toddlers.

INTRODUCTION

The typical infant and toddler occupations are the result of multiple factors influencing development. During this period of time, development follows a general sequence but with each individual child, the developmental rate will differ. Let's explore the richness of these age groups by analyzing the developmental influences on the occupations of Abby and Adam, full-term, first-born twins.

ABIGAIL AND ADAM:
NEWBORN TO 6 MONTHS

Parents were excited to have twins. During the first month, Adam and Abigail engaged in basic occupations of ADLs and social participation. They ate by bottle feeding, cried when they were hungry or tired, and engaged in social participation, interacting with their caregivers by gazing at their faces. Over the next two months they grew rapidly.

By 3 months of age, their capacity to engage in ADL, play, and social participation occupations expanded. They were sleeping through the night, crying when hungry or wet, and showing pleasure by cooing and smiling at caregivers. During feeding, they placed their hands on the bottle and they finished a bottle quickly. When

lying supine in the crib or on the floor, they swiped at the overhead mobile (Figure 5.1■); when lying prone, they lifted their heads and looked around the room. When seated in an infant chair, they held a rattle and explored objects by mouthing.

By 6 months of age, their ability to engage in their daily life occupations expanded further. Although the same chronological age, their parents observed some differences in how Abigail and Adam accomplished their daily life tasks.

In the areas of ADL, Abigail began to finger feed teething biscuits and held the bottle during feedings. She preferred to sit in an infant seat or high chair to engage

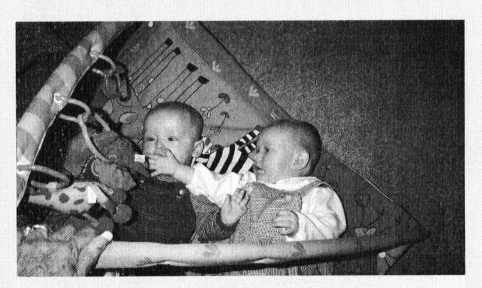

■ Figure 5.1
Abigail and Adam reach for overhead toys.

in play. Her favorite toys were noisy rattles that she would shake, bang, and transfer from one hand to another. Her parents gave her a wide variety of different types of rattles so if one dropped out of sight, she still had others available for play within her reach. When given a new toy, she would mouth and visually inspect it (Figure 5.2■). In social participation, Abigail smiled and cooed to familiar faces but would be quiet and scowl at unfamiliar people. For comfort, she preferred to be held firmly and expressed pleasure when hugged and cuddled.

In contrast, Adam accomplished the ADL of feeding by allowing the adult to hold the bottle. Although messier than Abigail, he also liked to finger feed with a teething biscuit. He preferred to engage in play while moving on the floor. He rolled from one place to another, stopping to explore by pulling on objects in the environment or mouthing a toy or object he found on the floor. Parents quickly learned that they needed to childproof the entire house! In social participation, Adam smiled and cooed at most people. He enjoyed being held and jiggled. For comfort, he preferred to be held and rocked.

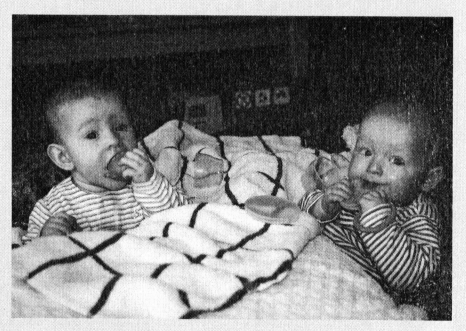

■ Figure 5.2
Abigail and Adam mouthing toys.

Recalling information from previous child development classes, earlier text chapters on occupation, and the Occupational Therapy Practice Framework, let's examine how the performance skills emerged that enabled Adam and Abigail to complete their tasks in different ways. Refer to Appendix B for an explanation of the reflexes that the infants integrated and Appendix A for a chart of developmental milestones they achieved to complete these tasks. Remember that even though both infants displayed different performance skills at the same age, each demonstrated skills that were age appropriate. A child's performance skills develop at different rates within the range of typical development.

To be able to perform the ADL occupation of eating, both infants integrated the primitive rooting **reflex**, coordinated the suck-swallow sequence, and developed muscular control to conform lips to the bottle nipple. By 6 months, both Abigail and Adam began self-feeding, which required developing the hand-to-mouth performance pattern. With practice this became a useful habit to perform more complex aspects of self-feeding. Abigail's ability to hold the bottle during feeding required motor strength and effort to grip the sides of the bottle and lift the bottle to her lips.

During the occupation of play, the children displayed a variety of performance skills which were influenced by the activity demands of objects used during play and the various contexts in which the play occurred. Abigail's play took place in a supported sitting position which allowed her to free her hands to manipulate objects. Similar to other 6 month old children, she integrated the grasp reflex and displayed consistent palmar grasp of the rattles, calibrating the amount of grip to shake and move the rattle in space (Alexander, Boehme, & Cupps, 1993). However, also typical for children 6 months of age, her equilibrium and righting reactions were not fully developed to allow her to sit independently without using hands for support (Bly, 1994).

Adam's play took place on the floor where he needed to work against the force of gravity to independently roll, push up to forearms and elbows, and free his arm and hand to reach in space. Because he had integrated the asymmetrical tonic neck reflex, tonic labyrinthine righting, and other primitive reflexes, he could assume symmetrical positions and coordinate his body parts to perform these complex movements (Cronin & Mandich, 2005). While moving on the floor, he also processed sensory information from his environment, such as texture of the carpet, hardness of the surface, and weight of objects that he encountered. He organized his space to navigate to different parts of the room and locate previously discovered objects. Since he was not in a supported sitting position while on the floor, he was unable to grasp and manipulate objects with the skills that his sister demonstrated and reverted to pulling at objects such as tablecloths. He needed to roll to his back when he wanted to stop to play with a small object. During the third to sixth month of development, typical children begin to develop symmetry in body postures and demonstrate a wide variety of movement patterns (Bly, 1994). At this age, asymmetry and stereotyped movement patterns are early warning signs of motor delays and possible neurological problems.

During these first six months, Abigail and Adam began to communicate with their caregivers. They engaged in conversation by making eye contact with the caretakers, developing a social smile, and making a variety of sounds that consisted of cooing and babbling. These early performance skills are important indicators of typical development. Children who are diagnosed with hearing impairment, communication disorder, or pervasive developmental disorder often lack these age appropriate communication skills.

Both Abigail and Adam displayed a variety of age appropriate client factors of global and specific mental functions. As highlighted in the vignettes, Abigail and Adam have two very different **temperaments** and personalities and interact with others in their unique fashion. Various psychological studies describe and name these personality types (Kail, 2002), but what is most important is to identify and accept that each infant interacts differently. Adults working with infants need to alter their adult behavior to engage with each infant as an individual. As described by Erickson, during this period of development, Abby and Adam developed basic trust versus mistrust through their interactions with their parents and caregivers (Kail). The adults met the children's basic needs and encouraged them to explore and interact with their environment.

Each infant displayed specific mental functions that are consistent with the sensorimotor stage of Piaget. Abigail engaged in **secondary circular reactions** when she accidentally shook the rattle, enjoyed the sounds, and repeated the movement pattern. When Adam pulled on the tablecloth and his dad's wallet fell to the floor, a parent quickly removed Adam from the area and distracted him with a new toy. Since

Adam had not yet developed **object permanence**, he was content with the replacement toy (Kail, 2002).

ABIGAIL AND ADAM: 6 TO 12 MONTHS

During the next six months, the children expanded and developed their areas of occupations. By 9 months of age, they devoted most of their day to play (see Figure 5.3■) and they took an active part in self-feeding. Individual differences were still noted between the two children, particularly in motor skills.

Abigail's means of locomotion was cruising around furniture, resorting to crawling when a supported surface was not available in the environment. Adam crept on all fours, occasionally pulling to stand in his crib or to explore items on the living room sofa. Both children responded to a caretaker's "no." However, because Adam often just paused and continued the activity, he required further intervention by the caretaker. Adam and Abigail enjoyed waving "bye-bye" and displayed voluntary release of objects during play. During feeding they held their bottles and tried to grab the spoon.

By 12 months, the children increased their involvement in ADL, play and social participation. Abigail was walking alone while Adam was cruising around furniture and taking steps with one hand held. In the area of ADL, both children were finger feeding, utilizing a pincer grasp, while sitting in a high chair. Communication skills were developing and both children were saying "dada," "mama," and responding with a gesture to simple requests such as "more juice?". Their favorite games were peek-a-boo and putting objects into containers. During a typical play time, Abigail walked around the room with a high guard position, finding objects on low tables and chairs, while Adam would seek out a toy, sit on the floor, and play by filling and dumping.

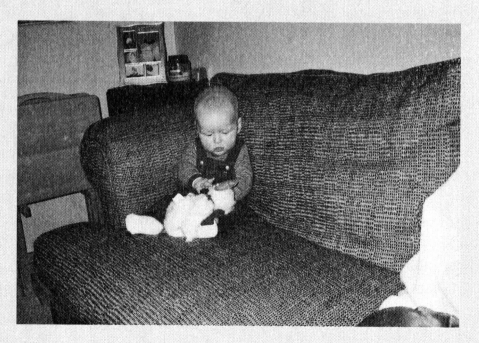

■ Figure 5.3
Abigail explores a toy.

During the prior six months, both children had demonstrated significant changes in motor skills. These new postural and mobility skills were the result of the development of righting, equilibrium, and protective reactions which allowed the children to develop balance and fluidity of movement for functional mobility and transitional movement patterns (Alexander, Boehme, & Cupps, 1993). While playing in prone, the children developed antigravity extension and flexion muscles which allowed them to stabilize and align the body during motor tasks. Their shoulder girdle muscles were strengthened during play in prone, pushing up off the surface, and mobile weight bearing over the joint. Stability in this proximal joint allowed the children to develop control of the arm, elbow, wrist, and hand (Bly, 1994). Weight bearing on the hands facilitated the development of palmar arches that are necessary for efficient grasp patterns (Alexander, Boehme, & Cupps).

Both Abigail and Adam enjoyed putting items into containers, which required both cognitive and motor development. In order to physically perform this task, the children had to automatically adjust the grasp and calibrate the grip while lifting the toy in space. **Voluntary release** of an object developed around the seventh month. By 9 months of age, the children were able to release an object into space without the support of the wrist (see Appendix C). These motor skills emerged due to the developed control of the shoulder, forearm, elbow, wrist, and hand (Alexander, Boehme, & Cupps, 1993), along with opportunities to manipulate objects and learn from sensorimotor experiences (Cronin & Mandich, 2005). Cognitive development also occurred and reflects the age appropriate sensorimotor stage described by Piaget. Adam engaged in goal directed behavior by purposefully placing the toy into a container, rather than randomly picking up and dropping the rattles. Piaget called this substage the coordination of secondary circular reactions (Feldman, 2004). During the sensorimotor stage, the children also began to develop object permanence, the ability to recognize that an object exists even though it is no longer seen. The children now dropped items into a lidded container and understood that the objects were still in the container, even though they were no longer visible (Feldman). Adam enjoyed filling the container, since he realized that the objects had not disappeared and he could always play the game again.

The children's ability to complete self-feeding skills was enhanced by the refinement of prehensile grasp patterns. Due to the development of the palmar arches and control of the thumb, Abigail and Adam were able to utilize a pincer grasp to pick up food pieces and complete finger feeding (Alexander, Boehme, & Cupps, 1993). Typically, pincer grasp develops in the following sequence:

- **Inferior pincer grasp:** Thumb against the volar surface of the index finger with first and second digits used as unit (Figure 5.4a■)

- **Pincer grasp:** Thumb in opposition to first digit with pad-to-pad contact (Figure 5.4b■)

- **Superior pincer grasp:** Thumb tip in opposition to first digit tip (Figure 5.4c■) (Cronin & Mandich, 2005).

Useful habits of **hand-to-mouth movements** and the ability to supinate the forearm (Cronin & Mandich, 2005) further assisted in the children's ability to self-feed. At this age, children usually are able to chew soft foods using a nonrotary movement (Cronin & Mandich). The advanced oral-motor skills are due to increased stability of the neck and head muscles that allow more refined tongue and jaw movements (Alexander, Boehme, & Cupps, 1993).

As Abigail and Adam advanced in cognitive skills and motor control, their ability to communicate also improved. The development of more precise tongue, lip, and

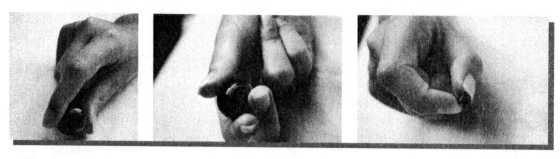

■ Figure 5.4
(a) Inferior pincer grasp; (b) pincer grasp; (c) superior pincer grasp.

jaw movements, and breath control allowed the children to produce a variety of sounds of varying length (Alexander, Boehme, & Cupps, 1993). Age appropriate cognitive skills allowed the children to begin to recall and label people and objects (Cronin & Mandich, 2005); they could use their first words of "ma-ma" and "da-da" appropriately. As with all developmental skills, each child progressed at an individual rate. Typically, children speak at least one word by 12 months of age (Feldman, 2004).

ABIGAIL AND ADAM: 12 TO 24 MONTHS

During the next year, Abigail and Adam continued to explore their environment and developed in the areas of ADL, play, and communication. Although all areas increased in skills, communication and social skill gains were most notable.

By 18 months, Abby and Adam were beginning to interact with one another during play. For instance, when Adam sat on the floor stacking graduated cups, Abigail intensely watched the play, and quickly picked up a discarded or unused cup and began to stack. As soon as Adam realized that he was losing his toy, he quickly and loudly verbalized "mine," gathered the cups, scooted a bit away, and began to restack. When Abigail loudly verbalized a protest, a parent resolved the situation by providing Abigail another suitable toy to stack (Allen & Marotz, 2006).

At 18 months, both children had about 8 to 10 words in their vocabulary and used words and pointing to communicate their wants and needs. Whenever they encountered a pencil or pen in their environment, they explored by putting it in the mouth and by spontaneously scribbling on any available surface. They began to assist in dressing by removing simple clothing items such as hats, mittens, and socks. They enjoyed feeding themselves using both their fingers and scooping with a spoon. They drank all liquids from a cup with occasional assistance, fascinated by a straw but unable to secure liquids through it.

At 24 months, Abigail and Adam displayed increased abilities in the area of communication, play, ADL, and social skills. During mealtime, they independently drank from a cup using a straw, proficiently used a spoon to eat their morning cereal, and a fork to stab the French toast. Since they were dry through the night, the parents began to introduce potty training. The children helped pull down their elastic waist pants and sat on a child-sized potty chair. Their vocabulary expanded and they used two to three words to express their thoughts; "car go," "more cookie," "baby drink bottle." They understood the prepositions "in" and "under" and were able to follow two-step directions.

Although both children enjoyed running, chasing, and throwing large balls in the yard, climbing on the outdoor play equipment, and being pulled in a wagon, each child preferred a different type of indoor play. Abigail liked to choose her favorite book off the shelf, climb up onto an adult lap, and command, "read book." While sitting on the adult's lap, she turned the pages of the book, pointed to pictures, and protested quite loudly if an adult attempted to shorten the story. Adam liked toys that he could pound and bang. He particularly liked to use a child hammer to force a small ball into an opening of a maze and watch it complete the path and reappear at the base of the toy. If his parents were working in the kitchen, he would play underfoot, opening drawers and cabinets, turning pots and lids into drums and cymbals as he sang his own tune. As he tired of this activity, he would line up the pots on the floor, locate a wooden spoon and pretend to cook his own dinner.

Although to the casual observer the children's new skills appeared overnight, careful consideration of the underlying aspects of development explains the emergence of all the new skills during this second year of life. The environment afforded opportunities for the children to practice skills until they no longer required conscious effort and became useful habits.

Even though Abigail's and Adam's most noticeable developed skills were in the areas of communication and social participation, it is necessary to consider how the acquisition of motor and cognitive skills enabled the children to acquire these receptive and expressive language skills. Although it is the primary responsibility of the speech and language pathologist to assess and plan intervention strategies for children with speech and language needs and delays, the occupational therapy assistant can influence these skills as the children are able to better explore their environment and engage in childhood occupation. Therefore, keep in mind that during typical development one skill can influence other skills and also areas of occupation. This is an important consideration when working as a pediatric occupational therapy assistant and selecting age appropriate activities to implement intervention strategies.

Abigail's and Adam's ability to communicate was due to their increased ability to both comprehend (**receptive language**) and speak (**expressive language**) words and sentences. Initially labeling nouns (cat, mama, doll) and then adding verbs (go, come, run), they now constructed simple sentences to express a want, need, or thought (Feldman, 2004). They could follow two-step commands and understand prepositions such as "in" and "on." They developed the understanding of these positional words as a result of interacting with the environment. Adam would climb into the kitchen cabinets to retrieve pots and pan, while Abigail would climb up on the sofa to sit in an adult's lap. Mastery in motor skills allowed the child to experience the sensation of directional movement, enhancing the ability to understand the concept.

Motor skills acquisition also impacted Abigail's and Adam's ability to perform age appropriate ADL. Their balance and coordination allowed them to keep the head and body erect while utilizing the oral muscles to chew and bite a larger variety of food textures. They successfully drank from a straw due to the ability to calibrate facial muscles to hold the straw tight enough to keep lip closure while coordinating the suck-swallow to draw the liquid up the straw. Due to improved jaw stability, they no longer used their teeth to stabilize an object, thereby no longer needing to bite on the straw to hold onto it while drinking (Alexander, Boehme, & Cupps, 1993). The children accomplished successful self-feeding by grasping and manipulating the spoon and fork. During toileting, they manipulated their thumbs and calibrated the grasp of the elastic waist band to successfully pull down and up their pants.

All areas of occupation were influenced by the children's cognitive abilities. When compared with Piaget's age appropriate sensorimotor stage, both Abigail and Adam displayed behaviors that suggested that they were developing the concepts of object permanence and **symbolic representation** (Kail, 2002). By purposefully looking for her favorite storybook on the bookshelf, Abigail demonstrated her knowledge of object permanence. Adam's pretend play with the kitchen pots and pans indicated that he understood the concept of symbolic representation. Both children also demonstrated their ability to use tools as functional objects, using utensils in place of fingers and toy hammers in place of the open palm to propel objects.

SUMMARY

In the short span of two years, Abigail and Adam significantly expanded the repertoire of occupations that they could accomplish as well as the performance skills and performance patterns necessary to engage in those occupations. As newborns, primitive reflexes and the effects of gravity influenced their movement patterns, and crying and smiles were their means of communication. They were dependent upon caregivers for nourishment and daily needs. By the time they were 2 years old, however, the children were able to perform complex motor tasks, feed themselves, and communicate their wants and needs to an adult with words. This change in the ability to participate in and perform their daily occupations came about because of the development, interdependence, and interrelations of the children's cognition, language, personal-social, and physical capacities, and the family and environmental supports they received. Abigail and Adam were able to expand their occupations and performance skills as they interacted with their caregivers and objects in their environment.

Though Abigail and Adam each developed differently, they followed a general pattern that can be seen in other children as they develop. Variances in these patterns of development occur because of differences in the innate capacities and health status of the children, family supports and influences, and environmental expectations and barriers.

Even though an occupational therapy assistant usually works with children who are older than Abigail and Adam and are no longer considered to be infants or preschoolers, it is important to understand early development of occupations and developmental skills. Often, older children with special needs lack the underlying foundation skills that allow further expansion of occupations. Understanding typical development principles enhances critical thinking skills needed to successfully design developmentally appropriate intervention strategies to achieve goals that are unique to the child.

REVIEWING KEY POINTS

1. Explain the influence of weight bearing on the development of upper extremity motor control.
2. Review Piaget's sensorimotor stage and define the following terms: object permanence, secondary circular reactions, and symbolic representation.
3. Give three examples of the interdependence and interrelations of cognition, language, personal-social, and physical capacities during typical development.
4. Describe the pincer grasp sequence of development. How would a delay in this grasp pattern effect processing, motor, and social interaction skills?
5. Describe receptive and expressive language of an infant and toddler. How do these skills impact development?

APPLYING KEY CONCEPTS

1. Using the Occupational Therapy Practice Framework as a guide, observe an infant or toddler. Identify the areas of occupation and performance skills that infant or toddler displays. Compare and contrast the observation with typical developmental milestones.
2. Visit a local store and choose a toy for either an infant or toddler. Determine what performance skills and body functions an infant or toddler would need to play with this toy.
3. Interview a parent of an infant or toddler who represents a different cultural background than you. Ask open-ended questions about how the parent interacts and plays with the child. Are these responses different from what you expect? Reflect on how culture and context influence parent–child interaction.

REFERENCES

Alexander, A., Boehme, R., & Cupps, B. (1993). *Normal development of functional motor skills*. Tucson, AZ: Therapy Skill Builders.

Allen, E., & Marotz, L. (2006). *Developmental profiles: Pre-birth through twelve* (5th ed.). Clifton Park, NY: Thomson Delmar Learning.

Bly, L. (1994). *Motor skills acquisition in the first year*. Tucson, AZ: Therapy Skill Builders.

Cronin, A., & Mandich, M. (2005). *Human development and performance throughout the lifespan*. Clifton Park, NY: Thomson Delmar Learning.

Feldman, R. (2004). *Child development* (3rd ed.). Upper Saddle River, NJ: Prentice Hall.

Kail, K. (2002). *Children*. Upper Saddle River: NJ: Prentice Hall.

Chapter 6

Developmental Influences on the Occupations of Young Children

Margaret J. Pendzick

Key Terms

Associative play
Chase games
Classification
Cooperative play
Cylindrical grip
Directed play
Dynamic balance
Egocentrism
Emergent literacy
Feedback
Feedforward
Finger-to-palm translation
Flow
Grammar
Hook grasp
In-hand manipulation

Initiative-versus-guilt stage
Lateral prehension
Lateral tripod grasp
Palm-to-finger translation
Power grasp
Pragmatics
Precision grasp
Preoperational stage
Shift
Simple rotation
Solitary play
Spontaneous play
Static balance
Syntax
Tripod grasp

Objectives

- Identify occupations and roles of young children.
- Identify factors that influence occupational performance.
- Understand the developmental and interrelated nature of factors that influence occupational performance.
- Explain how these factors influence the occupations of young children.

INTRODUCTION

During the preschool years, children rapidly gain new skills and engage in ever widening areas of occupation. As with all ages of development, the rate of development is unique to each child and greatly influenced by the opportunities and challenges of the contexts and social environments in which the child lives. These interrelated factors are illustrated when we reflect on Sweta's development through her preschool years.

SWETA: 3 YEARS OLD

Sweta is the oldest of two children, living with her mother and father. Her grandparents live in a nearby small town and she often talks with them on the telephone. Although she can carry on quite a conversation in person, Sweta usually just answers her grandparent's questions with one word and often nods her head and points to things when talking on the phone. Even though her parents will remind her that grandma can't see where she is pointing, she doesn't change her gestures while speaking.

Since her mother works full time outside the home, Sweta and her 2-year-old sister attend a daycare during weekdays. When given enough time in the morning, Sweta likes to dress herself, putting on a pullover shirt, elastic waist pants, socks, and shoes, even though she often puts the shoes on the wrong feet. Her mom puts her clothes out the night before so that Sweta can dress properly for the weather conditions. Although she likes to brush her own teeth and hair, she needs assistance, since she is not thorough enough. She is toilet trained during the day and night.

At daycare, Sweta sits with the rest of her class for a story, takes her turn dressing the weather bear, and sings songs with the class. Her favorite activities are painting at the easel, dressing up in costumes (Figure 6.1■), and playing in the housekeeping center. She likes

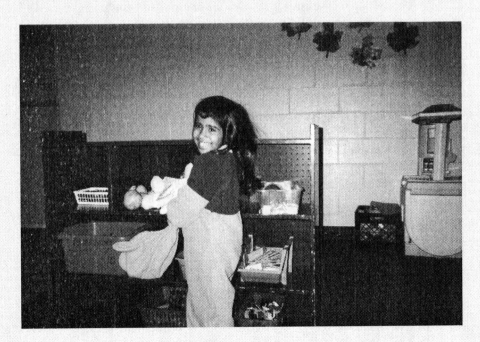

■ **Figure 6.1**
Sweta dons a costume while at daycare.

to pretend to cook at the stove and uses play dough for pretend food. She enjoys playing on the inside jungle gym—climbing up the child size ladder, sliding down the small slide, and swinging in the tire. Whenever the group is outside, she runs to get on a Big Wheel and pedal around the playground. When asked by a teacher, she allows another child to have a turn but usually waits on the side so that she can ride again.

At home, Sweta and her younger sister like to follow their mom while she is preparing dinner in the kitchen. Sweta helps by carrying dishes and silverware to the table and by setting the table with assistance from her dad. During her bedtime story, Sweta likes to sit on her parent's lap and help read a familiar story or guess the ending of a new one. She likes to be tucked in at night and sleeps with her favorite stuffed animal.

Typical of a 3-year-old, Sweta demonstrated characteristics of the **preoperational stage** in Piaget's theory of cognitive development. At this stage, preschoolers display **egocentrism**, which means preschoolers primarily see things through their own perspective. When Sweta nodded her head or pointed while talking on the phone, she didn't realize that her grandparent could not see her gesture or nod (Kail, 2002). Children at this age cannot fully conceptualize what another person is feeling or thinking, so they may not realize that their behaviors may not be acceptable to someone else. They have difficulty sharing a toy, since they are only beginning to take into consideration that another child may want to play, or they may only want to complete a task one particular way. The preschool teacher encouraged Sweta to share the Big Wheel tricycle by gently reminding her that another child wanted a turn. It is important when working with preschool children to realize that they only partially see another person's viewpoint, and to help them make the necessary social adjustments without viewing this as negative behavior.

As a 3-year-old, Sweta's ability to perform ADL skills increased as her motor and processing skills developed. Given enough time, she dressed herself, which required her to sequence dressing steps rather than just to don an individual clothing item, as she did as a toddler. She had begun to learn to organize her space when she helped to set the dinner table. With verbal assistance and reminders, she gathered the necessary dishes and cutlery and brought them to the table. When she duplicated the table setting pattern at each place, Sweta demonstrated developing premath concepts of matching and one-to-one correspondence (Feldman, 2004). She was establishing useful habits and routines when she repeated this and other daily chores and tasks. Typically children develop and expand their performance skills while completing simple, routine tasks. This is an important concept to remember when working with children who are developmentally challenged. Intervention strategies will be more effective if performance skills are addressed within the natural context.

As Sweta completes more tasks independently, she is developing a positive self-image (Feldman, 2004). Erickson called this the **initiative-versus-guilt stage**, where the child between the ages of 3 to 6 years begins to perform more tasks independently and has to deal with the outcomes of independent actions. When Sweta independently performed tasks that were pleasing to her parents, they rewarded her with praise and smiles, which boosted her self-esteem and self-concept. Sweta's parents encouraged her to act independently and gave guidance and correction when her choices were not acceptable (Feldman).

Sweta's ability to perform complex motor skills is the result of her development in the areas of **balance** and **flow** (Cronin & Mandich, 2005). As her basic automatic reactions of righting, equilibrium, and protection matured, she was able to complete motor tasks which required higher developed balance (Cronin & Mandich). Balance is either **static** or **dynamic**. Sweta utilized both forms of balance when she played on the indoor climbing bars. She used static balance to maintain an upright position while she reached for a bar that was out of her immediate reach. Although she kept both feet planted on the climbing structure, she needed to shift her weight off center and stretch to reach the next bar. When she pulled herself up to the next bar, she used dynamic balance, shifting her weight from one foot to the other while maintaining balance on the bar.

Flow describes smooth, controlled movement (AOTA, 2002). Sweta exhibited flow as she climbed on the bars. Although she constantly adjusted her balance to climb to the top of the bars, she demonstrated fluid rather than isolated, random movement. Given the opportunities that Sweta had in her daycare environment, she was able to perfect her motor skills throughout the day.

As Sweta played on the jungle gym, she maneuvered around objects in space and gained experiences and understanding of spatial concepts such as in, on, under, and over. She also completed simple puzzles, which gave her another early experience with spatial concepts and simple shapes. Although these spatial and geometric words will not be in her vocabulary until she is approximately 4 years old (Allen & Marotz, 2007), her experiences contributed to her future vocabulary and perceptual-motor development. Cognition and language are closely linked and interdependent on each other for child development (Kail, 2002). As a child uses language to express cognition, cognition advances and stimulates further language development. Sweta has grown up in a stimulating environment which has encouraged all areas of development.

SWETA: 4 YEARS OLD

As a 4-year-old, Sweta has increased her independence in areas of ADL. In the morning, she chooses clothes appropriate for the weather and dresses herself, needing assistance only for shoe tying. When she chooses cereal for breakfast, she can pour herself milk and juice out of small containers. She is able to use a spoon or fork to feed herself. She can spread butter over her toast and put the dirty dishes in the sink. She still needs supervision to brush her teeth and comb her hair but independently can wash and dry her face and hands.

At the daycare, she still enjoys art activities, painting pictures on the easel, coloring at the table, and

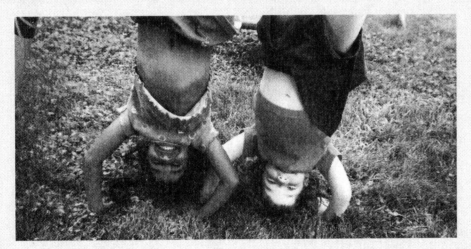

■ Figure 6.2
Sweta and her sister master standing on their heads!

assembling simple craft projects. She joins her friends in the housekeeping area and quickly assumes a make believe role within the group. If she is upset or frustrated, she usually can express displeasure with words rather than by crying or hitting other children. When outside, she enjoys riding the tricycles but also joins into group activities such as tag or climbing together on the jungle gym. Sweta and her sister like to perform tumbling tricks on the grassy areas (Figure 6.2■).

At home, Sweta plays with her younger sister and performs simple chores such as putting away her clothes, straightening up her room, and putting toys away at bedtime. Sweta and her sister like to help their mom cook in the kitchen and Sweta helps to wash vegetables or pour premeasured ingredients into the mixing bowl. She likes to wash dishes, but is easily distracted and turns the activity into water play.

As a 4-year-old, Sweta clearly displayed changes in her psycho-social skills. Her play activities frequently involved small groups of children rather than consistently engaging in solitary play. As Sweta and her friends played in the housekeeping corner, they spontaneously shared toys, even though the children assumed their own interests. On the outdoor jungle gym, the children simultaneously climbed the structure, verbally interacting with each other but not playing in an organized way. These are example of **associative play** which is developmentally appropriate for this age (Frost, Wortham and Reifel, 2005).

When outside with her friends, Sweta engaged in a **chase game** of tag. Chase games are a particular category of play that involves specific motor control and some strategy (Frost, Wortham and Reifel, 2005). As 4-year-olds, the game involved communication skills of exchanging information of who was playing and who was It. Running, stopping, and turning challenged both dynamic and static balance. The children determined their game strategies by frequently adapting their position to run away from the person who was It. Chase games become more complex and eventually develop into competitive sports such as soccer and football (Frost, Wortham and Reifel).

During art activities, Sweta demonstrated various aspects of motor performance. Her choice of painting at the easel allowed Sweta to develop basic strokes while keeping her wrist in a neutral or slightly extended position. Keeping her wrist in alignment is a useful habit that will enhance Sweta's ability to control the crayon. Since painting was an enjoyable activity, Sweta participated for an extended period of time. As Sweta prolonged the easel activity, she naturally strengthened her upper extremities as she worked against gravity (Myers, 1992). Although she switched hands often during activities, Sweta demonstrated a right-handed preference when using art supplies. She held the paint brush with a **lateral tripod grasp** pattern (Amundson, 1992). Although this grasp pattern is immature, it allows Sweta to hold either the paintbrush or crayon and make strokes on the paper. Within typical development, immature grasp patterns are refined as visual perceptual skills develop. Visual perceptual and hand skill development will be discussed further following the 5-year-old vignette.

When playing with her friends, Sweta displayed the typical difficulty that preschoolers have with Piaget's concept of conservation—the ability to understand that the amount remains unchanged if nothing is removed, even if materials are rearranged (McDevitt & Ormrod, 2004). When playing in the housekeeping corner, the children needed to share materials. Since conservation is not yet developed at this age, the children are not able to just visually inspect and decide that materials were divided equally. Since the divided materials may be arranged to occupy more or less space, a child may feel cheated and children may begin to fight over materials. It may be necessary for an adult to intervene and physically show the children how the portions are equal. This intervention not only avoids conflict but also helps the preschooler begin to master the understanding of conservation.

By organizing her toys and belongings, Sweta demonstrates Piaget's preoperational cognitive skill of **classification** (McDevitt & Ormrod, 2004). She is able to sort like things together. The Legos® will end up in one storage bin and her crayons in another, unlike a year earlier when toys were simply thrown into a toy box. She still has trouble sorting a pile by two attributes such as red, wheeled Legos and red, tall Legos. When giving verbal directions, it is important to consider the child's classification skills. Noncompliance may be due to lack of understanding, which is age appropriate for the circumstances.

When conflicts arise, Sweta has enough vocabulary to voice her displeasure or ask an adult for assistance. A typical 4-year-old's vocabulary consists of over 1,000 words; almost all of the speech is understandable. Since 4-year-olds can understand questions that ask who and why and relate to events in the past tense (Allen & Marotz, 2007), Sweta has the capability to tell an adult what happened and not revert to outbursts of crying or hitting. When children have a speech or language delay and are unable to communicate likes and dislikes to others, the children have difficulty playing and interacting, thereby developing typical social interaction skills.

SWETA: 5 YEARS OLD

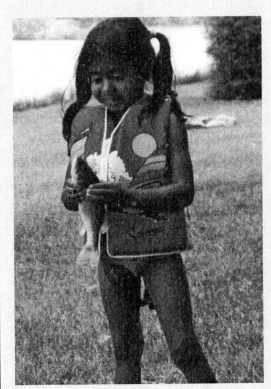

At 5 years of age, Sweta is a friendly and outgoing child. At the daycare, she eagerly joins group activities and can identify a specific best friend, even if this changes daily! At home, she engages her sister in play activities and willingly helps her mom in the kitchen or her dad with household chores. At the dinner table, Sweta likes to tell her family jokes and her day adventures.

Sweta likes to engage in preschool tasks such as cutting, pasting, and coloring. She often makes her own story books, drawing pictures on pages and writing some random letters. She is very proud that she can print her first name on paper and likes to make up stories when reading the comics with her dad.

Sweta and her sister often participate in different preschool recreational groups. Although she originally went to dance classes with her sister, Sweta prefers to participate in T-ball and soccer. She knows and follows the rules of the games but often gets distracted during structured practice. She likes to visit friends who live by a lake and is starting to learn to swim and fish (Figure 6.3■).

■ **Figure 6.3**
Sweta catches her first fish.

As a 5-year old, Sweta was able to participate in preschool arts and crafts activities due to increased motor and perceptual skills. Throughout Sweta's preschool years, she has developed the motor control and cognitive understanding to use her hands to manipulate objects and tools in her environment. Due to advances in cognition, she was able to follow multistep directions and attend to tasks to complete an age appropriate craft activity that required cutting, pasting, and coloring. Her hand skills included **power grasp**, **precision grasp** (Cronin & Mandich, 2005), and **in-hand manipulation** (Exner, 1992) skills along with controlled use of scissors, crayons and glue bottle. Table 6.1■ describes the combination of power grasp, precision grasp, and in-hand manipulation skills Sweta used to complete her various play and education occupations.

Sweta gathered her art supplies off the shelf and carried them to the small table. She used a variety of power grasps to achieve the task—a **hook grasp** to carry the buckets of crayons and craft accessories, a **cylindrical grip** to carry a glue stick, and **lateral prehension** to carry construction paper, tissue paper, and magazines (Cronin & Mandich, 2005). In-hand manipulation was observed when Sweta used the pads of thumb and fingers to separate two magazine pages (**shift**), moved the pompoms from fingers to palm of hand and back to fingers while gluing (**finger-to-palm translation and palm-to-finger translation**), and rolled tissue paper between pads of thumb and fingers to make raised dots (**simple rotation**) (Exner, 1992). Precision grasp patterns were used in a variety of different ways. **Tripod grasp** was used when Sweta used the crayons to draw on the paper. Lateral prehension was completed with the fingertips when Sweta grasped single sheets of paper. Pincer grasp patterns varied with object sizes—the smaller the object, the more precision grasp pattern was utilized. When Sweta used the scissors, she correctly donned the scissors, using her nondominant hand to hold the paper. Since she has not yet refined her bilateral hand skills, Sweta used shoulder, elbow, and forearm movement to direct the scissors rather than using the nondominant hand to adjust the paper. By calibrating the force and size of the scissor blades opening, Sweta successfully cut out items from the magazine.

When finished with the project, Sweta grasped the marker with a tripod grip and printed her name on the paper. As a 5-year-old, she has expanded her earlier scribbling, isolated strokes, and basic shapes to produce the letters of her first name. Since Sweta had an interest in printing her name, her parents and daycare providers have helped her to form the upper case letters. At this age, Sweta does not adhere to left-right orientation or letter-line positioning, so she randomly places her letters on the paper. Spatial orientation is not an area of concern for preschool printing, and for that reason preschoolers often use unlined paper.

Although it is often perceived as random play, when Sweta drew pictures and made her books, she was demonstrating **emergent literacy** (McDevitt & Ormrod, 2004). The understanding that written words are meaningful is the groundwork for future reading and writing skills (McDevitt & Ormrod). Even though Sweta is not yet reading, she can differentiate between storybooks, newspapers, and grocery lists, understanding that each has a different purpose. She understands that when printing the letters of her name, all the letters go together and have meaning. Even if she writes random letters on the papers of her homemade books, she is demonstrating that she realizes that pictures and letters can represent thoughts. Emergent literacy skills are important foundation skills and should be encouraged by everyone who works with preschool children.

Sweta simultaneously participated in a variety of different types of play. The art projects included **spontaneous** or **directed play**, depending upon the specific direc-

■ **Table 6.1**
Hand Skills

Type of Hand Skill	Description of Hand Skill
Power Grasp	**Gripping an object with full hand—provides maximum strength**
Cylindrical grasp	Wrapping fingers, thumb, and palm of hand around a tube-shaped object
Hook grasp	Inserting flexed fingers into the opening of a handle; thumb remains abducted
Plate or lateral prehension	Gripping a flat object between the thumb and fingers
Spherical grasp	Wrapping fingers, thumb, and palm of hand around a three-dimensional, round object
Precision Grasp	**Gripping an object with fingers while the wrist is extended—provides maximum control**
Chuck or tripod grip	Grasping an object with the pads of the thumb, middle, and index fingers
Pincer grasp	Grasping a small object with the tip of the thumb and index finger
Lateral or key prehension	Holding an object with the thumb and lateral side of the index finger
In-Hand Manipulation	**Adjusting the position of an object within one hand**
Finger-to-palm translation	Moving small object from fingers to palm of hand
Palm-to-finger translation	Moving small object from palm of hand to fingertips
Shift	Repositioning small object with pads of fingers
Simple rotation	Turning object held with finger pads 90 degrees or less
Complex rotation	Turning object held with finger pads 180–360 degrees

Adapted from Cronin, A., & Mandich, M. (2005). *Human development and performance throughout the lifespan*. Clifton Park, NY: Thomson Delmar Learning, and Exner, C. (1992). In-hand manipulation skills. In J. Case-Smith & C. Pehoski (Eds.), *Development of hand skills in the child* (pp. 35–45). Rockville, MD: American Occupational Therapy Association.

tions given to the children. If Sweta completed the art project alone at the table, she was engaged in **solitary play**. If other children were present sharing supplies, the project turned into associative play. And if all the children worked together to make one collage, they were beginning to engage in **cooperative play**. Through her experience in chase play, Sweta has learned to follow rules and is able to participate in T-ball and soccer, which are directive, physical play. Current research indicates that children engage in a wide variety of different types of social and physical play, with rules and activities increasing in complexity as the child grows and matures (Frost, Wortham & Reifel, 2005).

When playing recreational T-ball and soccer, Sweta demonstrates her increased abilities in gross motor skills. She balances on one foot, which enables her to kick the soccer ball. She also can catch a thrown ball, although her position in the outfield usually requires her to catch it rolling. Besides her increased abilities in dynamic balance and flow, Sweta also uses **feedback** and **feedforward** to accomplish these new skills (Shumway-Cook & Woollacott, 2006). Feedback is the sensory information that Sweta receives when she kicks or catches the ball. Feedback is both internal (information from joints, muscles, and tendons) and external (information on how well she completed the task). Feedforward is a mechanism that builds on previous feedback and helps Sweta anticipate the movement. When she sees the soccer ball propel forward, she knows to position her body so that her strong right kicking leg will be ready to kick.

When the ground ball rolls toward her, she bends at the waist and gets her hands ready to catch the ball (Shumway-Cook & Woollacott). Cognition and attention to task also play an important part in Sweta's sports games. Sweta must remember the rules in order to successfully play this organized sport and pay attention to the game that is happening around her. How preschoolers play organized games differs substantively from how older children play such games. The preschoolers are just beginning to build a repertoire of motor and attention skills. These are, however, the foundation skills that are later used to accomplish more complicated motorical tasks.

As a preschooler, Sweta increased her vocabulary to over 1,500 words (Allen & Marotz, 2007). She used complex sentences to relate events to her family and friends. Her understanding of **syntax** (combining words and phrases to make sentences) and **grammar** allowed Sweta to use the past tense of irregular verbs and produce sentences of over seven words (Allen & Marotz). Sweta also demonstrated her knowledge of **pragmatics** when carrying on a conversation by taking turns, staying on topic, and knowing she should use polite words of "please" and "thank you" when talking with adults. When a child has difficulty with syntax, grammar, or pragmatics of language, it can be an early indicator of developmental problems and the child should be referred to a speech and language pathologist for developmental testing.

Sweta was independent in the majority of her personal care ADLs. Except for hair washing, she completed her grooming, bathing, and toileting. Because of the complexity of the skill, shoe tying was the last dressing skill she learned. The shoe tying task required understanding of multistep spatial directions while performing a bilateral task involving both prehensile grip and strength. At 5 years old, Sweta was able to attend to the task for extended periods and emotionally handle the frustrations of not always being successful. Persisting at a task until completion contributed to Sweta's positive self-image and taught her a useful strategy for future learning encounters.

SUMMARY

By the age of 5, Sweta engaged in a variety of complex occupations. She carried on a conversation relating past events, participated in group recreational activities, and completed simple household chores. She no longer needed assistance in dressing, bathing, and toileting, and began to demonstrate early literacy skills. She used crayons, scissors, and glue to produce original artwork. The ability to participate in these various occupations expanded as she developed more complex language, motor, and cognitive skills. Likewise, her engagement in such activities facilitated the development of her linguistic, motor, cognitive, and social interaction capacities. As she anticipated beginning kindergarten, she exhibited self-confidence and a positive self-image—all important personal-social skills.

An occupational therapy assistant must understand the complex development that occurs within the preschool years. This information will help develop appropriate intervention strategies with this age group. Developmental problems are identified often during the preschool years, and occupational therapy intervention frequently is indicated. Knowing and understanding the complexity of typical development will enhance the ability to work with children of all ages.

REVIEWING KEY POINTS

1. Explain the difference among flow, static balance, and dynamic balance.
2. List and define the different types of grasp and in-hand manipulation skills observed in preschoolers.
3. Give an example of the following types of preschool play: solitary, associative, cooperative, directed, and spontaneous.
4. Describe Piaget's concept of conservation and explain why it is important for a child to understand the concept. Describe an activity that would foster the understanding of conservation.

APPLYING KEY CONCEPTS

1. Choose a group of preschoolers (3-, 4-, and 5-year-olds). Spend at least 30 minutes observing the children. Try not to interact with the children, and attempt to observe free play. What type of play occurred? Were all children engaged in the same type of play? Did any child switch his/her type of play during the observation? If an adult was present, how did that help or hinder play? How did the observations differ from what is described in the text?
2. Observe a 3-, 4-, or 5-year-old child during play. Look for instances of egocentrism, conservation, and classification. How do these concepts help or hinder the child's play and social interactions?

   Further investigate Piaget's cognitive skills by attempting to duplicate some of his original observation. Refer to your child development text or one listed in the reference section of this chapter to read about Piaget's tasks. Consult with the course instructor if unsure how to structure the tasks. Observe how the child problem solves each task. Is this consistent with Piaget's theories?
3. Observe a 3-, 4-, or 5-year-old level of language skills. Does the child use plurals or prepositions correctly? Can the child ask a question or make a negative statement? Is the child able to carry on a conversation with another person? Are the observations consistent with information on typical language development?
4. Interview a parent or caretaker and observe a 3-, 4-, or 5-year-old child. Find out whether the child enjoys being read stories and how often that takes place during the week. Does the child turn pages, comment on pictures, or attempt to "tell the story"? Does the child often take a picture book and "read to himself"? Does the child recognize any letters, like to label pictures, or make books? What does this reveal about the child's emergent literacy?

REFERENCES

Allen, E., & Marotz, L. (2007). *Developmental profiles: Pre-birth through twelve* (5th ed.). Clifton Park, NY: Thomson Delmar Learning.

American Occupational Therapy Association (2002). Occupational therapy practice framework: Domain and process. *American Journal of Occupational Therapy, 56*(6), 609–639.

Amundson, S. (1992). Handwriting: Evaluation and intervention in school setting. In J. Case-Smith & C. Pehoski (Eds.), *Development of hand skills in the child* (pp. 63–78). Rockville, MD: American Occupational Therapy Association.

Case-Smith, J., & Pehoski, C. (Eds.). (1992). *Development of hand skills in the child.* Rockville, MD: American Occupational Therapy Association.

Cronin, A., & Mandich, M. (2005). *Human development and performance throughout the lifespan.* Clifton Park, NY: Thomson Delmar Learning.

Exner, C. (1992). In-hand manipulation skills. In J. Case-Smith & C. Pehoski (Eds.), *Development of hand skills in the child* (pp. 35–45). Rockville, MD: American Occupational Therapy Association.

Feldman, R. (2004). *Child development* (3rd ed.). Upper Saddle River, NJ: Pearson Prentice Hall.

Frost, J., Wortham, S., & Reifel, S. (2005). *Play and child development* (2nd ed.). Upper Saddle River, NJ: Pearson Prentice Hall.

Kail, K. (2002). *Children*. Upper Saddle River, NJ: Pearson Prentice Hall.

McDevitt, T., & Ormrod, J. (2004). *Child development: Educating and working with children and adolescents* (2nd ed.). Upper Saddle River, NJ: Pearson Prentice Hall.

Myers, C. (1992). Therapeutic fine-motor activities for preschoolers. In J. Case-Smith & C. Pehoski (Eds.), *Development of hand skills in the child* (pp. 47–59). Rockville, MD: American Occupational Therapy Association.

Shumway-Cook, A. & Woollacott, M. (2006). *Motor control: Translating research into clinical practice.* (3rd ed.). Philadelphia, PA: Lippincott, Williams & Wilkins.

Chapter 7

Developmental Influences on the Occupations of School Age Children

Janet V. DeLany

Key Terms

Body schema
Classification
Cognitive maps
Coincidence-anticipation timing
Concrete operations
Conservation
Decentering
Gender cleavage
Home-schooling
Industry versus inferiority
Middle childhood

Motion hypothesis
Prosocial behaviors
Rapport-talk
Relational aggression
Report-talk
Reversibility
Social referencing
Spatial awareness
Temporal organization
Transformation

Objectives

- Identify occupations and roles of school age children.
- Identify factors that influence occupational performance.
- Understand the developmental and interrelated nature of factors that influence occupational performance.
- Explain how these factors influence the occupations of school age children.

INTRODUCTION

Children between the ages of 6 and 12 are in their **middle childhood** years of development. During this period, most enter and progress through a formal public or private school system, while a few remain home to receive their education as part of the **home-school** initiative. Though interspersed with periods of rapid change, the children's physical, cognitive, and social-emotional growth occurs gradually in their middle childhood years, allowing for mastery and integration of skills. As a result, they refine their ability to complete familiar occupations and receive opportunities to gradually participate in new ones. The environments in which they live and grow affect their exposure to and readiness to participate in these occupations. To illustrate middle childhood development, let us follow Jorge as he completes his elementary and middle school year occupations with particular interest in his development at ages 7, 10 and 12.

JORGE: 7 YEARS OLD

Jorge resides with his mother, grandparents, his 12-year-old brother, and his 3-year-old sister in a single family house in a small, rural town. His father is in the military and is stationed overseas. His grandparents communicate in Spanish, and his parents speak fluent English and Spanish. Jorge and his siblings' primary language is English, though they use Spanish when talking with their grandparents and older relatives.

Jorge dresses independently, needs monitoring for grooming tasks, and can prepare himself a simple snack or sandwich when he is hungry. Jorge is in second grade and rides the school bus to the public school. Since his mother works as a dietitian at the local hospital, Jorge leaves for the school bus as his mother leaves for work. His grandmother cares for him and his siblings after school. On Saturdays, Jorge participates in community sports programs—soccer in the fall and baseball in the spring. In the winter, he goes sledding and ice skating with his brother and friends.

Jorge likes to go to school but has some difficulty mastering the second grade routines. His teacher, Ms. Boggs, has a set procedure for the children to start their school day. Every morning Jorge must put his coat and lunch box in his cubby, place his completed homework assignments in the correct bin, and put his journal and pencil on his desk before the second bell rings. He also needs to check the bulletin board to see if he has a special chore such as leading the line, carrying the flag, or taking the lunch tickets to the office. Jorge takes his responsibilities very seriously, trying to earn a Good Citizen star for accomplishing his morning tasks on time.

Jorge's best friends are Ben and Marcus. Since they live on the same street, they walk to and from the bus stop together. Although they are in different second grade classrooms, they play at recess and eat lunch together. Sometimes Jorge's mother lets him go to one of their houses after school. When the family gets home, everyone has a job to do. His grandmother makes dinner while his mother checks the children's backpacks and sorts through the mail. Jorge and his brother set the table. After dinner, Jorge helps to clear the table. He then does his homework, watches TV, and plays with his sister. Jorge likes to build with his Legos and listen to his mother read a bedtime story. He shares a bedroom with his older brother, who reminds him to pick up his belongings before he goes to bed.

As highlighted in this story, Jorge participates in a variety of occupations at home, school, and in the community. Growing up in a bilingual, multigenerational home, he communicates in two languages, and has a mother and grandparents to care for him on a daily basis. He learns family social rules from interacting with his older brother; he teaches those rules to his younger sister. He must cope with the extended military absence of and constant safety concerns for his father.

Living in a small, rural town, he sometimes sees his classmates and teacher at the local grocery store and the library. He has access to open spaces for playing sports. Because his mother is a dietitian and is aware of the increased risk of obesity in children, she encourages Jorge to participate in these community recreational programs. His family, teacher, and coaches try to provide the necessary supports for him to be successful in his home, school, and community occupations. This social and physical environment, blended with his emerging physical, cognitive, and social-emotional development, contribute to Jorge's occupational performance.

At this age, boys and girls tend to have similar muscle mass and body size. They fluctuate between having periods of high energy and intermittent fatigue (Allen & Marotz, 2007). Physically, Jorge will grow 2 to 3 inches and gain 6 to 8 pounds each year until he is about 12 years old. Most of the growth will occur in his arms and legs, rather than in his trunk (Kail, 2002). As a result, his center of gravity will lower to his umbilicus, allowing him better to maintain dynamic and static balance, to move into and out of various sitting squatting, standing, and bipedal movement positions as he concurrently reaches for and manipulates his home and school belongings (Payne & Isaacs, 2001). His large muscles are developing rapidly, contributing to his increased postural control and the calibration of movements he needs to accomplish various tasks (Cronin & Mandich, 2005). As his movement patterns become more sophisticated, Jorge develops a **body schema,** an internalized sense of how his body occupies space (Gallahue & Ozmun, 2002). Consistent with the **motion hypothesis** proposed by Shaffer, Jorge's self-initiated, active movements likely contribute to development of his depth and spatial perception (Cronin & Mandich, 2005). The combination of lowered center of gravity, increased postural control, and maturing body schema enable Jorge and his friends to begin to participate in competitive sports such as soccer and T-ball that require dynamic balance, strength, and visiospatial perception. Like other boys his age, Jorge tends to excel in those sports activities requiring strength; the girls in his class are better at those sports involving balance and flexibility. Fortunately, Jorge's gym teacher, sensitive to cultural influences that may be contributing to these differences, encourages all of the boys and girls to sample a variety of sports activities.

Like his large muscles, Jorge's small muscles are developing, though more slowly. Because girls' small muscles develop more quickly than do boys', the girls in Jorge's class are about one year more advanced in their fine motor and in-hand manipulative skills than are the boys. For example, the girls print more legibly and cut more accurately than do the boys. They also are able to maintain spacing between words. However, because spatial awareness does not mature fully until they are about 10 years old, most of the boys and girls in Jorge's class struggle with maintaining constant size among letters (Cronin & Mandich, 2005).

In addition to muscle differences, brain studies show metabolic differences between boys and girls at this age. Boys have more metabolic activity in the areas of their brain associated with physical activity. In contrast, girls demonstrate more metabolic activity in the areas of their brains associated with emotions, audiovisual, and visuospatial working memory (Gur et al., 2005; Vuontela et al., 2003). Further research needs to be conducted to determine whether such physical and brain metabolism are inherited or culturally influenced by the type of sports, play, and household occupations deemed more appropriate for boys versus girls (Cronin & Mandich, 2005; Santrock, 1999).

Cognitively, Jorge is beginning to use **concrete operations** to solve problems. Thus he is developing rules and strategies to examine logically and mentally determine relationships among concrete, tangible objects. With this cognitive capacity, Jorge now understands the principle of **conservation.** That is, he understands that the quantity of something remains the same even if it is reshaped or put into a different container, such as when his grandmother gives him eight ounces of juice in a short, wide or in a tall, slender glass. Because he is able to **decenter,** he focuses on more than one aspect of the glass; he considers the width, depth, and height of the glass to arrive at his conclusion. He also is able to use the concepts of **transformation** and **reversibility** to understand that the size and shape of the juice transforms as it is poured from one glass to the other, and that the juice reverses to its original size and shape if it is poured back into the original glass. Cognitively, he also is able to use serial ordering to sequence the steps of his morning school routine and to grasp the relationship between day, week, month, and year. He uses **classification** to arrange his Legos into bins by their shape and color when he puts them away in the evening. Because of such cognitive abilities, Jorge understands and applies arithmetic strategies to manipulate numbers and draw simple graphs. He also uses symbols, such as letters, to represent concrete objects and sounds, skills needed for reading and writing (Allen & Marotz, 2007; Vander Zanden, 2003).

Socially, Jorge uses decentering skills to attend to and make judgments about people based on several of their characteristics, rather than just one, as he did when he was younger. Thus, though he finds his teacher, Ms. Boggs, strict about classroom procedures, he also thinks that she is funny and kind. However, instead of relying only on Ms. Boggs to learn all of the school rules, he attends to the emotional reactions of his friends and classmates, a strategy called **social referencing**, to determine how to respond to ambiguous situations (Vander Zanden, 2003).

Jorge's experiences with household chores, school tasks, sports programs, and play activities contribute to his sense of **industry versus inferiority** (Erikson, 1997). Through exploration of how things work and how his body moves, he develops a sense of his competencies. Because children who are encouraged to try many occupations within the range of their capacities develop positive self-esteem, his mother tries to expose him to developmentally appropriate challenges. Those children who are not afforded such opportunities, or expected to accomplish activities too difficult for them, are likely to develop low self-esteem (Vander Zanden, 2003).

This sense of industry versus inferiority often manifests itself at school. Wanting to be competent and to please his teacher, Jorge tries to remember and integrate all that he has learned, but he does not yet have sufficient practice to master the skills, or remember the details. When he does not succeed at the level he feels he should, he becomes frustrated, sad, and withdrawn (Allen & Marotz, 2003). Some early education specialists believe that schools place too high a level of academic expectation on children in primary grades for which they are not developmentally ready, contributing to this sense of failure (Vander Zanden, 2003). Signs such as bedwetting, nail biting, and behavioral problems may be indicators of when children are experiencing too much stress (Allen & Marotz, 2007).

JORGE: 10 YEARS OLD

As a 10-year-old, Jorge is more independent in his activities of daily living. Although he can complete all aspects of hygiene and dressing, he often needs reminders to wash his hair and put on clean clothes. He chooses his clothes based on what his friends are wearing. He also likes to wear logos of his favorite sports teams. He has more responsibilities at home, and his weekly chores include vacuuming the rugs, emptying the trash, and helping to prepare meals. Although things usually go smoothly at home, he battles with his mother over table manners—elbows on the table, talking with his mouth full, fisted grasp of spoon or fork. He tries to hang out with his older brother and his friends but usually is told to leave.

As a fifth grader, he is expected to complete his schoolwork in cursive handwriting and to learn to type with the computer. Classroom learning includes multiple opportunities for active experimentation and small group problem solving. He likes to complete science experiments and participate in class plays. His daily homework consists of routine assignments for spelling and math, independent pleasure reading, and social studies projects. As a member of the Best Buddies program, he helps a classmate who has autism to locate his school supplies and navigate around the building.

Jorge and his friends, Ben and Marcus, have built a fort and have developed a secret code for messages and a password for the door. They like to tell jokes, play computer games, and watch videos. Jorge remains active in the recreational sports at the local park; soccer in the fall, basketball in the winter, and baseball in the spring. He likes to play on teams and usually gets along with the coach and other members. If there is a disagreement, he uses harsh words rather than physical force.

Similar to many 10-year-olds, Jorge has entered a period of relative contentment. He feels comfortable at school and in his community, and has not begun to experience the tensions that surface in middle school. Continuing to grow gradually in height and weight, his body assumes a slimmer, long-legged appearance. His brain has reached almost its full adult size. In contrast to a few of the girls in his class, who are beginning to experience a rounding of their hips, a budding of their breasts, and a darkening of their hair color, his body is not showing any signs of hormonal changes. Running, climbing, biking, and skateboarding are daily activities. Because of his body growth and ongoing activity level, he eats frequently throughout the day. He remains unaware of his need for additional sleep, preferring to argue with his mother to allow him to stay up late at night (Allen & Marotz, 2003).

As he moves his arms, hands, and legs with increased precision, he is assigned specific positions on his sport teams. He can catch, throw, and kick a ball with accuracy and works to develop complex skills. He likes to build with his hands, attempting to construct and paint the fort with only minimal help from his grandfather. He has become skilled at manipulating the video game controls. Though he does not particularly like to do so, he is able to write in cursive and to use the computer to type short assignments. He prefers to experiment with the graphic features of the computer.

Cognitively, Jorge continues to use concrete operations to solve problems logically. Though he still sees answers to problems in terms of absolute yes or no responses, he is beginning to consider that more than one answer may be correct. His sense of fair play involves establishing and abiding by the rules for the game. He is able to recall a series of events in both forward and backward sequence to repeat and reconstruct multiple step tasks. Because he has mastered the concept of **conservation**, he can complete math problems involving weight, volume, and those involving time and distance (Allen & Marotz, 2007).

In addition, Jorge's sense of **spatial awareness** has expanded to include a dynamic sense of how objects move through space. He is starting to develop **cognitive maps,** that is, mental images of how to align various spaces and tasks in relation to one another, how to move around multiple spaces, and how to sequence a number of tasks. Jorge and his friends use their spatial awareness and cognitive maps to ride their bikes on dirt trails, to play their video games, and to understand the diagrams for their basketball competitions. Their classroom teacher has taught them to use cognitive maps to **temporally organize** the sequence of their science experiments and the events of their social study projects.

Jorge's auditory and visual figure-ground perception and movement perception have changed. The maturation of his figure-ground perception occurred when he was about 8 years of age, and the maturation of his movement perception occurred as he turned 10 (Cronin & Mandich, 2005). These auditory and visual figure-ground skills allow Jorge to attend selectively to the voices of and supplies used by the children in his group, in contrast to those of other groups, when working on collaborative tasks in the classroom. Movement perception allows him better to detect the change in position of his teammates during physical competitions.

Socially, Jorge has become more aware of his physical appearance, wanting to wear clothes that are deemed appropriate by his peers. He has learned to use language to express his thoughts and emotions. Seeing humor in the multiple meaning of words, he manipulates them to tell riddles and jokes. He uses harsh words and derogatory language to attack others, yet is offended when he is the recipient of such attacks. Sensitive to criticism, he feels them as personal hurts. He seeks friends who are his same gender and hold common interests, changing who he perceives to be friends and enemies based on concrete interactions with them. Consistent with the notions of **gender cleavage,** he seldom plays with girls unless required as part of an established program (Allen & Marotz, 2007; Kail, 2002).

Being bilingual, Jorge has an advantage over a number of his other classmates who are monolingual. Originally intermingling Spanish and English words and grammatical structures, he now easily thinks in and transitions from one language to the other. He uses his knowledge of the meaning of words in both languages to figure out the meaning of unfamiliar words. He better understands that concepts and ideas can be represented by various words and tonal inflections, and that he should adjust the expressions that he uses to fit the cultural context.

In contrast, he sees that his classmates who are first generation immigrants and whose primarily language is other than English struggle within the English speaking classrooms and sports programs. Socially, they misunderstand nuances of humor, thus become angry or victims of jokes. Academically, they miss key points to complex concepts, and misinterpret words on tests. During sports, they struggle to understand multistep directives that can not be demonstrated. Similar to national statistics, one-fifth of the students in Jorge's school do not speak English at home. Like other schools, his school struggles to procure fiscal resources and hire teachers competent to teach students for whom English is a second language (ESL). Three approaches have been used in schools: the ESL approach, the bilingual education approach, and the total immersion approach. When using the ESL approach, students learn English every day until they reach a basic standard of proficiency, then are fully integrated into the English speaking academic courses (Vander Zanden, 2003). Using this approach, children take between 3 to 5 years to reach grade level norms in English, if they receive formal education in their primary language, and 7 to 10 if they do not. They often score below national norms on standardized tests (Crawford, 1997). In bilingual education, students receive instruction in both languages by bilingually proficient teachers. They acquire knowledge of complex concepts in the primary language, while also learning English. Initially more expensive, these programs produce students who surpass monolingually schooled children in the upper grades and on standardized tests (Collier, 1997). In the total immersion approach, children are placed in English speaking classrooms for all of their instruction. This method works best when the environment is more social and learning occurs through active experimentation. When the classes are academically based, a number of children fall behind, and eventually withdraw from school (Vander Zanden, 2003). Fortunately for Jorge, his parents speak with him in English and Spanish, strengthening his ability to think conceptually and speak fluently in both languages.

JORGE: 12 YEARS OLD

As a seventh grader, Jorge attends the middle school where he has four different teachers and has to change classrooms (see Figure 7.1■). He also needs to use a locker, and take a shower after gym class. He no longer has recess. He is expected to work in cooperative groups in class and to complete reports and long term papers as part of his homework assignments. Respected by his teachers and classmates, he is a member of the peer conflict resolution team.

Since attending middle school, Jorge's circle of friends has expanded. Although he still plays with Ben and Marcus at home, he eats lunch with his school sports teammates. Since there is an after school activity bus, Jorge has joined the football and baseball teams. He enjoys practice and works hard on perfecting different skills of the game.

At home, Jorge has assumed more personal and family responsibilities. He walks his sister to the bus stop in the morning, and helps with the laundry and yard work on the weekends. He gets a weekly allowance, which he likes to use to go bowling with Ben and Marcus or save for a new video game. Given parental permission, Jorge uses his bike and skateboard to travel throughout the town. When he needs new clothes, he prefers to pick them out and dislikes having to wear his brother's hand-me-downs. During the weekend, he occasionally sleeps over at a friend's house and plans to attend an overnight summer sports camp. Though he resists it, he receives pressure from some of his peers to start smoking, drinking alcohol, and vandalizing property.

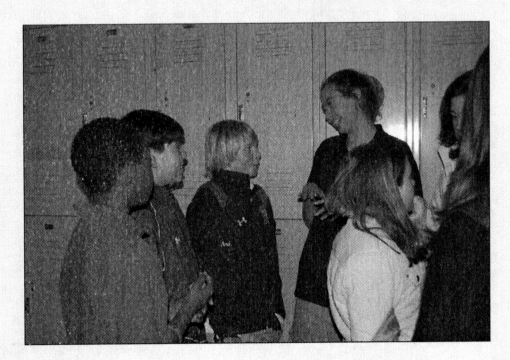

■ **Figure 7.1**
Middle school boys and girls.

Jorge has grown to about triple the length he was at birth. His posture has become more erect and the bones of his shoulder girdle are more prominent. His strength and muscle mass continue to increase. As he moves, he displays more coordination and control. He needs substantively more food and more sleep. Beginning to shows signs of a prepubescent growth spurt, his voice crackles and changes octaves when he speaks. Though unintended, he periodically experiences spontaneous erections that are stimulated by physical activity, pictures, or daydreaming. A number of the girls in his class also are experiencing prepubescent growth spurts and starting to menstruate (Allen & Marotz, 2007; Vander Zanden, 2003).

Additionally, Jorge's reaction time and perception of size constancy depth have improved, contributing to his **coincidence-anticipation timing** (Cronin & Mandich, 2005), and allowing him to better anticipate trajectory and speed, and thus run toward the thrown football and baseball. Both needing physical activity to release his built up energy and stimulated by physical activities that challenge him, he practices daily so that he can play on the school's sports teams.

Cognitively, he is able to remain focused on homework assignments to their completion. Because his memory for recalling details has expanded, he can solve multistep math problems. Accepting that questions may have various answers, he works in a sequential manner to find them. Better able to understand cause and effect relationships, he is able to follow the sequence of basic science experiments to identify factors that contribute to the final results. Grasping the concepts of sarcasm and irony, he uses them to entertain others, with the explicit intention of getting a reaction from them. He completes routine steps of school and home tasks without thinking about them (Allen & Marotz, 2007). Not wanting, but expected, to do household chores, he is not mindful of completing them carefully.

Socially, Jorge has become more self-conscious and aware of his responsibility for his own actions. Rather than reacting immediately to pressure from his peers, he considers the consequences of his decisions. He sees that those students who are more popular tend to be physically attractive, active, assertive, self-confident, and friendly (Vander Zanden, 2003). Recognizing that loyalty, trustworthiness, and honesty are important values among friends and teammates, he chooses to spend more time with them than with his family. Wanting to fit in with his classmates, he dislikes wearing five-year-old clothes that belonged to his brother.

As Jorge and his friends talk with one another at lunch, they notice students clustering themselves by the clothes they wear, and the activities they join. These outward symbols reflect the identity versus role confusion the students are experiencing. Studies conducted on middle schoolers indicate that they readily distinguish among themselves as being nerds, brains, skaters, dweebs, jocks, normals, goths, metal heads, druggies, preppies, and loners. These groups have pecking orders of prestige and power (Brown et al., 1994). Initially contributing to a sense of identity, pressure to be part of a particular group wanes as adolescents grow stronger in their sense of their own separate identities, form personal relationships with individuals across groups (Urberg et al., 1995), and engage in occupations most meaningful to them (Lashbrook, 2000; Ryan, 2001; Urberg et al., 1995). In their extreme, membership in or exclusion from groups can contribute to victimization of individuals and school violence.

As 12-year-old boys, Jorge and his friends frequently use **report-talk** to provide information and give directives to one another. Boasts and arguments about their talents and status dot their conversations. They may resort to making disparaging comments about one another's physical capacities or sexual orientation, or to fighting to resolve major conflicts. In contrast, the girls in their class more frequently use **rapport-talk** to negotiate relationships. Turn taking and sharing of feeling mark their conversations (Cronin & Mandich, 2005; Santrock, 1999). Though they may fight physically, more often they use **relational aggression,** a verbal form of bullying, to hurt one another. This form of bullying can occur face to face, over the telephone, or through cyberspace (Dellasega & Nixon, 2003). Because a sense of inclusion is important to children at this age, the victims of these verbal and physical attacks often experience a painful sense of exclusion.

To reduce the frequency of such aggressive behaviors, the teachers at Jorge's middle school have developed a program to encourage **prosocial behaviors** among the students. Through role playing, guided dialogues, and team building activities, they try to help the students recognize the effect of their words and actions on others. They encourage the students to examine issues from multiple perspectives, develop empathy for one another's feelings, learn cooperative skills, and care about one another. Realizing that social acceptance is related to the ability to read emotions, they teach the students how to read the facial expressions and detect the social intent of one another (Cronin & Mandich, 2005). Each student volunteers time at the library and animal shelter. As part of the program, Jorge serves on the peer conflict resolution team, modeling how to listen respectfully, to state positions in an assertive, nonaggressive manner, and to defuse potentially volatile situations. He also uses his bilingual skills to help resolve issues between Spanish speaking and English speaking youth.

SUMMARY

During the six years children are considered middle school age, they move from needing continual supervision to assuming a certain level of responsibility for their own care and the care of others. Physically, their body proportions change as they become taller and leaner; most growth occurs in their arms and legs. Balance skills, reaction time, and muscle strength improve. Concurrently, visual-spatial and auditory perceptual skills improve, allowing them to move their bodies with increased dexterity and fluidity, and contributing to the advancing capacity to explore various craft, art, sports, and dance occupations.

Cognitively, they advance from using preoperation to concrete operations to investigate and interpret their worlds. Using tangible evidence, they transition slowly from magical thinking and relying on adults for answers to reality based thinking and relying on their own experience for answers. This new way of thinking propels them to explore their environments with curiosity and enthusiasm, and to seek graduated levels of independence from authority figures.

Socially, they shift from seeking primary approval from adults to seeking approval from peers. Some succeed easily in achieving a status of popularity among their peers, while others struggle to gain acceptance and find friends. Physical appearance, self-assuredness, the ability to use social referencing skills to read the emotions and intentions of others, and the capacity to get along with others in organized activities contribute to the degree of peer acceptance. By the time they reach 12 years of age, participation in peer-related social occupations takes on primary importance for many of the boys and girls.

It is important to understand the development of middle school children, particularly when preparing to provide therapeutic services for those who are not able to participate fully in their daily living, educational, play, leisure, and social participation occupations. Spending time observing 6- through 12-year-old children provides insights about the various ways they perform their daily life activities, and the influence of the context in which they live and grow on that performance.

The theories and frames of reference presented in Chapter 3 offer a structure for organizing and explaining the physical, cognitive, and social-emotional growth of school age children. The occupation-based conceptual models discussed in Chapter 2 outline a framework for considering how the personal factors of the child, the properties of the task, and the complexities of the environment interact to affect the child's occupational performance. They enable occupational therapy practitioners to attend to the myriad of occupations the child needs and wants to perform at home, in school, and the community, so that services provided promote full participation in daily life.

REVIEWING KEY POINTS

1. Define each of the following words:

Body schema	Classification
Cognitive maps	Coincidence-anticipation timing
Concrete operations	Conservation
Decentering	Egocentric-cooperative play
Gender cleavage	Industry versus inferiority
Motion hypothesis	Prosocial behaviors
Rapport-talking	Relational aggression
Report-talk	Reversibility
Spatial awareness	Social referencing
Temporal organization	Transformation

2. Describe how a 7-year-old child might engage in daily life activities at home, school, and the community.
3. Explain how physical, social, cultural, personal, and virtual contexts influence the engagement of a 7-year-old child in these occupations.
4. Describe physical, cognitive, and psycho-social skills that 7-year-old children typically display.
5. Describe how a 10-year-old child might engage in daily life activities at home, school, and the community.
6. Explain how physical, social, cultural, personal, and virtual contexts influence engagement of a 10-year-old child in these occupations.
7. Describe physical, cognitive, and psycho-social skills that 10-year old children typically display.
8. Describe how a 12-year-old child might engage in daily life activities at home, school, and the community.
9. Explain how physical, social, cultural, personal, and virtual contexts influence engagement of a 12-year-old child in these occupations.
10. Describe physical, cognitive, and psycho-social skills that 12-year old children typically display.

APPLYING KEY CONCEPTS

1. Using the *Occupational Therapy Practice Framework,* with partners, role play Jorge engaging in one of his occupations with his friends or family members as

a 7-year-old. Refer to Chapter 1 of this text for a description of the *Occupational Therapy Practice Framework.*
   a. Role play Jorge engaging in that same occupation as a 10-year-old.
   b. Role play Jorge engaging in that same occupation as a 12-year-old
   c. For each age period, depict how the context influences how that occupation is performed.
2. With a partner, apply the language found in the performance skill section of the *Occupational Therapy Practice Framework* to describe six performance skills that the student demonstrates when performing at each of those ages. Describe any similarities and differences in the performance skills across the three ages.
3. With a partner, apply the language found in the task demand section of the *Occupational Therapy Practice Framework* to describe the tasks Jorge performs when engaging in that occupation. Discuss any changes in the demands of the task on across the three ages.
4. Select one of the occupation-based conceptual models to explain how and why Jorge engages in that occupation. Use bullet points, footnotes, word bubbles, or a paragraph to record the explanation. Refer to Chapter 2 to review the occupation-based conceptual models.
5. Select one of the non–occupation-based frames of reference or theories to explain how Jorge engages in that occupation. Use bullet points, footnotes, word bubbles, or a paragraph to record the explanation. Consider the developmental level of the occupation. Refer to Chapter 3 to review the non–occupation-based frames of reference and theories.

REFERENCES

Allen, E., & Marotz, L. (2007). *Developmental profiles: Pre-birth through twelve* (5th ed.). Clifton Park, NY: Thomson Delmar Learning.

American Occupational Therapy Association. (2002). Occupational therapy practice framework: Domain and process. *American Journal of Occupational Therapy, 56*(6), 609–639.

Brown, B. B., Mory, M. S., Kinney, D. (1994). Casting adolescent crowds in a relational perspective: Caricature, channel, and context. In R. Montenayor, G. R. Adams, T. P. Gullotta (Eds.), *Personal relationships during adolescence* (p. 123–167). Thousand Oaks, CA: Sage.

Collier, V. P. (1997). Acquiring a second language for school. *Directions in Language and Education, 1*, 4.

Crawford, J. (1997). *Best evidence. Research foundation of the Bilingual Education Act.* Washington, DC: Clearinghouse for Bilingual Educators.

Cronin, A., & Mandich, M. (2005). *Human development and performance throughout the lifespan.* Clifton Park, NY: Thomson Delmar Learning.

Dellasega, C., & Nixon, C. (2003). *Twelve strategies that will end female bullying: Girl wars.* New York: Fireside.

Erikson, E. H., & Erikson, J. M. (1997). *The life cycle completed.* New York: Norton and Company.

Feldman, R. (2004). *Child development* (3rd ed.). Upper Saddle River, NJ: Pearson Prentice Hall.

Frost, J., Wortham, S., & Reifel, S. (2005). *Play and child development* (2nd ed.). Upper Saddle River, NJ: Pearson Prentice Hall.

Gallahue, D., & Ozmun, J. (2002). *Understanding motor development* (5th ed.). Boston: McGraw-Hill.

Gur, R., Mosely, L., Resnick, S., Karp, J., Alvi, A., Arnold, S., & Gur, R. (2005). Sex differences in regional glucose metabolism during a resting state. *Science, 267*, 528–531.

Kail, K. (2002). *Children.* Upper Saddle River: NJ: Pearson Prentice Hall.

Lashbrook, J.T. (2000). Fitting in: Exploring the emotional dimensions of adolescent peer pressure. *Adolescence, 35*, 747–757.

McDevitt, T. & Ormrod, J. (2004). *Child development: Educating and working with children and adolescents* (2nd ed.). Upper Saddle River, NJ: Pearson Prentice Hall.

Payne, V. G. & Isaacs. L. D. (2001). *Human motor development: A lifespan approach* (5th ed.). Boston: McGraw-Hill.

Ryan, A.M. (2001). The peer group as the context for the development of young adolescent motivation and achievement. *Child Development, 2*(4), 1135–1150.

Santrock, J. (1999). *Life-span development* (7th ed.). Boston: McGraw-Hill.

Shumway, A., & Wollacott, M. (2006). *Motor control: Translating research into clinical practice applications* (3rd ed.) Philadelphia: Lippincott, Williams & Wilkins.

Urberg, K.A., Degirmencioglu, S.M., Tolson, J.M., & Halliday-Sher, K. (1995). The structure of adolescent peer networks. *Developmental Psychology, 33,* 834–844.

Vuontela, V., Steenari, M., Carlson, S., Koivisto, J., Fjallberg, M., & Aronen, E. (2003). Audiospatial and visuospatial working memory in 6–13-year-old school children. *Learning and Memory, 10,* 74–81.

Vander Zanden, J., Crandell, T., & Crandell, C. (2003). *Human development* (7th ed. revised). Boston: McGraw-Hill.

White, S., Duda, J., & Keller, M. (1998). The relationship between goal orientation and perceived purposes of sport among youth sport participants. *Journal of Sport Behavior, 21*(4), 474–483.

Chapter 8

Developmental Influences on the Occupations of Adolescents

Janet V. DeLany

Key Terms

Anorexia
Bulimia
Conventional
Ethnic identity
Exercise bulimia
Foreclosure
Formal operations
Hypothetico-deductive reasoning
Identity achievement
Identity diffusion

Identity status
Metacognition
Metamemory
Moratorium
Moral development
Obesity
Postconventional
Preconventional
Sensation seeking

Objectives

- Identify occupations and roles of adolescents.
- Identify factors that influence occupational performance.
- Understand the developmental and interrelated nature of factors that influence the occupational performance and occupations of adolescents.

INTRODUCTION

During their adolescence, teens undergo significant changes in their physical, cognitive, and social development that affect their ability to perform their daily life occupations. As with all ages, adolescents develop at individual rates in response to hereditary factors, task and occupational demands, and opportunities and challenges within the environment or performance context. However, in contrast to earlier stages of development, the breadth and diversity of the context that influences how the adolescents select and engage in various occupations often stretches beyond the immediate family into the larger community. Typically, girls change more rapidly in their development in early adolescence, whereas boys demonstrate more profound changes in their development in mid to late adolescence. The following stories about the daily life occupations of Saburi, Galit, Maher, and Zach highlight the similarities and differences in the growth and maturation between adolescent boys and girls. The occupation-based conceptual models reviewed in Chapter 2 help to elucidate the interrelatedness of the person factors, the occupation and task demands, and the environment or context that influence how these adolescents perform their occupations. Similarly, the non–occupation-based frames and theories discussed in Chapter 3, such as Erikson's psychosocial theory of development and Piaget's cognitive theory of development, provide a backdrop for understanding the changes in body functions that adolescents experience. The ability to use occupation-based with non–occupation-based models to direct services is central to occupational therapy practice.

Occupations of 14-Year-Old Adolescents

SABURI, GALIT, MAHER, AND ZACH: 14-YEAR-OLDS

Saburi and Galit, two teenage girls, and Maher and Zach, two teenage boys, live in a large city. Each of these friends resides in a different type of home. Saburi resides in a single house, Galit in a duplex, Maher in an apartment complex, and Zach above a storefront. They meet one another at the bus stop every morning on their way to high school. At the beginning of middle school, the two girls and the two boys were the same size. Now the girls are taller than the boys. They have begun menarche and developed breasts. In contrast, the boys are just beginning to notice changes in their voices.

They use public transportation to get to school. Their bus ride usually is noisy and filled with people from all aspects of life. On their way, they pass by homeless people and professional people, laborers, shopkeepers, and tradesmen. They see young children with their parents and elderly citizens doing their weekly shopping. They hear some people speaking in English and others speaking in Spanish, Chinese, Yiddish, and Arabic; occasionally they see some using sign language. Though most of these people wear western garb, a few wear dress and head coverings reflective of various ethnic and religious heritages.

Once they arrive at their high school, the four friends see each other for only a few of their classes. During the first few months of high school, they must learn to find their way around their four-story school. The first story contains administrative and counseling offices, the cafeteria, auditorium, gymnasiums, athletic facilities, vocational classes, and music rooms. Most of their freshman classes are on the left wing of the second and third floors, along with classes for sophomore students. Most of the classes for the juniors and seniors are in the right wing of the second and third floor. The specialty art, lab, and science classes are located on the fourth floor. Saburi, Galit, Maher, and Zach must manage their time and plan their schedules to get to each class on time and with the necessary supplies.

The four friends also must decide which extra curricular activities interest them. Unlike with the open enrollment policy of their middle school, they now must compete for slots in these programs. Saburi, who has played the violin and flute for several years, wants to join the orchestra and band. Graphic arts and journalism interest Maher, while student government and basketball excite Galit, and lacrosse and school plays appeal to Zach.

During lunch, Saburi and Galit sit together with other freshman girls and talk about their classes, their families, boys, pop culture, and their weekend plans. Maher and Zach sit with other freshman boys and talk about video games, girls, sports, and action movies. They take turns trying to tell the most outrageous jokes and embellish stories about their real and imagined exploits. To learn peer rules for dressing, behaving, talking, and socializing, they carefully watch the older students.

At home Saburi, Galit, Maher, and Zach are expected to assume additional household responsibilities. Saburi is responsible for the yard work; Galit prepares the evening meals; Maher babysits his younger siblings; and Zach does the grocery shopping. Sometimes they want to sleep all day; at other times they want to stay awake all night. Finding their moods fluctuating frequently and in emotional intensity, they question their parents' actions and disagree with the household rules. Sometimes they feel positive about themselves, want to be with other people, and risk new challenges; at other times they believe that no one understands or likes them, and want to hide in their rooms. Relying more on peers for advice and approval, they increasingly confront choices about socially approved and risky behaviors.

Becoming 14 years old and entering high school afford the four friends new occupational opportunities and new occupational responsibilities. At school they now have the opportunity and the responsibility to choose some classes and to join some extracurricular activities that interest them. At home, they are trusted and expected to carry out instrumental activities of daily living with little supervision.

The environments where they live and go to school influence how they engage in their home and school related occupations. For example, Saburi, the only one who lives in a detached house, does yard work. Zach, who lives above the store, does the daily grocery shopping. They have the opportunity and the obligation to learn to use public transportation to commute between home and school. During the commute they can interact with people from multiple backgrounds, but need to learn to be respectful of these differences and to be vigilant about personal safety. Their large city high school allows them to take an array of specialty courses, but also demands that they learn to find their way around the multistory complex and to compete for slots in extracurricular activities. Only those students with more developed and coordinated bodies will be selected for the sports teams. As the four friends continue through high school, the type of occupational opportunities and responsibilities available to them will expand in response to their developing performance capacities, body structures, and body functions. These developmental changes influence the occupational performance of the students within the context of their school and home.

Physically, their bodies are metamorphosing into their adult sizes and shapes. Because twenty percent of their adult bodies develop during adolescence (Cronin & Madish, 2005), they require extended periods of sleep. Their physical development allows the students to participate in occupations that require more complex and integrated performance skills. The girls' bodies change more quickly than the boys'. Saburi and Galit accomplish occupations requiring advanced fine motor manipulation, such as writing and craft projects for their classes, more easily than the boys because their wrist joints mature by midadolescence. Likewise, the girls' other joints mature more quickly, resulting in their ability to perform more coordinated athletic tasks than the boys, such as in their gym and dance classes (Tanner, 1990).

Like most of their female classmates, Saburi's and Galit's bodies have produced estrogen and adrenal androgen, resulting in the development of their ovaries, uterus, vagina, breasts, and pubic hair. The level of estrogen will increase eightfold in the girls' bodies throughout puberty (Nottelmann et al., 1987). Maher's and Zach's bodies are just beginning to show signs of adult development. In response to increased levels of testosterone, their testes and penises are starting to enlarge, and their pubic and auxiliary hair is starting to grow. Throughout puberty, the boys will experience an eighteenfold increase in their testosterone levels (Biro, Lucky, Huster & Morrison, 1995). The change in the girls' and the boys' hormonal levels contributes to their dramatic mood swings, and the additional quarrels they have with their parents. In the United States, most adolescents believe they will go through puberty sometime between the ages of 12 and 14 years. The timing of puberty affects the adolescents' perceptions of themselves. Girls who experience puberty early tend to have a negative self-image; those who go through puberty later do not experience the same self-image difficulties. In contrast, boys who go through puberty early tend to have a positive self-image; boys who go through puberty late tend to have a negative self-image (Dick, Rose, Viken, & Kaprio, 2000; Reirdan, & Koff, 1993). As Saburi, Galit, Maher, and Zach go through puberty, they spend additional time in grooming, shopping, sleeping, and eating occupations to adapt to their changing bodies and self-images.

In addition to their bodies, the function and structure of their brains also change. Between the ages of 13 and 15 years their cerebral cortexes become thicker and their neuronal pathways become more efficient, particularly in the areas that control spatial perception and motor functions (Fischer & Rose, 1994). As a result, they find that they can complete spatial and motor tasks more efficiently than they could previously. Their ability to complete bilateral motor tasks fully matures, enabling them to use two different body parts to stabilize and manipulate their school, music, and athletic equipment. Saburi and Maher easily isolate and synchronize finger movements to play their musical instruments and draw intricate patterns. Galit and Zach shift quickly between dynamic movement and static balance positions, calibrate the strength of their movements, and judge spatial distances to play basketball and lacrosse (Cronin & Mandish, 2005). Similarly, Saburi simultaneously can march and play her band instrument because of her advancing spatial and motor skills.

Consistent with Bandura's social learning theory, the four friends carefully watch the older students during lunch. Through vicarious reinforcement they learn about socially accepted behaviors for each of the various groups, and determine which ones to follow. For example, they learn about the types of jokes and stories to tell, clothes to wear, language patterns to use, and codes of silence, honesty, and dishonesty to practice. Likewise, as they use public transportation, they observe the social and cultural behaviors of people throughout the city. Issues related to personal and family belief systems, safety, finances, prestige, and peer acceptance influence their decisions as to the social behaviors they copy. Consistent with Skinner's theories of operant conditioning, they modify their behaviors in response to positive and negative feedback they seek and receive from their peers, teachers, family, and community members regarding those behaviors they demonstrate. At times, feedback from their peers is most crucial. The feedback may boost their sense of competency and willingness to risk new challenges; conversely, it can contribute to sense of isolation and belief that no one understands them.

Occupations of 16-Year-Old Adolescents

SABURI, GALIT, MAHER, AND ZACH: 16-YEAR-OLDS

Saburi, Galit, Maher, and Zach successfully have completed two years of high school. As they enter their junior year, they notice additional physical changes in one another. Though not much taller than they were as 14-year-olds, the girls' bodies have shifted in proportion and have more defined breasts, waists, and hips. The boys have grown substantively in height, and have gained some weight and muscle mass. They now have pubic and auxiliary hair; their penises and testicles have enlarged. Fewer of their classmates are wearing braces; more are wearing glasses and contact lenses. Some have tattoos and body piercing.

The four friends notice changes in their classroom environment. They have fewer classmates this year than they had when they started high school; some of their former classmates have transferred to specialty focused schools for the arts, sciences, or engineering. Others entered vocational and alternative high schools, while others dropped out of high school, or have been incarcerated. Some of the female students are pregnant. The high school has a daycare program attached to it for those teens who have children, and who want to remain in school to complete their high school education.

Academic expectations have shifted. The four friends need to manage their time to complete longer term projects that require them to integrate information from their literature, social studies, and government classes. Rather than taking one side of a controversial topic, they need to explain competing views. In science and math classes they must memorize and determine when to use multistep formulas. Guidance counselors approach them about scheduling for aptitude tests and planning for post secondary occupations in education, military service, and the workforce.

During lunch, they sit with clusters of friends from their classes or extra curricular programs. Some of the cafeteria tables have only girls sitting at them; some have only males; others have a mixture of males and females who socialize together or who have begun dating. Students at the various tables distinguish themselves from one another by their particular style of clothing, body art, codes of behavior, and topics of conversation. (See Figure 8.1■.)

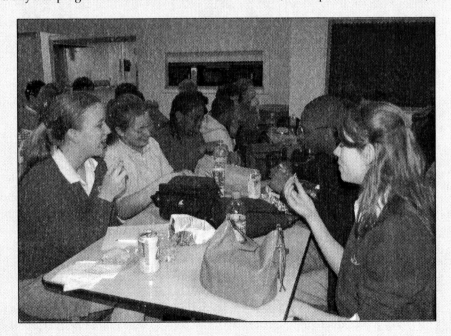

■ **Figure 8.1**
High school cafeteria.

At home, the four friends still find themselves questioning their parents and quarreling with their siblings. They fluctuate between feeling competent and overwhelmed, cheerful and depressed, genial and irritable. As they prepare to get their drivers' licenses, they procure part-time jobs to pay for their car insurance as well as some of their food, clothing, and leisure activities. Saburi clerks at a local music store; Galit supervises children at the day care center, Maher waits on tables at the pizza shop, and Zach referees at lacrosse games. During their free time they make plans to watch the sports games and theater productions at the school, shop, attend impromptu parties with their friends, and go to the movies. As they spend less time with their families and more time with their peers, they make additional decisions about money management, eating behaviors, sexual practices, peer and gang membership, alcohol and drug usage, and potentially violent or illegal activities.

As 16-year-olds, Saburi, Galit, Maher, and Zach experience new ways of engaging in familiar social and education based occupations, and attempt new work occupations. Social relationships take on additional sexual aspects. School presents more cognitive challenges. Work schedules compress time for extracurricular activities. Responsibility for personal decisions and exposure to illegal activities increase. The types of occupations in which they engage as 16-year-olds affect and are affected by changes in their physical capacities, social-emotional and cognitive capacities, and by the changes in their environment.

The girls have reached almost their full adult height. The boys will continue to grow for a few more years. They find that others treat them differently and make sexual references as their bodies take on more adult features. During their lunch breaks, the four friends talk about this. Consistent with national norms, approximately 1 percent of adolescent boys and 0.4 percent of adolescent girls in their school identify themselves as homosexual. A large percentage of students are not clear as to their sexual orientation (Remafedi, Resnick, Blum, & Harris, 1998). By eleventh grade, approximately 50 percent of high school students state that they have had sex at least once; the male students boast that they have had more sexual partners than have the female students. When their classmates discuss boyfriend and girlfriend relationships, they often confuse their physical capacity to engage in sexual activity with the stage of intimacy versus social isolation as defined by Erikson. Only 58 percent of the students share that they used condoms during their most recent sexual intercourse, and only 20 percent of the females report using birth control pills, placing them at risk for sexually transmitted diseases and unintended conception (CDC, 2000). Saburi, Galit, Maher, and Zach notice that some of their classmates are more sexually active than others. Across cultures, they tend to be the teens who physically develop and date early, perform poorly in school, drink alcohol, do not participate in supervised extracurricular activities, have permissive family attitudes about sexual experimentation, have little adult supervision, or are victims of sexual and physical abuse. The greater number of risk factors, the greater is the likelihood that the teen will be sexually active (DeLany & Spottswood, 2000; Herrenkohl et al., 1998; Kirby, 1997; Koniak-Griffin et al., 2003). In an effort to encourage adolescents to delay intercourse and to use contraceptives once they become sexually active, Saburi, Galit, Maher, and Zach's school introduced multisession abstinence programs in 7th and 8th grades. Their high school expanded these endeavors by offering a combination of programs to address abstinence, sexual protection, reproduction, relationship and esteem development, and community activism. Their school also connected with community agencies to address the occupational and developmental needs of their pregnant and parenting teenage classmates through multifaceted home visitation programs, and high school connected child care programs. These programs focus on the adolescents' parenting and educational occupations, and on their family, financial, psychological, social, safety, and health needs (DeLany & Spottswood, 2000).

In addition to sexual exploration, the four friends find that they and their peers engage in **sensation seeking** occupations and behaviors as they try to establish their own sense of autonomy and peer acceptance. Acquisition of drivers' licenses and access to cars allow the students to explore their physical environments and participate in sensation seeking occupations beyond their immediate neighborhoods. Such activities further contribute to the students' sense of identity versus role confusion. Those teens who are successful in their school related occupations, participate in extracurricular activities, and have a supportive network of family and friends are more likely to participate in healthy sensation seeking behaviors and occupations. Those adolescents who have less structured time and participate in more non–goal directed leisure occupations tend to engage in more risky behaviors that involve compulsive actions, alcohol and drug usage, petty crime, violence, and sexual promiscuity (Carpenter, 2001; Farnworth, 2000; Stein, Roesner, & Markus, 1998).

Marcia (1980) expanded upon Erikson's work to propose four different **identity statuses: identity achievement, moratorium, foreclosure,** and **identity diffusion.** As they look around their school and observe their classmates with body piercing, tattoos, and various styles of hair and dress, Saburi, Galit, Maher, and Zach find examples of students in each of these stages. Those classmates who are in the identity achievement status have experienced a sense of personal turmoil and have come to a resolution about their belief systems and occupational roles. Some of these students already have transferred to specialty programs that focus on the arts and sciences. Those in the moratorium status still are experiencing personal turmoil and have not yet arrived at a resolution. These students find themselves testing out different life style options, some that are healthy and some that are risky. A few are thinking about dropping out of school. Those students in foreclosure status have accepted familial or culturally defined occupations or belief systems without reassessing the choices. Those in identity diffusion status have neither experienced the turmoil nor have come to a resolution about belief systems and occupational roles. It is as if they do not yet have a sense of their own identity. Participation in occupations within a variety of contexts contributes to students' sense of identity. Conversely, self-identity influences the occupations they choose to perform (Kielhofner, 2002).

As part of their self-identity, the four friends also formulate notions about their sex-role identity and **ethnic identity.** Sex-role identity reflects socially prescribed occupations and behaviors deemed as more appropriate for males or females (see Figure 8.2■). Within a number of cultures in the United States, it is considered more appropriate for girls to perform masculine tasks than it is for boys to perform feminine tasks (Bee & Boyd, 2002). Ethnic identity involves self-identification with and acceptance of the values, attitudes, and occupational roles of a specific group of people. This group may be based on ancestry or religion, and is set apart in some way from the dominant culture. Because of societal biases, adolescents may struggle between belonging to their ethnic community and the dominant culture. Consistent with social learning theory, if Saburi, Galit, Maher, and Zach have positive role models, they will be more successful in developing bicultural competencies to navigate between both cultures and form their self- and ethnic identities. During adolescence, girls tend to resolve their identity status earlier than boys by consolidating internal beliefs about themselves with those learned through social relationships (Moretti & Wiebe, 1999) that occur as part of their

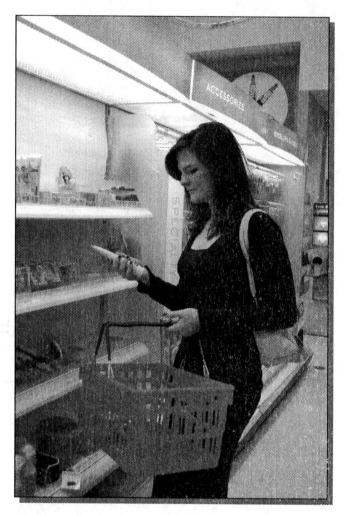

■ **Figure 8.2**
Adolescent choosing personal care products to reflect
her sense of personal identity.

daily occupations. In contrast, boys are more likely to delay identity achievement until
later adolescence or adulthood, and base their decisions more on internal than social
perspectives. It is important to note that adolescence is only one of the time periods
during which people examine their self-identity. People may do so several times
throughout the course of their lives (Bee & Boyd, 2002).

In school, as a result of the brain growth that occurred between the ages of 13 and
15, the four friends find they are required to complete longer term projects by using
inductive and deductive reasoning to examine issues from alternative perspectives
and to solve multistaged problems. In addition, their teachers expect them to use
metacognition and **metamemory** strategies to contrast and compare science and math-
ematic formulas, and to learn essential information from texts. Piaget believed that
adolescents begin to develop the ability to engage in these **formal operations** to solve
problems some time between the ages of 12 and 16 (Piaget, 1977). Later studies found
that only some adolescents use formal operations to solve future oriented and logic
problems (Bradmetz, 1999). Those adolescents whose levels of education and life

situations foster it develop the ability to use formal operations. The ability to use formal logic is necessary for college level course work, and for nonroutinized jobs such as those associated with managerial, administrative, and professional careers.

When using formal operations, adolescents employ **hypothetico-deductive reasoning** to generate a hypothesis and logically deduce viable conclusions about abstract concepts. Hypothetico-deductive reasoning involves if-then logic to generate plausible hypothesis and systematic problem solving to change and measure the effect of one variable at a time to solve abstract problems. In contrast, students who use a concrete level of thinking change and measure the variables in a haphazard trial and error manner (Bee & Boyd, 2002). The ability to use formal operations contributes to the ability to use metacognitive and metamemory strategies. Metacognitive strategies help the students think about, plan, and modify what they are doing before, during, and after the task. Metamemory strategies enable the students to devise systems for memorizing and recalling multiple details. Galit and Saburi use metacognitive strategies to plan and modify the long-term interdisciplinary projects their teachers assign them. They use metamemory strategies to recite passages from texts and to recall details from their Internet searches.

The four friends each have paid jobs outside of their homes. Those who advocate for teens working believe it helps them to develop positive work habits, personal accountability, and time and money management responsibilities. Studies conducted by Mael, Morath, and McLellan (1997) and McNeal (1997) found that those students who had positive work experiences developed increased sense of competency and worth. However, others are concerned that working detracts from time the students commit to studying and extracurricular activities. A number of studies have discovered negative correlations between the hours teens work and the grades they earn, particularly when teens work more than 20 hours per week (Steinberg, Fegley, & Dornbusch, 1993). Other studies have found that alcohol and illicit drug consumption increases as the adolescents work more, possibly because of the strain, additional money to purchase alcohol and illicit drugs, and access to older adolescents who can purchase the substances for them (Valois, Dunham, Jackson, & Waller, 1999). Teens in other industrialized countries work fewer hours than do those in the United States, but spend twice as much time completing their schoolwork. Some suspect that these factors contribute to the lower academic performance of United States versus European and Asian students (Larson & Verma, 1999).

Occupations of 18-Year-Old Adolescents

SABURI, GALIT, MAHER, AND ZACH: 18-YEAR-OLDS

Saburi, Galit, Maher, and Zach now are in the last semester of high school. Physically, the girls' faces have become more angular. They move easily and gracefully in their bodies, and possess the stamina and strength to participate in a variety of physical activities. The boys' faces have become more angular and have facial hair. They have gained additional muscle mass, particularly in their arms and torso. Moving their bodies with agility, power, and speed, they feel impervious to injury or accidents.

At school, they serve in various leadership positions. Saburi is the first violin chair in the orchestra and section leader in the band. Galit is treasurer of the student counsel and captain of the basketball team. Maher is the graphic editor for the yearbook. Zach is co-captain for the lacrosse team and has a supporting role in the school play. As part of their senior requirement, they volunteer at the community homeless shelter once a month. There, they use their talents to help run music, art, photography, and sports programs for the children and youth.

At lunch, conversation centers on the upcoming school proms, regional music and sports competitions, graduation ceremonies, and class trips. Some of the students have taken scholastic and skill based aptitude tests, and have spoken with college and military recruiters. Other students have submitted employment applications with local businesses. While some of the students are clear about their post–high school plans, others struggle about whether to attend community colleges, private colleges, state universities, or technical and art institutes. Debates about whether to enroll in the military, look for full time work, or travel throughout the country fill the air. As part of this, the students find themselves in a dilemma about the moral righteousness of war and their moral obligation to protect their homeland.

Periodically, during these lunch conversations, the four friends talk about classmates who will not be graduating with them. (See Figure 8.3■.) Suicide, drug overdose, and street violence have claimed the life of a few of their peers. Long term hospitalizations because of eating disorders, psychiatric difficulties, and automobile accidents have postponed the graduation date for others. A few students dropped out of school because they felt academically and socially unsuccessful, or because they needed to work to contribute to the family finances. Still others left school and their homes because of familial discord and abuse.

At home, Saburi, Galit, Maher, and Zach are better able to clarify their viewpoints and to discuss issues with their parents. Their moods are more predictable and stable, and they can use effective coping mechanisms to control them. They divide their free time between going out with a group of friends and being alone with a particular friend. Some weekends they go to the beach, the amusement park, or community festivals. Though they love their families, they find themselves increasingly restless to become independent of them.

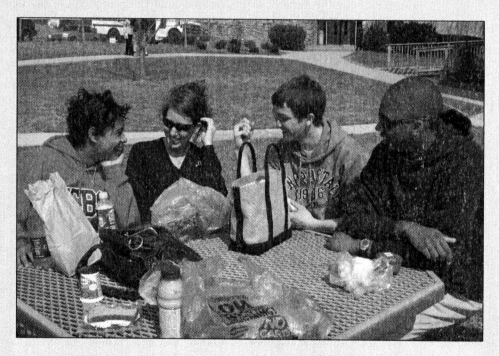

■ Figure 8.3
Saburi, Galit, Zach, and Maher sharing their experiences.

By their senior year, the four friends hold leadership roles in their school related occupations, and contribute to their community through civic engagement activities. As they begin to transition from the adolescent to the young adult stage of their lives, they examine their future occupational options, and the decisions they and their peers have made. Their ability to do so reflects the continuing evolution of their physical, cognitive, and psychosocial development and the changing supports and demands from their environment.

Maher and Zach continue to grow and will reach their full adult height between the ages of 18 and 20. During this time, their joints will reach full maturity and muscle mass will increase to 40 percent, enabling them to demonstrate more coordinated and powerful movements, and greater endurance than the girls (Bee & Boyd, 2002; Cronin & Mandish, 2005; Tanner, 1990). Though not as much difference is noted in leg strength, the boys demonstrate considerably more abdominal, upper arm, and grip strength, allowing them to excel in contact sports (see Figure 8.4■) (Payne & Isaacs, 1999). Because of these physical changes in his athletic abilities, Zach is cocaptain of his lacrosse team. Recruiters have come to the high school to watch him play.

The boys' bodies tend to decrease in their percentage of body fat, whereas the girls' bodies tend to increase in the percentage of body fat as measured by Body Mass Index, *BMI* (Murphy, 1990). Some of Saburi and Galit's female classmates and a few of Maher and Zach's male classmates try to control their body weight through unhealthy eating and dieting patterns. Students in sports and performing arts programs where low body weight is deemed critical, such as wrestling, ballet, and horse racing, experience additional pressure to consume unhealthy small amounts of calories. Other students undereat, overeat, purge, or overexercise to cope with self-image and other psychosocial issues. When done persistently, this leads to **anorexia, obesity, bulimia, or exercise bulimia.** Unhealthy family eating and exercise patterns, parental and cultural beliefs about desired body size, fashion trends, television and video images, fast-food availability, and sedentary life styles also contribute to under- and overeating behaviors (Bee & Boyd, 2002; Gallahue & Ozmun, 2002; Hill & Franklin, 1998; Rabasca, 1999; Vander Zanden, Crandell, & Crandell, 2003).

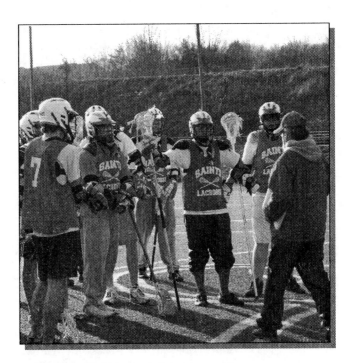

■ Figure 8.4
Lacrosse practice.

Along with bodily changes, brain size continues to change. The frontal lobe of the cerebral cortex, which controls logic and thinking, begins to expand from around 17 years of age through early adulthood, allowing adolescents to use more complex strategies to solve problems (Davies & Rose, 1999). Expanding on the work of Piaget, Kohlberg outlined stages of **moral development**, based on questions related to justice. He enumerated three levels, with each level having two stages. The three levels are **preconventional, conventional,** and **postconventional**. At the preconventional level, adolescents make moral decisions based on an external source of authority that is powerful and near to them, such as parent, school principal, or police. They are more likely to make decisions about legal and illegal activities based on reward and punishment expectations from those who hold power over them. For example, some students make decisions to join the military or enroll in college based on praise and rewards they will receive from their parents. At the conventional level, students make decisions based on the norms and rules of the group. The group might be the family, church, peer group, gang, or government. Students internalize but do not question these external sources of authority. For example, some students will believe in the correctness or wrongness of the war efforts based on governmental or church related positions about it. Because students frequently hold membership in several groups, they must decide which group norms to follow when the norms of the groups conflict with one another. At the postconventional stage, students make decisions based on principles that address the needs of the larger society and transcend the needs of any particular individual. They make decisions based on issues such as justice, equality, and compassion across groups of people. As related to the war efforts, these students will weigh the immediate and long-term good that results from the war in relationship to the immediate and long-term devastation that it causes. Saburi, Galit, Maher, and Zach volunteer at the homeless shelter because of their postconventional beliefs about equality and compassion. Whereas younger children make decisions at the preconventional level, most adolescents make decisions at the conventional level. Only a very few of the older adolescents demonstrate postconventional moral decision making (Bee & Boyd, 2002). Those students who demonstrate more advanced prosocial behaviors and are less tolerant of violence also demonstrate more advanced levels of moral decision making. Conversely, those who tolerate violent behaviors and demonstrate more antisocial behavior often use lower levels of moral decision making (Schonert-Reichl, 1999; Sotelo & Sangrador, 1999).

Given the body related and social changes, occupational adjustments, and family and contextual pressures they have faced during their high school years, some adolescents experience episodes of depression; some commit suicide. About 5 to 8 percent of adolescents experience longstanding depression, with girls twice as likely as boys to report it. One in 13 adolescents attempt suicide, with boys 5 times more likely than girls to be successful in their attempts (NCIPC, 2000; Nolen-Hoeksema & Girgus, 1994). Adolescents who feel depressed, display aggressive behaviors, grow up in households where parents feel depressed or have committed suicide, or have family histories of drug and alcohol abuse, are more likely to attempt suicide. Often these adolescents undergo a triggering stressful event such as rejection, isolation, or humiliation. Concurrently, they experience an altered mental state such as new and overwhelming feelings of hopelessness or rage, and have access to objects such as guns or pills, just before committing suicide. As Saburi, Galit, Maher, and Zach reflect on their classmates who died or required long-term hospitalizations, it is clear that depression was an underlying cause of the eating disorders, drug and alcohol use, automobile accidents and suicide attempts. Hotlines provide support to these students to continue to live (Garland & Zigler, 1993). Students who engage in a combination of healthy occupations, and have a support network of friends and family, develop a better sense of their capacities and more positive coping mechanism to cope with the challenge of adolescence.

SUMMARY

A transition from childhood to adulthood, adolescence is an intense period of physical, cognitive, and social development. Twenty percent of a person's growth into an adult body occurs during adolescence. Physical development occurs in height, weight, muscle mass, fat composition, hormonal levels, joint formation, brain size, and neuronal connections. Cognitive development is reflected in the ability to organize and process information, evaluate situations, abstract, and make judgments. Social development manifests itself through moral decision making, group membership, personal relationships, leadership roles, and emotional connections. Non–occupation-based theories and frames of reference reviewed in Chapter 3 provide clues as to how these developmental changes occur. These include Erikson's psychosocial theory of development, Piaget's cognitive theory of development, Skinner's behavioral theories, and Kolberg's moral development stages.

Concurrently, the contexts in which adolescents live, work, and play expand beyond the family control to include larger community influences. Adolescents travel further from home, spend less time under their parental influence, spend more time with peers, and expose themselves to other societal influences through electronic media, books, coaches, teachers, co-workers, employers, religious leaders, and community members.

The occupation-based conceptual models reviewed in Chapter 2 provide a structure for understanding how personal development couples with these contextual changes to affect the occupations that adolescents choose and must perform, and the way they perform these occupations. Such knowledge enables occupational therapists and occupational therapy assistants to provide interventions that promote full community participation for those adolescents who may be struggling to engage in their daily occupation. How this occurs will be explored in more detail in Sections III and IV.

REVIEWING KEY POINTS

1. Define each of the following words:

Anorexia	Bulimia
Conventional	Deductive reasoning
Ethnic identity	Exercise bulimia
Foreclosure	Formal operations
Hypothetico-deductive reasoning	Identity achievement
Identity diffusion	Identity status
Metacognition	Metamemory
Moratorium	Moral judgment
Obesity	Postconventional
Preconventional	Sensation seeking

2. Describe how a 14-year-old adolescent might engage in daily life activities at home, school, and the community.
3. Explain how physical, social, cultural, personal, and virtual contexts influence engagement of a 14-year-old adolescent in these occupations.
4. Describe physical, cognitive, and psycho-social skills that 14-year-old adolescents typically display.
5. Describe how a 16-year-old adolescent might engage in daily life activities at home, school, and the community.
6. Explain how physical, social, cultural, personal, and virtual contexts influence engagement of a 16-year-old adolescent in these occupations.
7. Describe physical, cognitive, and psycho-social skills that 16-year-old adolescents typically display.
8. Describe how an 18-year-old adolescent might engage in daily life activities at home, school, and the community.
9. Explain how physical, social, cultural, personal, and virtual contexts influence engagement of an 18-year-old adolescent in these occupations.
10. Describe physical, cognitive, and psycho-social skills that 18-year-old adolescents typically display.

APPLYING KEY CONCEPTS

1. Select Saburi, Galit, Maher, or Zach.
   a. Using the *Occupational Therapy Practice Framework,* list five occupations in which that student engages. Refer to Chapter 1 for a description of the *Occupational Therapy Practice Framework.*
   b. For each of those occupations, describe the context that influences how that occupation is performed.
   c. Applying the language found in the performance skill section of the *Occupational Therapy Practice Framework,* describe six performance skills the student demonstrates when performing for each of those occupations. Note any similarities in the performance skills across the five occupations.
   d. Applying the language found in the task demand section of the *Occupational Therapy Practice Framework,* describe one of the tasks the student performs when engaging in each of those occupations.
2. Draw a picture of that student engaging in one of the occupations.
   a. Select one of the occupation-based conceptual models to explain how and why the student engages in that occupation. Use bullet points, footnotes, word bubbles, or a paragraph to record the explanation. Refer to Chapter 2 to review the occupation-based conceptual models.
   b. Select one of the non–occupation-based frames of reference or theories to explain how the student engages in that occupation. Use bullet points, footnotes, word bubbles or a paragraph to record the explanation. In the explanation, consider the developmental level of the occupation. Refer to Chapter 3 to review the non–occupation-based frames of reference and theories.

REFERENCES

Bee, H., & Boyd, D. (2002). *Lifespan development* (3rd ed.). Boston: Allyn and Bacon.

Biro, F. M., Lucky, A. W., Huster, G. A., & Morrison, J. A. (1995). Pubertal stages in boys. *Journal of Pediatrics, 127,* 100–102.

Bradmetz, J. (1999). Precursors of formal thought: A longitudinal study. *British Journal of Developmental Psychology 17,* 61–81.

Carpenter, S. (2001). Teens' risky behavior is about more than race and family resources. *APA Monitor, 32,* 22–23.

Centers for Disease Control (2000). Youth risk behavior surveillance. United States, 1999. *Morbidity and Mortality Weekly Report, 49*, 1–96.

Cronin, A., & Mandish, M. (2005). *Human development and performance through the lifespan.* Clifton Park, NY: Thomson Delmar Learning.

Davies, P., & Rose, J. (1999). Assessment of cognitive development of adolescents by means of neuropsychological tasks. *Developmental Neuropsychology, 15,* 227–248.

DeLany, J.V., & Spottswood, A. (2000). *Pregnancy prevention and support programs for adolescent parents.* Chambersburg, PA: Summit Health.

Dick, D., Rose, R., Viken, R., & Kaprio, J. (2000). Pubertal timing and substance use. Association between and within families across late adolescence. *Developmental Psychology, 36,* 180–189.

Farnworth, L. (2000). Time use and leisure occupations of young offenders. *American Journal of Occupational Therapy, 54*(3), 315–324.

Gallahue, D. L., & Ozmun, J. C. (2002). *Understanding motor development.* New York: McGraw-Hill.

Garland, A. F., & Zigler, E. (1993). Adolescent suicide prevention: Current research and social policy implications. *American Psychologist, 48,* 169–182.

Herrenkohl, E. C., Herrenkohl, R. C., Egolf, B. P., & Russo, M. J. (1998). The relationship between early maltreatment and teenage parenthood. *Journal of Adolescence, 21,* 291–303.

Hill, A., & Franklin, J. (1998). Mothers, daughters, and dieting: Investigating the transmission of weight control. *The British Journal of Clinical Psychology, 37,* 3–13.

Kielhofner, G. (2002). Model of human occupation. Theory and application. (3rd ed.). Baltimore, MD: Lippincott, Williams & Wilkins.

Kirby, D. (1997). *No easy answers: Research findings on programs to reduce teen pregnancy.* Washington, DC: National Campaign to Prevent Teen Pregnancy, Task Force on Effective Programs and Research.

Koniak-Griffin, D., Lesser, J., Uman, G., & Nyamathi, A. (2003). Teen pregnancy, motherhood, and unprotected sexual activity. *Research in Nursing and Health, 26*(1), 4–19.

Larson, R., & Verma, S. (1999). How children and adolescents spend time across the world; Work, play, and developmental opportunities. *Psychological Bulletin, 125,* 701–736.

Marcia, J. E. (1980). Identity in adolescence. In J. Adelson (Ed.), *Handbook of adolescent psychology* (pp. 159–187). New York: Wiley.

Mael, F., Morath, R., & McLellan, J. (1997). Dimensions of adolescent employment. *Career Development Quarterly, 45,* 351–368.

Moretti, M., & Weibe, V. (1999). Self discrepancy in adolescence: Own and parental standpoints on self: *Merrill-Palmer Quarterly, 45,* 624–649.

McNeal, R. (1997). Are students being pulled out of high school? The effect of adolescent employment on dropping out. *Sociology of Education, 70,* 206–220.

Murphy, J. M. (1990). The pediatric and adolescent athlete. In B. Saunders (Ed.), *Sports physical therapy* (pp. 151–157). East Norwalk, CT: Appleton and Lange.

National Center for Injury Prevention and Control (NCIPC) (2000). *Fact book for year 2000.* Washington, DC: Author.

Nolen-Hoeksema, S., & Girgus, J. S. (1994). The emergence of gender differences in depression during adolescence. *Psychological Bulletin, 115,* 424–443.

Nottelmann, E. D., Susman, E. J., Blue, J. H., Inoff-Germain, G., Dorn, L. D., Loriaux, D. L., Cutler, G. B. Jr., & Chrousos, G. P. (1987). Gonadal and adrenal hormone correlates of adjustment in early adolescence. In R. M. Lerner & T. T. Foch (Eds.), *Biological-psychosocial interactions in early adolescence* (pp. 203–324). Hillsdale, NJ: Erlbaum.

Payne, V. G., & Isaacs, L. D. (1999). *Human motor development. A lifespan approach.* Mountainview, CA: Mayfield Publishing Company.

Piaget, J. (1977). *The development of thought: Equilibrium of cognitive structures.* New York: Viking.

Rabasca, L. (1999). Ultra thin magazine models found to have little negative effect on adolescent girls. *APA Monitor Online 30.* Http://www.apa.org/monitor/oct99.

Reirdan, J., & Koff, E. (1993). Developmental variables in relation to depressive symptoms in adolescent girls. *Development and Psychopathology, 5,* 485–496.

Remafedi, G., Resnick, M., Blum, B., & Harris, J. (1998). Demography of sexual orientation in adolescent. *Pediatrics, 89,* 714–721.

Schonert-Reichl, K. (1999). Relations of peer acceptance, friendship adjustment, and social behavior to moral reasoning during early adolescence. *Journal of Early Adolescence, 19,* 249–279.

Sotelo, M., & Sangrador, J. (1999). Correlation of self-rating of attitudes towards violent groups with measures of personality, self-esteem, and moral reasoning. *Psychological Reports, 84,* 558–560.

Stein, K., Roesner, R., & Markus, H. (1998). Self-schemas and possible selves as predictors and outcomes of risky behaviors in adolescent *Nursing Research, 47,* 96–106.

Steinberg, L., Fegley, S., & Dornbusch, S. M. (1993). Negative impact of part-time work on adolescent adjustment. Evidence from a longitudinal study. *Developmental Psychology, 27,* 304–313.

Tanner, J. (1990). *Fetus into man. Physical growth from conception to maturity.* Cambridge, MA: Harvard University Press.

Valois, R., Dunham, A., Jackson, K., & Waller, J. (1999). Association between employment and substance abuse behaviors among public high school adolescents. *Journal of Adolescent Health, 25,* 256–263.

Vander Zanden, J., Crandell, T., & Crandell, C. (2003). *Human development* (7th ed. rev). Boston, MA: McGraw-Hill.

Evaluation of Children and Adolescents: General Principles

Janet V. DeLany

Key Terms

Active participant observation
Analysis of occupational
    performance
Assessment
Ceiling effect
Close-ended questions
Criterion referenced
Distant observation
Evaluation
Floor effect
Measurement tool
Natural environments
Nonstandardized

Norm referenced
Occupational profile
Open-ended questions
Psychometric properties
Re-evaluation
Reliability
Screening
Sensitivity
Service competency
Standardized assessments
Structured environments
Validity

Objectives

- Understand the evaluation process.
- Clarify the role of the occupational therapist and the occupational therapy assistant in the evaluation process.
- Articulate the steps of the evaluation process.
- Differentiate among the various types of assessments.
- Understand how the selection of measurement tools is influenced by the client's level of development, the client's roles and occupations, and the specific delivery model.

INTRODUCTION

The occupational therapy **evaluation** is a comprehensive process that involves the collection and analysis of information necessary to determine appropriate and effective interventions for the children and adolescents. Information consistent with the domain of occupational therapy is gathered and analyzed. This includes information about the children's and adolescents'

- Occupations
- Performance skills
- Performance patterns
- Performance context
- Task demands
- Body structures and functions

Specific **assessments,** including chart reviews, observations, interviews, and measurement tools, are used to gather this information (AOTA, 2002; AOTA, 2004b; Hinojosa, Kramer, & Crist, 2005).

The evaluation often starts at the beginning and continues throughout the delivery of occupational therapy services. It is a dynamic process, responsive to changes in the children and adolescents, the environment, and the task. Terms such as **screening,** initial evaluation, and **re-evaluation** differentiate among the various times that formal evaluations occur.

The screening often involves an introductory review of available data, a brief observation of the child or adolescent, and the administration of quick measurement tools (Hinojosa et al., 2005). The purpose of the screening is to look for possible signs of performance problems that may warrant a fuller evaluation. Because screenings are relatively brief, they can be administered to a larger number of children or adolescents in an efficient manner. For example, in some school districts, occupational therapists collaborate with other professionals such as school psychologists, nurses, and educators to conduct screenings on all children as they enter the school. The information gleaned from these screenings helps to determine which children should be evaluated more fully for potential occupational performance problems. In other situations, particularly when the need for a fuller evaluation is apparent, it is not necessary to conduct a screening.

The initial evaluation involves comprehensive chart reviews, observations, interviews, and administration of measurement tools. Through these assessments, information is gathered about the children's or adolescents' occupational interests and expectations, performance capacities, environmental supports and barriers, and tasks demands. The initial evaluation

- Establishes a baseline to describe current level of performance
- Focuses the direction of occupational therapy intervention
- Furnishes justification for the need for and reimbursement of occupational therapy services (Law et al., 2001)

The re-evaluation can occur at various intervals during and at the end of the intervention process. Re-evaluations may be conducted when a change in occupational performance is noted. The type of information collected during the re-evaluation should be consistent with the type collected during the initial evaluation to be able to measure the effect of the occupational therapy intervention. For example, to be able to state that occupational therapy intervention positively affected the child's eating and sleeping patterns, measurable data about the child's eating and sleeping patterns need to be collected during the initial and the re-evaluation. When systematically collected in this manner, the data from the re-evaluation can be used to

- Adjust the focus of the intervention
- Measure the outcomes of occupational therapy intervention
- Justify reimbursement for occupational therapy services
- Develop a database for evidence based practice (Law et al., 2001)

When conducting the screening, initial evaluation, or re-evaluation, it is crucial to be sensitive to the children's and adolescents' developmental levels. Developmental levels involve the capacity to perform tasks that are consistent with a particular age as well as the chronological age. Children and adolescents who are developmentally advanced accomplish tasks at a level above what is expected for their chronological age. Children and adolescents who are developing more slowly accomplish tasks at a level below what is expected for their chronological age. Chronological age is determined by subtracting the child's or adolescent's birth date from the evaluation date. For example, let us suppose the child was born in May 7, 1998 and date of the observation was July 10, 2006. To find the chronological age, set up the dates in the following manner and subtract:

2006 yr	7 mos	10 days
−1998 yr	5 mos	7 days
8 yrs	2 mos	3 days

In this scenario, the child's age is 8 years, 2 months, and 3 days. Assume, however, that the child was born on August 26, 2000 and the date of the observation was March 15, 2005. Again, set up the dates in the following manner:

2005 yr	3 mos	15 days
−2000 yr	8 mos	26 days

As written, it is not possible to subtract 26 days from 15 days, nor is it possible to subtract 8 months from 3 months. To do the subtraction, first do the following conversions as demonstrated in Table 9.1■. In the table, one year is converted to 12 months, and one month is converted to 30 days.

■ **Table 9.1**
Converting Years to Months and Months to Days

DIRECTIONS	ORIGINAL DATE	CONVERTED DATE
Change the number of months from 3 to 2 months and 30 days	2005 yr 3 mos 15 days =	2005 yr (2 mos + 30 days) 15 days
Add the 30 days to the 15 days to make 45 days	2005 yr (2 mos + 30 days) 15 days =	2005 yrs 2 mos 45 days
Change the year from 2005 to 2004 and 12 months.	2005 yrs 2 mos 45 days	(2004 yr + 12 mos) 2 mos 45 days
Add the 12 months to the 2 months	(2004 yrs + 12 mos) 2 mos 45 days =	2004 yrs 14 mos 45 days

Now subtract:

	2004 yr	14 mos	45 days
−	2000 yr	8 mos	26 days
	4 yrs	6 mos	19 days

In this scenario, the child's age is 4 years, 6 months, and 19 days. Typically, when the number of days is 15 or less, the age is stated in years and months, and the number of days is dropped. When the number of days is 16 or more, the days are dropped and the age is rounded up to the next month. Thus, the child whose age is 8 years, 2 months, and 3 days would be considered 8 years, 2 months old. A child, whose age is 4 years, 6 months and 19 days would be considered 4 years, 7 months old.

It also is important to be respectful of the cultural context that influences the children's and adolescents' occupational performance during the evaluation. Cultural norms influence developmental patterns, language patterns, and ways of interacting and behaving. For example, in some cultures, children are expected to converse in full sentences and maintain eye contact when interacting with adults. They are encouraged to actively initiate playing with various materials. In other cultures, children are to listen and to divert their gaze when in the presence of adults. They are to wait to touch materials until they receive permission to do so from their caregivers (Wells and Black, 2000). It would be as inaccurate to judge such children in the first culture setting as being rude and impulsive as it would be to judge the children in the second culture setting as having difficulty maintaining eye gaze and initiating play.

In addition to developmental level and culture, it is essential to be mindful of the external context where the evaluation occurs. External contexts include the physical, virtual, and social contexts. Since these contexts can provide support for or barriers to occupational performance, when feasible, it is better for the evaluation to occur in the natural rather than a simulated or contrived setting. For example, it is better to observe the play skills of children in the natural environment of the playground with peers, then in the simulated environment of the clinic with staff. Doing so provides a more accurate picture about how the children actually participate in their daily life occupations and how these settings enable or prevent occupational performance. In order to identify successfully the children's and adolescents' areas of occupational performance strength and difficulties, evaluations should be grounded within an appreciation of the context of the children's and adolescents' developmental, cultural, and environmental influences (AOTA, 2002; AOTA, 2004b; Law, Baum, & Dunn, 2001).

ROLE OF THE OCCUPATIONAL THERAPIST AND OCCUPATIONAL THERAPY ASSISTANT IN THE EVALUATION PROCESS

The occupational therapist is responsible for initiating and directing the evaluation process, interpreting the data, and determining the intervention. What is evaluated and how the evaluation is conducted is based on the expectations and needs of the children, the adolescents, and their families, the domain of occupational therapy practice, and the laws regulating occupational therapy services in that practice setting. The occupational therapist must be involved actively in all aspects of the evaluation process. The occupational therapist:

- Defines the occupational challenges the children and adolescents are experiencing
- Clarifies their goals and priorities
- Establishes intervention priorities
- Determines the type and level of occupational therapy service to address these challenges

When using a client-centered approach, such decisions are made in collaboration with the children and adolescents, their family members and caregivers, educators, health professionals, and social service professionals (AOTA, 2004a, 2005a, 2005b).

Occupational therapy assistants contribute to the evaluation process. They do so by carrying out particular aspects of the assessment delegated to them by occupational therapists, and for which they have demonstrated **service competency.** Service competency means that the occupational therapy assistant

- Understands the purpose, scope, and bounds of the assessment
- Knows the language to use and the procedures to follow when conducting the assessment
- Obtains the same information as would the occupational therapist when conducting the assessment (Hinojosa et al., 2005)

After completing the delegated assessments, the occupational therapy assistant provides verbal and written reports of the information to the occupational therapist. Since laws and regulatory requirements vary among states and practice settings, they must be checked to determine to what extent occupational therapy assistants can contribute to the evaluation process at the place where they work (AOTA, 2004a, 2005a, 2005b).

STEPS IN THE OCCUPATIONAL THERAPY EVALUATION PROCESS

The evaluation process involves two parts: the development of an **occupational profile** and the **analysis of occupational performance**. As part of the occupational profile, the occupational therapist and the occupational therapy assistant gather information about what the children or adolescents could do previously, currently have difficulty doing, and need and want to be able to do. To accomplish this, the occupational therapist and the occupational therapy assistant collect information about the children's and adolescents'

- Occupational history and experiences
- Patterns of daily living, interests, values, and needs
- Problems about performing occupations and daily life activities
- Occupational priorities (AOTA, 2002)

They gather this information through chart reviews, and through conversations with the children and adolescents, their family and caregivers, their educators, and other professionals who work with them.

The second part of the evaluation, the analysis of occupational performance involves

- Synthesizing information from the occupational profile
- Observing the children and adolescents perform their occupations and activities
- Noting the occupations they choose and need to perform at home, school, and in the community
- Learning the meaning and purpose of those occupations
- Recording the skills and patterns they employ to perform them
- Learning what motivates the children and adolescents to perform and their level of satisfaction with their performance
- Selecting and administering assessments that are developmentally appropriate and occupationally relevant
- Assessing the environment and the performance tasks
- Considering barriers and supports to occupational performance
- Interpreting the assessment data, and considering what is relevant to the children's and adolescents' immediate condition and those relevant to their future activity and participation level
- Reaching conclusions about the appropriateness of occupational therapy services for addressing the occupational challenges, based on best practice and evidence (AOTA, 2002; Crepeau, Cohn, & Schell, 2003; Finch, Brooks, Stratford & Mayo, 2002; Law et al., 2001; WHO, 2001).

Clinical reasoning, based on occupation and nonoccupation theories and conceptual models, guides the judgments made during the evaluation process. To determine which theories and conceptual models to use, the occupational therapist considers the scientific knowledge and evidence about the diagnostic conditions of the children and adolescents, their developmental and life stages, and the occupational challenges confronting them (AOTA, 2002). Initially, the occupational therapist should consider which occupation-based conceptual model most effectively organizes the occupational therapy services at the particular practice setting, facilitates interdisciplinary communication and collaboration, and matches the children's and adolescents' goals. Guided by this occupation-based conceptual model, the occupational therapist uses clinical reasoning to make judgments about which

- Measurement tools to administer
- Interviews, chart reviews, and observations to conduct
- Temporal, fiscal, and personnel resources to allocate
- Data synthesis and analysis processes to follow

Likewise, occupational therapy assistants apply clinical reasoning to guide their thinking and actions as they administer various measurement tools, gather information from interviews and observations, and report their findings.

As preliminary data is gathered, the occupational therapist further considers which non–occupation-based practice models add to the evaluation process. The inclusion of these non–occupation-based models contributes to the collection of core information about performance capacities, performance context, and body functions and structures. The clinical reasoning process, guided by these occupation and non–occupation-based conceptual models allows for the

- Identification of cues to understand the challenges and capacities of the children and adolescents
- Formulation of hypothesis about factors contributing the occupational challenges the children and adolescents are experiencing
- Interpretation of the cues
- Evaluation and reformulation of the original hypotheses
- Construction of an effective intervention plan (Humbert, 2004; Mattingly & Fleming, M., 1994; Schell & Cervero, 1993)

TYPES OF ASSESSMENTS

Occupational therapists and occupational therapy assistants use a variety of assessments to conduct the evaluation and make decisions about occupational therapy services. Assessments are the specific chart reviews, observation procedures, interviews, and measurement tools used during the evaluation process (AOTA, 2005b). Some assessments are **nonstandardized**. Nonstandardized assessments do not have a specified administration, content, or scoring procedure to follow. They also do not have a specific physical or emotional environment where they must be administered. Because of this nonspecificity, they are relatively easy to administer and can be tailored to respond to needs of the children and adolescents and the context where the assessment is conducted. Checklists, informal observations, interviews, chart reviews, and site developed questionnaires are examples of nonstandardized assessments. However, the data gathered from the nonstandardized assessment cannot be compared across individuals. Thus, such information does not contribute to the database needed for evidence based practice. A dressing checklist is an example of a nonstandardized assessment (Hinjosa et al., 2005).

Other assessments are **standardized.** Standardized assessments have specified administration and scoring procedures, and are based on established **norms** or **criteria** that allow comparison of performance across individuals.

Norms are behaviors that have been measured across many individuals to determine what is and what is not typical. For example, it is the norm that children in the United States sit at approximately 6 months of age, and crawl between 7 and 9 months of age. Norm referenced assessments use norms to compare the performance of one individual to that which is typically expected of most individuals within the normal population. The *Peabody Motor Development Scale II* (Folio & Fewell, 2000) is an example of an assessment that uses age norms of when infants and young children typically display certain fine motor and gross motor skills such as scribbling, cutting, printing, walking, running, and jumping.

Criteria are lists of behaviors an individual is expected to demonstrate. However, these behaviors have not been measured across many individuals to determine the typical distribution of the behavior across a given group of people. Some criteria for adolescents to be able to drive an automobile include: stopping at a red light, obeying the speed limits, wearing seatbelts, and using turn signals. Criterion-referenced assessments use the criteria to compare the performance of an individual in relation to an established standard or level of expectation of performance. The *School Functional Assessment* (Coster et al., 1998) is an example of an assessment that uses criteria regarding expected classroom behaviors such as organizing class supplies, following directions, and navigating around the school.

Norm and criterion referenced assessments have published **psychometric properties.** Frequently cited psychometric properties are **validity, reliability,** and **sensitivity.** They are used to judge whether the assessment accurately and reliably measures the specified behaviors, and can be used to detect varying levels of difficulties with performance. Specifically, the validity score is used to determine how accurately the assessment tool measures what it purports to measure (Lyman, 1998; Silverlake, 1999). For example, the validity score for the *Sensory Profile* (Dunn, 1997) gives an indication of how accurately that assessment measures sensory processing behaviors. The reliability score measures how likely the child would receive the same score if the assessment were to be given at a different time or by different a person. The higher the reliability, the more likely the child's assessment results would remain the same regardless of who administers the assessment or when it is administered. Sensitivity gives an indication of how much change in behavior a child or adolescent needs to demonstrate before the assessment registers that change (Lyman, 1998). For example the *Denver Developmental Screening Test II* (DDST) (Frankenberg et al., 1992) measures changes that occur in the development of young children over a period of months. It is not sensitive to changes in development that occur within a day or a week.

Validity and reliability scores are stated statistically in terms of correlation, that is, how likely the achieved scores are consistent with what is expected. Because there are different types of validity and reliability, and because a measurement tool may have subsections, several validity and reliability scores may be recorded. A score of 1.0 indicates a perfect one to one correlation. A score of -1.0 indicates a perfect inverse correlation. Validity or reliability scores between .07 and 1.0 are considered excellent. Those between .04 and .06 are considered acceptable. Those between .00 and .03 are considered weak. Table 9.2■ provides a sampling of validity scores. Sensitivity measures may be described rather than stated in statistical terms. Reading the manual and reviewing the scoring sheet give indicators of how sensitive the measurement tool is for recording change in behavior.

■ **Table 9.2**
Sample of Validity and Reliability Scores of Measurement Tools Used to Assess Children and Adolescents

MEASUREMENT TOOL	VALIDITY SCORE	RELIABILITY SCORE
Assessment of Motor and Process Skills	R = 0.50 to 0.70 for concurrent validity	R = 0.81 to 0.91 for motor skill test-retest reliability; R = 0.71 to 0.90 for process skill test-retest reliability
Peabody Development Motor Scales, 2	R = 0.84 to 0.98 for internal consistency	R = 0.73 to 0.98 for test-retest reliability; R = 0.96 to 0.98 for interrater reliability
Pediatric Evaluation of Disability Inventory	R = 0.70 to 0.97 for Concurrent validity	R = 0.95 to 0.99 for Caregiver Assistance and Modifications; R = 0.79 to 1.00 for agreement between parents and professionals

Standardized assessments follow specified administration, data recording, and scoring protocol. The occupational therapist and the occupational therapy assistant must follow the protocol to gather meaningful, accurate information and to compare the results of one child or adolescent with those of a larger, comparable sample of children or adolescents. The *Bayley Scale of Infant Development III* (Bayley, 2006) is a standardized assessment used in occupational therapy to measure cognition, receptive and expressive communication, social emotional and adaptive behavior skills, and gross motor and fine motor skills of young children. It is best to use standardized assessments to compare performance over time, because they provide a uniform method for measuring changes in performance. However, it is not always feasible to use standardized measurement tools. Standardized measurement tools have not been developed to address all of the diverse occupations in which children and adolescents engage, nor the diverse skills levels, contexts, and body functions and structure that influence their performance capacities. For example, there are no standardized assessments to measure the capacity of young adolescents to accomplish instrumental activities of daily living. Only a few have established protocols that can be used for children who speak a language other than English, or who have vision and auditory difficulties that limit their ability to see and hear directions.

Regardless of whether a standardized or nonstandardized assessment is administered, it is important to report the

- Assessment results
- Assessment procedures
- Context where the assessment occurred
- Behaviors and adaptations of the children and the adolescents during the assessment

Having such information is critical for understanding whether the changes that are recorded during the occupational therapy interventions actually measure real changes and the outcomes of these services, or reflect temporary changes resulting from the assessment procedures, context, and adaptive behaviors (Hinjosa, et al., 2005).

Chart Reviews

Through chart reviews, occupational therapists and occupational therapy assistants can review essential information about the child or adolescent that was obtained and recorded by other professionals. Each practice setting follows a particular protocol for organizing and entering information. Medical charts often contain information about the types and results of daily interventions, background and intake history, and evaluations conducted by various members of the health team, lab results, and permissions forms. School related charts contain information about academic programs and progress, counseling and other support services, individualized education plans, evaluations conducted by various members of the educational team, and permission forms. Charts in community settings may have information related to family supports, living situation, economic status, social service agency contacts, and program provision. In most practice settings, these charts are confidential, and are stored in a central location. Practice settings have established procedures that must be followed regarding who can access these files, and how information can be added to or copied from them. Parents may access these records, if their children are younger than 18 years of age.

Observations and Site-Specific Checklist and Forms

Observations allow the occupational therapist and occupational therapy assistant to record information about the performance capacities of the children and adolescents in a multitude of situations and settings, particularly when standardized assessments procedures may not apply. Observations can occur in **structured** or **natural environments.** In structured settings, also known as contrived or simulated settings, the occupational therapist and occupational therapy assistant set up the environment in a particular manner to elicit certain behaviors. In natural environments, the occupational therapist and the occupational therapy assistant examine how the children and adolescents typically engage in their familiar occupations (Hinojosa et al., 2005). Both types of environments can provide supports and barriers for performance. For example, the structured environment of the therapist's distraction-reduced office may allow the student to focus better on a task of dressing than the natural environment of the busy locker room. As likely, the structured environment of the therapy room may not provide the clues to aid dressing that may be found in the locker room. It is important to note how the environment affects the skills, performance patterns, and task demands.

At times, it is best for the occupational therapist and occupational therapy assistant to observe but not interact, or only minimally interact, with the child or adolescent. Called **distant observation**, this approach allows for minimal influence by the occupational therapist and the occupational therapy assistant on the behaviors of the child or adolescent, and on the surrounding environment. To gather information through distant observation, the occupational therapist or occupational therapy assistant might sit quietly at the back of the classroom. At other times, it is best for the occupational therapist and occupational therapy assistant to directly interact with the child or adolescent. Called **active participant observation,** this approach allows the occupational therapist and the occupational therapy assistant to facilitate and respond to specific behaviors of the child or adolescent, and to adjust the task and the environment to encourage various adaptive responses. The occupational therapist or occupational therapy assistant might sit on the floor and play with the child during active participant observation. However, whether making observation at a distance or through active participation, the occupational therapist and the occupational therapy assistant must be vigilant about how their presence and their intended and unintended cues affect occupational performance. Children and the adolescents quickly learn to interpret facial cues such as smiles and frowns, verbal cues such as praises and sighs, and body cues such as gestures and note taking as indicators to continue with or to alter their behaviors.

The value of the information gathered from these observations depends on the thoroughness and objectivity of the observation skills of the occupational therapist and occupational therapy assistant. The information needs to be based on demonstrated behaviors and observable facts, rather than judgments about those behaviors, or assumptions about the capacities of the children and adolescents, and the context influencing them. When recording demonstrated behaviors it is helpful to include details about the frequency and the rate of performance. Stating that the adolescent completed his homework for five days in a row is an example of frequency. Stating the adolescent completed his homework within 30 minutes is an example of the rate of performance.

When recording the observations, the occupational therapist and occupational therapy assistant should write in active voice and in past tense. Using active voice clearly indicates who performed the activity. Using past tense clarifies that the behavior was observed at least once, but does necessarily occur all of the time (Hinojosa et al., 2005). The following are examples of statements based on observable behaviors and written in active voice, past tense. They also contain information about the rate and frequency of performance.

> **The child printed her letters within the boundaries of the lines, and maintained equal spacing among words to complete a three-paragraph paper within 30 minutes on two different assignments.**

> **The student stood quietly for three minutes when at the rear of the line on two occasions, but fidgeted and hugged himself after 30 seconds when in the middle of the line on three other occasions during the day.**

In contrast, the following are examples of statements based on judgments or assumptions. They do not contain information about the frequency and rate of performance.

> **The child printed beautifully and was motivated to do her best.**

> **The student was constantly disruptive when standing in line.**

Such statements should not be included in written or verbal report. They are not verifiable, and do not provide a clear reference point from which to measure change in performance over time.

Site-Specific Checklists and Forms

To structure the observations, the occupational therapist and occupational therapy assistant might use a checklist developed at the site (see Figure 9.1■). These site-specific checklists provide guidance about what to observe and how to record those observations. Some checklists focus on a specific occupation such as a dressing or meal preparation. Some focus on a specific context such as a home safety or a work safety. Others provide a method for recording body functions and performance skills such as physical strength, range of motion, mobility, and concentration. Often, site-specific checklists provide a quick method to record basic information about demographics, performance capacities, and body functions. The child or adolescent may be scored as able or not able to perform the task or skill, or as needing minimum, moderate, or maximum assistance to perform the task or skill. Minimum assistance implies help with approximately 25 percent of the task; moderate assistance implies helps with 50 percent of the task; and maximum assistance implies help with at least 75 percent of the task. The categories of minimum, moderate, and maximum are ordinal ratings. Ordinal ratings are subjective. They provide a way to rank the level of assistance needed based on the judgment of the rater. However, they do not provide a way to measure precisely the level of assistance needed, nor do they describe for what aspect of the task the child or adolescent needs assistance. For example, one child may need moderate assistance with organizing and sequencing the task, while the other child may need moderate assistance with physically manipulating the supplies. Because of this limitation, some checklists include a comment section where additional details can be added. Videotaping the child or adolescent performing the task also helps with this imprecise scoring and provides a method to compare initial and re-evaluation results.

Site-specific forms provide another method for structuring informal observations. These forms allow the occupational therapist and occupational therapy assistant to describe their observations using single words, phrases, or more detailed sentences. Similar to the checklists, these site-specific forms may direct the occupational therapist and occupational therapy assistant to attend to specific occupations and performance skills. Because these forms often do not have predetermined rating scales,

	Independent	Min A	Mod A	Max A	Not Able	Not Applicable	Comments
Name:							
DOB: DOA							
Workplace Site:							
Evaluator:							
1. Completes daily self-care routine in preparation for work							
2. Dresses appropriately for work							
3. Arranges transportation to and from work							
4. Uses transportation							
5. Adheres to time schedule for starting work							
6. Adheres to schedule for days to work							
7. Checks "clock in" upon arrival							
8. Knows the tasks to accomplish							
9. Completes task in a timely manner							
10. Maintains steady work pace							
11. Follows verbal directions							
12. Follows written directions							
13. Communicates							
a. With co-workers							
b. With supervisors							
c. With customers							
14. Adheres to workplace safety rules							
15. Asks for assistance when needed							
16. Displays positive attitude							
17. Follows procedures for requesting time off							
18. Completes all job responsibilities for the day							
19. Reports unfinished tasks to supervisor before leaving when applicable							

■ **Figure 9.1**
Sample Work Readiness Checklist
Compiled by Amy Mateer, OTS Towson University.

occupational therapists and occupational therapy assistants use precise language that provides a clear, concrete image of what was observed. Figure 9.2■ is an example based on the Occupational Therapy Practice Framework (AOTA, 2002: AOTA, NO). Because this form allows for more open-ended responses, it requires astute observation skills and more time to use it competently.

Interviews

Assessment information also can be gathered through interviews with the children and adolescents, their family members and caregiver, and other professionals who work with them. Depending on whether the practice setting is in the community, at a hospital or clinic, or in a school, these professionals may include social workers, speech and language therapists, physical therapists, nurses, physicians, psychologists, counselors, and educators. Before beginning the interview, it is important to review the reports already written about the child or adolescent. Doing so helps to ensure that the interview builds upon existing information rather than repeats questions already answered. When conducting interviews, the occupational therapist and the occupational therapy assistant consider two central questions:

- What information do I need to gather that relates to the child's or adolescent's capacities to participate in their daily life activities?
- How do I conduct the interview in a therapeutic and client-centered manner?

Reflecting on the domain of occupational therapy helps to answer the first question. The questions asked should provide clues about:

- What occupations are necessary for and important to the child or adolescent to perform?
- Why are these occupations necessary and important?
- What performance skills, performance patterns, contexts, and body functions are necessary to engage in the occupations? How does the child or adolescent perform these occupations?
- What performance skills, body functions, and performance patterns of the child or adolescent promote or hinder participation in the occupations?
- How does the capacity of the child or adolescent to engage in these occupations change over time?
- What contexts support or hinder participation in the occupations?
- What task and environmental adaptations support or hinder participation in the occupations?

Information to answer these questions can be gathered through open-ended or closed-ended questions. **Open-ended questions** allow the respondents, that is, the people answering the interview questions, to talk about the topic in their own words, adding important and meaningful details. This can lead to a fuller understanding of the topic, the contexts surrounding it, and the feelings and values of the respondents about it. Below are two examples of open-ended questions. The first may be appropriate to ask of a 10-year-old child; the second may be appropriate to ask of his parent.

Tell me what you do to get ready for school before you leave the house in the morning.

Describe what your child does by himself and the assistance you provide him to get ready for school in the morning.

Occupations observed	Performance skills demonstrated	Performance patterns demonstrated	Context for performance
Making a poster with three other children of equipment used to play various sports; 20 minute observation	Recognized basic equipment (helmet, ball or puck, nets, stick) used in popular sports Cut out pictures by cutting within ½ inch of straight lines drawn by aide around the picture Cut using loop scissors and palmar grasp. Leaned on elbows and placed trunk against edge of table when cutting Glued by pressing glue stick on dots marked by aide on reverse side of picture Printed name on poster by coping from a model Spoke using simple sentence structures sentences five times. Usually spoke in two- or three-word phrases. Directed comments about own work toward aide; did not make comments about peers' work.	Flipped through pages of several sports magazines quickly without locating a picture Needed verbal prompts from aide five times to remember and focus on the task. Found equipment related to particular sport when pictures were clearly spaced, and when given only one page at a time Stopped working after finding, cutting, and pasting one picture Followed two-step direction of aide to look for and cut out second, then third, picture	In an inclusion classroom with 20 children, teacher and aide Seated in a child size chair at a table with three other peers and an aide Children talked quietly and remained in their seats
Eating in the school cafeteria; 30 minute observation	Stood in and follows cafeteria lunch line Made food selections given two choices verbally	Ate one type of food at a time Ate with open mouth; food spillage occurred	School lunchroom with ten round tables and eight children at a table; three aides provided supervision Cafeteria accommodated special diets

■ **Figure 9.2**
Sample Observation Form

	Used pictures of food items and eating utensils on placemat to get necessary items from lunch line	Rocked in chair when noise level in the cafeteria increased	
	Carried non-liquid foods on tray to table independently; needed lids for containers with liquids	Covered his ears when he heard sudden or loud noises	
	Ate independently with fork and spoon; held them with a cylindrical grasp	Wiggled in chair when he needed to use the bathroom	
	Tore bread as he attempted to butter it with a knife		
	Ate softer type foods; pushed chewy type foods (meats, raw vegetables) to side of plate		
Playing at recess; 20 minute observation	Ran with a wide based gait and forward slanted trunk; stopped to catch breath after running 25 yards	Stayed by best buddy when in a group	Grassy, enclosed lot in the back of the school with outdoor climbing equipment
	Followed actions of a best buddy (a peer volunteer who helps him at recess) to know when and where to run during kick ball	Played on the swings or in sand pile when alone	
	Waited for large ball to stop rolling before kicking it	Crossed his arms and sat on the ground when required to come back into school	
	Kicked the ball 15 feet but not toward a specific target		

■ **Figure 9.2**
Sample Observation Form (cont.)

Interviews that use open-ended questions can take more time to complete. They require the occupational therapist or the occupational therapy assistant to word the questions skillfully so that the discussion remains focused. For example, the above questions to the child and the parent direct focus on morning preparations for school. Questions such as "Tell me what you do during the day" and "Tell me how you are feeling" may be so broad as to elicit short nondescriptive answers such as "Not much," or "fine" or lengthy answers containing a mixture of relevant and tangential facts.

Close-ended questions allow the respondent to answer with a single word, such as yes or no, or with short phrases. Close-ended questions are useful for structuring the interview and obtaining an easily recordable answer. It is easier for children and adolescents who have limited cognitive abilities or language processing difficulties to answer close-ended rather than open-ended questions. Below are examples of close-ended questions.

What articles of clothing can the child remove independently?

Does the student cry when she does not get what she wants?

Are you responsible for managing a weekly allowance?

How long does your child sleep at night?

Occupational therapists and occupational therapy assistants may use a combination of close- and open-ended questions during the interview to get short answers to specific questions as well more detailed answers to more general questions. Sometimes they follow a script containing a series of specifically worded questions; other times they refer to an outline of general topics to covers. The script allows for consistency among the interviews; the outline allows for flexibility within the interview. However, regardless of whether the occupational therapists or occupational therapy assistants ask open- or close-ended questions, or follow a specific script or general outline, they must word questions in a developmentally appropriate, understandable, nonjudgmental, and nondirective manner. Developmentally appropriate and understandable questions match the cognitive, social, and chronological levels of the respondent. A question such as "Show me your dolls" may be appropriate to ask a 3-year-old child; a questions such as "How does the child play with toys and with the other children?" may be appropriate to ask the preschool teacher. Nonjudgmental and nondirective questions allow the respondent to answer honestly without expectations about what that answer should be. "Tell me what you feel when riding the school bus" is an example of a nonjudgmental and nondirective question. In contrast, "Why can't you sit still like the other children when riding the school bus?" can be interpreted as a judgmental question. "You like to ride the school bus, don't you?" can be interpreted as a directive question.

Throughout the evaluation process, occupational therapists and occupational therapy assistants are to establish a positive relationship with the child, adolescent, and family members through the therapeutic use of self. This means that occupational therapists and occupational therapy assistants are to use their personal and professional traits to interact with the children, adolescents, and their families in an open, honest, collaborative, empathic, and supportive manner (Peloquin, 2003). They are to interact in a respectful manner by considering how the culture of the children, adolescents, and other people interviewed frames the interview process. A few pointers to consider:

- Before beginning the interview, find out which family members should be included in the discussions

- Before beginning the interview, find out if the people wish to be addressed by their first name, last name, or titles
- Before beginning the interview, find out if there are cultural norms for the types of questions to ask
- Before asking the interview questions, find out if it is more appropriate to engage in social conversation, and share some food and drink, or to ask the questions immediately
- Determine if it is best to first observe or engage in a success-oriented activity with the child before asking questions
- If using an interpreter, direct the questions and eye gaze to the person being interviewed, not the interpreter
- Ask for clarification rather than assume understanding of what is said or seen
- Pace the rate of speech and adjust the vocabulary level to that of the person being interviewed
- Consider how body language, dress, and phrasing of questions promotes openness and trust, or generates caution and mistrust
- Consider if and what types of physical contact and humor are acceptable
- Consider how much personal information to reveal to promote open dialogue, but not distract from the intent of the interview

Measurement Tools

Measurement tools are instruments for systematically gathering and recording information about the child or adolescent. The information is gathered by following a prescribed procedure for:

- Observing specific behaviors demonstrated by the child or adolescent and the context in which these behaviors occur
- Interviewing the child, adolescent, or their caregivers and others professionals who work with them
- Obtaining written responses from the child or adolescent
- Completing questionnaires about the child or adolescent

Often, measurement tools use a combination of two or three of these methods. The *Developmental Test of Visual Perception* is an observation based tool to measure visual perception and visual motor skills of children ages 4 to 10 years (Hammill, Pearson, & Voress, 1998). The *Gardner Social Development* Scale is a questionnaire designed to gather information from parents about the social skills of their children (Gardner & Gardner, 1994). The *Pediatric Evaluation of Disability Inventory (PEDI)* is an example of a measurement tool that uses a combination of structured interviews and observations to assess self-care, functional mobility, and social functioning of children ages 6 months through 7 years who have significant motor or cognitive disabilities (Haley, Coster, Ludlow, Haltiwanger, & Andrellos, 1998).

Manuals that frequently accompany the measurement tool provide written directions regarding administration, recording, and scoring procedures (Hinojosa et al., 2005). They specify competency standards a person must demonstrate before administering the measurement tool. To administer some measurement tools, the person must: understand its purpose and psychometric properties, have knowledge of child and adolescent development, and become familiar with the administration and scoring procedures by reading the manual and practicing the procedures. To administer other measurement tools, the person must complete a required course, pass a written and practical examination, and become certified.

Unless the measurement tool manual specifies how and what modifications are permissible, occupational therapists and occupational therapy assistants are to adhere to the administration, recording, and scoring procedures. Doing otherwise invalidates the resulting scores. Specifically, they are to administer all of the sections, not just some of the subsections of the measurement tool, and to adhere to the prescribed verbal, written, and demonstrative directions, not modifications of the directions. They are to administer the measurement tool only to those children and adolescents for whom it was intended, for example only to children and adolescents within the specified age range.

In addition, they are to guard against inadvertently cueing the children and adolescents as to expected behaviors and correct answers. Smiling and praising a child every time he gets a correct answer, while remaining silent or encouraging the child to try again every time he gets an incorrect answer unintentionally lets the child know how he is performing and what he might do to modify his responses. Occupational therapists and occupational therapy assistants are to be cautious about scoring errors and personal biases that too easily or too harshly rate the child's or adolescent's performance. Numerous studies have found that children who are viewed as attractive and friendly are more likely to benefit from positive scoring biases; whereas, children who are viewed as unattractive and unfriendly are more likely to confront negative scoring biases (Vander Zanden et al., 2003).

Finally, occupational therapists and occupational therapy assistants are to be cognizant of the floor and ceiling effects inherent in some measurement tools. The **floor effect** is the lower limit of the test where there is not room to detect further deterioration. The **ceiling effect** is the upper limit of the test where there is no room to detect further improvements (Finch et al., 2002). Tests that measure visual perceptual skills and visual motor skills often have a floor effect. That is, they do not distinguish well between young children who have and do not have visual motor and visual processing skills, because young children need to get only a few of the easiest items correct to be considered as functioning within the expected norm. Tests that measure motor development in older children often have a ceiling effect. That is, they contain so few challenging items that the older children are likely to get most of the items correct, even if they are not functioning within expected norms.

In most settings, occupational therapists assume the responsibility for administering and scoring the measurement tools. In some settings, occupational therapy assistants may administer some of them, after demonstrating service competency. Occupational therapy assistants are expected to be able to use the results from the measurement tools to provide appropriate occupational therapy interventions. Table 9.3■ provides a list of measurement tools commonly used when working with children and adolescents. The first column lists the name and author of the measurement tool. The section column highlights its purpose. The third column provides information about the type of data collected, and the fourth column lists the age range of the children for whom the measurement tool is appropriate. Some of these measurement tools are used to gather information about the occupations of the children and adolescents. Others address the children's and adolescents' performance skill, performance patterns, and the context affecting the occupation.

■ Table 9.3
Measurement Tools

MEASUREMENT TOOL AND AUTHOR	PURPOSE (OT DOMAIN)	TYPE OF DATA (NORM REFERENCED, CRITERION REFERENCED, STANDARDIZED, NONSTANDARDIZED)	AGE RANGE	AUTHORS, CORPORATION, CITY, STATE
Activities Scale for Kids (ASK)	Self-report measure of the affect of a musculoskeletal disorder on personal care, dressing, eating and drinking, locomotion, stairs, play, and standing	Criterion referenced	5 years to 15 years	N. L. Young, The Hospital for Sick Children, 555 University Avenue, Toronto, Ontario, Canada M5G 1X8
Ages and Stages Questionnaire	Communication, gross-motor, fine-motor, problem-solving, and personal-social	Norm referenced	Birth to 5 years	Diane Bricker, Ph.D., & Jane Squires, Ph.D.; Brookes Publishing, Baltimore, MD
Alberta Infant Motor Scales (AIMS)	Motor development	Norm referenced	Birth to 18 months	Martha C. Piper, Ph.D. & Johanna Darrah, M.S.C., P.T., The Psychological Corporation, San Antonio, TX
Assessment of Motor and Process Skills (AMPS)	Motor and process skills in ADLs	Standardized	3 years and older	Ann Fisher, AMPS International, Hampton Falls, NH
Battelle Developmental Inventory (BDI)	Personal-social, adaptive, motor, communication and cognition	Standardized	Birth to 8 years	Jean Newborg, Riverside Publishing, Itasca, IL
Bayley Scales of Infant Development III	Cognition, language, social skills, gross motor and fine motor skills, sensory integration, perceptual-motor integration, orientation with environment and objects	Norm referenced	Infants 1 to 42 months	Nancy Bayley, PhD, Harcourt Assessment, San Antonio, TX
Bruininks-Oseretsky Test of Motor Proficiency 2	Gross motor and fine motor skills	Norm referenced	4.5 to 14.5 years	Robert H. Bruininks, & Brett D. Bruininks, AGS Publishing, Circle Pines, MN
Child Health Questionnaire	Physical, social, and emotional well-being as perceived by parent or guardian	Norm referenced	5 years and older	Jeanne M. Landgraf, & John E. Ware, Jr., HealthAct Inc., Boston, MA

Instrument	Areas Assessed	Type	Age Range	Authors/Publisher
Childhood Autism Rating Scale	Observation of child's behavior, ability, and characteristics, and information from parent & other reports to indicate how much child's behavior deviates from typically developing child of the same age	Norm referenced	Children over 2 years with autism	Eric Schopler, Ph.D., Robert J. Reichler, M.D., & Barbara Rochen Renner, PhD. AGS Publishing, Circle Pines, MN
Children's Assessment of Participation and Enjoyment and Preferences for Activities of Children (CAPE/PAC)	Occupational performance, participation and preferences in daily activities outside of mandated school activities	Criterion referenced; standardized	6 to 18 years	Gillian King, Mary Law, Susanne King, Patricia Hurley, Peter Rosenbaum, Steven Hanna, Marilyn Kertoy, Nancy Young, Harcourt Assessment, Inc., San Antonio, TX 78259
Canadian Occupational Performance Measure (COPM)	Occupational performance	Criterion referenced; standardized	Children of all ages	Mary Law, Sue Baptiste, Anne Carswell, Mary Ann McColl, Helene Polatajko, Nancy Pollock, Canadian Occupational Therapy Association, Ottawa, Ontario, Canada
Denver Developmental Screening Test (Denver-II)	Personal-social, fine motor adaptive, language, and gross motor skills	Standardized screening	1 month to 6 years of age	W. K. Frankenburg; Josiah Dodds; Phillip Archer; Beverly Bresnick; Patrick Maschka; Norma Edelman; Howard Shapiro, Denver Developmental Materials, Denver, CO
Developmental Test of Visual Motor Integration	Visual perception, motor coordination	Norm referenced; standardized	3 to 8 years of age (short form) and 3 to 18 years of age (long form)	Keith E. Beery, PhD, Norman A. Buktenica, and Natasha A. Beery, Pearson Assessments, Minneapolis, MN
Developmental Test of Visual Perception	Visual perceptual skills: eye motor coordination, figure ground, constancy of shape, position in space, spatial relationships	Norm referenced; standardized	4 to 10 years of age	Don Hammill, Nils Pearson, & Judith Voress, Pro-Ed, Austin, TX

■ Table 9.3
Measurement Tools (cont.)

Measurement Tool and Author	Purpose (OT domain)	Type of Data (Norm Referenced, Criterion Referenced, Standardized, Nonstandardized)	Age Range	Authors, Corporation, City, State
Early Coping Inventory	Sensorimotor organization, reactive behaviors, self-initiated behaviors	Standardized	4 to 36 months of age	Dr. Shirley Zeitlin, Dr. G. Gordon Williamson, & Margery Szczepanski, Scholastic Testing Service, Inc., Bensenville, IL
Erhardt Developmental Prehension Assessment	Arm & hand development	Standardized	Children who have cerebral palsy or other neurodevelopmental disorders (all ages and cognitive levels)	Erhardt, Rhoda P, Therapy Skill Builders—A Division of The Psychological Corporation, San Antonio, TX
Erhardt Developmental Vision Assessment	Motor components of visual development, cognitive levels	Standardized	Individuals of all ages and cognitive levels with neurodevelopmental disorders	Erhardt, Rhoda P, Therapy Skill Builders—A Division of The Psychological Corporation, San Antonio, TX
Evaluation Tool of Children's Handwriting (ETCH)	Cursive and manuscript handwriting, legibility, pencil grasp and pressure, hand preference, manipulative skills with writing tools, and classroom performance	Criterion referenced	Children grades 1 through 6	Susie Amundson, Ph.D., OTR/L, FAOTA O.T., Kids, Inc., Homer, AK
First STEP: Screening Tools for Evaluating Preschoolers	Cognition, communication, motor, social-emotional, and adaptive behavior	Standardized	2 years 9 months to 6 years 2 months	Lucy Miller, Harcourt Assessment, Inc., San Antonio, TX
Gesell Preschool Test	Motor, adaptive, language, and personal/social areas	Norm referenced	2.5–6 years	Jacqueline Haines, Louise Bates Ames, Clyde Gillespie, Modern Learning Press, Inc., Rosemont, NJ
Gross Motor Function Measure (GMFM)	Gross motor functions in children with cerebral palsy	Criterion referenced; standardized	5 months to 16 years	D. Russell, P. Rosenbaum, L. Avery, & M. Lane, CanChild: Centre for Childhood Disability Research, McMaster University, Hamilton, Ontario, Canada

Instrument	Description	Type	Age Range	Author/Publisher
Hawaii Early Learning Profile	Cognition, language, gross-motor, fine-motor, social-emotional, self-help, regulatory, sensory organization	Curriculum based assessment, nonstandardized	Birth to 3 years	Setsu Furuno, Katherine O'Reilly, Carol Hosaka, Takayo Inatsuka, Barbara Zeisloft-Falbey, & Toney Allman, VORT Corporation, Palo Alto, CA
Home Observation for Measurement of the Environment (HOME)	Daily routine, home environment	Standardized	Birth to 14 years	Bettye Caldwell & Robert Bradley, Home Inventory LLC, Little Rock, AR
Infant-Toddler Developmental Assessment	Gross and fine motor, Cognition, language/communication, self-help skills, psychosocial, and emotional	Standardized	Birth to 36 months	Sally Provence, Joanna Erikson, Susan Vater, Saro Palmeri, Riverside Publishing, Itasca, IL
Infant/Toddler Sensory Profile	Sensory processing on functional performance	Standardized	Birth to 3 years	Winnie Dunn, PhD, OTR, FAOTA, Harcourt Assessment, San Antonio, TX
Miller Assessment for Preschoolers (MAP)	Measures sensory and motor abilities	Norm referenced	Children ages 2 years 9 months to 5 years 8 months	Lucy Jane Miller, PsychCorp, San Antonio, TX
Motor-Free Visual Perception Test (MVPT-3)	Visual perception	Norm referenced; standardized	Individuals 4 years to 70 years of age	Ronald Colarusso, & Donald Hammill, Pro-Ed, Inc., Austin, TX
Parenting Stress Index	Child domain/parent domain; assesses stressful parent-child systems and impact of intervention	Norm referenced	Parents of children ranging in age from 1 month to 12 years	Richard Abidin, EdD, Psychological Assessment Resources, Inc., Lutz, FL
Peabody Developmental Motor Scales	Gross motor and fine motor skills	Norm referenced	Birth through 5 years 11 months	Rhonda Folio & Rebecca Fewell, Pro-Ed, Inc, Austin, TX
Pediatric Activity Card Sort (PACS)	Self rate of frequency of participation in personal care, school/productivity, hobbies/social, and sports activities	Criterion referenced	6 years to 12 years	Canadian Occupational Therapy Association, CAOT Publications, ACE CTTC, Building 3400-1125, Colonel By Drive, Ottawa, Ontario, Canada K1S 5R1, www.caot.org

■ Table 9.3
Measurement Tools (cont.)

Measurement Tool and Author	Purpose (OT domain)	Type of Data (Norm referenced, Criterion referenced, Standardized, Nonstandardized)	Age Range	Authors, Corporation, City, State
Pediatric Evaluation of Disability Inventory (PEDI)	Social function, self-care, mobility	Standardized	Children between 6 months and 7.5 years	Stephen Haley, Wendy Coster, Larry Ludlow, Jane Haltiwanger, & Peter Andrellos, Center for Rehabilitation Effectiveness, Boston University, Boston, MA
Pediatric Interest Profiles: Survey of Play for Children and Adolescents	Assists in identify risk of play related problems for children and adolescents; collects information on participation in activities and individual's feelings and competence while performing activities	Standardized	Children and adolescents between 6 and 21 years	Alexis Henry, Harcourt Assessment, Inc., San Antonio, TX
Posture and Fine Motor Assessment of Infants	Posture, fine motor skills	Criterion referenced	Infants 2 to 12 months	Jane Case-Smith, & Rosemarie Bigsby, Harcourt Assessment, Inc., San Antonio, TX
Quality of Upper Extremity Skills Test (QUEST)	Dissociated movement, grasp, protective extension, and weight bearing	Standardized	18 months to 8 years	DeMatteo, C., Law, M., Russell, D., Pollock, N., Rosenbaum, P., & Walter, S., Can Child: Center for Childhood Disability Research, McMaster University, Hamilton, Ontario, Canada
School Function Assessment	Participation, task supports, activity performance	Criterion referenced; standardized	Children in elementary school	Wendy Coster, Theresa Deeney, Jane Haltiwanger, Stephen Haley, Harcourt Assessment, Inc., San Antonio, TX
Sensory Integration and Praxis Tests (SIPT)	Sensory processing of perception and praxis	Norm referenced; standardized	4 to 9 years	Jean Ayres, Ph.D., Western Psychological Services (WPS), Los Angeles, CA

Assessment	Areas Measured	Type	Age Range	Author/Publisher
Sensory Profile	Measure children's responses to sensory events in daily life	Standardized	3 to 10 years	Winnie Dunn, Ph.D, OTR, FAOTA, Harcourt Assessment, Inc., San Antonio, TX
Test of Sensory Functions in Infants (TSFI)	Sensory processing and reactivity	Standardized	Infants 4 to 18 months	Georgia A. DeGangi, Ph.D., OTR, & Stanley I. Greenspan, M.D., Western Psychological Services (WPS), Los Angeles, CA
Toddler and Infant Motor Evaluation (TIME)	Motor	Norm referenced; standardized	4 to 18 months to 3 1/2 years	Lucy Miller & Gale Roid, Harcourt Assessment, Inc., San Antonio, TX
Transdisciplinary Play-Based Assessment (TPBA)	Cognitive, social-emotional, communication and language, and sensorimotor	Standardized	Birth to 6 years	Toni Linder, Ed.D, Brookes Publishing, Baltimore, MD
Vineland Adaptive Behavior Scales	Communication, Daily Living Skills, Socialization and Motor Skills	Standardized	Birth to 18 years	Sara S. Sparrow, David A. Balla, & Domenic Cichetti, AGS Publishing, Circle Pines, MN
WeeFIM	Self-Care, Mobility, and Cognition	Norm referenced	6 months to 7 years	B.B. Hamilton & C.U. Granger, Uniform Data System for Medical Rehabilitation, Amherst, NY

Compiled by Amy Mateer, OTS Towson University.

SUMMARY

The occupational therapy evaluation is a comprehensive process that involves the collection and analysis of information necessary to determine appropriate and effective interventions for children and adolescents. Evaluations are essential for establishing a baseline to describe current level of performance, focusing the direction of occupational therapy intervention, and providing justification for the need for and reimbursement of occupational therapy services. The American Occupational Therapy Association has published guidelines regarding the roles and responsibilities of occupational therapists and occupational therapy assistants during the evaluation process.

The evaluation process involves two parts: the development of an occupational profile and the analysis of occupational performance. Terms such as screening, initial evaluation, and re-evaluation differentiate among the various times that formal evaluations occur. Clinical reasoning, based on occupation and nonoccupation theories and conceptual models, guides the judgments made during the evaluation process. When conducting the evaluation it is crucial to be sensitive to the children's and adolescents' developmental levels, cultural context, and the external context where the evaluation occurs.

Specific assessments are used to gather this information during the evaluation process. Some of these assessments are nonstandardized. Nonstandardized assessments do not have a specified administration, content, or scoring procedure to follow. They also do not have a specific physical or emotional environment where they must be administered. They are relatively easy to administer and can be tailored to respond to needs of the children and adolescents and the context where the assessment is conducted. Other assessments are standardized. They have established administration, recording, and scoring procedures. They are based on established norms or criteria that allow comparison of performance across individuals. Norm-referenced assessments use norms to compare the performance of an individual to that which is typically expected within the normal population. Criterion-referenced assessments use the criteria to compare the performance of an individual in relation to established standard or level of expectation of performance.

Types of assessments include chart reviews, observations, interviews, and measurement tools. Through chart reviews, occupational therapists and occupational therapy assistants can collect essential information about the child or adolescent that was obtained and recorded by other professionals. Observations allow the occupational therapists and occupational therapy assistants to record information about the performance capacities of the children and adolescents in a multitude of situations and settings, particularly when standardized assessments procedures may not apply. Observations can occur in structured or natural environments.

Assessment information also can be gathered through interviews with the children and adolescents, their family members and caregiver, and other professionals who work with them. Before beginning the interview, it is important to review the reports already written about the child or adolescent. Doing so helps to ensure that the interview builds upon existing information rather than repeats questions already asked. Occupational therapists and occupational therapy assistants may use a combination of close and open-ended questions during the interview to get short answers to specific questions and more detailed answers to more general questions. Sometimes they follow a script containing a series of specifically worded questions; other times they refer to an outline of general topics to covers. The questions asked must be worded in a developmentally appropriate, understandable, nonjudgmental, and nondirective manner.

Measurement tools are instruments for systematically gathering and recording information about the child or adolescent. Some of these measurement tools are used to gather information about the occupations of the children and adolescents. Others address the children's and adolescents' performance skills, performance patterns, and the context affecting the occupation. Manuals that frequently accompany the measurement tool provide written directions regarding these administration, recording, and scoring procedures, as well as the specific competency standards a person must demonstrate before administering the measurement. In most settings, occupational therapists assume the responsibility for administering and scoring the measurement tools. In some settings, occupational therapy assistants may administer some of them, after demonstrating service competency. Unless the measurement tool manual specifies how and what modifications are permissible, occupational therapists and occupational therapy assistants are to adhere to the published administration, recording, and scoring procedures. Doing otherwise invalidates the resulting scores.

REVIEWING KEY POINTS

1. What are the two parts of an occupational therapy evaluation and what type of information is gathered during them?
2. Explain the similarities and differences in the roles of the occupational therapist and the occupational therapy assistant when conducting an evaluation.
3. What is the difference between an evaluation and an assessment?
4. List and describe the different kinds of assessments.
5. Distinguish between standardized and nonstandardized assessments.
6. Explain the value of conducting an observation in a natural and in a structured setting.
7. Explain the difference between open-ended and close-ended questions.
8. Explain cautions that should be observed when conducting an interview.
9. Explain the floor and ceiling effect in some measurement tools.
10. Explain cautions that should be observed when using a measurement tool.

APPLYING KEY CONCEPTS

1. Calculate the age of a child who was born on May 21, 2000 and who is participating in occupational therapy evaluation on March 6, 2005.
2. Use Figure 9.1 to interview an adolescent who has just procured part time work. Record and critique the interview. Ask a classmate to critique the interviewing skills.
3. Observe an elementary age child for 45 minutes. Use Figure 9.2 to record the observations. Use objective, observable, and measurable terms. Ask a classmate to critique the language used for recording the observations.
4. Write a list of five close-ended questions and five open-ended questions to use when interviewing a 12-year-old student about his school day. Ask a classmate to review those questions, and circle those that might be interpreted as judgmental or directive. Rewrite those questions.
5. Investigate three different measurement tools for children and adolescents. List the materials contained in each of the measurement tools. Explain the purpose and scoring procedures for each of these measurement tools. Explain the qualifications necessary to administer the measurement tool.

REFERENCES

American Occupational Therapy Association (2002). Occupational therapy practice framework: Domain and process. *American Journal of Occupational Therapy, 56,* 609–639.

American Occupational Therapy Association (2004a). Guidelines for supervision, roles, and responsibilities during the delivery of occupational therapy services. *American Journal of Occupational Therapy, 58* (November/December).

American Occupational Therapy Association (2004b). Occupational therapy services in early intervention and school-based programs. *American Journal of Occupational Therapy, 58* (November/December).

American Occupational Therapy Association (2005a). Model State Regulation for Supervision, Roles, and Responsibilities during the Delivery of Occupational Therapy Services. (Available from the State Affairs Group, American Occupational Therapy Association, 4720 Montgomery Lane, PO Box 31220, Bethesda, MD 20824-1220.)

American Occupational Therapy Association (2005b). Standards of Practice for Occupational Therapy. *American Journal of Occupational Therapy, 59* (November/December), 663–665.

American Occupational Therapy Association (ND). Occupational Therapy Practice Framework: Domain and Process (2nd ed.). draft.

Bayley, N. (2006). *Bayley Scale of Infant Development III.* San Antonio, TX: Harcourt Assessment.

Crepeau, E., Cohn, E., & Schell, B. (2003). *Willard and Spackman's occupational therapy* (10th ed.). Philadelphia: Lippincott, Williams & Wilkins.

Coster, W., Denney, T., Haltiwanger, J., & Haley, S. (1998). *School Functional Assessment (SFA).* San Antonio, TX:. The Psychological Corporation.

Dunn, W. (1997). *The Sensory Profile.* San Antonio, TX: Psychological Corporation, Therapy Skill Builders.

Finch, E., Brooks, D., Stratford, P. W., & Mayo, N. E. (2002). *Physical rehabilitation outcome measures: A guide to enhanced decision making* (2nd ed.). Baltimore: Lippincott, Williams & Wilkins.

Folio, R., & Fewell, R. (2000). *Peabody Development Motor Scales 2.* Austin, TX: Pro-Ed.

Frankenberg, W. K., Dodds, J., Archer, P. et al. (1992). *The Denver II Training Manual.* Denver, CO: Developmental Materials, Inc.

Gardner, M., & Gardner, A. (1994). *Gardner Social Development Scale.* Hydesville, CA: Psychological and Educational Publications.

Haley, S., Coster, W., Ludlow, L., Haltiwnager, J., & Andrellos, P. (1992). *Pediatric Evaluation of Disability Inventory.* San Antonio, TX: Psychological Corp.

Hammill, D., Pearson, N. A., & Voress, J. K. (1998). *Developmental Test of Visual Perception (DVPT-2).* Austin, TX: ProEd.

Hinojosa, J., Kramer, P., & Crist, P. (2005). (Eds.). *Evaluation: Obtaining and interpreting data* (2nd ed.). Bethesda, MD: AOTA Press.

Humbert, T. K. (2004). The use of clinical reasoning skills by experienced occupational therapy assistants. Dissertation thesis. The Pennsylvania State University.

Law, M., Baum, C., & Dunn, W. (2001). *Measuring occupational performance:Supporting best practice in occupational therapy.* Thorofare, NJ: SLACK.

Lyman, H. B. (1998). *Test scores and what they mean* (6th ed.). Boston: Allyn and Bacon.

Mattingly, C., & Hayes Fleming, M. (1994). *Clinical reasoning: Forms of inquiry in therapeutic practice.* Philadelphia: F. A. Davis.

Peloquin, S. M. (2003). The therapeutic relationship. Manifestations and challenges in occupational therapy. In E. B. Crepeau, E. S. Cohn, & B. Schell (Eds.), *Willard and Spackman's occupational* therapy (10th ed., pp. 157–170). Philadelphia: Lippincott Williams & Wilkins.

Schell, B., & Cervero, R. (1993). Clinical reasoning in occupational therapy: An integrative review. *American Journal of Occupational Therapy, 47*(7), 605–610.

Silverlake, A. C. (1999). *Comprehending test manuals: A guide and workbook.* Los Angeles: Pyrczak.

Vander Zanden, J., Crandell, T., & Crandell, C. (2003). *Human Development* (7th ed. revised). Boston: McGraw-Hill.

Wells, S., & Black, R. (2000). *Cultural competency for the health professional.* Bethesda, MD: American Occupational Therapy Association.

World Health Organization (2001). *International classification of functioning, disability, and health (ICF).* Geneva, Switzerland: Author.

Chapter 10

Interventions for Children and Adolescents: General Principles

Margaret J. Pendzick

Key Terms

Adapt
Backward chaining
Consultation process
Create
Depth perception
Downgrade
Establish
Extrinsic feedback
Far transfer
Figure ground
Form constancy
Form perception
Forward chaining
Full physical assistance
Generalization
Gesture
Hand-over-hand assistance
Hand-to-mouth pattern
Imitate
Intermediate transfer
Intrinsic feedback
Knowledge of performance (KP)
Knowledge of results (KR)
Maintain
Memory notebook

Metacognition
Mirror image
Modeling
Multicontext treatment approach
Near transfer
Observational prompt
Occupation-based activity
Parallel image
Partial physical assistance
Position in space
Preparatory methods
Prevent
Promote
Purposeful activity
Restore
Self awareness
Spatial perception
Therapeutic use of occupation
    and activities
Therapeutic use of self
Topographical orientation
Transfer
Upgrade
Verbal directions
Verbal cues

Verbal hints	Visual closure
Verbal prompts	Visual discrimination
Verbal rehearsal	Visual imagery
Very far transfer	Visual memory
Visual attention	Written directions

Objectives

- Understand the goal of occupational therapy interventions.
- Understand that interventions may be directed to the person, task, or environment.
- Identify types of occupational therapy interventions and factors that influence their selection.
- Explain the use of preparatory activities, occupations, and the therapeutic use of self in OT intervention.
- Describe and apply teaching principles used in occupational therapy.

INTRODUCTION

After an occupational therapy evaluation is completed and it is determined that intervention is required, client-centered outcomes goals and objectives are defined. Interventions are based on what is important to the client and what the client needs to do. When working with children, the client also involves the caregivers such as family members. Interventions are used to strengthen existing capacities and to develop new capacities. Intervention plans need to be designed carefully in collaboration with the children, adolescents, and their caregivers since the interventions may need to address the children's and adolescents' areas of occupation, performance skills, performance patterns, and body functions and structures. Intervention plans should be carefully designed to respect the occupational context of the children and adolescents, that is, their physical, social, cultural, temporal, virtual, and developmental context.

In order for intervention to be effective, however, it is necessary to consider a wide range of issues that affect intervention strategy selection. Regardless of the uniqueness of the outcome, there are general principles of intervention to consider when designing an intervention plan.

GOALS AND METHODS OF INTERVENTION

As identified in the Occupational Therapy Practice Framework, there may be different overarching goals for designing and implementing occupational therapy intervention (AOTA, 2002). These overarching goals were examined in Chapter 2 of this text. When working with children and adolescents overarching goals may focus on:

- Creating or promoting their ability to participate in daily life occupations
- Establishing, restoring, and maintaining their capacity to perform their occupations

- Modifying or adapting tasks and environments so that they can participate in their daily life tasks
- Preventing the development of barriers that limit their occupational participation
- Designing occupationally enriched environments (AOTA, 2002; Dunn, 2000).

It is important for the occupational therapist and the occupational therapy assistant to identify these goals, in collaboration with the children, adolescents, or their caregivers, since they influence intervention strategy choices. To illustrate these overarching goals and possible intervention methods, let's consider an example of Tonya, a girl whose occupations are challenged due to juvenile rheumatoid arthritis (JRA). Refer to Chapter 18 for further information on JRA. Since JRA is a chronic disease, different goals are considered at various stages of the disease process and at different ages of the child.

- **Create** or **promote:** Adhering to physician's advise to avoid physical activities that increase stress to the joints, the occupational therapist, and the occupational therapy assistant help Tonya and her family choose age appropriate recreational activities that promote Tonya's physical and social well-being.
- **Establish** or **restore:** Following an extended stay in the hospital, the occupational therapy assistant, in collaboration with the occupational therapist, design an age-appropriate exercise program and a series of craft activities to restore Tonya's muscle strength and endurance.
- **Maintain:** In order to maintain Tonya's present joint movement, the occupational therapist designs a hand splint to wear at night that the occupational therapy assistant constructs.
- **Adapt:** Upon entering first grade, Tonya's intervention goal is to be as independent as possible in her classroom environment. The occupational therapy assistant installs larger handles and knobs so that Tonya can open the doors and cabinets independently.
- **Prevent:** In order to prevent further joint damage, the occupational therapy assistant, under the supervision of the occupational therapist, instructs Tonya and her high school home and family science teacher in joint protection techniques to utilize during cooking tasks.

Reflecting upon the above examples, there are four different types of intervention approaches. These included **therapeutic use of self**, **therapeutic use of occupations and activities**, **consultation process**, and **education process.** For example, during construction of the night hand splints, the occupational therapy assistant answered Tonya's and her parent's questions and concerns about the splints. During the dialogue, the occupational therapy assistant used therapeutic use of self to encourage discussion to dispel current apprehensions about splints and understanding of the importance of use. Therapeutic use of occupations and activities are utilized within the home program of exercises and craft activities.

Also, these examples illustrate that the intervention is not directed always at the person. Rather, interventions also may be directed to the task or the environment, as appropriate. When providing a strengthening program and constructing a splint, the occupational therapy assistant directs the intervention to the person. By adapting the first grade classroom so that Tonya easily can access and manipulate classroom supplies, the occupational therapy assistant addresses the environment to affect the occupational outcome. In order to prevent further joint damage, the occupational therapy assistant instructs Tonya and her home and family science teacher in methods to alter the cooking task within the high school curriculum. The occupational therapist and the occupational therapy assistant utilize clinical reasoning to determine the best type of and direction for intervention. They take into consideration the task that needs to be accomplished and the context of where the task will be completed. The occupational therapist and occupational therapy assistant use evidence based practice principles and personal knowledge to determine what overarching goal is attainable and whether the outcome will best be achieved by addressing the person, task, or environment. The following sections consider the type of and directions for intervention in more detail.

Types of Intervention

As delineated in the Occupational Therapy Practice Framework (AOTA, 2002), there are four different types of intervention that are used in occupational therapy. Regardless of the practice setting, interventions can be categorized as one of the following: therapeutic use of self, therapeutic use of occupations and activities, consultation process, and education process. Referring to the overarching goals and methods for Tonya, each type of interventions is utilized. The following section discusses the types of interventions in more detail.

Therapeutic Use of Self

The occupational therapist and the occupational therapy assistant take a holistic view of an individual and family, recognize each individual and family as unique, and design specific interventions to meet their identified client outcomes. In the midst of intervention, occupational therapists and occupational therapy assistants often engage in therapeutic use of self. This is more than a friendly conversation, but a planned part of intervention. Based on judgment and personality (AOTA, 2002), dialog and interaction are used in a therapeutic way. For instance, when working in the home setting, the occupational therapy assistant notices that that the parent is disinterested in the therapy sessions. She discusses this with the mother to ascertain whether there is dissatisfaction with the focus of the occupational therapy intervention. The mother indicates that she is not dissatisfied, but that she is overwhelmed with taking care of the child and the rest of the family. The occupational therapy assistant asks insightful questions and allows the mother to talk about the problem and voice solutions. The mother comes to the conclusion that she needs to delegate some household responsibilities to other family members. With that resolved she begins to show more interest in the intervention session and willingly participates in a home program. Therapeutic use of self is an intervention that occupational therapists and occupational assistants incorporate into every aspect of intervention.

Therapeutic Use of Occupation and Activities

When working with children and adolescents, it is important to choose occupations and activities that are age, developmentally, and socially appropriate. Occupational therapists and occupational therapy assistants collaborate with the children and adolescents to select occupations and activities that are meaningful to them, and that focus on achieving specific outcomes. For instance, even though an adolescent may have limited hand skills and only can push a button, it would be more appropriate to help her learn to activate a switch on a video recorder than on an infant musical toy.

As identified in the Occupational Therapy Framework, occupational therapists and occupational therapy assistants use occupation-based interventions, **purposeful activity**, and **preparatory methods**. When working with children and adolescents

- Occupation-based interventions engage the child or adolescent in age appropriate and meaningful pursuits which address overall therapeutic goals. This type of approach requires an element of creativity in intervention planning and directly relates to the occupational profile developed during the evaluation. Because of the meaning attached to them, occupation-based interventions are unique to each individual and specific to the environment in which they are performed. For instance, if a teenager's goal is to increase social participation at school, an occupation-based intervention would be to investigate various school clubs and decide which ones to join. For a younger child whose lack of social participation skills interferes with his ability to join appropriate play groups during recess, an intervention might include the child requesting to join his peers in kickball and remaining a member of the group for five minutes.

- Purposeful activities permit the child or adolescent to participate in activities that will contribute to the overall attainment of the specific goal. Many times this requires the goal to be broken down into small steps so that each step can be achieved. For example, if independent dressing is a goal for a 5-year-old child, a purposeful activity would be to practice manipulating fasteners on a child sized doll or dress up clothes.

- Preparatory methods may be used prior to purposeful or occupation-based activities. In isolation, preparatory methods have no functional purpose but often need to be performed or applied before beginning a task. Consider the two above examples. The teenager who experiences high anxiety in groups engages in relaxation techniques prior to attending a social event. The 5-year-old, who had been burned in a house fire, performs finger stretching exercises before beginning to work on the fasteners. Both the adolescent and the child are engaged in preparatory activities that enable them to participate in the occupation-based and purposeful activity.

When planning an intervention session, the occupational therapist and the occupational therapy assistant choose activities and occupations that challenge without overwhelming the child or adolescent. Although practicing a skill is beneficial, intervention approaches should be planned so that the child or adolescent makes some gain after each session. In order to provide the correct challenge during an intervention session, the occupational therapy assistant may need to **upgrade** or **downgrade** an activity or occupation. For example, while working in the lunchroom with a group of children, the occupational therapy assistant notices that one boy is getting very frustrated opening his milk carton. In order to make the task easier but still allow him a measure of success, he downgrades the task by partially opening the carton and letting the child finish by himself. Another child easily scoops his applesauce with a spoon. He upgrades the scooping task by offering the child cereal and milk that easily can slip off the spoon. In both examples, the occupational therapy assistant makes slight changes in the activities so that the child is successful and correctly challenged for his present abilities.

Consultation Process

To best achieve particular outcomes, the occupational therapist and the occupational therapy assistant may engage in collaborative consultation with the client. Since this process involves dialogue and insight, consultation primarily involves an adult or adolescent. Consultation is an effective means of intervention when an outcome requires establishing a new habit or routine. Consultation frequently is used in the school setting.

Consultation is a collaborative and a multistep process. Consider how consultation would take place in the school setting.

- *Define the Problem:* An occupational therapy assistant, providing consultative services to a third grade special education teacher, has scheduled a monthly consultative meeting. The students in this class have cognitive limitations that affect their ability to accomplish their school related tasks. This month, the teacher indicates that the students need assistance in the lunchroom. She would like them to independently carry their trays from the end of the lunch line and sit down at the classroom designated lunch table.

- *Observe the Problem:* The occupational therapy assistant schedules a lunchtime observation to view the context of the problem. She takes notes on how each child carries the full tray, the distance from lunch line to table, and the distractions that occur while walking.

- *Discuss Solutions and Develop a Plan:* After discussing her observations and intervention strategies with the supervising occupational therapist, the occupational therapy assistant meets again with the teacher. She discusses a wide variety of solutions, including the use of some adaptive equipment, reconfiguration of the lunchroom table, and ways to decrease environmental distractions. The occupational therapy assistant engages the teacher in a collaborative discussion and agrees on what strategies to implement. In order to ensure consistency, a plan is written which includes specific steps, as appropriate.

- *Implement the Plan:* The occupational therapy assistant provides the necessary adaptive equipment and any necessary training to the classroom aide. The classroom aide implements the plan and records daily progress.

- *Review Progress:* At the next scheduled meeting, the teacher, aide, and occupational therapy assistant review the class progress. If necessary, the occupational therapy assistant makes adjustments to the plan, after consulting with the occupational therapist. The teacher determines whether she requires further occupational therapy consultation.

In order for the students to achieve the desired outcomes, the teacher, occupational therapist, and occupational therapy assistant recognize that the students need to establish new habits. Given their cognitive limitations, they require consistent instruction and frequent opportunities to practice and refine the skills. Because the classroom aide could assume these responsibilities, consultation by occupational therapy was an effective and appropriate intervention method to achieve the desired outcome.

Educational Process

Occupational therapists and occupational therapy assistants who work with children and adolescents often provide occupational therapy services that include educational process (AOTA, 2002). An occupational therapist might give an in-service to day care workers on how to encourage age appropriate self-care skills for 3 years. An occupational therapy assistant might instruct high school teachers in the proper chair and seat height for optimum keyboarding performance. In both of these instances, intervention took place although neither the occupational therapist nor the occupational therapy assistant worked directly with the children or adolescents. Rather, the occupational therapist and the occupational therapy assistant informed the teachers of insights or procedures that impact lives of the children and adolescents they encounter.

Direction of Intervention

Consistent with occupation-based conceptual models, interventions can be directed at the person, the environment, or the task. The occupational therapist, with the occupational therapy assistant's input, determines how to provide intervention best to achieve the determined occupation-based outcomes. The decision is based on a number of considerations, including information from the occupational profile, analysis of the occupations and activities required, and the contextual environment of the outcome. Clinical reasoning determines what direction of intervention will impact the successful achievement of the child's or the adolescent's occupation-based outcomes. In the following sections, let's consider each of the intervention directions.

Interventions Directed at the Person

During the evaluation process, the occupational therapist determines the strengths and challenges of the child or adolescent and decides if interventions directed towards performance skills, performance patterns, body functions, or body structures successfully will achieve the determined occupation-based goals. As identified by the Occupational Therapy Practice Framework (AOTA, 2002) and consistent with ICF classifications, performance skills include motor, processing, and communication/interaction skills, while cognition and perception are classified under mental body functions.

Motor Skills.   As defined by the Occupational Therapy Practice Framework (AOTA, 2002), this category includes small units of observable action categorized according to posture, mobility, coordination, strength and effort, and energy. If the evaluation results indicate that a desired outcome best can be achieved by directing intervention to these performance skills, an intervention plan, based on a chosen model of practice, might include activities that improve strength, coordination, or posture so that the child or adolescent is able to complete an area of occupation such as dressing or grooming. Time and effort is spent to improve the motor skills directly so that the child or adolescent can meet the desired occupation-based outcomes.

Processing Skills.   As defined by the Occupational Therapy Practice Framework (AOTA, 2002), processing skills are small units of observable action categorized according to the energy, knowledge, temporal organization, spatial organization, and adaptation used while completing a daily life task. An intervention plan directed toward developing or strengthening these performance skills might focus on helping the child or adolescent to inquire about, choose, organize, and use the appropriate school supplies to complete a classroom assignment. The intervention plan might also foster the ability of the child or adolescent to notice, accommodate to, and respond to nonverbal and perceptual cues in the classroom environment to initiate and terminate classroom assignments at the designated times.

Communication/Interaction Skills.   At times, children or adolescents may have immature or ineffective interaction performance skills that interfere with their ability to complete social interaction. For instance, a school age child may have difficulty playing with children at recess and become physically aggressive when he does not always win while playing an age appropriate game. Occupational therapy intervention may be designed to teach the child nonviolent ways to express his anger. The outcomes of the intervention are directed toward providing the child with performance skills to handle stressful situations. Through intervention, the child develops new interactions, performance patterns, and habits. The child acquires coping skills to handle his anger and learns how to use those new skills in everyday situations.

Mental Body Functions.   The ability to process information involves both cognition and perception, as well as other mental functions. Although occupational therapy is not able directly to affect one's innate cognitive ability, improvement in the way information is processed so that functional skills can be accomplished is often an identified outcome of intervention. Specific therapeutic intervention often is directed to four visual-cognitive functions:

- **Visual memory**, which includes both short and long term memory
- **Visual attention**, which includes alertness, selective attention, visual vigilance, and divided attention
- **Visual discrimination**, which involves being able to recognize, match, and categorize differences in visual features
- **Visual imagery**, which involves visualizing objects, actions, and ideas without really seeing them (Schneck, 2005).

Visual discrimination skills are used to detect difference between objects and spatial relationships. Object or **form perception** can be classified as:

- **Form constancy**, which recognizes that a form is the same regardless of size, position, or background
- **Visual closure**, which is the ability to identify a form even though it is incompletely drawn
- **Figure ground**, which is the ability to identify an object within a distracting background

Spatial perception involves the following abilities:

- **Position in space**, which is the ability to recognize the direction that an object is turned
- **Depth perception**, which is the ability to judge the distance between two objects
- **Topographical orientation**, which is the ability to determine a route to a location (Schneck, 2005).

Based on the model of practice chosen, intervention strategies may create activities that allow the child or adolescent to acquire the ability or to establish compensatory strategies. Either approach provides intervention directed to the individual person to develop skills to overcome the deficit area and thereby be able to perform the desired occupation-based outcome.

Interventions Directed at the Task

Occupational therapists and occupational therapy assistants working with children and adolescents may find that interventions directed to the task achieve the determined occupation-based outcomes. For instance, the occupational therapy assistant may work with a first grade child whose occupations are challenged due to congenital anomalies of the hand and who is unable to manipulate the fasteners on his coat. Since the determined occupation-based goal is to enable the child to become independent in all school ADL skills, the occupational therapy assistant installs a larger zipper and zipper pull so that the child can zip and unzip independently. The task has been altered in a way that the child is able to successfully perform an age-appropriate ADL skill.

Interventions Directed at the Environment

Interventions also can be directed to the environment. In the previous example of the first grader, the occupational therapy assistant may discuss ways to adapt the classroom environment so that the child can retrieve classroom supplies independently, access the computer, and write at the board.

TEACHING PRINCIPLES

During the intervention process, occupational therapists and occupational therapy assistants often give instructions to the child, adolescent, or family. In order to provide optimum instruction, the occupational therapist and occupational therapy assistant consider which approach is most appropriate for the individual and the desired outcome. There is a wide variety of teaching strategies to consider and apply. The following section examines different teaching techniques and considers when and where to implement these strategies.

Context

Context plays an important part in intervention teaching strategies. Occupation-based outcomes involve performance of a skill in contexts specific to the child or adolescent. Desired outcomes often require performance of the same skill in a variety of settings and with a variety of materials or **generalization** of the skill. For example, even though an adolescent learns to set a table at home, he can generalize the skills and set restaurant tables as a busboy. A kindergartener initially may learn to tie school gym shoes but generalizes the skill to tie other types of shoe laces, along with bows on packages.

When working toward generalization of a skill, it is necessary to vary the setting and activity to allow the child or adolescent to learn to **transfer** the skill to new situations (Toglia, 2003). Based on cognitive and learning research, the **multicontext treatment approach** (Toglia) considers the complexity of situation and how multiple contexts influence one's ability to generalize a skill. Although this approach was designed to address cognitive difficulties in individuals with brain injuries, it identifies different issues related to generalization that could be used during any intervention plan. Toglia suggests that there are four types of transfers: **near transfer, intermediate transfer, far transfer,** and **very far transfer**. The different types are based on the number of changes in context and materials that an individual encounters in order to generalize a skill. In order to understand the different transfer levels, let's consider the example of a child standing at a table and finger painting.

- A near transfer of the skill would be for the child to stand at an easel and paint with a brush. The child has not changed his posture but the surface is now vertical rather than horizontal. The paint still is being applied to paper but the child now grasps a brush and strokes across the paper.

- An intermediate transfer would be for the child to sit down at a table and spread butter on French toast. He now grasps a new object to spread the butter.

His posture has changed from standing to sitting and his nondominant hand is stabilizing the plate or piece of toast.

- A far transfer of the original skill would be for the child to hold a fork and feed himself French toast. He remains in the same posture at the table but he now is required to stab at the food rather than spread. He is using a new utensil and his movement pattern is more precise to bring the fork to the mouth.

- A very far transfer would be for the child to feed himself the French toast after cutting it with a knife and fork. The child now is required to use both hands to grasp different utensils and perform different functions and movements. Using the American system of cutting, he is required to switch the fork from one hand to another between cutting and eating.

Although the child still is able to perform all the earlier transfer skills, the ability to transfer the early finger painting experiences to the complex use of eating utensils required many new learning steps. When helping children and adolescents to generalize skills into new contexts, it is important to consider how many variables are changed at a time in each situation. If a child or adolescent has difficulty transferring skills, it may be necessary to limit the number of changes or initially teach the skill in the environment where it will be used.

Directions

Before initiating intervention, it must be decided what specific type of instruction promotes optimum understanding of the child or adolescent. Each child and adolescent possesses specific strengths, limitations, and feels different levels of motivation toward a task. The occupational therapy assistant uses this information to choose a strategy that promotes success for the child or adolescent. The occupational therapy assistant, in consultation with the occupational therapist, decides whether the instructions should be verbal or nonverbal, complex or simple, or a combination of both.

Verbal Directions

Although **verbal directions** frequently are given when providing occupational therapy, they take thought to compose. The occupational therapy assistant matches the vocabulary used to the child's or the adolescent's verbal comprehension and the number of steps given to their cognitive ability. Before initiating verbal directions, the occupational therapy assistant gains the attention of the child or adolescent and monitors the directions complexity by eliminating unnecessary phrases. After giving the direction, it is helpful for the occupational therapy assistant to pause and allow the child or adolescent to process the information and respond. Adding unnecessary or unrelated information may distract and confuse them. If the children or adolescents have hearing impairments, it is important to allow them to attend visually to verbal and signed instructions without requiring them to simultaneously attend to other printed or visual materials. This allows them to watch the mouth movements of the speaker.

Written or Pictorial Directions

Written or pictorial **directions** may be used when the children or adolescents have difficulty processing verbal instruction, speak in a different language, or have a hearing impairment. Written words and pictures are helpful to use when providing directions for use outside of the intervention session such as for home programs and or equipment directions. It is useful to review the written or pictorial directions verbally with the children or adolescents and their caretakers. Care must be taken in wording the directions so that they are stated clearly and are consistent with the cognitive and language comprehension level of the children, adolescents, and their caregivers. It also is important to draw and label any pictures and diagrams clearly and make sure that they are culturally sensitive.

Demonstrated Directions

Depending on the children's or adolescents' ability to process information, demonstrations may be given with or without verbal directions. If verbal and demonstrated directions are given simultaneously, time the verbal direction to coincide correctly with the demonstrated step.

When performing the demonstration, it is important to consider the instruction from the viewpoint of the child or adolescent. The occupational therapy assistant makes sure that the demonstration can be viewed and that environmental distractions are minimized. The occupational therapy assistant considers whether the child or adolescent will view the demonstration as a **mirror** or **parallel image**. Although a clear, nondistracted view may be achieved by sitting directly in front of the child or adolescent, a mirror image may be confusing if spatial directions are involved. Instruction also may be video taped and reviewed by the child, adolescent, or caretaker for initial or review of instructions.

Complexity of Directions

Before accurate directions can be given to the children, adolescents, or their caregivers, the occupational therapy assistant needs to understand their abilities and the complexity of the task being performed. There often are numerous ways to complete a task but the occupational therapy assistant chooses a method that is most compatible with the habits, patterns, and routines of the children or adolescents and their caregivers. Multi-step directions and environmental distractions may contribute to the complexity of the task. At times, it may be necessary to simplify steps or eliminate distractions so that the children or adolescents can attend to and successfully complete the task. The occupational therapy assistant needs to assess which steps of the task are essential and must be completed in specific order, and which may be altered or skipped. When a task can be accomplished may different ways, consistent directions are established in order for new habits and routines to be learned.

When initiating multistep directions, the occupational therapy assistant also considers whether it will be helpful to use **forward** or **backward chaining**. Forward chaining is the process whereby the steps of a task are taught in the order in which they occur. For instance, when teaching a child to tie his shoe, the child would first learn to cross and tie the initial shoe knot before proceeding to the next step of making a bow. Backward chaining is a technique whereby the child or adolescent watches the initial steps but complete the last step. Using the shoe tying as an example, in backward chaining, the occupational therapy assistant demonstrates tying the initial knot, making the bow and loops, and then have the child learn to pull the loops to complete the shoe tying. Once the child could do this independently, she then would have the child complete the last two steps. This would continue until the child is able to complete all steps of the task. Although both techniques are used, backward chaining has the advantage of allowing the child or adolescent to complete the product which is often a helpful teaching strategy.

Prompts

In order to ensure success, it may be necessary to provide prompts before or while a task is being accomplished. Prompts are physical, verbal, or observational stimulations to assist children or adolescents to complete a certain task (Orelove & Sobsey,

1996). The frequency and amount of detail of prompts should be decreased gradually during instruction until the children or adolescents no longer need them. While prompts may help the child or adolescent to complete the task, they also may be distracting. Over use of prompts may not allow the child or adolescent to develop problem solving skills and mastery.

Physical Prompts

Depending on the amount of prompt needed, it often is necessary to give **full physical assistance** or **partial physical assistance** (Snell & Brown, 2000). Initially the occupational therapy assistant may use hand-over-hand guidance to provide full assistance to the child or adolescent. For example, he might provide **hand-over-hand assistance** to a child who needs help in both holding the spoon and bringing the spoon to the mouth. Initially, she would grasp the child's hand and wrist, and assist with the grasping while guiding the spoon to the mouth. As the child improved, she would decrease the full physical prompt to a partial physical prompt. The occupational therapy assistant might help the child by lightly guiding his hand to his mouth, briefly touching his hand to stimulate the grasp pattern, or slightly tapping his forearm to facilitate the **hand-to-mouth patterns**. Although physical prompts may be most helpful in teaching new skills, it is important to eliminate them as soon as possible. If the child or adolescent always needs physical assistance to complete a task, the occupational therapist and occupational therapy assistant may consider the use of assistive technology to eliminate the need for constant physical assistant prompting.

Verbal Prompts

Verbal prompts may be required to initiate a skill or complete a specific step of the skill. **Verbal cues** often involve a word or phrase that helps refresh the child's or adolescent's memory. For example, a preschooler who is learning to use scissors may need the teacher to give the verbal cue of "thumb up" to reminder to hold the scissors in the proper spatial orientation. Usually phrased as questions, **verbal hints** are prompts that encourage the child or adolescent to problem solve a solution. For example, the occupational therapy assistant might prompt a ninth grader who is having difficulty balancing a checkbook improve his organizational skills by asking "What is the first thing you need to do?"

Observational Prompts

Throughout development, children and adolescents learn by watching others perform a skill and attempting to copy what they have observed. The occupational therapy assistant may use different types of **observational prompts** to assist children or adolescents in learning new tasks. He may perform a step of a task and ask the child or adolescent to **imitate** his performance. He might **gesture** to alert or emphasize a particular step. He also may **model** a particular behavior that the child or adolescent needs to perform in later social situations.

Feedback

When learning or performing a skill, children and adolescents receive both **intrinsic** and **extrinsic feedback** (Shumway-Cook & Woollacott, 2006). Intrinsic feedback is sensory information that comes from the body, such as feeling the movement or seeing the results, while extrinsic feedback comes from the environment or another person.

During intervention, occupational therapists and occupational therapy assistants give two different kinds of extrinsic feedback to children and adolescents. **Knowledge** of results **(KR)** alerts the child or adolescent to the results or outcomes of the performance. **Knowledge of performance (KP)** is external feedback that comments on the quality of the movement pattern (Shumway-Cook & Woollacott, 2006). For instance, while instructing an adolescent to operate a new electric wheelchair, the occupational therapy assistant may make many different comments during the intervention session. "Look straight ahead" or "Speed up when going up the ramp" are KP comments since they reflect specific performance of the skill. "You were able to turn without bumping into the wall. That's a real improvement from yesterday!" is KR feedback since it reflects the entire outcome. It is important to realize what type of feedback is given in order compose clear and concise statements. As with instructions, the occupational therapy assistant must match KR and KP comments to the cognitive and developmental level of the child or adolescent.

When giving feedback, it also is essential to consider the frequency and timing of the comments. Initially, it may be necessary to give frequent KP feedback but then decrease the frequency over time. It is important for the children or adolescents to monitor their own performance and to judge their own success without outside feedback. It also is important to consider when feedback is given. Although simultaneous KP feedback may be helpful, it also can be distracting. The occupational therapy assistant must monitor each child's or adolescent's response to feedback and adjust input to optimize individual success.

Learning Strategies

A variety of different strategies are used to enhance learning. Internal learning strategies involve techniques that are intrinsic to the child or adolescent. Some examples of internal strategies include **verbal rehearsal** and **self-awareness**. In verbal rehearing, the child or adolescent verbally repeats instructions without performing the skill. For example, when an adolescent is learning to line dance, she may practice by repeating the instructions while visualizing but not actually performing the dance. In self-awareness strategies, children or adolescents ask themselves questions to ascertain whether the task is completed correctly. For instance, when a child is getting his backpack ready for school, he might ask himself whether he has his school supplies, homework, and lunch. It is important that the child or adolescent be able to identify when to repeat a step. For instance, it is important for a child to know how to tie his shoe but it is just as important to realize that the shoe lace is tied too loosely and needs to be adjusted.

Often, external learning strategies can be useful in learning or remembering a task. A **checklist** allows the child to make sure that his backpack contains all necessary items for school. A **memory notebook** helps children and adolescents to recall a variety of tasks. Classroom teachers often require the students to have a daily planner that serves as a memory aid for homework, assignments, and special events. A pocket notebook can be used to record important information or specific steps of a skill for later recall. There are a variety of different external tools that can be used. Occupational therapists and occupational therapy assistants who work with children and adolescents often are responsible for identifying external learning strategies that can be helpful for the individualized needs of the child or adolescent.

Another type of learning strategy involves **metacognition**, the ability to recognize and monitor how one successfully learns (McDevitt & Ormrod, 2004). As children and adolescents mature, they begin to recognize that there are many ways to learn tasks and recognize ways that are successful for them. For instance, a young grade school student is exposed to various types of learning strategies. The classroom teacher helps the children learn their weekly spelling words by assigning various structured assignments such as writing out the words multiple times, composing sentences with the words, and completing workbook games and activities. As cognitive and processing skills mature, children and adolescents begin to recognize what learning strategies work best for them and consciously choose techniques that they find successful. Helping the child or adolescent to identify successful problem solving strategies is another learning tool used by occupational therapists and occupational therapy assistants. Rather than providing a checklist to follow, they help the child or adolescent develop their own organization list by asking reflective questions such as "What will you do first? What will you do if (blank) happens?" When playing a board game, they encourage the child or adolescent to consider multiple options before making a move, discouraging random trial and error responses. When employing these techniques, the occupational therapy assistant considers the child's or adolescent's developmental age and cognitive ability, matching problem solving demands accordingly.

Summary

There are five overarching occupational therapy goals for working with children and adolescents. These include creating or promoting opportunities to engage in occupation; establishing, restoring, and maintaining their capacity to perform their occupations; modifying or adapting tasks and environments so that they can participate in their daily life tasks; preventing the development of barriers that limit their occupational participation; and designing occupationally enriched environments (AOTA, 2002; Dunn, 2000). Each of these goals can be achieved by directing intervention to the person (child, adolescent, or caretaker), the activity, or the environment in which the occupation-based outcomes occurs.

Regardless of the selected occupation-based outcomes, there are four types of occupational therapy interventions. These include therapeutic use of self, therapeutic use of occupations and activities, consultation process, and education process. When implementing therapeutic use of occupations and activities, occupation-based interventions, purposeful activities, and preparatory methods also may be used.

A variety of teaching principles can be utilized when implementing interventions. Some of these techniques involve selecting the appropriate type of directions, prompts, or feedback. The activity context may need to be altered or new learning strategies may need to be introduced. Use a strategy that is developmentally appropriate, meaningful, and culturally sensitive to the child and adolescent and environment where it will be implemented.

Reviewing Key Points

1. List the five overarching goals of occupational therapy intervention and give pediatric example of each goal.
2. Define and give an example of the following visual discrimination skills: depth perception, figure ground, form constancy, topographical orientation, position in space, and visual closure.
3. Explain and give example of how intervention can be directed to the person, environment, or task.

4. Explain and give examples of how physical, verbal, and observational prompts can be used during an intervention session that involves a child or adolescent.
5. Describe the multicontext treatment approach.

APPLYING KEY CONCEPTS

1. With a partner, choose a multistep activity such as macramé knotting or preparing a meal from scratch. Complete a brief analysis of the activity and determine what steps are necessary or optional. Demonstrate and give verbal directions to assist your partner with learning the task. Have your partner give feedback on your clarity of directions.
2. Learn a new game or sport that requires memory of multiple rules or complicated sequences of steps. What learning strategies did you employ to learn the new skill? Compare your strategies with another classmate.
3. Observe an occupational therapy intervention session. Based on your observation, determine the overarching outcome and occupational therapy interventions utilized in the session. Identify the occupation-based activity, purposeful activity, or preparatory methods used during intervention. Note any teaching or learning strategies that you observe. Compare your observation with a peer or practitioner who conducted the intervention session.

REFERENCES

American Occupational Therapy Association (2002). *Occupational therapy practice framework: Domain and process.* American Journal of Occupational Therapy, *56*(6), 609–639.

Dunn, W. (2000). *Best practice occupational therapy: In community service with children and families.* Thorofare, NJ: SLACK.

McDevitt, T. M., & Ormrod, J. E. (2004). *Child development: Educating and working with children and adolescents (2nd ed.).* Upper Saddle River, NJ: Pearson Prentice Hall.

Orelove, F. & Sobsey, D. (1996). *Educating children with multiple disabilities: A transdisciplinary approach* (3rd ed.). Baltimore, MD: Paul H. Brooks.

Schneck, C. (2005). Visual perception. In J. Case-Smith, *Occupational therapy for children* (5th ed.) (pp. 412–445). St. Louis, MO: Elsevier Mosby.

Shumway-Cook, A., & Woollacott, M. (2006). Motor control: Translating research into clinical practice. (3rd ed.). Baltimore: Lippincott, Williams and Wilkins.

Snell, M. & Brown, F. (2000). *Instruction of students with severe disabilities.* (5th ed.). Upper Saddle River, NJ: Pearson Prentice Hall.

Toglia, J. (2003). Multicontext treatment approach. In E. Crepeau, E. Cohn, & B. Boyt Schell (Eds.), *Willard & Spackman's occupational therapy.* Philadelphia, PA: Lippincott, Williams & Wilkins.

Chapter 11

Documenting the Occupational Therapy Process and Outcomes

Margaret J. Pendzick

Key Terms

Evaluation report
Goals
Individualized Education
    Program (IEP)
Individualized Family Service
    Plan (IFSP)
Intervention plan

Narrative note
Objectives
Outcome
Progress note
Referral
SOAP note

Objectives

- Understand the purpose of documentation.
- Clarify the roles of the client, occupational therapist, occupational therapy assistant, and other team members in the documentation process.
- Examine how to use documentation to identify and measure the outcomes of occupational therapy intervention.
- Identify and describe various forms of documentation.
- Learn how to write occupation-based documentation.

INTRODUCTION

Throughout the occupational therapy process, the occupational therapist and occupational therapy assistant are required to document services. This chapter introduces the purpose of documentation and examines types of documentation specific to settings that service children and adolescents. It is important to remember that within these settings the concept of client may refer to the specific child or adolescent, a group of children or adolescents, or a caregiver such as a parent, guardian, or teacher.

PURPOSE OF DOCUMENTATION

Accurate written records reflect the services provided by an occupational therapist or occupational therapy assistant. In the practice setting, the occupational therapists and occupational therapy assistants use accurate documentation to:

- Measure a client's progress on occupationally based goals
- Make intervention decisions based on the measured progress
- Communicate client's status to other team members
- Request reimbursement from funding sources for occupational therapy services
- Evaluate the effectiveness of occupational therapy

Occupational therapists and occupational therapy assistants also may use documentation notes when working on research projects to gather data to support *best practice* or when serving in an official capacity within the legal system. Regardless of the use, it is important that documentation accurately and clearly reflect the occupational therapy services provided to the client and the outcomes of those services. The language used in the documentation must be professional, specific, objective, and understandable for the intended audience.

ROLE DELINEATION

Throughout the occupational therapy process, the occupational therapist and the occupational therapy assistant often are responsible for different aspects of documentation. Although the occupational therapy assistant may contribute to the report, the occupational therapist has the primary responsibility for composing the initial evaluation of the client, which includes an occupational profile, an analysis of occupational performance, and intervention goals, as appropriate.

An occupational therapy assistant often is involved in the intervention process and is responsible for documentation that reflects the current **intervention plan** and the client's progress in that plan. In collaboration with the occupational therapist, the occupational therapy assistant makes intervention decisions based upon the recorded observations during intervention sessions. Documentation provided by other team members provides information on areas outside the scope of the occupational therapy intervention. In turn, the occupational therapy documentation alerts team members to the occupational therapy intervention **outcomes** of the client. Documentation serves as a communication tool between all members of the team.

TYPES OF DOCUMENTATION

Documentation is required throughout the occupational therapy process and in a variety of different contexts. Though the specific names of these documents may vary according to the practice setting, their essential functions are to explain evaluation results, outline intervention plans, document progress during therapy, and summarize the outcomes of therapy. In addition, written documents are needed for parental consent, and for **referrals** to and from physicians and other professionals.

Evaluation reports contain a summary and analysis of standardized and nonstandardized assessments conducted on the child or adolescent, the occupational profile of the child or adolescent, and outcomes and intervention plan, if appropriate. Although the report is composed by the occupational therapist, an occupational therapy assistant may contribute to the process. When working with children and adolescents, the evaluation reports may be used to determine the need for occupational therapy services within medical, school, community, or home settings. The occupational therapist and occupational therapy assistant use the information in the evaluation report to develop intervention strategies that address the occupational challenges, contextual needs, and interests of the children and adolescents.

Intervention plans provide written documentation of the desired intervention outcomes, and the specific long term goals and short term objectives to achieve those outcomes. Depending on the setting, the occupational therapy intervention plan may be included in the evaluation report or be a separate document. In school settings, an occupational therapy intervention plan can be part of the **Individualized Education Program (IEP).** Within early intervention programs for infants and toddlers, it is part of the **Individualized Family Intervention Plan (IFSP),** and in medical settings, it is part of the interdisciplinary treatment plan. Because of federal laws regulating IEPs, and IFSPs, they will be discussed in more detail later in this chapter.

Progress notes are used to record the progress of the intervention process. They document the child's or the adolescent's current status on projected outcomes and interventions implemented by the occupational therapist and occupational therapy assistant. Depending on the setting, funding source, and duration of the intervention, an occupational therapy assistant may write progress notes on a daily, weekly, or monthly basis. In medical settings, they may write the progress notes daily or weekly. In educational settings, they may write the progress notes quarterly to correspond with the report card cycle of the school. The occupational therapist is responsible for providing supervision and determining what parts of the progress notes the occupational therapy assistant will write.

A discharge summary is written at the completion of occupational therapy services, and provides a summary of the occupational therapy intervention strategies, outcome attainment, and length of intervention. This report also includes recommendations for continued occupational therapy services in another setting, when appropriate.

OUTCOME DEVELOPMENT

In order to design an occupation-based intervention plan, the occupational therapist analyzes and synthesizes information gained through the evaluation process and develops a client-specific occupational profile. To assist with the evaluation process, the occupational therapist may request the occupational therapy assistant to complete specific assessment procedures, and provide verbal and written reports related to performance capacities of the children and adolescents (AOTA, 2004). In collaboration with the children, adolescents, their caregivers, and other professionals, the occupational therapist and occupational therapy assistant identify appropriate outcomes that relate to engagement of occupations. In the *Occupational Therapy Practice Framework: Domains and Process*, various types of outcomes appropriate to occupational therapy are described (AOTA, 2002). These include the children's or adolescents':

- Improved or sustained level of occupational performance
- Satisfaction with occupational therapy services
- Increased or sustained ability to perform occupational roles
- Additional ability to adapt to occupational challenges
- Improved or sustained state of health and wellness
- Improved or sustained quality of life

For example, for a child or adolescent who has a developmental delay, improvement in occupational performance of skills may be the outcome of the intervention. For a child or adolescent with a degenerative condition, maintaining the present level of performance may be the desired outcome. For a child or adolescent with psychosocial issues, improved health and wellness may be an appropriate outcome. Client satisfaction based on feedback from the child, parent, or caregiver, may also be the targeted measure.

Outcomes are best evaluated by well written individualized **goals**. Although it is the responsibility of the occupational therapist to write the goals, an occupational therapy assistant often contributes to the process, particularly when providing the direct intervention.

When writing a goal, it is important to keep in mind the:

- Client's cognitive, physical, and emotional levels of functioning
- Client's developmentally appropriate skill expectations
- Context in which the skill will be performed

Goals need to address specific outcomes that relate to the child's or adolescent's needed occupations to be successful in given roles.

The intervention plan includes two outcome measures—goals and **objectives**. Although the words goal and objective often are used interchangeably, there actually is a distinct difference between the two terms.

Goals reflect outcomes that are global in scope and usually take an extended period of time to accomplish. Often these are referred to as long term goals. An example of a long term goal could be: Client will complete morning dressing independently within twenty minutes.

In order to measure progress towards the long term goal, short term objectives are written to support the goal. Short term objectives are benchmarks of the steps necessary to accomplish the desired outcome of the long term goal. A minimum of two short term objectives should support a long term goal. Objectives help design intervention sessions that will impact the outcome of the long term goal.

Although several children and adolescents may have the same long term goals, their short term objectives will be unique. Objectives reflect the specific strengths and difficulties of each child or adolescent along with the contextual demands of the long term goal. Consider the previously stated long term dressing goal for two different adolescents.

Peter attends a high school with a dress code that requires a conservative school uniform: button-down shirt, necktie, and tied dress shoes. His difficulty with hand coordination interferes with his ability to dress himself independently for school in the morning. His intervention plan may include the following:

Short term objective 1: Peter will fasten six out of seven ½″ shirt buttons independently, within five minutes.

Short term objective 2: Peter will knot his tie independently, within five minutes.

Short term objective 3: Peter will tie his shoes independently each morning, five out of seven days per week.

In collaboration with the occupational therapist, the occupational therapy assistant develops an intervention plan to improve the hand coordination Peter needs to accomplish his dressing occupation. Peter's speed, accuracy, and frequency of performance would be used to measure progress.

Marko attends a high school with no specific dress code and he prefers to wear jeans, T-shirt, and sneakers to school. He needs assistance with his dressing due to difficulties sequencing tasks and recognizing the front–back of items. Like Peter, Marko's long term goal is to become independent in dressing; however, his objectives focus on sequencing and alignment.

Short term objective 1: Marko will recognize front of T-shirt and put on correctly, three out of five attempts.

Short term objective 2: Marko will follow picture sequence to independently fasten shoes, four out of eight attempts.

To achieve these objectives the occupational therapist and occupational therapy assistant select intervention methods to address Marko's cognitive difficulties with front–back recognition, alignment, and sequencing.

EVALUATION OF GOALS AND OBJECTIVES

Many different authors have suggested ways to write and evaluate a goal. The acronym SMART is one approach for constructing a well written pediatric occupation-based goal (Sames, 2005). The term SMART stands for **S**pecific, **M**easurable, **A**ttainable, **R**elated, and **T**ime-lined. The following questions serve as a guide for developing well written goals.

Specific: Is the goal precise and explicit so that all readers understand what is being measured? If any adaptations or conditions need to be considered, are they included in the goal?

Measurable: Do the words of the goal provide a method for calculating the progress? Instead of vague words such as *improve* does the goal include measurable terms, such as two out of four attempts?

Attainable: Is this goal within the physical, emotional, or cognitive level of the child or adolescent?

Related: Does this goal relate to the child's or adolescent's engagement in occupation? Is the goal appropriate for the contexts in which the child participates in these occupations?

Time-lined: Does this goal indicate when the child or adolescent is expected to achieve the goal?

Here are some examples of SMART goals.

- By the end of the school year, the student will be able to complete her morning routine (removing and hanging up outdoor clothing, placing lunchbox in cubby) within five minutes after entering the classroom, four out of five days per week.
- Within six months, the child will initiate play with a peer during recess or free time, four out of five days per week.
- Within two months, the child will put on and remove lower extremity bracing, 8 out of 10 times.
- Within four months, without verbal prompts, the child will legibly copy 12 out of 15 weekly spelling words from blackboard.
- Within three months, the child will express anger verbally rather than utilizing physical force, three out of four incidents.

FORMAT OF DOCUMENTATION NOTES

Though various practice setting and funding sources may outline different formats to follow, all require accurate and clear documentation notes. Facilities that follow the medical model such as hospitals, outpatient clinics, or home health agencies often require a **SOAP note** or **narrative note** to document occupational therapy services. School-based practices need to follow the guidelines of an individualized education program (IEP). Early intervention programs for infants and toddlers require adherence to individualized family service plan (IFSP) guidelines.

SOAP Note Format

The SOAP format is designed to organize medical records and is regularly used in medical settings. Each section of the note is labeled with the appropriate letter and contains the following:

S stands for subjective. It contains nonobservable information or opinions provided by nonmedical personnel such as the child, adolescent, family member, or caregiver. It often will contain relevant quotes that relate to the intervention outcomes such as "It hurts when I move my arm" or "I don't like to touch that!"

O stands for objective. It contains observable information about the child's or adolescent's performance during the intervention session, goals that were addressed and what the therapist did in order for the child or adolescent to attain the level of achievement.

A stands for assessment. It contains statements that reflect judgments about the progress that a child or adolescent has made on specific goals. It also is the place in the documentation to identify a problem that is interfering with the child's or adolescent's ability to master a goal.

P stands for plan. The plan contains clear and specific information that details the determined occupation-based outcome and the next intervention session. It often states the frequency and duration of occupational therapy services.

Narrative Note Format

A narrative note contains all pertinent information, written in a concise paragraph. Unlike the SOAP format, objective and subjective information may be combined in the same paragraph; and judgment statements may be embedded in the body of the note. To enhance clarity, information is linked according to topics or areas of occupational performance.

GENERAL GUIDELINES

Regardless of the format, it is important to write in third person. Third person language includes such words as therapist, child, parent, teacher, they, and their. Avoid using first person words such as I, me, my, and our. Also avoid second person language such, as you and your. Each facility approves acceptable abbreviations that can be utilized to keep notes as brief as possible. Required frequency of notes is dictated by the major funding sources of each facility. This may be daily, monthly, quarterly, or yearly.

No matter what format is chosen, the same information is provided in the documentation. Here is an example of an intervention session followed by appropriate documentation in both the SOAP and narrative format:

OCCUPATIONAL THERAPY INTERVENTION SESSION

Nakoma, a six-year-old child with a diagnosis of moderate cerebral palsy, has just received a custom built electric wheelchair. The physician has written a prescription for occupational therapy intervention to instruct the child in wheelchair mobility. Nakoma's parents decided to utilize occupational therapy services at the local children's hospital outpatient clinic. The occupational therapist conducted an evaluation and determined that adaptations for the wheelchair were appropriate for Nakoma's physical and cognitive abilities, but that Nakoma currently lacked the skill to maneuver the chair successfully.

Parents, child, and chair arrive in the clinic for the first intervention session with the occupational therapy assistant. The parents immediately explain that they thought the chair was unsafe. When they tried to have Nakoma use it at home, she constantly crashed into furniture, walls, and family members. The occupational therapy assistant explains that she will be working with Nakoma to ensure that she safely operates the wheelchair and invites the parents to stay for the intervention session.

After introductions, the occupational therapy assistant explains that today they will be working on safely stopping and making simple turns with the chair. The therapist shows the parents how to set the chair speed to low and plays games with Nakoma that require her to stop the chair before crashing into obstacles. Initially, Nakoma needs hand-over-hand assistance to remove her hand from the joy stick, but after seven repetitions, Nakoma is able to stop the chair consistently before crashing into an obstacle. As the session progresses, the therapist gradually changes the obstacle course so that Nakoma begins to alter the direction of the chair and make wide right and left hand turns. At the end of the session, the parents are given handouts on how to adjust chair speed, and how to provide the verbal and physical prompts during instruction sessions. The parents are encouraged to provide Nakoma practice time with the chair and to make a follow-up appointment for next week.

Intervention Documentation

SOAP Format

S: Parents indicated that child was unsafe with wheelchair, "crashing into walls, furniture, and people" at home.

O: Parents were in attendance during the skilled OT intervention session, which focused on wheelchair safety and simple maneuverability skills. Wheelchair safety and maneuverability are deemed necessary for the child to participate in age appropriate daily life activity roles in and around the house. After guided instruction, the child learned to stop forward motion of chair and make wide right and left hand turns. Engine speed was adjusted. Parents were given handouts on wheelchair adjustments and reinforcement of introduced skills. Suggestion was made to provide child with daily practice in wheelchair.

A: Following instructional practice, the child has improved her ability to safely maneuver the power wheelchair. She now is able to stop the chair's forward motion and make wide turns. With additional instruction, she should become independent in age appropriate wheelchair mobility skills.

P: Schedule follow-up session in seven days to introduce tighter turning and backing up and safety rules for inside and outside of the home. Anticipate discontinuation of outpatient services in two weeks.

Narrative Note

Child and parents were seen this date for skilled occupational therapy intervention to address child's inability to safely maneuver newly purchased custom wheelchair. Wheelchair safety and maneuverability are necessary for the child to participate in age appropriate daily life activity roles in and around the home. Initially parents were concerned about safety since child has been unable to stop the chair and crashes into objects and people in the home. Therapist adjusted chair speed and provided parents with handout on chair adjustments.

After guided instruction, child learned consistently to stop forward motion of chair and has begun to make wide turns safely. Parents were provided with written instructions to reinforce intervention session and were encouraged to allow child daily practice time in the wheelchair.

Follow-up session was scheduled for one week to continue to address wheelchair maneuverability and skills—tighter turns, backing up, and safety rules in and around the home. Anticipate discharge from outpatient OT services in two weeks.

INDIVIDUALIZED EDUCATION PROGRAM (IEP)

Documentation in the school setting is dictated by federal legislation, which provides guidelines and laws for implementation of services for children and adolescents with special needs. In a school based setting for children 3 to 21 years of age, occupational therapy is considered a related service. This means that a child first qualifies for special education services before occupational therapy services can be included in the school program.

An Individualized Education Program (IEP) is developed by a team consisting of educators (regular classroom, resource, and special education teachers, principal, school administrators), school psychologist, school therapists (speech, physical therapist, and occupational therapist), parents and/or guardians and the student. Although initial testing results qualify a student for special education services for three years, an IEP is written at least yearly to reflect the particular needs of that school year.

As with all evaluations, the school based occupational therapy evaluation is written by the occupational therapist but the occupational therapy assistant may contribute to this report, if appropriate. The child's annual goals are curriculum driven so that they reflect the child's role as a student and the occupational performance skills needed to be successful in that role. There often is confusion over this issue but simply stated, the areas of intervention by occupational therapy should reflect what the child is required to perform as a student in that particular school setting for a given school year.

Figure 11.1■ contains an IEP written for Nikki, a child whose vignette is given in Chapter 22. Notice that the annual goals and objectives are written in measurable terms, reflecting Nikki's needs as a second grade student. Occupational therapy is included as a related service and primarily addresses annual goals 3 and 4.

Individualized Education Program

Student Name: Nikki
Age: 8 years   **Grade:** second
School: Kennedy Elementary School
Date of Meeting: 1/12/07

IEP Team Members
Mrs. Johnson, grandmother and legal guardian
Mr. Hazel, second grade classroom teacher
Ms. Alvarez, second grade learning support teacher
Mr. Bell, Kennedy Elementary School Principal
Ms. Schmidt, Occupational Therapist

Present Levels of Educational Performance
Nikki, an 8-year-old second grader, receives learning support services for math and reading within the classroom setting. Current math skills are at a first grade level—she can count to 100, skip count by 10 to 50, and complete addition and subtraction without regrouping. All current reading skills are at a first grade level. She recognizes all letters and consonant sounds but has difficulty with short and long vowels. Reading comprehension requires frequent repetition to remember story facts. Nikki struggles with printing, often producing illegible work and frequent frustration. Nikki works cooperatively in the classroom but does not join peers in recess games or attend after-school activities.

Measurable Annual Goals (Including Benchmarks or Short Term Objectives)
Goal 1: Student will demonstrate second grade reading skills.
    Objective 1a: Student will decode words with long vowels, 7/10 attempts.
    Objective 1b: Student will decode words with short vowels, 5/10 attempts.
    Objective 1c: Student will answer correctly reading comprehension questions appropriate to reading
            level, 7/10 attempts.

Goal 2: Student will demonstrate second grade math skills.
    Objective 2a: Student will add two digit numbers requiring regrouping without uncorrected errors, 4/5 attempts.
    Objective 2b: Student will subtract two digit numbers requiring regrouping without uncorrected errors,
            3/5 attempts.
    Objective 2c: Student will skip count by 2 and 5 to 50 without uncorrected errors, 4/5 attempts.

■ **Figure 11.1**
Sample IEP.

Goal 3: Student will demonstrate legible printing on class assignments.
  Objective 3a: Student will print upper and lower case letters with correct formation, 9/10 attempts.
  Objective 3b: Student will produce upper and lower case letters in proportion to printed lines, 8/10 attempts.
  Objective 3c: Student will erase mistakes without tearing paper, 5/7 attempts.

Goal 4: Student will demonstrate age-appropriate social competency skills.
  Objective 4a: When arriving at the playground, student will initiate participation in a group, 3/5 days per week.
  Objective 4b: When conversing with others, student will use appropriate voice volume and maintain eye contact, 3/5 attempts.
  Objective 4c: Student will participate in group decision making by expressing her opinions or contributing an idea, 2/5 attempts.

Special Education and Related Services:
Special Education
- Start Date   1/16/07
- Location   regular education classroom
- Frequency   5 day/wk
- Duration   1 3/4 hours per day

Occupational Therapy
- Start Date   1/16/07
- Location   regular ed classroom, playground, lunchroom, club room
- Frequency   2×/week
- Duration   60 minutes per week; individual, group session, or consultation, as appropriate

How will the child's parents be regularly informed of child's progress toward annual goals and extent to which child's progress is sufficient to meet goals by end of year?
Child's progress or lack of progress will be recorded each grading period. Report will be inserted into student's progress report.

Is child included in regular education classroom? YES
If no, give justification:

Will student participate in districtwide student achievement assessments? YES
If no, give justification:

Will accommodations to districtwide achievement assessment be required? YES
If yes, list accommodations:
1. Reading comprehension section will be read to student.
2. Written responses will be recorded for student.

Is child at or over age 16? NO
If yes, are transition goals included in IEP? n/a

■ **Figure 11.1**
Sample IEP (cont.)

INDIVIDUALIZED FAMILY SERVICE PLAN (IFSP)

Infants and toddlers between the ages of birth and 3 years of age often are provided occupational therapy interventions through an early intervention program. Based upon the results of a multiteam evaluation and parents' input, an IFSP is developed to address the occupational demands and developmental needs of the infant or toddler who displays delays in development or is at risk to develop delays. Goals and objectives are child centered and prioritized by the family. The IFSP is a legal document and needs to be revised at least every six months.

Figure 11.2■ is an IFSP. Notice that the format and language of this document reflects family-centered practice. It is designed to prioritize the family's and child's strengths and needs first, followed by how the early intervention team will assist the family to achieve their goals.

County Birth to 3 Services

Individualized Family Service Plan

Birth to 3

CHILD: _____

BIRTHDATE: _____

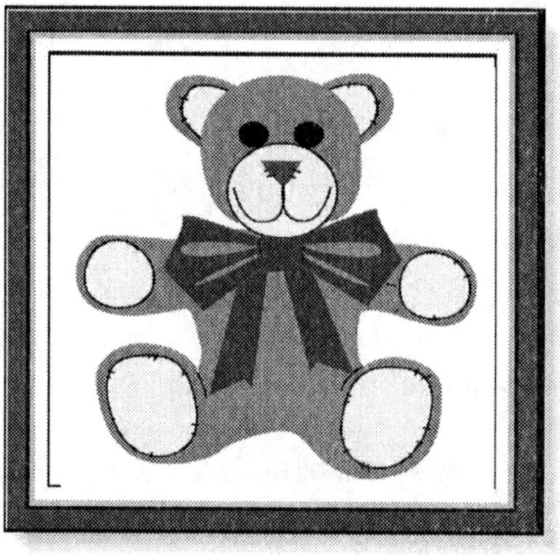

Service Coordinator: _____

Phone Number: _____

Referral Date: _____

Initial IFSP Date: _____ Next IFSP Review Due: _____

IFSP Review Date(s)*: 1) _____ 2) _____ 3) _____

4) _____ 5) _____ 6) _____

7) _____ 8) _____ 9) _____

HFS 90.10(7); HFS 90.10(5)(c)
Revised: 6/06

■ **Figure 11.2**
Individualized Family Service Plan.
Copied with permission of Wisconsin IFSP Work Group and the Waisman Center, University of Wisconsin-Madison with funding from the Wisconsin Birth to Three Program, Wisconsin Department of Health and Family Services.

Birth to 3

ALL ABOUT _____ Date: _____

Child lives with: Relationship:	Other parent/guardian name: (if applicable)
Address:	Address:
Home phone:	Home phone:
Alternate phone:	Alternate phone:

Email:

Other parent/guardian: (if different from above)
Address: Phone:

Primary Language of Parents: Primary Language of Child:

Spends day with:
- ☐ Mom   ☐ Childcare Provider: _____
- ☐ Dad   ☐ Other (Specify): _____

Siblings:

Other important people or information:

Primary Medical Care Provider/Medical Home:

Services and programs my child/family currently use:

☐ Badger Care	☐ Health Dept.	☐ SSI
☐ CYSHCN	☐ Healthy Start	☐ Support Groups
☐ Dept. of Human Services	☐ Katie Beckett	☐ W2
☐ Family Resource Center	☐ Library	☐ WIC
☐ Family Support	☐ Medical Assistance	☐ YMCA
☐ Head Start	☐ MUMS	☐ Other _____

We want more information about the following programs: _____
_____
_____

■ **Figure 11.2**
Individualized Family Service Plan (cont.)

Birth to 3

TELL US ABOUT YOUR FAMILY · Date: _____

What is going well for your child and family right now? (e.g., activities, routines, times of day, relationships)	What is your family concerned or interested in learning more about?
People or supports that are helpful to your family:	What are some activities you enjoy doing with your child and family?
What would you like to see happen for your child and family in the next six months?	What activities or times of day are difficult or stressful for your child and family?

*HFS 90.09 (2)

■ **Figure 11.2**
Individualized Family Service Plan (cont.)

Birth to 3

SUMMARY OF ALL DEVELOPMENTAL AREAS*

(For use with the Early Intervention Team Report and IFSP. Include tools, strategies, and locations.)

Name _____   Date: _____

Birth date _____

Age at evaluation _____   Adjusted Age _____

PHYSICAL DEVELOPMENT

HEALTH (Includes Medical, Dental, Nutrition):

VISION/HEARING (Screening, Glasses, Hearing Aids, History of Ear Infections):

FINE MOTOR (Use of Hands and Upper Body, Sensory):

GROSS MOTOR (Quality and Function of Movement, Equipment/Devices):

* HFS 90.08(7)(h); HFS 90.08(7)(c); HFS 90.08(7)(h)(1); HFS 90.10(5)(a)

■ **Figure 11.2**
Individualized Family Service Plan (cont.)

SUMMARY OF ALL DEVELOPMENTAL AREAS*

(For use with the Early Intervention Team Report and IFSP. Include tools, strategies, and locations.)

COMMUNICATION (Understanding, Expression, Intelligibility, Use of Language)

COGNITION (Thinking, Play Skills, Sensory)

SOCIAL EMOTIONAL (Engagement, Response to Caregivers, Coping, Sensory)

SELF-HELP (Feeding, Dressing, Toileting, Sleeping)

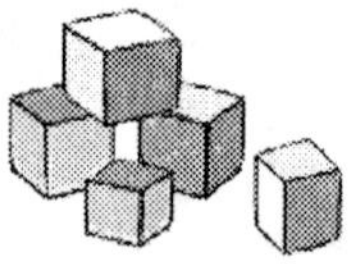

* HFS 90.08(7)(h); HFS 90.08(7)(c); HFS 90.08(7)(h)(1); HFS 90.10(5)(a)

■ **Figure 11.2**
Individualized Family Service Plan (cont.)

EARLY INTERVENTION TEAM REPORT*

Birth to 3

WISCONSIN EARLY INTERVENTION ELIGIBILITY DETERMINATION

Child's Name: _____ Date: _____

(Check A or B)

☐ A This child meets the eligibility criteria for early intervention services (Check 1 or 2)*:

    ☐ 1 a) A developmental delay of 25% or greater or -1.3 standard deviation in the following area(s):

        _____

        b) Atypical development based on:

        _____

    ☐ 2 A diagnosed physical or mental condition exists which has a high probability of resulting in a developmental delay. Specify condition(s) and source of diagnosis: _____

Comments:

_____

_____

☐ B This child does not meet eligibility criteria for Birth to 3 services:

Offer to re-screen the child within 6 months.

    Notes: _____

The following community resources might benefit the family:

_____

The following information was given to the family:

_____

PARTICIPANTS IN EARLY INTERVENTION TEAM MEETING

Signature	Title
	Parent/Guardian
	Parent/Guardian
	Service Coordinator

* HFS 90.08(5); HFS 90 08(6); HFS 90 08(7); HFS 90.08(4)

■ **Figure 11.2**
Individualized Family Service Plan (cont.)

Birth to 3

CHILD AND FAMILY OUTCOME* Date: _____

We want: (What will happen or change?)

So that: (Why is this important?)

What is already happening? (What is the child doing now? What has been tried? What is working?)

We will know we are successful when: (What can we measure?)

What will happen within the child and family's everyday routines and activities and places?	Notes

Date(s) Reviewed: _____

Describe progress toward outcome:

Check one: ☐ Accomplished ☐ Continue ☐ Other: _____

* HFS 90.10(5)(c)

■ **Figure 11.2**
Individualized Family Service Plan (cont.)

Birth to 3

EARLY INTERVENTION SERVICES TO HELP
_____'S DEVELOPMENT

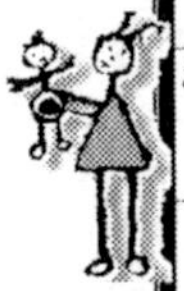

BIRTH TO 3 SERVICES			Date:		
Services	**Start/End Dates**	**Location**	**Frequency***	**Intensity**	**Funding Sources**
Service Coordination					

If a service will not be provided in a natural environment, please attach a plan with steps to be taken to get back to a natural environment.

NEEDED MEDICAL AND OTHER SERVICES
(These are resources, supports or services that assist the family but are not funded by Birth to 3.)

SUPPORTS NEEDED	WHO WILL HELP	STEPS TAKEN	FUNDING SOURCE

☐ IFSP Team discussion found that no medical or other services were identified at this time.

Comments:
_____
_____
_____

* HFS 90.10(5)(d)

■ **Figure 11.2**
Individualized Family Service Plan (cont.)

TEAM SIGNATURE PAGE*

Birth to 3

▶ I/We have received a copy of and understand the parent and child rights.

▶ This plan reflects the outcomes that are important to my child and family.

▶ I/We give consent for the services described in this IFSP for my child and family.

▶ I understand that this plan will be shared with all team members listed below so we can work in partnership on behalf of my family.

Parent/Guardian Signature	Date
Parent/Guardian Signature	Date
Parent/Guardian Signature	Date Reviewed

We have worked together with the family to create this Individualized Family Service Plan and agree that this plan will guide our work.

OTHER IFSP TEAM MEMBERS NAMES & SIGNATURES   Date

Service Coordinator:	
Team Member:	
Team Member:	
Team Member:	
Team Member:	
Team Member:	

* HFS90.12(2)(b)

■ **Figure 11.2**
Individualized Family Service Plan (cont.)

TRANSITION PLAN FOR _____ Date: _____

Birth to 3

A transition is any major event that impacts a child and family, such as moving out of county or state, moving into or between programs, coming home from the NICU, changing a child care situation, or turning 3.* For children turning 3, this page is to be filled out by 2 years 3 months.

What kind of transition is this? _____

What does your family want and hope for your child for this transition?
_____
_____
_____

Date(s) of transition planning discussions: _____

Who participated in these discussions and what options were discussed?
_____
_____
_____
_____
_____
_____
_____

NEXT STEPS

Who will do what?	When?

If referring to public school system:
☐ Family given "Step Ahead at Age 3".
☐ Non-identifying, confidential information forwarded to school district. Date: _____
☐ Transition Planning Conference held and Preschool Options discussed. Date: _____
Comments: _____
☐ Referral made at least 90 days before 3ʳᵈ birthday. Date: _____
Comments: _____

* HFS 90.10(5)(f)

■ **Figure 11.2**
Individualized Family Service Plan (cont.)

JUSTIFICATION FOR SERVICES PROVIDED IN LOCATIONS OTHER THAN NATURAL ENVIRONMENTS*

Child's Name: _____ Date: _____

List services and activities provided in a setting other than the child's natural environment:

Team recommendation, explaining why this outcome cannot be met in the child's natural environment:

How will the outcome be met in this setting?

What activities will be provided to include this outcome in the child's home and community environment?

When will services be provided in the child's home and community environment (time frame)?

* HFS 90.11(5)(a)

■ **Figure 11.2**
Individualized Family Service Plan (cont.)

SUMMARY

Documentation of occupational therapy process and outcomes is an important part of the occupational therapist's and the occupational therapy assistant's work tasks. Documentation provides a chronological and legal record of occupational therapy services and justification for intervention and reimbursement. It holds the occupational therapist and the occupational therapy assistant accountable for the outcomes of their services and facilitates communication with the family and other service providers. Types and frequency of documentation vary depending on the practice setting and include evaluation reports, intervention plans, progress notes, discharge summaries, and referral forms. However, regardless of setting, format, or frequency, documentation needs to be accurate and clearly written. It needs to address the current and needed capacities of the child or adolescent to engage in contextually relevant daily life activities at home, school, or in the community. The language used in the documentation must be specific, objective, professional, and understandable by the intended audience.

REVIEWING KEY POINTS

1. Explain the purposes of documentation of occupational therapy services.
2. Describe the different types of documentation.
3. Outline strategies for providing clear and accurate documentation of occupational therapy services and for writing occupational therapy goals.
4. Describe how documentation is used to measure occupational therapy outcomes.
5. Describe each section of a SOAP note.
6. Explain the differences between: narrative and SOAP notes, objectives and goals; IEP and IFSP.

APPLYING KEY CONCEPTS

1. Reexamine the examples of Peter and Marko. What additional short term objectives can you develop to address their long term goals? Make sure you write a SMART objective.
2. In the Nakoma case study and examples of narrative and SOAP documentation, determine what details of the intervention session were not recorded in the documentation record. Determine why these details were not included in the documentation. In what circumstances might it be important to include this excluded information?
3. Design the second intervention session for Nakoma. Document your session using both a SOAP and narrative note format.
4. With a partner, observe an intervention session. Write an intervention note based on these observations. Compare your note with your peer. Make appropriate comments on style and content.

REFERENCES

American Occupational Therapy Association (2002). Occupational therapy practice framework: Domain and process. *American Journal of Occupational Therapy, 56*(6), 609–639.

American Occupational Therapy Association (2004). Guidelines for supervision, roles and responsibilities during the delivery of occupational therapy services. *American Journal of Occupational Therapy, 58*, 663–667.

Sames, K. (2005). *Documenting occupational therapy practice.* Upper Saddle River, NJ: Pearson Prentice Hall.

Chapter 12

Interventions for Activities of Daily Living (ADL)

Janet V. DeLany

Key Terms

Activities of daily living (ADLs)
Arms first method
Asymmetrical bilateral
   movements
Backward chaining
Bite reflex
Bridging
Capacity
Cephalocaudal
Developmental norms
Dynamic balance
Eating
Establish

Extensor positions
Feeding
Flexor positions
Forward chaining
Metacognition
Modeling
Restore
Static balance
Swallowing
Symmetrical bilateral
   movements
Tongue thrust

Objectives

- Clarify the role of the occupational therapist and occupational therapy assistant in the intervention process for activities of daily living.
- Explain intervention approaches that promote the ability of children and adolescents to engage in activities of daily living.
- Examine intervention strategies for caregivers to assist with or complete the activities of daily living.

- Examine ways to modify the task and adapt the environment to support the ability of children and adolescents to engage in activities of daily living.
- Develop developmentally and contextually relevant intervention strategies that promote the ability of children and adolescents to engage in activities of daily living.

INTRODUCTION

This chapter describes interventions to support the participation of children and adolescents in **activities of daily living (ADL)** occupations. The ability of children and adolescents to perform their activities of daily living contributes to their ability to engage in other areas of occupations, such as education, school, and social participation. Rogers and Holm (1994) define ADLs as activities directed at caring for one's body. ADLs include bathing, personal hygiene and grooming, bowel and bladder management, toilet hygiene, dressing, eating and feeding, functional mobility, personal device use, sexual activity, sleep, and rest (AOTA, 2002). Occupational therapists and occupational therapy assistants play key roles in designing, implementing, and measuring interventions that focus on these ADL occupations. Occupational therapists and occupational therapy assistants use their critical reasoning and clinical skills to:

- Facilitate the ability of children and adolescents to perform their own activities of daily living
- Outline strategies that caregivers can use when assisting with or completing the activities of daily living for the children and adolescents
- Modify tasks and environments to support children, adolescents, and their caregivers in the performance of ADLs

GENERAL PRINCIPLES

Regardless of the specific ADL, some general principles apply. Some focus on the skills and abilities of the children, adolescents, family members, and caregivers to perform the ADL. Other principles apply to tasks, task modifications, the environment, and environmental modifications. Though examined separately below, there is overlap among these principles.

Ability of the Children and Adolescents to Perform Their ADLs

Because the physical, social, and cultural contexts strongly influence when and how children and adolescents perform their ADLs, occupational therapists and occupational therapy assistants need to understand and respect these factors. For example, in some communities young children are permitted to breastfeed in public places until they are 5 years of age; in other communities, infants are allowed to breastfeed only in the privacy of the family home and only for a few months. Some families encourage children to finger feed, while other families only permit children to eat with utensils. In some cultures, children learn to use toilet paper, while in others they learn to use water to cleanse themselves after toileting. Similarly, some children and adolescents learn to bathe outdoors using rainwater and streams, whereas others learn to bathe indoors using bathtubs and shower stalls. Prior to initiating interventions, it is important for occupational therapists and occupational therapy assistants to observe carefully and to speak with family and community members about available physical resources, socioeconomic conditions, and cultural norms influencing the ADL occupations of the children and adolescents.

When helping children and adolescents master the skills to perform ADLs, occupational therapists and occupational therapy assistants focus on **establishing** new skills and **restoring** previously learned skills. The term establish refers to those skills that children and adolescents learn for the first time, while the term restore refers to those skills that children and adolescents lost and need to relearn. For example, a 4-year-old girl with cerebral palsy, who has been fed by her caregivers, may receive occupational therapy intervention to establish the ability to feed herself with a spoon and to drink from a cup. In contrast, a 10-year-old boy who sustained a closed head injury due to a car accident may require occupational therapy intervention to restore his ability to successfully feed himself.

Occupational therapists and occupational therapy assistants consider **developmental norms** and children's and adolescents' current **capacities** when addressing ADLs. Developmental norms provide guidelines, not strict benchmarks, for explaining and measuring the progression of skill acquisition. They are useful for creating intervention plans that focus on establishing age appropriate ADL skills or on restoring previously learned ADL skills within a typical developmental sequence. Sometimes, it takes young children longer to establish their ability to perform ADL occupations than it takes older children to restore their ability to perform previously learned ADL occupations. This occurs because young children concurrently need to develop the cognitive, sensory, motor, physiological, social, and emotional capacities to perform the task (Christiansen, Baum, & Bass-Haugen, 2005). In contrast, the older children already may have acquired some of those capacities. Capacities are the level of ability the child or adolescent possesses to perform the ADL without any assistance or adaptations to the task (WHO, 2001). This capacity level can be affected by illness, injury, environmental influences, and ability status. A 5-year-old child with severely limited motor, sensory, and cognitive capacities has a different level of ability to perform ADLs than a child the same age who is talented in these areas. Similarly, a child who eats only fast foods may not master the use of eating utensils at the same developmental age as a child who consistently eats more formal meals.

Based on their assessment of the child's or adolescent's developmental readiness and current capacities, the occupational therapist and the occupational therapy assistant select various approaches to help establish or restore the ability to perform ADLs. For example, the occupational therapist and occupational therapy assistant might use cognitive approaches such as **forward** or **backward chaining, modeling,** or **metacognition** strategies to help the children and adolescents learn how to perform the occupations. The occupational therapist and the occupational therapy assistant consider the number and complexity of directions, the type of prompts and feedback mechanisms, and the learning strategies that best match the children's and adolescent's cognitive capacities. These strategies are described in Chapter 10.

The occupational therapist and the occupational therapy assistant also consider motor and sensory approaches when promoting the learning of ADLs, particularly for children with neuromusculoskeletal challenges. Guided by neurodevelopmental, biomechanical, and sensory integration principles that are outlined in Chapter 3, occupational therapists and occupational therapy assistants:

- Facilitate motor coordination and control to complete ADLs following a **cephalo** to **caudal** (head to tail), and proximal to distal (midline to peripheral) muscular development sequence
- Foster pelvic, trunk, and shoulder girdle stability to promote controlled movements of the head, arms, and legs when performing ADLs
- Encourage performing ADLs using **static balance** and control (keeping head, shoulders, hips, and feet aligned when not moving) prior to **dynamic balance** and control (keeping head, shoulders, hips, and feet aligned when moving) in the prone, crawling, kneeling, sitting, and standing positions
- Promote placement of feet shoulder width apart on a flat, solid surface when performing ADLs in the sitting or standing position to provide stability
- Encourage 90 degrees of flexion at hips, knees, and ankles when sitting
- Promote the development of **symmetrical bilateral movements** (both hands and arms perform the same movement), prior to the development of **asymmetrical bilateral movements** (arms and hands on one side of body performing coordinated but different movements of arms and hands on other side of the body) to complete bimanual ADL activities
- Follow the developmental sequence for grasp and release patterns and for in-hand manipulation skills related to ADLs (see Appendix C)
- Use deep pressure and slow, rhythmic movements to relax hypertonic or contracted muscles, and use light touch and quick movements to facilitate the contraction of hypotonic muscle fibers when performing ADLs
- Keep the joints warm and the muscles stretched to maintain flexible movement while completing ADLs
- Adjust the amount of sensory input from objects and environment based on the children's and adolescents' ability to modulate and generate motor responses

In addition, occupational therapists and occupational therapy assistants utilize social and emotion based approaches when addressing the ADLs with children and adolescents. Incorporating a client-centered and a family-centered approach, they focus on those ADLs that the child, the adolescent, and the family members deem meaningful and central to their lives. Guided by occupation based models of practice and psychosocial frames of reference, they consider how the ability of the children and the adolescents to complete the ADLs and the assistance from their family members and caregivers influence self-esteem, self-concept, emotional regulation, family dynamics, peer relationships, and inclusion within the larger community. Care is taken to grade the level of challenge of the activity to match the children's and adolescents' capacity, and thus maximize their feeling of autonomy and sense of relative mastery.

Strategies for Caregivers

Depending upon the child's level of cognitive, physical, or psychosocial difficulties, their family members and caregivers may assist with or complete the ADLs. It is useful for occupational therapists and occupational therapy assistants to discuss with family members and caregivers the immediate and long term consequences of their involvement with performing the children's and adolescents' ADLs. Some critical questions to ask include:

- Does the current level of assistance provide an appropriate or inappropriate level of support to encourage the child or adolescent to master those parts of the task that are within his capacity?
- Does the current level of assistance positively or negatively affect the time the child or adolescent has to participate in those occupations that are more meaningful or important to her?
- Does the current level of assistance positively or negatively affect the caregiver's or family member's ability to complete other tasks and occupations that he or she wants or needs to accomplish?
- Does the current level of assistance positively or negatively affect the growth and development of the child or adolescent, the family interactions, and participation in community life?
- How do the family's and community's values systems, resources, expectations, and traditions affect the level of assistance the family member or caregiver can, wants to, or is obligated to provide?
- Is the family member or caregiver capable of or willing to continue that level of assistance over an extended period of time?

There are not correct or incorrect answers to these questions. The questions are complex; the answers depend upon the family members' and caregivers' cultural and social beliefs, role expectations, resources, energy level and health status, competing obligations, and temporal demands. For example, a single parent who has several children with special needs, who is the primary caregiver and breadwinner for the family, and who also has health complications, may seek options that support immediate expediency and efficiency, rather than those that promote the long term independence of the child. In contrast, a family with several adult members or fiscal resources to procure additional help, and which is able to devote time and energy to focus on the occupational choices of the child, may choose to focus on long term options that promote the independent functioning of the child. Occupational therapists and occupational therapy assistants need to attend carefully to what family members and caregivers say and do not say to interpret what is important to them, and what is possible for them to do, given their life circumstances.

In addition to helping family members and caregivers resolve these questions, occupational therapists and occupational therapy assistants can work with family members and caregivers to determine the most effective approaches for teaching the children and adolescents how to learn to complete ADLs. These include the cognitive, motor, sensory, social, and emotional approaches previously discussed. The occupational therapist and occupational therapy assistant also can recommend handling and positioning techniques that make it easier and safer for the family members and caregivers to provide assistance with or to complete the ADLs for children and adolescents with neuromusculoskeletal challenges. General techniques are based on neurodevelopmental and biomechanical principles:

- Provide just enough external support to the hips, trunk, and shoulder girdle regions to provide the midline stability that the child or adolescent needs to accomplish ADL tasks with control
- Center the ADL materials near the midline of the child's or adolescent's body
- Pick up and hold the child by the trunk rather than the limbs
- Use bolsters, firm pillows, and firm surfaces to help the child or adolescent maintain alignment of the head, shoulders, and hips, if necessary, when lying and sitting

- Place the child or adolescent in **flexor positions** (flexed shoulders, hips, knees, and ankles) if primitive extensor tone persists when lying or sitting
- Place the child in side lying positions if primitive extensor tones persist when he is prone, and primitive extensor tones persist when he is supine
- Engage in activities with the child or adolescent at his eye level and at midline
- Use slow, rhythmic movements, deep pressure stroking, soft voices, muted lights and sounds, or swaddling techniques to calm the child or adolescent
- Use quick movements, light touch, varied voice patterns and sounds, bright lights, and strong smells to increase the child's or adolescent's level of arousal
- Use firm manual pressure and steady joint compression to provide joint stability
- Use firm, steady pressure and gentle rotation movements to relax tight muscles
- Respect the child's or adolescent's sensitivity to tactile input; provide strong tactile stimulation for those who are sensory seeking; slowly introduce tactile stimulation for those who are sensory sensitive

Figure 12.1■ includes a series of drawings that illustrate various handling and positioning techniques that family members and caregivers may incorporate when assisting with or encouraging their children to perform bathing, dressing, and feeding activities. Figure 12.2■ shows pictures of different seating devices that provide additional external support the child may need to accomplish the ADL task. The specific techniques and position selected depend on the child's age and size, degree of muscle tone and muscle strength, and capacity to perform the task. The occupational therapist determines which handling and positioning techniques to use based on knowledge of motor control theory and neurodevelopmental principles.

Regardless of the specific handling or position technique used, it is important to inform the child or adolescent where and how he will be touched before touching him. This helps the child or adolescent to prepare for the touch or movement and to maintain some control over what happens.

Task and Environmental Modifications

Since children and adolescents often prefer to perform tasks in a manner similar to their siblings and peers, the occupational therapist and occupational therapy assistant recommend task modifications and adaptive equipment only when it is necessary to accomplish the ADLs. Built up handles and enlarged objects are useful for those children and adolescents with limited grasp patterns. Weighted objects help those who have muscle coordination problems, but adequate muscle strength and tone. Soft, stretchy materials, such as terry cloth, and pliable containers with large openings, such as plastic cups, are easier to handle than resistive materials, and nonpliable objects, such as glass. Wraparound handles, universal cuffs, and wooden frames for objects provide external stability for those who cannot sustain grasp. Additional time benefits those children who are slower or more deliberative at processing information. It also benefits those who are slower at planning and executing their motor movements.

The occupational therapist and occupational therapy assistant also consider the impact of the environment on the performance of ADLs. When feasible, the occupational therapist and the occupational therapy assistant help the children and adolescents to acquire ADL skills within a natural rather than a contrived or simulated environment. For example, when providing interventions related to feeding and eating, the occupational therapist and occupational therapy assistant try to work in a cafeteria or kitchen rather than in the occupational therapy clinic. When working on toileting activities,

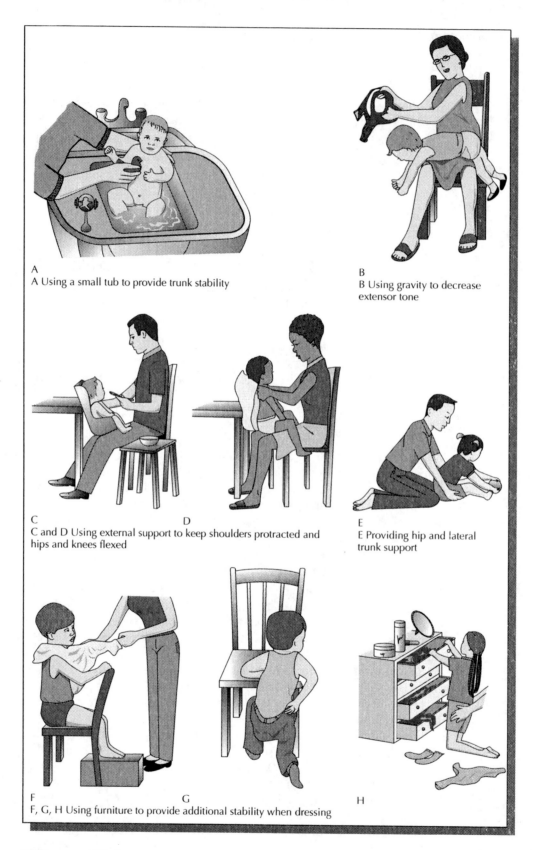

A
A Using a small tub to provide trunk stability

B
B Using gravity to decrease extensor tone

C   D
C and D Using external support to keep shoulders protracted and hips and knees flexed

E
E Providing hip and lateral trunk support

F   G   H
F, G, H Using furniture to provide additional stability when dressing

■ **Figure 12.1**
Handling and position strategies during ADLs.

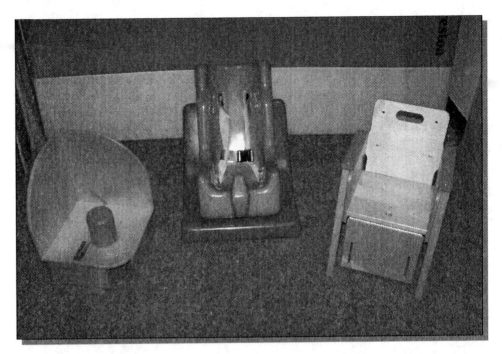

■ **Figure 12.2**
Examples of adaptive seating for young children.

they try to accommodate their schedules to coincide with when the child or adolescent may need to use the bathroom facilities or lavatories at home and school. Using natural rather than contrived environments promotes better transfer of learning from the practice sessions to the actual times when the children and adolescents perform the ADL as part of the daily routine.

The occupational therapy and occupational therapy assistant also assess how the light, noise, smells, and activity level, and degree of privacy within the environment create barriers or supports for the children and adolescents. Some children and adolescents work more comfortably on ADLs within the noisy and busy environment of the school classroom and locker rooms. Others need calm, quiet, work areas. Privacy issues may take on additional importance for older children and adolescents, particularly when addressing intimate dressing, toileting, and hygiene tasks.

In addition, occupational therapists and occupational therapy assistants concern themselves with the accessibility of the environment. They provide recommendations regarding the size, height, type, and placement of equipment and supplies used to perform ADLs, and the accessibility of pathways to those locations for performing the ADLs. Since current Americans with Disabilities (ADA) guidelines do not include provisions that accommodate children and adolescents, the occupational therapist and occupational therapy assistant need to consider the children's and adolescents' body size, height, strength, and mobility, and their auditory, visual, and perceptual skills to ensure environmental accessibility. Appendix F provides a list of online resources for purchasing adaptive equipment and environmental modifications. Through accessing these online resources and related product catalogs, occupational therapists and occupational therapy assistants can view detailed photographs of commercially available adaptive equipment and environmental modifications. Some of them can be custom fitted to accommodate the particular needs of the child or adolescent.

BATHING

Bathing involves the ability to gather, manage, and use supplies and facilities to cleanse the body; wash, rinse, and dry various body parts; and enter and exit places and facilities used for cleansing the body. These places and facilities might include bedrooms, bathrooms, kitchens, showers, bathtubs, washbasins, public and school shower stalls, and outdoor water sources. Infants may begin to participate in the bathing process by splashing in the water. Toddlers cooperate by moving body parts and assisting with some of the washing, rinsing, and drying. During the next several years, they learn to open and close bottles, use cleaning supplies such as washcloths and soap, and to wash some of their body parts. By the time they reach 4 or 5 years of age, most children can cleanse their bodies given supervision to make sure they clean all body parts, and regulate the water temperature (Allen & Marotz, 2007). However, some children and adolescents, because of physical, cognitive, or sensory challenges, or because of limited opportunities and access to resources, may need additional time to develop or relearn these skills, assistance from caregivers, or modifications made to the task and the environment. Table 12.1■ provides examples of adaptive equipment.

■ **Table 12.1**
Examples of Adaptive Equipment Used for Bathing

TYPE	NAME	DESCRIPTION
Shower chair	Rifton Blue Wave Bathing System® from Rifton Equipment	These bath chairs include a tub stand or shower stand version. They are made of lightweight plastic and mesh seating and have a lap tray, removable headrest, and adjustable trunk, lap, and feet straps.
Bath chair	High-Back Corner Bath Chair® from FlagHouse; Special Populations	This is a small bath chair with high back, full side-wings and pommel, and optional suction handrail. It is used frequently with toddlers and young children.
Tub transfer bench	Norco Tub Transfer Bench® from Functional Solutions Catalog	This is a lightweight, aluminum tub bench with adjustable backrest and nonslip seating surface. The bench height also is adjustable and supports up to 250 lbs.
Hand held shower	Carex Hand Held Shower with Diverter Valve® from Functional Solutions Catalog	The showerhead converts into a hand held unit through the converter valve. It includes a wall mount and on/off valve.
Long handled sponge	Long Scrub Sponges® from Sammons Preston Rolyan; Pediatrics Catalog	These sponges have extended handles to aid in reaching and cleaning the back, legs, feet, and toes for those individuals with limited reach.
Bath mat	Safety Bath Mat® from Sammons Preston Rolyan; Pediatrics Catalog	The plastic bath mat has suction cups to help prevent falls by providing a nonslip surface.
Suction soap holders	InterDesign Forma Suction Soap Holder®	These soap holders attach to the side of a sink or bathtub with a suction cup. They can be placed at various heights for those with limited reach.

■ **Table 12.1**
Examples of Adaptive Equipment Used for Bathing (cont.)

TYPE	NAME	DESCRIPTION
Bath mitts	Norco Wash Mitts® from North Coast Medical Rehabilitation Catalog	The terry cloth mitts fit over the hand and close with a hook and loop Velcro® strap. They aid with bathing for those children and adolescents with limited hand grasp.
Water temperature control devices	Kohler K-669-KS MasterShower XVII® 3/4" thermostatic valve	This plumbing device sets water temperature at precise levels to avoid scalding. They are useful for those children and adolescents with sensory deficits, visual limitations, or cognitive challenges.

Table 12.2 ■ describes different strategies that might be used when working with a child or adolescent on bathing. It is important to incorporate these strategies in a way that assists the child or adolescent to perform the skills, and in a manner that is acceptable to the child, adolescent, and family members.

■ **Table 12.2**
Bathing Occupations and Intervention Strategies

OCCUPATION	OCCUPATIONAL CHALLENGE	INTERVENTIONS
Rahm receives a bath by his caregiver.	Because of spastic cerebral palsy, Rahm is unable to sit independently in the bathtub.	Use a supported seating system in the bathtub to position Rahm. Depending on Rahm's age, options include placing: • Rahm's buttock inside a flotation ring and draping his legs and arms over the edge of the ring • Rahm in a round or rectangular shaped plastic basket with sides that come just below his axilla • Rahm in a low, semireclined beach chair that has webbing • Rahm in a shower chair with supported size, head, and foot rests, seat belt, and chest strap. Use these options to bathe Rahm in a shower stall with a hand held shower spray. Use nonslip strips in and around the bathtub and shower stall to minimize slippage. Install heat lamps in the bathroom to minimize increased muscle tone and muscle contraction resulting from temperature changes.

■ **Table 12.2**
Bathing Occupations and Intervention Strategies (cont.)

OCCUPATION	OCCUPATIONAL CHALLENGE	INTERVENTIONS
Moshe bathes himself in a tub.	Because of sensory sensitivity, Moshe has difficulty tolerating the shower spray, changing temperatures, and hair washing.	Encourage Moshe to: • Rub his hair and body with a dry towel before bathing to desensitize his skin • Use a hand held shower spray with pressure sensor to control the flow and force of the water • Install water temperature controls that keep temperature in the midrange of tolerance • Wash his hair when taking a bath by tilting his head backward into the water, using the palms of the hands with firm pressure to rub shampoo into the hair, and placing a dry towel around his shoulders immediately after lifting his head out of the water.
Sarada bathes with supervision.	Because of cognitive limitations, Sarada does not consistently select the correct supplies to use, determine the appropriate amount of soap to use, wash all body parts, and regulate the temperature.	Laminate and post visual cue cards around the bathtub or shower stall to provide step by step directions. Color code shampoo, conditioner, and body soap containers to match visual directions on the cards. Use soap containers that have a pump. Teach Sarada to pump the container one time for each body part she washes. Install a water temperature control device on the faucet. Mark a spot on the faucet to indicate the appropriate temperature setting.
Li receives assistance to wash parts of her body.	Because of arthrogryposis, Li cannot reach all body parts.	Teach Li to use long handled sponges, soap on a rope, and towels with handles when washing and drying.
Josh needs to find a place to bathe himself on a routine basis.	Because of his living situation, Josh comes to school dirty and with soiled clothing.	Invite Josh to serve as an aide to the physical education teacher. As part of this role, have him be responsible for washing the gym balls and other equipment several times a week in the gym showers. While in the shower, he can wash his own clothes. Have a second set of clean dry clothes for him to wear.

Figure 12.3■ shows examples of two tub chairs, one for a younger and one for an older child. These tub chairs provide maximum sitting support. Figure 12.4■ contains pictures of a tub transfer bench and a shower chair that an older child or adolescent who has some limited physical mobility or endurance can use.

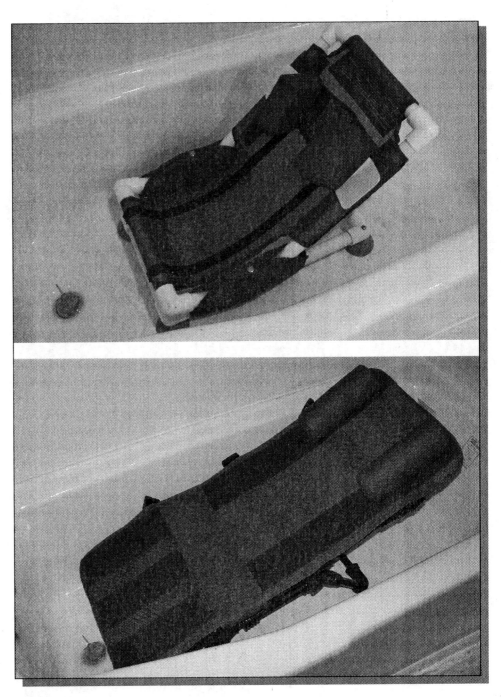

■ **Figure 12.3**
Tub chairs.

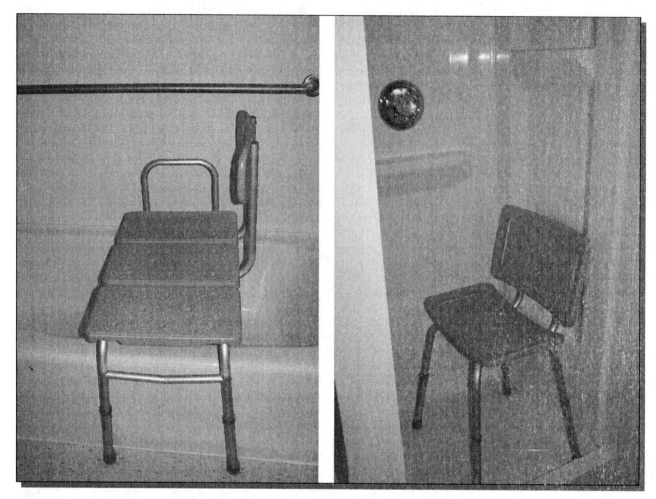

■ **Figure 12.4**
Tub bench (a) and shower chair (b).

PERSONAL HYGIENE AND GROOMING

Personal hygiene and grooming involve the ability to gather, manage, and use supplies to care for teeth, eyes, ears, nose, nails, skin, and hair. Brushing and flossing teeth, using mouthwash, rinsing eyes, cleaning ears, wiping the nose, clipping and filing nails, applying lotions and deodorant, applying and removing cosmetics, shaving, tweezing, and cutting, brushing, combing, and styling hair are personal hygiene and grooming activities. Young children learn to accomplish these activities through direct instruction and observation. Older children and adolescents also learn how to perform these activities by talking with peers, experimenting, reading magazines, and watching television. Cultural and social norms within the family and larger community create expectations regarding acceptable and nonacceptable personal hygiene and grooming practices. Access to resources also affects how children and adolescents complete personal hygiene and grooming activities. For example, by observing adults in their families, boys and girls may learn how to shave and trim body hair in manner that is consistent with community and religious practices. As the boys and girls grow older, receive input from peers and the media, and access different types of razors and hair trimming devices, they may experiment with what body parts they will shave and how they will manage their body hair. The ability to manage and use various personal hygiene and grooming supplies such as toothbrushes, floss, tissues, cotton swabs, clippers, nail files scissors, applicators, razors, tweezers, combs, pics, and styling brushes develops over time.

To enable those children and adolescents who have difficulty completing personal hygiene and grooming tasks, occupational therapists and occupational therapy assistants consider strategies for teaching the skills, or modifying the task or environment. Table 12.3■ lists some adaptive equipment that may be useful. Table 12.4■ outlines some strategies for teaching the skills or modifying the task and environment. The developmental age, abilities, and preferences and needs of the child or adolescent influence when and what skills to teach.

■ Table 12.3
Examples of Adaptive Equipment Used for Personal Hygiene and Grooming

TYPE	NAME	DESCRIPTION
Inspection mirror	Quad Inspection Mirror, Hand-Held Inspection Mirror (Large and Small), and Stand Mirror from North Coast Medical Rehabilitation Catalog	The mirrors have adjustable-length hand loops, finger loops, and extended handles that enable self-examination and skin inspection to identify skin breakdown.
Long handled brush and comb	Long Handled Brushes and Combs from Sammons Preston Rolyan; Pediatrics Catalog	Extended handles enable access of hard-to-reach areas due to limited arm reach or hand movement.
Nail board	Nail Clipper Board from Functional Solutions Catalog	The nail clipper and the nail file are attached to a plastic base with two to three suction cups on the bottom to secure it to a surface. Children and adolescents who have the use of one hand or who have limited pinching ability can use them.
Built-up handled toothbrush	Easy-Grip Toothbrush® from Beyond Play Catalog	Toothbrushes with large, colored built-up handles are helpful for children and adolescents with limited grasp strength.
Toothpaste dispenser	Tooth Paste Dispenser from Sammons Preston Rolyan; Pediatrics Catalog	The plastic dispenser holds the toothpaste tube. Children and adolescents can dispense paste by pressing down on a long arm lever.
Hands-free hair dryer	Hands-Free Hair Dryer Pro Stand 2000® from Sammons Preston Rolyan; Pediatrics Catalog	The stand rests on a tabletop and holds the hair dryer in place with a clamp. It is helpful for children and adolescents with decreased strength, range of motion, or joint stability.

Compiled by C. Torres, COTA/L, OTS, Towson University.

■ **Table 12.4**
Hygiene and Grooming Occupations and Intervention Strategies

OCCUPATION	OCCUPATIONAL CHALLENGE	INTERVENTIONS
Tzivia wants to care for her nails.	Because of limited vision, Tzivia has difficulty cutting her nails safely and polishing them with control.	Encourage Tzivia to use a magnifying glass with 10× or greater power that is on a self-supporting stand and can be positioned over her fingers.
		Have Tzivia use a nail file or emery board to trim her nails, using her sense of touch to follow the shape of her fingers.
		Have Tzivia experiment with the following options to polish her nails: • Use a fine grit polishing stone and oil rather than colored enamel. • Use clear color polish that does not require precise application. • Create cut out forms from masking tape or other pliable material to go around the outside of each nail. Use the cut out form to provide boundaries for where to apply the polish.
Alfredo's parents need to care for his teeth.	Because of a bite reflex, Alfredo bites objects when placed into his mouth. Because of medication to control seizures, his gums are swollen, and bleed easily.	Apply firm, constant pressure to the mandible joint to relax jaw muscles.
		Holding a water pick external to the mouth, use warm water and constant pressure to clean teeth and gums.
		Use a cloth around a piece of flexible tubing to massage gums. Based on recommendations from the dentist, medication may be placed on the cloth to reduce the swelling and bleeding.
Rudy wants to learn to shave.	Rudy routinely cuts himself and misses sections of his face when shaving.	Encourage Rudy to use a battery powered rather than a manual razor.
		Using the image of a clock, teach Rudy to shave his face in quadrants that correspond to the number placements.
Clarisse's parents need to style her hair.	Because of tactile defensiveness, Clarisse cries when her parent tries to comb, brush, or trim her hair.	Prior to the parent styling the hair, have Clarisse firmly press then rub her scalp for several minutes.
		When possible, first have Clarisse use her fingers to detangle her hair before using a brush, or comb, or scissors.
		Warm the brush, comb, or pick to a temperature that Clarisse tolerates.

■ **Table 12.4**
Hygiene and Grooming Occupations and Intervention Strategies (cont.)

OCCUPATION	OCCUPATIONAL CHALLENGE	INTERVENTIONS
		Have Clarisse hold the shaft of her hair, while the parent brushes, combs, or cuts it.
		Have Clarisse place her hand over her parent's hand to control the speed, direction, and force of combing and brushing.
		Help Clarisse select an easy maintenance hair style, either one that is short, or one that is long and can be tied in place.

BOWEL AND BLADDER MANAGEMENT AND TOILET HYGIENE

Bowel and bladder management requires awareness of bowel and bladder pressure, control of sphincter muscles, and awareness of voiding cycles. Toilet hygiene involves transferring to and from and maintaining the toileting position; cleansing after toileting and menstruation; and managing clothing and supplies such as toilet tissue, tampons, sanitary napkins, catheters, colostomy bags, and suppositories (AOTA, 2002). Most children develop daytime bowel and bladder control by 3 years of age, though they may continue to have occasional accidents for several years because of rushing or waiting too long to use the toilet. Consistent control of nighttime bladder functions and consistent management of most toilet routines, except menstrual care, occurs by the age of 6 or 7 (Allen & Marotz, 2007).

Diminished ability to feel bladder and bowel pressure, to control the sphincter muscles, or to know how to interpret such pressure and how to control the sphincter muscles interfere with development of the bladder and bowel management. In addition, humans do not have sensory receptors for wet or dry, but only for temperature, pressure, light touch, and pain. Since the plastic in disposable diapers keeps the urine at body temperature, children and adolescents who wear them receive fewer sensory cues as to when they have voided.

Prior to initiating toilet training, it is useful to keep a record for a week or more of the times throughout the day when the child or adolescent typically voids. This can be accomplished by checking the child's or adolescent's undergarment every half hour. To establish a routine for voiding, have the child or adolescent eat and drink at approximately the same time each day. Switch from plastic disposable diapers to cotton underwear to help the child or adolescent feel the temperature difference that occurs with wet clothing. Take the child or adolescent to the bathroom 30 to 60 minutes after he has drunk an increased amount of liquids to increase the likelihood that he will associate voiding in the toilet with feeling added bladder pressure. Turning on the water faucet sometimes stimulates urination. Encouraging boys to aim at Cheerios or sheets of toilet paper in the toilet bowl when urinating helps them develop directional control. Pommels and splashguards help reduce the amount of urine that is sprayed outside of the toilet bowl. To promote nighttime dryness, have the child stop drinking fluids at least one hour before bedtime. Then escort the child to the bathroom several times through the night.

Toilet training can be complicated by fears the child or adolescent has of using the toilet. Placing the toilet seat at the height that allows the child or adolescent to position his feet firmly on the floor and spread shoulder width apart when seating or standing offers security. Footstools and side rails provide added stability. Some children prefer to sit backwards on the toilet seat and to use the toilet tank as a base of support. Other children prefer to use a potty chair that positions them closer to the floor. Since the sound of the flushing toilet frightens some children, allowing them to practice flushing the toilet at nonvoiding times can help them to accommodate to the noise. For some children, playing familiar music makes them feel more secure in the bathroom. For others, turning off the buzzing fluorescent lights helps reduce auditory and visual discomfort.

Cleansing after toileting is an essential aspect of bowel and bladder management. It is easier for some children and adolescents to cleanse themselves by spreading their legs and bending forward. Others prefer to shift their body weight to one side and to reach behind themselves. Children and adolescents need to learn to use different toilet tissue when wiping away the urine and when wiping away the feces. Girls especially need to learn to wipe in a forward to backward direction to prevent urinary tract infections. In addition, some children and adolescents may require hand-over-hand assistance to practice applying the correct amount of pressure during the cleansing process. They also may need guidance regarding how much toilet tissue to use, and how frequently to get new tissues to wipe themselves. Alcohol-free wipes initially may be easier to manage than dry toilet tissue. Backward chaining is more effective than forward chaining when teaching children or adolescents with cognitive limitations to cleanse themselves because it reduces the chance for smearing the feces and urine to other body parts. Using water-filled squirt bottles or bidets are alternative options for cleaning after toileting, particularly for those with limited range of motion or who can clean themselves more effectively with water than a dry tissue. Washing hands thoroughly after voiding is an essential part of toileting hygiene. Children and adolescents should learn to wash their hands under a running faucet for at least 25 seconds, rubbing from the wrists down to the fingertips. Frequent verbal and visual reminders may be necessary for hand washing to become a habit. Caregivers also should abide by universal precautions and glove and wash their hands when providing toileting hygiene training and assistance.

Some children and adolescents use catheters and colostomy bags to manage their bowel and bladder waste. This involves knowing how and when to empty their bags to prevent spillage, how and when to clean their ports to prevent infection, and how to use lubricants to insert tubing. Some children and adolescents also learn the daily voiding schedule their body follows. Using this information, they can use the catheter and the colostomy bags on an intermittent rather than a continuous basis. Occupational therapists and occupational therapy assistants frequently collaborate with nursing staff to provide such training and to plan environmental accommodations within the school or community settings.

Sometime between the age of 9 and 15 years, most girls begin menstruating and need to learn to use tampons or sanitary napkins. Tampons with applicators are more manageable to use than applicator free tampons for girls who have limited upper extremity control. Placing a small amount of a vaginal lubricant on the tip of the applicator helps with insertion into the vaginal tract. Girls who use tampons should choose the smallest size that is necessary for the level of protection they require, and should understand the warning signs for toxic shock syndrome. Sanitary napkins are easier to manage than tampons for those girls who need visual cues to determine how much protection they need. Sanitary napkins with winged sides afford additional security. Those girls with limited cognitive abilities can be instructed to change their sanitary napkin every time they see bloodstains on it, or every time they go to the bathroom.

These girls also may benefit from instruction on how to clean their clothing, if leakage should occur. Encouraging girls to keep a calendar of the frequency and length of their menstrual cycles helps them to predict when they should carry tampons, sanitary napkins, and a change of underwear with them.

Table 12.5■ provides examples of adaptive equipment used for bowel and bladder management, and toilet hygiene. Table 12.6■ describes different strategies that might be used when on these activities.

■ Table 12.5
Examples of Adaptive Equipment Used for Bowel and Bladder Management, and Toilet Hygiene

TYPE	NAME	DESCRIPTION
Toilet chair	Blue Wave Toileting System® from Rifton Equipment	The chair can be used as a freestanding commode, over the toilet, on the toilet, or as a shower chair. It comes in large and small sizes. It is made of plastic with mesh backing, and includes a lap tray, removable headrest, and adjustable trunk, lap, and feet straps.
Potty chair	Smirthwaite Adjustable-Height Potty Chairs® FlagHouse; Special Populations	The adjustable potty chair comes with a seat, back pads, side pads, and a quick-release toggle handrail. It is made of hardwood with a molded plastic potty within the seat. It provides support for those with limited motor control.
Toilet tissue aid	Toilet Tissue Aid® from Functional Solutions Catalog	A spring clamp opens to release the tissue paper. It comes with an open vertical handle or horizontal clamp, and is useful for those with limited grasp or reach.
Splash guard	P Splash Guard® from Sammons Preston Rolyan Pediatrics Catalog	The splashguard sits on the anterior portion of the toilet seat and deflects urine into toilet for those with limited control.
Bowel stimulator and suppository inserters	Digital Bowel Stimulator and Suppository Inserter® from North Coast Medical Rehabilitation Catalog	The bowel stimulator is inserted with an extended tip. It helps to stimulate a bowel movement. The suppository inserter has a spring-loaded tip that pushes suppository into the rectum. Both items are held with an adjustable hook and loop handle and can be used by children and adolescents with limited hand usage.
Self-catheterization mirror	Clinic/Self-Cath Mirror® from Sammons Preston Rolyan; Pediatrics Catalog	The adjustable mirror locks into position providing visual feedback during self-catheterization.
Portable urinals for men and women	SPIL-PRUF Urinals® from Functional Solutions Catalog	The urinals can be transported or used at bedside. They come in regular or clear models.
Bidet systems	Hygenique Plus Bidet/Sitz Bath System® from North Coast Medical Rehabilitation Catalog	The bidets have a spray wand with glycerin cartridges for self-cleaning after toileting. Children and adolescents with limited reach or movement can use them.

Compiled by C. Torres, COTA/L, OTS, Towson University.

■ **Table 12.6**
Bowel and Bladder Management and Toilet Hygiene Occupations and Intervention Strategies

OCCUPATION	OCCUPATIONAL CHALLENGE	INTERVENTION
Priyadarshini wants to use the toilet independently.	Due to decreased postural stability and muscle control, Priyadarshini is unable to transfer to and sit safely on a standard toilet seat.	Have Priyadarshini use a toilet chair over the toilet that provides adequate head, trunk, leg and foot support. The toilet chair can be used as a commode and placed near her bed for nighttime use. Place grab bars on the walls on both sides of the toilet to provide stable support for Priyadarshini when she transfers to and from the toilet.
Heinrick wants to cleanse himself after toileting.	Heinrick is unable to reach his buttocks in order to cleanse after toileting.	Have Heinrick use a toilet tissue aid for easier reach and apply the tissue to a long-handled sponge in order to wipe. Install a bidet system onto a toilet at home and at school that Heinrick can use to cleanse himself.
Diana wants to self-catheterize.	Diana uses a catheter in order to rid herself of urine waste. Due to limited trunk mobility, she has difficulty seeing herself when performing this task.	Instruct Diana to use a self-catheterizing mirror that provides the best angle for her to see.
Stephen wants a way to perform toileting when he travels with his family.	Stephen uses a specialized toilet chair at home and school due to limited balance and stability; however he is unable to use standard toilets in public places in the community.	Have Stephen carry a portable urinal with him to be used and emptied in a public restroom while sitting in his wheelchair. Teach Stephen how to estimate the time cycle between drinking and voiding fluids that his body follows. Using this knowledge, encourage him to allot sufficient time to void at home or school prior to traveling, when feasible.

Compiled by C. Torres, COTA/L, OTS, Towson University.

Figure 12.5■ illustrates two examples of adapted toilet seats with side supports that may be used by older children and adolescents.

DRESSING

Dressing involves the ability to retrieve, put on, take off, and adjust clothing, shoes, and accessories; manipulate fasteners; select clothing appropriate for the activity, weather, and time of day; and put on and remove personal devices, orthotics, and

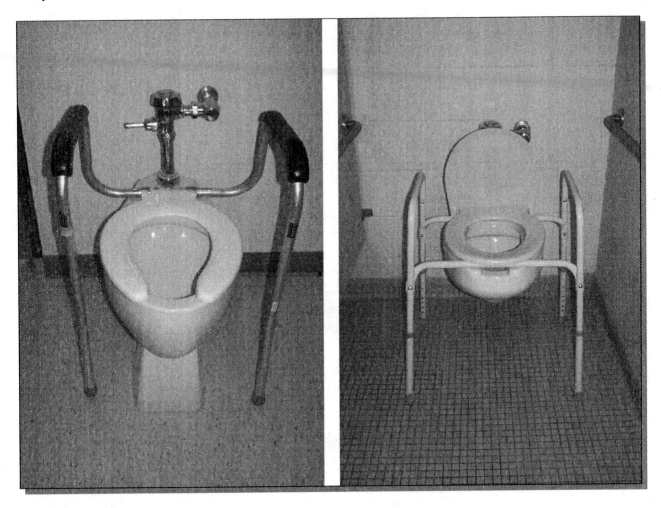

■ **Figure 12.5**
Adapted toilet seats.

prostheses (AOTA, 2002). Children learn to undress before they learn to dress. Between the ages of 4 to 8 months, babies begin to engage in the dressing process by pulling off their hats and socks. Enjoying being free of clothing restraints, their first undressing actions often are unplanned. Between 8 and 12 months of age the children begin to cooperate in dressing by pushing their limbs into or pulling their limbs out of clothing as their caregivers dress and undress them. Entering toddlerhood, they start to take off their own shoes, and attempt to put on their shirts and pants, though often incorrectly. Two and three-year-old children learn to remove simple clothing independently, excluding fasteners. Four-year-olds can dress themselves, lace their shoes, and manage large buttons and buckles. Playing dressup helps to foster dressing skills and allows for role experimentation. By 5 years of age, children have mastered most of the basic dressing skills, manipulate medium size fasteners, tie their shoes, and judge when their clothes are on backwards. During the next several years, they become more explicit about the types of clothes they prefer to wear, though they may need occasional guidance regarding the appropriateness of their choices. As the children enter middle school, they become more concerned with how their clothing compares with those of their peers, often wanting to fit in with the norms of a particular group (Allen

& Marotz, 2007). They begin to wear more accessories such as jewelry and scarves, and to carry wallets and purses. As adolescents, they may experiment with different styles of clothing, seeking to establish their identities within and separate from subgroups of peers. Their clothing serves as an outward manifestation of their sense of self, their sexuality, interests, values, socioeconomic status, spiritual and religious beliefs, political views, and gendered roles.

Similar to other ADL occupations, the physical, cognitive, and sensory challenges that the children and adolescents confront, and life situations that they experience, may alter the typical sequence for mastering dressing skills. Asking the following questions helps occupational therapists and occupational therapy assistants to determine if they should focus their interventions on improving the child's or adolescent's performance skills and performance patterns, modifying the task demands and the environment, or training the caregivers on strategies to assist with or complete the dressing task.

- Does the child or adolescent possess the physical, cognitive, and sensory capacities to learn or relearn how to dress independently or with assistance?
- What teaching methods will enable the child or adolescent to learn to dress?
- Will modifications to the task demands, or the physical and social environments, make it easier for the child or adolescent to dress independently?
- Will alternative strategies make it easier for the caregiver to perform or assist with dressing tasks?

Teaching Strategies

If the child or adolescent has the physical, cognitive, and sensory capacities to learn to dress, then the occupational therapist and the occupational therapy assistant consider how to create multiple practice opportunities within the natural environment. In the hospital or rehabilitation setting, practice sessions can be incorporated into the morning and evening routines. In the home and preschool settings, practice opportunities can be blended into dress up play sessions and into bathroom and nap time routines. At school, preparations for gym and swimming classes and for outdoor recreation afford natural opportunities for practice.

It is beneficial for all of the adults who are involved in teaching the dressing task to a specific child or adolescent to agree upon a consistent set of instructions and cueing strategies to minimize confusion. When feasible, the method selected should build upon the child's existing flow of movements for dressing and undressing. In addition, because children and adolescents typically spend most of their time with their families, dressing expectations and instructional methods should incorporate family values and dressing routines.

Various teaching strategies make it easier for children and adolescents to learn to dress and undress. Common strategies include verbal and visual instruction using a backward chaining sequence, and gentle guidance of hand motions initially to accomplish the task. Verbal and visual instructions and tactile cues are kept simple so as not to distract the child's or adolescent's attention from the central task. The number of these prompts is adjusted in response to the amount of assistance needed. The goal is to eliminate all prompts for those steps of the dressing sequence that the child or adolescent can initiate independently. Sometimes, visual cue cards serve as supplemental teaching aids.

Clothes that have elastic or stretchy waistbands, cuffs, and collars, and that are made of stretchy fabric are easier to put on and remove. Clothes with short sleeves or legs, and without fasteners are easier to manage. Practicing with oversized buttons, buckles, snaps, and hooks that contrast with the colors of the fabric to which they are attached provides additional tactile and visual cues to help children and adolescents learn how to manipulate them. Using two contrasting colors of shoelaces helps children and adolescents visually to follow the sequence for lacing and tying.

In addition, there are various sequences that children and adolescents can learn to follow to put on and remove shirts and jackets, and to tie their shoes. For shirts, some of these include the head first method, **arms first method,** and over the shoulder method. Shoes can be tied using the standard looping method, the double loop or bunny ear method, and the square knot method. If they are not able to maintain their balance while standing or sitting, children and adolescents can learn to use a side rolling and **bridging** method to put on or remove their pants while lying in bed.

Head-first Method

The head first method can be used for pull on shirts, sweaters, and jackets (see Figure 12.6■). Using this technique, the child or adolescent gathers the back of the garment in his hands, then pulls the garment over his head. When putting on the garment, the child or adolescent gathers the material from the waist to the collar. Sometimes, to start the process, he may lay the garment face down on his lap, with the waist of the garment near his own waist, and the collar of the garment near his knees. When removing the garment, he gathers the material from the collar to the waist.

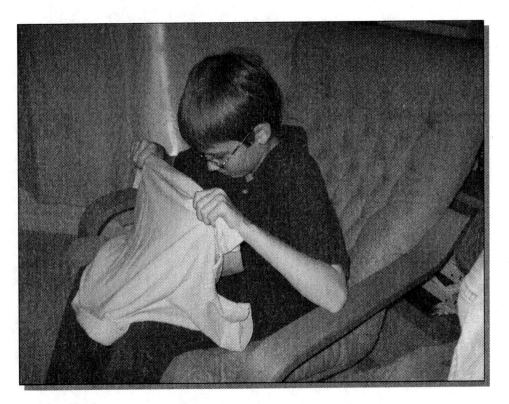

■ **Figure 12.6**
Head first method for putting on a shirt.

Arms First Method for Pull On Shirts, Sweaters, and Jackets

To use this method to put on the garment, the child slips his arms into the waistband and through the sleeves. The child then flings his arms over her head, inserts his head into the opening at the waistband of the garment, and pulls the garment down over his head and torso. To start the process, the child or adolescent may place the garment on his lap in a manner similar to that described in the head first method. To remove the garment using the arms first method, the child tugs the shirt sleeves from the arms by pulling at the sleeve cuffs. Once the arms are removed from the sleeves, the child gathers the garment at the waistband and lifts it over his torso and head. This method works best when the garment fits loosely or is made of stretchy material.

Arms First Method for Front Opening Shirts, Sweaters, and Jackets

To use this method, the child places the garment front side up across the legs, with the collar near his waist, and the waistband near his knees (see Figure 12.7■). The child slips his arms into the sleeves, then flings his arms over his head. He tugs at the sides and back of the garment to adjust it. This technique more commonly is taught to younger than to older children.

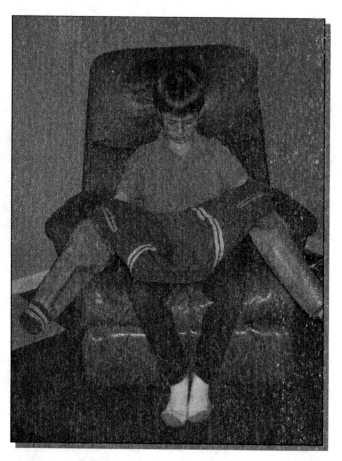

■ **Figure 12.7**
Arms first method for putting on a jacket.

Over the Shoulder Method

Using this method to put on a jacket or shirt that opens down the front, the child inserts his arm into one sleeve (see Figure 12.8■). Holding the collar in his other hand, he brings the rest of the garment across the back of his neck and onto his other shoulder. He then inserts his second arm into the second sleeve. To remove the garment, he pushes the jacket off of one shoulder, removes that arm from the garment sleeve, and then pushes the garment off of the second shoulder and arm. If the child has one arm that is less mobile than the other, he puts the jacket on the less mobile arm first, and removes the jacket from the less mobile arm last.

Standard Loop Method

This method is the one used most commonly to tie shoes. It involves (a) crossing and knotting the two sides of the laces, (b) making a loop with one lace, (c) wrapping the second lace around the base of the loop, and (d) forming a bow by pushing the second lace through an opening at the intersection where the loop and the wrapped lace cross. (See Figure 12.9■.)

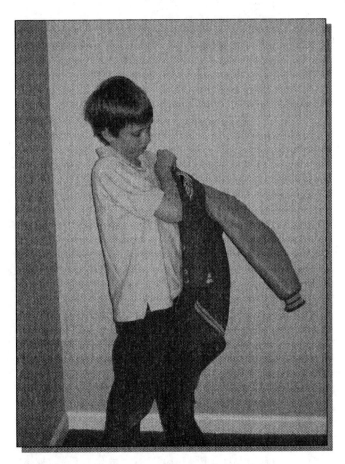

■ **Figure 12.8**
Over the shoulder method for putting on a jacket.

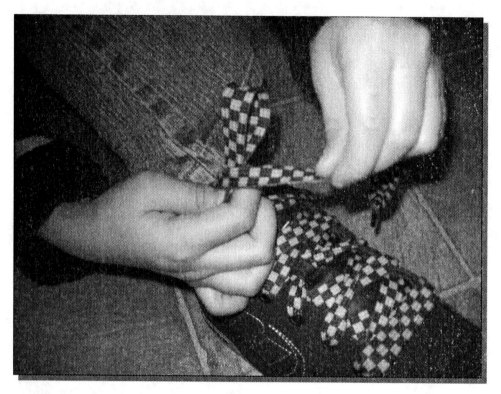

■ **Figure 12.9**
Standard loop method for tying shoes.

Double Loop Method

This method often is taught to young children who are beginning to learn to tie their shoes. Also known as the bunny ear method, it involves (1) crossing and knotting the two sides of the laces, (2) making two loops, one from each lace (see Figure 12.10■), (3) crossing both loops, (4) pushing the first loop behind the second loop, and (5) forming a bow by pulling the first loop through an opening at the intersection where the two loops cross.

Square Knot Method

This method can be used to tie shoes using one or both hands. It involves (1) crossing and knotting the two sides of the laces, (2) crossing and knotting the two sides of the laces a second time to form a square knot, (3) adjusting the tension on the knot until it is secure, and (4) pushing the tips of both laces through the opening at the middle of the square knot until the correct size bow is formed. (See Figure 12.11■.)

Bridging Method

This technique provides an alternative for those who have difficulty standing or sitting in a chair to put on their pants. The child or adolescent puts on his pants by (1) placing the pants on top of and to the side of the bed at about knee height, (2) rolling to one side and bending the hip and knee of the leg that is on top toward the chin, (3) inserting the foot of that leg into the corresponding leg of the pants, (4) rolling to the other side of the bed and bending the hip and knee of the leg that is on top toward the chin, (5) inserting the foot of that leg into the corresponding leg of the pants, (6) rolling onto his back and bending his hips and knees by placing the soles of his feet

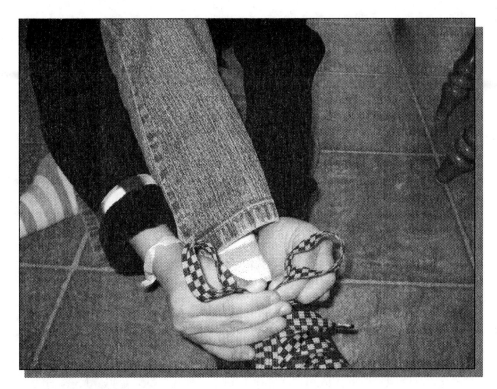

■ **Figure 12.10**
Double loop method for tying shoes.

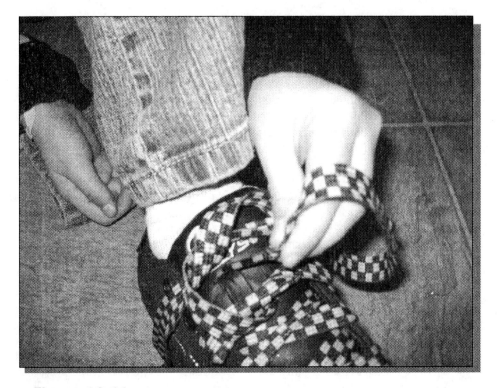

■ **Figure 12.11**
Square knot method for tying shoes.

flat on his bed, (7) lifting his buttock off of the bed by pushing against the top of the bed with the soles of his feet, and (8) simultaneously pulling the waistband of the pants over the hips and toward the waist. The child or adolescent can straighten the pant legs by using a long handled dressing stick or shoehorn, and by sitting or standing once the pants are zipped and fastened. (See Figure 12.12■.)

As part of the teaching process, children's and adolescents' sensitivity to various textures needs to be respected. Those children who are hypersensitive to touch tend better to tolerate clothing with few seams, no tags, and made from breathable, pliable fabrics such as cotton blends. Some of these children prefer to wear an under layer of firm fitting clothing that covers their arms, legs, and torso; others prefer to wear non-binding clothing. In contrast, those children who like to receive tactile input (sensory seeking) may want to wear clothing constructed from mixed or multitextured fabrics. They may favor clothing that sparkles, makes noise, and swishes against their arms and legs as they move. Chapter 21 discusses sensory avoiding and sensory seeking behaviors in more detail.

Clothing and Task Modifications

Modifications to the clothing and the dressing task also aid children and adolescents with dressing. For those children challenged by physical, cognitive, or sensory limitations, the modifications are especially helpful. The modifications can be used in conjunction with or separate from the teaching strategies previously discussed. Velcro® can substitute for clothing fasteners. Elastic laces and pretied bows can replace cloth laces. Pants with snap or Velcro openings on both sides from the waist to the hips are easier to manipulate than front opening pants, especially during catheter use or diapering. For those children and adolescents who sit in a wheelchair most of the day, pants with elongated seats and shirts with shortened backs are more comfortable. Ponchos with wide neck openings are an alternative to jackets and sweaters. Bras that are fastened in the front by slipping a long strip of Velcro through a D-ring and then back onto itself are more manageable than those with back fasteners or that slip over the head. Dressing aids such as long handled shoehorns, dressing sticks, reachers, and button-hooks are useful for children and adolescents with limited grasp and reach. For children and adolescents with limited vision, sewing textured tags onto clothing provides tactile clues for matching clothing. Using Velcro or safety pins to keep matching socks or clothing together during the washing and drying process also is a useful technique. Table 12.7■ provides additional examples of adaptive equipment used for dressing.

Figure 12.13■ shows dressing and bathing equipment. Starting at the top then continuing clockwise are a reacher, dressing stick, sock aid, button hook and washing mitts.

Dressing children and adolescents with severe physical limitations presents additional challenges for caregivers. Sometimes it is more efficient to put on and remove pants and shorts while these children are lying on the bed, and to put on and remove their shirts, jackets, and sweaters while they are sitting. When dressing children in bed who are hypertonic and who display residual primitive reflexes, it is easier to place them on their sides or to flex their hips and knees. Placing such children in supine position and with straight legs exacerbates the exaggerated muscle tone and primitive reflexes. When dressing such children in a seated position, it is better to position their hips, knees and ankles at least 90 degrees of flexion, to move their arms symmetrically, and to work from the midline of their bodies. Tumble forms and other positioning devices help to maintain the child in these positions during dressing and other ADL activities. Slow, gentle rocking movements are more effective than fast

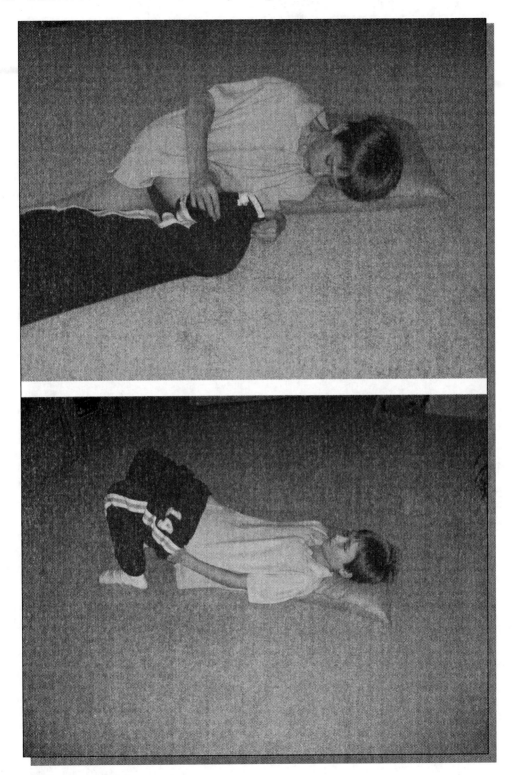

■ **Figure 12.12**
Bridging method for putting on pants.

Examples of Adaptive Equipment Used for Dressing

TYPE	NAME	DESCRIPTION
Dressing stick	Dressing Stick™ from Functional Solutions Catalog	Dressing sticks typically have long, wooden shafts and plastic coated hooks on each end, one a "C shaped" hook and one "push-pull" hook. They can be used to reach and grasp shirts, pants, and socks when dressing and are helpful for children and adolescents with limited hip flexion and grasp strength.
Reacher	Easireach II Reacher® from Sammons Preston Rolyan; Pediatrics Catalog	The reacher has a long, aluminum shaft with a pulling lug (trigger) on one end and a clamp jaw on the other end. Only one finger is needed to activate opening/closing the clamp. The reacher is useful for picking up lightweight objects that are out of reach. It also can be used to help put on pants or shirts when dressing.
Button hook	Good Grips Button Hook® from North Coast Medical Rehabilitation	Buttonhooks have a hook or wire loop attached to a built up, rubber handle. They enable the child or adolescent to manipulate buttons with a cylindrical rather than a pincer grasp.
Zipper grip	Zip Grips® from Sammons Preston Rolyan; Pediatrics Catalog	A plastic grip with ring attaches to a zipper. It is useful for those who have difficulty grasping and pulling small zipper tabs.
Shoe remover	Shoe Remover® from North Coast Medical Rehabilitation Catalog	The plastic shoe pedal sits on the floor for hands free removal of shoes. It is beneficial for those with limited range of motion, dynamic sitting balance, or hip flexion.
Sock aid	Pediatric Sock and Stocking Aid® with Built-Up Foam Handles from Sammons Preston Rolyan	The sock aid assists with donning socks. It is made of plastic material and an extended built up handle.
Elastic shoelaces	Coilers® from Functional Solutions Catalog	The coiled shoelaces eliminate the need for tying shoes. They can be tightened or loosened by pulling on them.
Long handled shoehorn	Stainless-Steel Shoehorn from Sammons Preston Rolyan; Pediatrics Catalog	The long handle shoehorn is used to put on and push off shoes. It has an extra long, stainless steel curved surface attached to a built up handle.
Dressing vest	I Can Dress Myself® from FlagHouse; Special Populations	The child wears the vest to practice snapping, buttoning, lacing, and zipping using oversized fasteners.
Tumble forms	Tumble Forms 2 Tadpole Pediatric Positioner® from Southwest Medical Online	Tumble forms are used to help children with excessive or low tone to maintain a prone, seated, or side lying position while they are performing ADLs, playing, or resting .The tumble forms used for prone lying have a tray and mirror.

Compiled by C. Torres, COTA/L, OTS, Towson University.

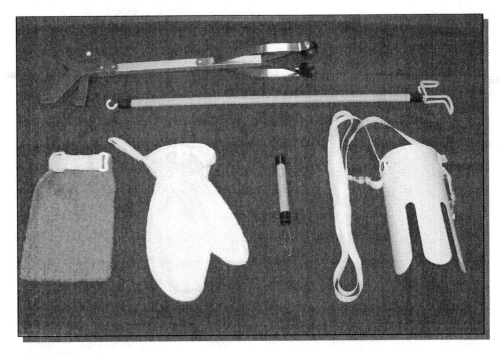

■ **Figure 12.13**
Dressing and bathing aids.

pulling or pushing movements for easing children's body parts into and out of the clothing. Table 12.8■ outlines other examples of dressing challenges and possible intervention strategies.

■ **Table 12.8**
Dressing Occupations and Intervention Strategies

OCCUPATION	OCCUPATIONAL CHALLENGE	INTERVENTION
Philipe wants to dress himself independently.	Since his spinal cord injury several months ago, Philipe has been unable to dress himself without his mother's help.	Have Philipe use a button hook and zipper grip to put on his shirts and fasten his pants.
		Encourage Philipe to put his pants on in bed using a side to side rolling method. Sew extended loops on his pants to assist him with pulling up his pants.
		Teach Philipe to use a sock aid to put on his socks. Use larger, stretchy socks for easier placement on the sock aid.
		Have Philipe wear pants with elastic waistbands and pull-over shirts. Replace buttons and snaps with Velcro fasteners.
		Have Philipe use a dressing stick to help pull up and/or push off socks and pants.
Sarah wants to tie her shoes and select the clothing she wears.	Due to cognitive limitations, Sarah has difficulty tying her shoes and selecting clothes that match.	Have Sarah wear slip-on shoes and shoes with Velcro closures, or use elastic shoelaces rather than string laces.

■ **Table 12.8**
Dressing Occupations and Intervention Strategies (cont.)

OCCUPATION	OCCUPATIONAL CHALLENGE	INTERVENTION
		Teach Sarah how to tie her shoes using backward chaining and two different colors of shoelaces.
		Use fabric swatches and cut-out samples from magazines to teach Sarah how to match basic colors and pattern of clothes.
		Insert color-coded tags into Sarah's clothes that indicate which ones match.
		Help Sarah to arrange her closet according to clothes that match. Have her put a shirt and a skirt or a pair of pants that match on the same hanger.
Rosalie wants to put on her bra.	Rosalie developed a tumor that caused hemiplegia. She is unable to put on her bra by herself.	Have Rosalie use a front-opening bra with loops, rather than a back opening. She also might use a bra without fasteners that can be pulled overhead.
Awotwi needs to dress himself before school each morning.	Awotwi has difficulty learning new motor tasks and has not yet learned to tie his shoes, or button or snap his clothes.	Use dressing vests with oversized fasteners to let Awotwi practice the necessary skills. Utilize forward or backward chaining techniques to teach the skills in a systematic, sequential manner.
		Encourage Awotwi to wear clothes with only a few buttons, zippers, and snaps and until he develops additional competency to manipulate fasteners.
Ming's mother needs to dress her.	Because of spasticity, Ming's mother has difficulty dressing her.	Place Ming in a side lying position with a firm pillow under her head, and with her arms placed forward and her hips and knees slightly bent to help decrease spastic tone when dressing.
		Have Ming's mother place Ming on her lap when dressing. Place Ming in a sitting symmetrical position, facing forward with her hips and knees flexed, and with her feet flat on a stool to help decrease tone and increase stability.
		Have Ming wear clothes that can be easily pulled over the head, and have minimal closures and elastic waistbands.
		Use inhibitory techniques prior to and during dressing to help decrease tone, such as applying firm, deep pressure to joints, rocking or rolling Ming in a linear direction, and singing to her with a calm, soothing voice.

Compiled by C. Torres, COTA/L, OTS.

EATING AND FEEDING

Feeding is the process of providing liquid and food that is nutritional and adequate for the self or another person. **Eating** involves a series of coordinated tasks including opening containers, manipulating eating utensils, bringing the liquid and food to the mouth, and managing the liquid and food within the mouth. **Swallowing** involves bringing the saliva, liquid, and food from the mouth, through the esophagus, and to the stomach (WHO, 2001). Eating and swallowing are essential for human survival (AOTA, 2002).

Typically, newborns nourish themselves by sucking milk from their mother's breast or from a bottle using a rhythmic suck-swallow-breathe pattern (Frick et al., 1996). They may eat 6 to 10 times a day. During the next four months, the infants begin to use their hands to guide the nipple to their mouths. Between the ages of 4 and 8 months, they progress from fluids, to thickened fluids, to soft solids. They accept small amounts of pureed food from a spoon, demonstrate food preferences, and reach for the spoon or cup (Allen & Marotz, 2007). Initially demonstrating munching or vertical chewing, they advance to diagonal chewing by 8 months of age (Morris & Klien, 2000). They are more successful at swallowing food that is placed toward the back of the tongue. Because of a residual reflex pattern, they will push the food placed on the tip of their tongue back out of their mouths. During the 9th through 12th months of life, their diet expands to include small pieces of hard solids. They start to chew, finger feed, and drink from a cup. From 12 to 24 months of age, they continue to refine their ability to drink from a cup, and practice feeding with a spoon or other eating utensil, though the results often are messy (Allen & Marotz). By age 2 years, they use rotary chewing to masticate their foods (Morris & Klien). As 3-year-olds, the children start to spear food and drink using straws. Four-year-old children can eat independently with a fork and spoon, or chopsticks, and can use a knife to spread or cut soft foods (Allen & Marotz). During the next several years, through practice and observation of others, most children refine their ability to utilize all of the eating utensils and to adhere to their family and community norms for feeding and eating.

The way children learn to feed and eat is influenced by their physical, sensory, and cognitive capacities, by their social and physical environments, and by their cultural beliefs (AOTA, in press). The types of food they eat and the eating rituals they perform also are influenced by these factors. American children learn to use knives, forks, and spoons. Chinese children learn to use chopsticks. Sans children use wooden sticks and cups made from the hard shells of some fruits. They include monkey oranges, roots, and tuber in their diet (Arlon, Mack, & Shalev, 2003). Children who abide by conservative Jewish or Muslim traditions keep meat and dairy products separate, and avoid eating meat from a pig. Ritual washing and a prayer of thanks often precede eating food for those children whose families observe religious practices.

Though they may be slower to master the skills, with practice, children with cognitive challenges typically learn to eat independently or with assistance. Children and adolescents who are hypersensitive to touch may develop a narrow range of tolerance for food textures, temperatures, and tastes. Depending on the degree of severity, children with physical challenges may learn to eat independently, eat using modified techniques and adaptive equipment, or require assistance to eat and feed.

Children with physical challenges may have difficulty bringing food to the mouth because of coordination problems, restricted range of motion, sensory limitations, or missing upper hands and arms. They also may have difficulty controlling their oral musculature. For example, they may have difficulty maintaining lip closure and using their tongue to push liquid food to the sides and back of the mouth. They also may exhibit **tongue thrust** or **bite reflex**. Tongue thrust is an exaggerated, uncontrolled pushing of the food or fluid forward out of the mouth with the tongue; bite reflex is an exaggerated, uncontrolled clamping down with the jaws when an object is inserted into the mouth.

Because of the complexity of eating, the risks associated with aspiration or choking, and malnourishment, the AOTA has established guidelines regarding entry level knowledge and skills necessary to provide basic or general feeding and eating interventions. In the same document, the AOTA describes advanced knowledge and skills to provide specialized feeding, eating, and swallowing interventions (in press). Occupational therapy assistants with entry level knowledge and skills who have demonstrated service competency can:

- Promote oral motor and upper extremity motor control for eating and feeding
- Teach how to time eating and breathing, and where to place food in the mouth
- Encourage visual perceptual and attending skills for feeding and eating
- Encourage olfactory awareness, and oral sensitivity or insensitivity
- Promote social interactions that encourage eating
- Promote healthy mealtime habits and routines
- Recommend adjustments to the lighting, noise level, timing, and location to support eating and feeding
- Provide appropriate seating and mealtime positioning of the child
- Modify the type and position of foods, and utensils used to compensate for motor and visual limitations, and visual field neglect
- Teach caregivers appropriate feeding techniques, including jaw and lip control and the placement of food within the mouth (AOTA, in press)

Table 12.9■ provides examples of adaptive equipment that can facilitate feeding and eating. Table 12.10■ outlines some strategies to promote eating and feeding.

■ Table 12.9
Examples of Adaptive Equipment Used for Feeding and Eating

Type	Name	Description
Automated self-feeder	Winsford Feeder® from Sammons Preston Rolyan; Pediatrics Catalog	This automated feeding device is operated by a slight move of the head. A chin switch or plug-in rocker switch controls feeding. The automated spoon/fork gathers food and brings it to the mouth as the plate/bowl rotates. The feeding device includes a cup holder whose height can be adjusted to mouth level.
Adapted feeding chair	Toddler Chair from Rifton Equipment	This is a wooden chair with backrest, arm, leg, and foot supports. It comes with an optional feeding tray, support vest, and wedge, and provides additional trunk stability.
Adapted plates/bowls	Scooper Bowl® from Beyond Play Catalog	The plastic bowl has a high rim on one side to help protect food from spilling. It is held in place on the table or tray with suction cup base.

Examples of Adaptive Equipment Used for Feeding and Eating (cont.)

Type	Name	Description
Built up handle utensils	Good Grips Utensils® from Functional Solutions Catalog	The built up handle is made of flexible ribbing that is easy to grip. It is available on forks, teaspoons, tablespoons, small spoons, rocker knives, and pediatric spoons.
Angled utensils	EasieEaters Curved Utensils® from Beyond Play Catalog	The angled utensils are designed for those with minimal forearm pronation or supination. The handle is built up. Models are available for left and right handed individuals. An optional safety shield is available to keep utensil from going too far into the child's mouth.
Universal cuff	Universal Cuff® from Sammons Preston Rolyan	The elastic cuff is worn around the palm of the hand and is fastened with a Velcro® closure. A small insert in the palm of the cuff allows children and adolescents with limited grasp to hold silverware, writing utensils, combs, or brushes. The insert can be stretched to fit a variety of handles.
Nose cutout Glass	Flexi Cut Cups® from Beyond Play Catalog	Made from flexible plastic, the drinking glass has a cut out nose section. It allows children and adolescents with limited neck extension or neck muscle control to drink from a glass.
Drinking cup with handles	Two Handle Mugs® from Sammons Preston Rolyan	The drinking cup has one or two handles and a spouted lid to aid with grasping and control the flow of liquid.
Rocking knife	Rocking "T" Knife® from Functional Solutions Catalog	The T-shaped knife has a large handle. It enables a child or adolescent with the use of one hand to cut her food using a rocking motion.
Apron	Tulip Apron® from Community Playthings Catalog	The nylon apron is designed to protect regular clothing during feeding or messy play. It fastens in the back with a hook and loop.
Haberman feeder	Haberman® and Mini-Haberman Feeder® from Beyond Play Catalog	The Haberman feeder is a bottle with slit-valve nipple that dispenses liquid when squeezed. It is designed for young children with a cleft palate or other oral/facial abnormalities who have decreased sucking abilities. It is not appropriate for children who have swallowing difficulties.
Supported stationary chair	Stationary Chair from Rifton Equipment Catalog	The supported seating chair provides minimum to moderate external support for children who need assistance maintaining their posture. It comes with a lap strap, adjustable high arm rests, and foot rests with straps.

■ **Table 12.9**
Examples of Adaptive Equipment Used for Feeding and Eating (cont.)

TYPE	NAME	DESCRIPTION
Supported mobile chair	Low Back and High Back Mobile Chairs from Rifton Equipment Catalog	This seating chair provides support at the trunk, head, leg, and foot for children who need moderate to maximum assistance to maintain their posture. It comes in either a low back or high back model, and with an optional wedge and tray. It can be used as an alternative to table seating.
Supported toddler chair	Toddler Chairs from Rifton Equipment Catalog	This toddler size chair offers additional trunk and leg support. It comes with an optional tray, chest support vest, and wedge.
Arm anchor	Arm Anchor® from Rifton Equipment Catalog	The forearm stabilizer provides external support for the involved arm so that a child or adolescent with hemiplegia can use the noninvolved arm to feed himself. The armrest attaches to the table surface with a large industrial strength suction cup; the forearm and hand are kept in place with Velcro attachments.
Floor sitters	Tumble Forms Deluxe Floor Sitter® from Allegro Medical Online	The tumble form floor sitter enables children with motor impairments to sit in a supported position on the floor. It comes in various sizes from infant to adult, and includes an abductor strap, hip strap, and an H strap to maintain hip alignment and chest support.

Compiled by C. Torres, COTA/L, OTS, Towson University.

■ **Table 12.10**
Feeding and Eating Occupations and Intervention Strategies

OCCUPATION	OCCUPATIONAL CHALLENGE	INTERVENTION
Kristofer's parents want to use a bottle to feed him.	Due to a cleft lip and palate, Kristofer is unable to form a tight seal around the nipple and to use a normal suck-swallow pattern.	Teach Kristofer's parents how to use a Haberman® feeder to squeeze small amounts of liquid at a time into Kristofer's mouth. Recommend that Kristofer's parents try a calf nipple rather than standard baby nipple to provide a larger surface area for sucking. Encourage lip closure by lightly stroking the skin between the nose and upper lip several times.

■ **Table 12.10**
Feeding and Eating Occupations and Intervention Strategies (cont.)

Occupation	Occupational Challenge	Intervention
Tulio's parents want to help him transition from a bottle to a cup and straw.	Tulio has difficulty pursing his lips to suck from a straw and drink from a cup.	Encourage Tulio's parents to experiment with cups with different types of spouts. To encourage lip pursing to drink from a spout, experiment with placing small amounts of sour juice such as lime or lemon on his lips and the tip of the spout. Place the spout in the center rather than the side of his mouth. Start with a short, rather than a long spout. Gradually transition to narrower spouts and then to a straw. When using a cut out cup, instruct Tulio's parents to thicken the liquid with pureed fruits and vegetables or a commercial thickener.
Eli's caregivers want to feed him with a spoon.	Eli was born with cerebral palsy and has fluctuating tone. He exhibits tongue thrust, asymmetrical tonic neck reflex, and symmetrical tonic neck reflex. He has difficulty maintaining lip closure when eating.	Teach Eli's caregivers to position Eli in a chair that provides adequate head, trunk, and leg support. The chair should allow him to flex his neck slightly, maintain his trunk in an erect and symmetrical position, and flex his hips, knees, and ankles at approximately 90 degrees. Encourage caregivers to use a front tray, and a seat belt placed at a 45 degree angle around his hips to maintain proper positioning. To facilitate jaw stability and mouth closure when eating and drinking, teach Eli's caregiver to provide external jaw control from the front or side. They should apply pressure with their fingers under the upper lip and around the lower jaw. To inhibit the primitive asymmetrical and symmetrical tonic neck reflexes, instruct the caregivers sit in front of and slightly below eye level when feeding Eli. To inhibit tongue thrust, teach the caregivers to apply gentle pressure under the chin near the neck and to apply downward pressure to the center of Eli's tongue when inserting the spoon into his mouth. Direct them to use a rubber coated spoon to minimize damage to the enamel on his teeth.

■ **Table 12.10**
Feeding and Eating Occupations and Intervention Strategies (cont.)

Occupation	Occupational Challenge	Intervention
Ayla's parents want to transition her from liquids to solid foods	Because of low muscle tone and mild oral motor planning problems, Ayla has some difficulty chewing food.	Start with pureed or soft foods such as pudding, or mashed bananas. Gradually add bits of crunchier food such as cracker bits, noodles, or semipureed foods.
		To facilitate chewing, place a piece of juicy food wrapped in a cheesecloth onto the molar teeth, then apply pressure on the jaw, directly under the lower molars (Solomon & O'Brien, 2006).
Kimeran's caregivers want to feed him nutritional meals.	Kimeran is hypersensitive to various food textures, temperature, and tastes.	Encourage Kimeran to play with nonedible oral-motor toys to decrease oral sensitivity.
		Slowly expose Kimeran to the smells of different foods. Let him hold the food items in his hands and smell them without initially encouraging him to eat them.
		Rub or have Kimeran rub the inside and outside of his mouth with the oral motor toys or glycerin swabs. Dip them in foods or juices that he likes. As Kimeran increases his tolerance for them, gradually change their temperature, texture, and taste.
		Expand the food items that Kimeran will eat by gradually changing the temperature, texture, and taste. Change only one of these at a time, and in small increments.
Olivia wants to be a more active participant in her feeding.	Olivia has a congenital limb deficiency and was born without arms. Her grandmother feeds her.	Have Olivia use an automated self-feeder. Adjust the feeder to match Olivia's height. Teach her how to activate the head switch to gather food on the utensil and bring the utensil to her mouth.
		Teach Olivia how to hold utensils with her toes to feed herself.
Pankaja wants to feed herself.	Pankaja was born with arthrogryposis and has joint contractures in her arms and hands that make it difficult for her to self-feed.	Have Pankaja use utensils that are angled and have built up handles, to increase her ability to grasp the utensil and reach it to her mouth.
		Encourage Pankaja to drink from cups that have handles on both sides so she can lift the cup by inserting her fingers in the handles without having to grasp the cup.
Jahed wants to develop better upper extremity motor control when feeding.	Jahed has difficulty scooping food from his plate and grasping utensils with narrow handles.	Attach a plate guard to the edge of Jahed's plate, or use scooper bowls, to reduce spillage.

■ **Table 12.10**
Feeding and Eating Occupations and Intervention Strategies (cont.)

OCCUPATION	OCCUPATIONAL CHALLENGE	INTERVENTION
		Place large foam handles on utensils, or use built up utensils to give Jahed a larger, pliable surface to grasp when feeding with a fork or spoon.
		Have Jahed practice scooping foods that tend to stick to the spoon such as oatmeal or applesauce, before attempting more challenging foods such as pasta and vegetables.
		Use a rocker spoon to reduce spillage of food between plate and mouth.
Genevieve wants to know where her food is on her plate	Because of her limited vision, Genevieve has difficulty seeing her food.	Establish a system for placing food in a particular order on the plate, for example, salad in the upper right quadrant, vegetables or fruit in the lower right quadrant, meat or fish in the lower left quadrant, and bread in the upper left quadrant.
		Provide Genevieve with a plate that contrasts in color to the food she is eating. Consider using a plate that has two colors, dark on one side and light on the other. Place dark colored foods on the light side of the plate, and light colored food on the dark side of the plate.

Compiled by C. Torres, COTA/L, OTS, Towson University, and J. DeLany, DEd, OTR/L.

Figure 12.14■ shows examples of adapted cups that the children and adolescents may use to aid with drinking. Figure 12.15■ depicts adapted plates, knives, forks, and spoons that children and adolescents may use to eat.

SEXUAL ACTIVITY

Sexual activity involves actions that contribute to sexual gratification (AOTA, 2002). How children and adolescents learn about their sexuality and the manner in which they seek sexual gratification is strongly influenced by the norms and practices of their family, peers, and community. During the first year of life, infants typically experience nurturing types of affection and touch from their caregivers. Between 3 and 5 years of age, depending upon the culture in which they live, the children learn names for their genitalia, show interest in the genitalia of others, and start to practice rules for privacy while dressing and toileting. They also begin to learn boundaries for acceptable touch and affection. During the next several years, they continue to

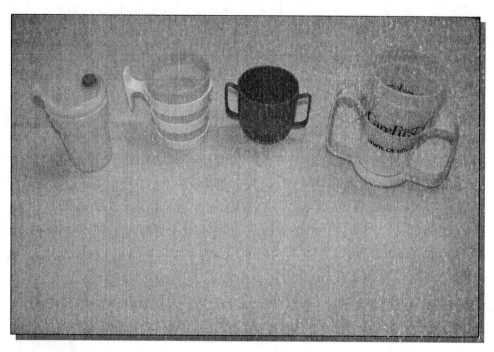

■ **Figure 12.14**
Adapted cups.

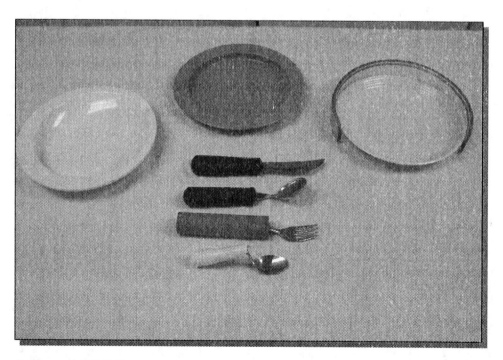

■ **Figure 12.15**
Adapted plates and utensils.

differentiate between boys and girls, and learn about friendships. They also start to internalize family and cultural norms to distinguish between acceptable and nonacceptable social and sexual behaviors. Depending upon the standards for conversation within their families and schools, children ages 9 through 11 years may participate in adult-directed discussions about body image, puberty related body changes, and reproduction. They also may participate in discussions and learning activities about personal boundaries, self-esteem, assertiveness and refusal skills, and sexual abuse. As they progress through their adolescence, the youth may explore their own sexuality through their dress and body movements, discuss sexual practices with their friends, use values to make decisions about their sexual actions, learn about sexually transmitted diseases, and investigate birth control and safe sex options. They may attempt to date, experiment with how to communicate and express love, and consider birth options (American Academy of Pediatrics, 2001; Couwenhoven, 2001; DeLany & Spottswood, 2000; Suner, Nakamura, & Caulfield, 2003). By the age of 18 years, 50 percent of teens experience sexual intercourse at least once, though they may continue to clarify their sexual beliefs and their sense of self as sexual beings for the next several years (Albert, Brown, & Flanigan, 2003.)

Because of their physical, cognitive, or psychosocial challenges, children and youth with special needs may have additional concerns related to sexual activities that are not addressed within typical sexual education programs. In the process of addressing other personal activities such as dressing, toileting, menstrual care, and social participation, occupational therapists and occupational therapy assistants may help children and adolescents learn about sexual activities. Schools and communities also may seek the expertise of occupational therapists and occupational therapy assistants to tailor their sexual education programs for these children and adolescents. Given family and cultural norms associated with sexual activities, parental approval is needed to provide education and interventions related to sexuality. It is important that these education and intervention programs are sensitive to family and community values.

Because children and adolescents with physical, psychosocial, and learning challenges are more vulnerable to sexual abuse than are other children and adolescents, additional vigilance to protect them is needed. As health care professionals, occupational therapists and occupational therapy assistants are responsible for reporting their suspicions of sexual abuse to the proper authorities within their practice or community setting. Warning signs of sexual abuse include: promiscuity, vaginal and rectal bleeding, urinary track infections, bedwetting, sexually transmitted diseases, unexplained acts of aggression or withdrawal, fear of being alone with or seductive actions toward a particular person, over compliance to a particular authority figure, and runaway behaviors (Child Welfare Information Gateway, 2006).

Occupational therapists and occupational therapy assistants may employ various teaching strategies to help children and adolescents learn about sexuality. Engaging in pretend play with stuffed animals or dolls can help young children learn about and practice accepted bounds for affection and touch, and rules for privacy. Using puppets to modify and dramatize scripts from books about friendships, school age children can practice assertiveness and refusal skills, and differentiate between acceptable and non acceptable social behaviors. Through dramatization they also can learn how to define personal boundaries and to report inappropriate sexual advances. Critiquing movies and writing plays about social relationships can help adolescents to distinguish between healthy and unhealthy practices, explore their emerging sexuality, examine their value systems, and reflect on the consequences of their behaviors.

Children and adolescents with learning challenges, such as those with a cognitive developmental disability or head trauma, may need very explicit instructions and multiple practice sessions to distinguish between acceptable and unacceptable physical contact and sexual behaviors. Using a color coding system of green-yellow-red circles provides a visual system to help some children and adolescents identify appropriate, cautionary, and inappropriate contact and sexual behaviors. For example, to learn who is appropriate to kiss, the occupational therapy assistant might have the child put pictures of his parents and siblings in the green circle, pictures of family friends in the yellow circle, and pictures of store clerks in the red circle. Similarly, to learn where it is appropriate to masturbate, the occupational therapy assistant might have the adolescent put pictures of her bedroom in the green circle, and pictures of a school bus or classroom in the red circle. The occupational therapy assistant would adjust the complexity of the visual cuing system to match the children's and adolescents' cognitive capacities.

In contrast to this concrete training method, adolescents with physical and sensory challenges and chronic health conditions may benefit from small groups discussions about sexual activities. Given their limitations, they may want an opportunity to discuss personal issues such as how they can engage in physically intimate relationships, practice safe sex, procreate, and care for their offspring. Online support groups can provide a forum for these youth to pose their questions to other individuals who have coped with such concerns. Caution is necessary, however, to determine the legitimacy and purpose of online discussion groups because of the risk of sexual exploitation.

SLEEP AND REST

Sleep and rest are periods of inactivity (AOTA, 2002). They allow the body and brain to recuperate and heal. Infants sleep an average of 14 to 18 hours a day, divided into four to six intervals. Young children sleep approximately 12 hours a day, often taking a nap in midday. Adolescents benefit from a minimum of 8 hours of sleep per day, though may fluctuate between getting only a few hours of sleep one night and extended hours of sleep another night because of the many activities in which they become involved (Allen & Marotz, 2007).

Some children and adolescents struggle with getting to sleep. Regular daily routines that incorporate periods of physical activity and rest help promote sleep. Some children benefit from a 30-minute period of quiet time before going to bed to sleep. Others may need a 2-hour interval of quiet time. For some children, a warm bath, followed by reading, or listening to instrumental, rhythmic, soothing music in a darkened room encourages sleep. Pressure and neutral warmth generated from a weighted blanket, a firm fitting blanket, or a quilt can have a calming affect. Eliminating caffeine from the diet, avoiding eating foods several hours before bedtime, and drinking a warm cup of mild herbal tea also are useful strategies. Background white noise, such as that created by an overhead fan, may help children who are hypersensitive to household noises. For those who are hypersensitive to touch, flannel cotton sheets without any nap may feel most comfortable. They also may sleep better in pajamas that cover their entire body and form a layer of protection between their body and the bed covers.

Positioning and safety are concerns for other children. Children and adolescents with little mobility need to be rotated in their beds every few hours to prevent pressure sores. Lying on sheepskin also may help to minimize pressure ulcers. Children and adolescents with severe spasticity should be positioned on their side with firm pillows. Children who are congested benefit from sleeping with their head and trunk slightly elevated or in a semireclining position. While young children may remain safe in cribs with railings, adaptations may be necessary for older children with physical and cognitive limitations. Hospital bed rails may suffice for some children. Others may need to have their mattress on the floor to eliminate the risk of falling out of bed. For children who roam during the night, Dutch doors that allow the top half to be opened and the bottom half to remain locked may be an appropriate solution. Motion detectors may need to be installed around windows and doors to warn the parents if the child starts to leave the house. A family dog, trained to bark when the child attempts to roam from the house, provides added safety.

SUMMARY

Occupational therapists and occupational therapy assistants design, implement, and measure interventions that focus on the ability of children and adolescents to participate in their ADL occupations. Using their critical reasoning and clinical skills, occupational therapists and occupational therapy assistants (1) help children and adolescents to perform their activities of daily living; (2) advise caregivers how to provide necessary assistance; and (3) modify tasks and environments to support the efforts of the children, adolescents, and their caregivers.

Occupational therapists and occupational therapy assistants consider the developmental capabilities of the children and adolescents and the physical and social context of their families and communities when designing and implementing ADL interventions. They consider the number and complexity of directions, the type of prompts, and the feedback mechanisms that best match the children's and adolescents' learning capacities. Guided by neurodevelopmental, biomechanical, and sensory integration principles they select motor and sensory approaches to promote skill acquisition. Directed by occupation based models of practice and psychosocial frames of reference, they also consider how the ability of the children and the adolescents to complete the ADLs influences their sense of self, and their relationship with their family and peers. Care is taken to grade the level of challenge of the activity to match the capacity of the children and adolescent to succeed at the task.

As part of the intervention process, the occupational therapist and occupational therapy assistant may recommend handling and positioning techniques that make it easier and safer for the family members and caregivers to provide the necessary assistance. Recognizing that children and adolescents often prefer to perform tasks in a manner similar to their siblings and peers, they recommend task modifications and adaptive equipment only when it is necessary to accomplish the ADLs. When feasible, they help the children and adolescents to acquire ADL skills within a natural rather than a contrived environment.

The occupational therapy and occupational therapy assistant also assess how the light, noise, smells, and activity level, and degree of privacy within the natural or contrived environment create barriers or supports for the children and adolescents. Concerned with the accessibility of the environment, but recognizing that the current Americans with Disabilities (ADA) guidelines do not include provisions that accommodate children and adolescents, they consider the children's and adolescents' body size, height, strength, mobility, and perceptual skills to ensure environmental accessibility.

REVIEWING KEY POINTS

1. List and define the ADL occupations.
   a. Describe how an infant participates in each of the ADL occupations.
   b. Describe how a young child participates in each of the ADL occupations.
   c. Describe how a school age child performs each of the ADL occupations.
   d. Describe how an adolescent performs each of the ADL occupations.
2. Describe teaching strategies to consider when helping children and adolescents learn to perform their ADL occupations.
3. Describe sensory and motor principles to consider when helping children and adolescents learn to perform their ADL occupations.
4. Describe psychosocial principles to consider when helping children and adolescents learn to perform their ADL occupations.
5. Outline handling and positioning strategies for caregivers to consider when providing assistance or completing ADL occupations for children and adolescents.
6. Describe four difficulties that children and adolescents with physical, learning, or psychosocial challenges might experience when trying to complete each of the ADL occupations. For each of the challenges describe and justify two possible solutions.
   a. Bathing
   b. Personal hygiene and grooming
   c. Bowel and bladder management and toileting hygiene
   d. Dressing
   e. Eating and feeding
   f. Sexual activity
   g. Sleeping and resting
7. Describe five pieces of adaptive equipment and five task modifications to assist children and adolescents in the performance of the following ADL occupations. Explain the purpose of each piece of adaptive equipment and how to use it. Explain the purpose for each task modification.
   a. Bathing
   b. Personal hygiene and grooming
   c. Bowel and bladder management and toileting hygiene
   d. Dressing
   e. Eating and feeding

APPLYING KEY CONCEPTS

1. Choose an ADL occupation that a young child performs. List 10 approaches that you could provide to assist a young child who is having difficulty performing this occupation. Include approaches that focus on the child, task modifications, and adaptive equipment.
2. Using the same ADL, list 10 approaches that you would provide to assist an adolescent who is having difficulty performing this occupation. Compare the differences and discuss the expanded contexts.
3. Examine three different catalogs. Find and describe 10 pieces of adaptive equipment for each of the following ADL occupations. List the cost for each piece of adaptive equipment.
   a. Bathing
   b. Personal hygiene and grooming
   c. Bowel and bladder management and toileting hygiene
   d. Dressing
   e. Eating and feeding

4. Observe a child or adolescent performing an ADL occupation. Write down all of the steps she performs to complete the task. Instruct a classmate to perform that ADL task, following only the steps that you wrote. Evaluate the clarity and precision of your written instructions. Rewrite those that were not clear or precise. Consider additional steps you should have written. Add them to your list of instructions.

5. Observe a child or adolescent with a physical, learning, or psychosocial challenge who is having difficulty completing an ADL occupation that is important to him. Make a piece of adaptive equipment or propose a modification to the task to make it possible for him to complete the ADL occupation.

REFERENCES

Albert, B., Brown, S., & Flanigan, C. (Eds.) (2003). *14 and younger: The sexual behavior of young adolescents.* Washington, DC: National Campaign to Prevent Teen Pregnancy.

Allegro Medical Online (2006). Tumble forms deluxe form sitter. Retrieved December 12, 2006, from http://www.allegromedical.com/tumble-forms-deluxe-floor-sitter-medium-includes-feeder-seat-and-floor-sitter-wedge-186416.html.

Allen, K. A., & Marotz, L. (2007). *Developmental profiles: Prebirth through twelve* (4th ed.). Clifton Park, NY: Thomson Delmar Learning.

American Academy of Pediatrics (2001). Care of adolescent parents and their children. *Pediatrics, 107*(2), 423–435.

American Occupational Therapy Association (AOTA) (2002). Occupational therapy practice framework: Domain and process. *American Journal of Occupational Therapy, 56,* 609–639.

American Occupational Therapy Association (AOTA) (in press). Specialized knowledge and skills in eating, feeding, and swallowing for occupational therapy practice. *American Journal of Occupational Therapy.*

Arlon, P., Mack, L., & Shalev, Z. (2003). *How people live.* New York: DK Publishing.

Beyond Play LLC (2005). *Beyond play: Early intervention products for young children with special needs,* 2005/2006 catalog. Berkeley, CA: Beyond Play.

Child Welfare Information Gateway (2006). *Recognizing child abuse and neglect: Signs and symptoms.* Retrieved December 21, 2006 from http://www.childwelfare.gov/pubs/factsheets/signs.cfm.

Christiansen, C., Baum, C. M., & Bass-Haugen, J. (Eds.) (2005). *Occupational therapy: Performance, participation, and well-being* (3rd ed.). Thorofare, NJ: SLACK.

Community Products, LLC. (2005). *Special education: Classroom furniture for exceptional students,* 2005 catalog. Chester, NY: Community Playthings.

Couwenhoven, T. (2001). Sexuality education. Building a foundation of healthy attitudes. *Disability Solutions, 4*(6) 1–8.

DeLany, J.V., & Spottswood, A. (2000). Pregnancy prevention and support programs for adolescent parents. Chambersburg, PA: Summit Health.

FlagHouse. (2005). *Special Populations* summer 2005 catalog. Hasbrouck Hts., NJ: FlagHouse.

Frick, R., Frick, S. M., Oetter, P., et al, (1996). *Out of the mouths of babes: Discovering the developmental sequence of the mouth.* Hugo, MN: PDP Press.

Morris, S.E., & Klein, M.D. (2000). *Pre-feeding skills.* Tucson, AZ: Therapy Skill Builders.

North Coast Medical, Inc. (2004). *Rehabilitation* catalog 2004/2005. Morgan Hill, CA: North Coast.

North Coast Medical, Inc. (2005). *Functional Solutions* catalog 2005. Morgan Hill, CA: North Coast.

Patterson Medical Products, Inc. (2006). *Sammons Preston Rolyan: Pediatrics: Special needs products for schools and clinics* Fall 2006 catalog. Bolingbrook, IL: Sammons Preston Rolyan.

PlumberSurplus.com, LLC (2006). *Shower and tub rough-in valves.* Retrieved November 20, 2006, from http://www.plumbersurplus.com/ProductDetail.aspx?Prod=46004&Cat=281.

Rifton Equipment (2005). Rifton equipment catalog 2004–2005. Chester, NY: Rifton Equipment.

Rogers, J., & Holm, M. (1994). Assessment of self care. In B. R. Bonder & M.B. Wagner (Eds.), *Functional performance in older adults* (pp. 181–202). Philadelphia: F. A. Davis.

Solomon, J., & O'Brien, J. (2006). *Pediatric skills for occupational therapy assistants* (2nd ed). St. Louis: Mosby

Southwest Medical Online (2006). Positioning products: Tumble forms 2 tadpole pediatric positioner. Retrieved December 12, 2006, from http://www.southwestmedical.com/Pediatric_Products/Positioning_Products/Tumble_Forms_2_Tadpole_Pediatric_Positioner/16673p0.

StorageWorks. (2005). Products: Bathroom and shower organization. Retrieved November 20, 2006, from http://www.storageworks.com/bath.html#.

Suner, J., Nakamura, S., & Caulfield, R. (2003). Kids having kids: Models of intervention. *Early Childhood Education Journal, 31,* 71–74.

World Health Organization (2001). *International classification of functioning, disability, and health.* Geneva, Switzerland: Author.

Chapter 13

Interventions for Instrumental Activities of Daily Living (IADL)

Margaret J. Pendzick

Key Terms

Accessibility options	Meal preparation and cleanup
Augmentative and alternative communication methods	Personal safety
	Pet care
Calibrate	Posture
Communication device use	Shopping
Community mobility	Support walker
Computers	Telecommunication devices
Depth perception	for the deaf (TDD)
Hand-held walker	Topographical orientation
Instrumental activities of daily living (IADL)	Universal design
	Visual figure-ground perception

Objectives

- Clarify the role of the occupational therapist and occupational therapy assistant in the intervention process for IADL.
- Explain intervention approaches that address children's and adolescents' IADL needs and are developmentally and contextually relevant.
- Develop intervention plans to address IADL.

INTRODUCTION

This chapter focuses on specific interventions that are used to address children's and adolescents' **instrumental activities of daily living (IADL)** occupations. Since children and adolescents perform these occupations in a variety of different environments, it is important to consider how they generalize these skills in different contexts.

Occupational therapy interventions may be directed toward the person, task, or environment in order to achieve the goals of establishing, modifying, preventing, or enriching a child's or adolescent' ability to engage in IADL. When designing interventions for IADL, occupational therapists and occupational therapy assistants utilize therapeutic use of self, therapeutic use of occupation and activities, consultation services, and education. These are the same type of intervention strategies utilized for ADL. However, IADL occupations, by their nature, usually are more complex than ADL occupations; thus interventions directed toward them may require additional planning and time to accomplish.

IADL

As defined by the Occupational Therapy Practice Framework (AOTA, 2002), IADL include activities that are complex in nature and involve the child or adolescent interacting with the environment. This section focuses on a few of them and include age and developmentally appropriate intervention strategies that are specific to the IADL of **pet care**, **communication device use**, **community mobility**, **meal preparation and clean-up**, **personal safety**, and **shopping**. These intervention strategies also can be generalized to other IADL occupations.

Pet Care

A family pet gives many children and adolescents the opportunity to experience daily responsibilities. Since there are numerous types of pets that require a variety of different categories of care, this section focuses on the establishment of a generic routine for care of any pet rather than specific care that may need to be given to a particular pet. Establishing a routine task often requires intervention strategies to be directed to the child's or adolescent's processing performance skills and body functions. Interventions also may be directed to adapting the task or modifying the environment.

In order to perform routine tasks in pet care, the children or adolescents demonstrate a variety of different performance skills, performance patterns, and body functions. For instance, when a child puts out food and water for her pet, she demonstrates performance skills by selecting what type of food to put in the bowl and how often to provide the food and water. She might choose to use a step stool to reach the pet food on the shelf or ask her parents for help. If she spills food over the rim of the bowl, she follows procedures to clean up the floor. She uses performance patterns to accomplish the task by routinely returning the pet bowls to their designated place on the kitchen floor and placing empty pet food containers in the trash. Her neuromusculoskeletal and movement-related body functions allow her actively to move her joints to reach items and perform the eye-hand coordination task of pouring items into the pet bowls.

If a child or adolescent has difficulty performing the task, the occupational therapist analyzes the task and determines what is limiting the child's or adolescent's participation. Supervised by an occupational therapist, the occupational therapy assistant provides specific interventions that facilitate the development of the needed performance skill, performance pattern, or body function deficit. The occupational therapy assistant might adapt the task or the environment to support the child's or the adolescent's existing capacities. For instance, if the child has difficulty organizing and locating objects, she might adapt the environment by color coding all of the necessary supplies. Thus, when the child looks for them on the shelves and in the cabinets, she can locate them more easily. If the child or adolescent has difficulty remembering to clean the cat litter box every day, the occupational therapy assistant might provide a large reminder poster on the refrigerator door. If a motor skill limitation hinders the child's or adolescent's ability to lift heavy items, the occupational therapy assistant might exchange individually wrapped servings for the original bulk bags of dog food.

Table 13.1■ provides additional interventions to consider when helping a child or adolescent engage in pet care occupations. The table is divided into columns. The first column presents a brief description of the child or adolescent engaging in a specific type of pet care. The second column lists occupational challenges that the child or adolescent might confront. The third column provides suggested interventions.

Communication Device Use

Communication device usage includes a wide variety of equipment with various degrees of complexity (AOTA, 2002). Although speech and language pathologists and

■ **Table 13.1**
Pet Care

Occupation	Occupational Challenges	Interventions
Alex, a 14-year-old who has limited vision, needs to groom and exercise his horse in the pasture.	Unable to visually locate grooming supplies in the barn.	Place grooming supplies in a bucket and store in a consistent designated area.
	Unable to lead horse from barn to pasture.	Install a handrail from the barn to pasture gate. Instruct Alex to glide hand along handrail as he walks his horse to gated pasture.
Perdita, a 10-year-old, who has spina bifida, wants to feed and groom her dog.	Unable to reach supplies from her wheelchair.	Provide a long handled reacher and place items on low shelves.
	Unable to bend over and reach dog for grooming and bathing.	Instruct Perdita on how to train dog to fetch grooming and bathing supply bucket, to sit on a low table to be groomed, and to sit on a shower chair to be bathed using hand held controls.
Terrel, a 12-year-old who has Down syndrome, needs to assume responsibility for feeding the gerbil and cleaning the cage in his classroom.	Unable to remember all steps to clean the cage.	Construct a cue card that provides pictures or words of each task in sequence.
	Unable to open all food and cleaning supplies.	Place food and cleaning supplies in easy opening containers. Instruct Terrel in efficiently opening and closing new containers.

audiologists are the team members responsible for comprehensive evaluation, selection, and training in the use of sophisticated communication devices for children and adolescents with hearing and speech impairments, occupational therapists and occupational therapy assistants may need to address this IADL if the child or adolescent is having trouble performing the task or needs adaptations for independent usage.

Augmentative and **alternative communication methods (AACs)** are used by children and adolescents who have limited or absent verbal communication skills. Communication methods can be nonaided or aided. Nonaided methods include gestures, facial expressions, body postures, and sign language. Aided methods include the use of devices that are categorized by their level of technical sophistication. They range from low level technical devices such as a simple communication board with a few objects or pictures that represent a child's or adolescent's daily needs, to high level technical devices such as a sophisticated electronic speech synthesizer. The speech and language pathologist, in collaboration with the child or adolescent, family members, educational staff, and occupational therapy personnel, designs an AAC system. Using the SETT Framework, they consider the student (S), the environment (E), the task demands (T), and the tools available (T) (Cook & Hussey, 2002). They take into account the child's or the adolescent's developmental, physical, and cognitive abilities; the environment where the ACC method will be used; the communication needs and wants of the child or adolescent; and the usability, costs, and durability of the method. Young children often use communication methods that involve real objects. As the children grow in their cognitive communication capabilities, pictures, the drawing may replace the real objects. Symbols, then words eventually replace the pictures. With advances in computerized technology, a wide variety of sophisticated systems have become available. A few of these are described in Table 13.2■. Children and adolescents can access some of these aided AAC devices through the state assistive technology lending libraries. The location of these lending libraries is published on the web at http://www.usatechguide.org.

Supervised by the occupational therapist, the occupational therapy assistant may provide adaptations that allow the children and adolescents to use their augmentative communication device. For instance, the occupational therapy assistant might place pictures on a vertically positioned Plexiglas® communication board to enable a child with severe motor limitations to use his eyes to gaze at a picture of an idea he wishes to convey. Separating the pictures or words sufficiently from one another on the board allows the person communicating with the child to determine the focus of the child's gaze. If a child has some control of his arm movements but is unable to isolate a finger to point to a picture or turn multiple pages of a communication book, the occupational therapy assistant might provide a universal cuff or construct a hand splint to hold a pencil for pointing and turning. The occupational therapy assistant also might replace the standard switch with an alternative device the child or adolescent can use to activate an electronic based augmentative communication system. For example, if a switch is too small or requires too much pressure to activate, the occupational therapy assistant may replace it with a larger switch or one that requires less force to activate. Often the occupational therapy assistant needs to redesign the system so that the child or adolescent can activate the switch with a different body part. If a child or adolescent cannot use his hands to push down a switch, the occupational therapy assistant may change or position the switch so that it can be activated by a shrug of a shoulder or tap of an elbow.

Children and adolescents whose occupations are challenged due to inefficient or limited motor, cognitive, or sensory skills also may have difficulty using everyday communication devices such as writing utensils, telephones, and computers.

■ **Table 13.2**
Aided AAC

COMMUNICATION SOFTWARE	DESCRIPTION
EZ Keys™	The software provides dual word prediction, abbreviation expansion, rapid text-to-speech voice output. Users can use software to communicate with others.
Talking Screen™	The screen is designed for individuals who prefer using pictures and symbols to communicate. The user is able to use a customized display board to assist with communication. Furthermore, the user is able to select pictures and symbols to communicate feelings, ideas, and thoughts to others.
Quickpage™	The preprogrammed symbol pages are available to use with Talking Screen™ software. The user selects a symbol or picture to use when communicating with others. Once the symbol is selected, another page with similar topics/content will appear for individual to incorporate into conversation. Using QuickPage™, the user quickly can build and speak complete sentences by selecting symbols in the appropriate order.
Abbreviate!™	The abbreviation expansion program assists users in typing/communicating with others. Once abbreviations are established for common words or phrases, the user types in the abbreviation and the word/phrase will appear on the screen.
Boardmaker®	The communication and learning tool has over 3,000 picture symbols; it is designed to enhance the language and learning process.
Writing with Symbols	The word processing program allows users to type words with picture symbols.
COMMUNICATION SYSTEMS	DESCRIPTION
PEC—™ Picture Exchange Communication	Child selects a picture or symbol to communicate a want or need. The adult acknowledges the child, verbally names the picture, and encourages the child to repeat the word.
Communication boards	The user manually points to or electronically selects a picture, Bliss symbols™, Rebus™, or PicSyms™ from a series of options to communicate. The number of options can be adjusted from 2 to 128 to correspond to the child's capacities. Different boards can be designed to correspond with various topics of interest, such as one for ADLs, one for food, and one for play and leisure.
Big Mac™	The user presses the circular disk to activate a standard recorded message.
Talk Trac™	The user presses a wrist size device to activate a recorded message.
Voice Pal™	The user presses a switch connected to real objects.
Delta Talker™	The child uses direct touch to activate an electronic speaking communication board.
Light Talker™	The child can use direct selection, optic scanning, row or column scanning, or Morse code to activate an electronic speaking communication board.

■ Table 13.2
Aided AAC (cont.)

COMMUNICATION SYSTEMS	DESCRIPTION
Dyna Vox System™	The adolescent can activate the device through direct contact, single or dual switches, visual or auditory scanning. The device offers graphic and text options and synthesized speech output.
DynaWrite™	Speech-output and communication device. Users use the keyboard to type messages and the voice technology creates the automated output.
Say-It SAM Tablet/Say-It SAM Communicator™	PDA communication and programming tool. Users can use software to create communication boards with over 6,000 symbols.

Source: Compiled by Amy Mateer, OTS, Towson University.

Occupational therapy intervention may focus on establishing skills or adapting the tasks to enable the children or adolescents to access these devices independently. A comprehensive evaluation conducted by the occupational therapist identifies the occupation based outcomes that are appropriate to the individual child or adolescent. An occupational therapy assistant can contribute to the evaluation and provide intervention strategies that address the child's or adolescent's performance skills, performance patterns, client factors, and contexts in which the communication devices will be utilized. This chapter offers examples of intervention strategies for computer usage, telephone, and writing utensils. Additional handwriting interventions are discussed in Chapter 14 of this text.

Computers

Children and adolescents use **computers** for written and oral communication, as well as for leisure time pursuits. An occupational therapy assistant may be part of an assistive technology team that makes recommendations on the appropriate types of computer program options and accessories that allow children and adolescents to use computers successfully.

There is a wide selection of options that allow children or adolescents with physical and cognitive impairments to independently access a computer. Most computer control panels have **accessibility options** that allow adjustments or configurations for mobility, vision, and hearing needs. For instance, activating the sticky key command eliminates the need for a child or adolescent with motor difficulties to press down two or more keys concurrently. Adjusting the computer's color displays, font size, and cursors may make the characters on the screen easier to see for a child or adolescent with visual acuity or visual processing challenges. As well, the toggle key option that links the capital and number lock selection with an audible tone is useful for those with low vision difficulties. A comprehensive listing of products, options, and tutorials available for computers can be viewed at http://www.microsoft.com/enable and http://www.apple.com/accessibility.

Changes also can be made to computer accessories such as the mouse, keyboard, screen, microphone, or sound system to improve a child's or an adolescent's ability to access and successfully use a computer. Since there is a wide variety of computer accessories available, the occupational therapy assistant considers the child's and the adolescent's performance skills, performance patterns, and body functions as well as the context of where the computer will be used. Table 13.3■ provides examples of how computer accessories are used to enhance access and use of a computer.

The addition of specific software packages also can improve communication skills. For example, voice activated word processing systems can eliminate the need to physically manipulate a keyboard. When considering these systems, however, it is important to assess breath control and energy level that can impede the ability to successfully operate the program. There also are word prediction software programs available that decrease the number of keystrokes required to produce a word. Word prediction software enables the child or adolescent to select from a menu of predicable words based on the first few letters they enter on the screen. With the everyday advances in software technology, it is necessary to remain informed about new software options that may enhance the children or adolescents you encounter.

■ Table 13.3
Computer Accessories

OCCUPATION	OCCUPATIONAL CHALLENGES	INTERVENTIONS
Logan, a 16-year-old with a spinal cord injury, needs to use the computer to complete academic schoolwork.	Due to paralysis in the upper extremities, Logan is unable use a keyboard to type school assignments.	Instruct Logan on using an eye gaze or sip and puff system of access to the computer. Provide word recognition software and onscreen keyboard to select words and text.
Hakeem, a 13-year-old who has muscular dystrophy, wants to communicate with friends and play games on the computer.	Unable to isolate finger movements to type email or instant message to friends.	Provide Hakeem with a voice recognition device that allows him to speak into the computer to communicate with friends.
	Unable to press enter and arrow keys on keyboard to play computer game.	Incorporate a modified keyboard with custom overlays to enable selection of large arrow and enter key.
Malvina, a 12-year-old who has a traumatic brain injury, limited hearing, and decreased cognition, wants to listen and to watch storybooks on the computer.	Unable to remember steps to turn on computer and access web site.	Create a shortcut card to place on the side of the monitor screen that provides pictures of the task and buttons for Malvina to press.
	Unable to hear stories through speakers within computer monitor.	Install external amplified speakers at computer workstation and instruct Malvina in using personal headphones.
Sekou, an 18-year-old who has a learning disability and ADHD, uses the computer to complete data entry at a work-training program he attends three days a week.	Unable to attend to single task for long periods of time.	Install a timer or screensaver on Sekou's computer that provides a visual cue after a designated period of time to allow for a break.
	Easily distracted with letter keys and other computer applications on workstation.	Provide Sekou with a numeric keyboard at her workstation that eliminates the need for a letter keyboard.

Source: Compiled by Amy Mateer, OTS, Towson University.

Telephone Usage

Children and adolescents are frequent users of the telephone. By the age of 5, most children can answer the phone appropriately, call another person to the phone, or take a brief oral message (Allen & Marotz, 2007). Caregivers often help young children to talk with relatives on the phone. By the time children reach their teen years, they often use the telephone as a major means of peer communication. Therefore, if a child or adolescent is unable to successfully utilize the telephone due to occupational challenges, intervention by occupational therapy is appropriate.

With the common use of cell phones, the occupational therapist or occupational therapy assistant also may need to investigate available features that would allow access to these devices. For instance, the phone book option on the cell phone may need to be preprogrammed for either manual selection or voice commands, or the ring tones may need to be changed to vibration or louder volume to accommodate limited hearing. The occupational therapy assistant may help those children and adolescents with hearing impairments learn how to use the text messaging options on their cellular phones, and instant messaging options on their computers to communicate in real and virtual time with one another. In addition, **Telecommunication Devices for the Deaf (TDD)** also are available for children or adolescents with hearing impairments. These systems allow children and adolescents to send typed messages to one another through the telephone network. The TDD generates a visual and paper copy of the typed message. Messages can be sent back and forth as long as the telephone lines remain open. There is a wide variety of different reasons that a child or adolescent is unable to use a telephone. With the introduction of **universal design**, an array of adaptations is available to meet many of these needs. Table 13.4■ illustrates some of the ways current features can be used.

Writing Utensils

Depending upon the age and developmental level of the child or adolescent, specific writing utensils are used. For a young child, this would include large circumference crayons, markers, and paint brushes; for an elementary school child this would include standard pencils, crayons, and markers; for an adolescent this would include pens and pencils. If the child or adolescent has difficulty writing due to physical challenges, the occupational therapy assistant might provide interventions to improve grasp of the utensil or alter the activity demand by adapting the utensil to accommodate to the child's or adolescent's grasp pattern. By analyzing evaluation results and utilizing clinical reasoning, the occupational therapist and the occupational therapy assistant decide which approach best achieves the child's or adolescent's occupation based goals and outcomes.

In addition to grasp, it is also important to consider the child's or adolescent's **posture** when attempting the task. Since a stable base of support is necessary to grasp and manipulate objects, the occupational therapy assistant makes sure that the child or adolescent is seated symmetrically in a chair that allows feet to be flat on the floor. Table height should be at low chest level. Hips, knees, and ankles should be at approximately 90° of flexion, with elbows resting comfortably on the table and with back supported by the chair. When working at an easel or a chalkboard, the child should position the materials at or around midline and keep symmetrical alignment of the head, trunk, and extremities. With the adjustment in posture and stabilization of extremities, grasp of writing utensils often improves without further intervention required. The occupational therapy assistant can provide age appropriate activities that encourage the child or adolescent to practice automatically adjusting his or her posture to accommodate different activity contexts. For instance, the occupational

■ **Table 13.4**
Telephone Usage

OCCUPATION	OCCUPATIONAL CHALLENGES	INTERVENTIONS
Aiyana, a 12-year-old who has Down syndrome, needs to assume responsibility for calling her parents when she arrives at an after-school day program.	Unable to remember her parents' number at work.	Create a cue card with important numbers next to the phone or utilize a programmable touchpad and designate one number for each parent.
	Unable to use small keypad on cellular phone to contact her parents.	Work with Aiyana in creating a contact list within her cell phone that she can access using voice recognition (if her cell phone is compatible with this software) or create one-touch button contacts for family members and 911.
Hakim, a 9-year-old who has limited vision, wants to use the telephone to speak with his grandparents every weekend.	Unable to visually identify the small numbers on the telephone receiver.	Provide a large, illuminated button phone, with or without pictures for Hakim to access. Provide Hakim with a keypad with tactile marking.
	Unable to locate phone in time to answer a phone call.	Set telephone to extended number of rings and place a noncorded telephone in designated area that is accessible for Hakim.
Ilse, a 15-year-old who has muscular dystrophy, wants to use her cell phone and house phone to keep in touch with her parents and friends as well as for emergencies.	Unable to press individual buttons on telephone keypad to dial a call.	Work with Ilse to put phone numbers into a contact list and instruct Ilse to use the voice-activation option with all her phones.
	Unable to get to the phone in time when it is ringing due to decreased endurance.	Place phones on each level of Ilse's home and select option for longest number of rings. Install an answering machine and have Ilse record a message.
Rafal, a 16-year-old who has limited hearing, talks with friends and his girlfriend on the telephone on a regular basis.	Unable to hear when the phone is ringing.	Install a light activated switch on telephone to signal to Rafal when the phone is ringing.
	Sometimes unable to hear friends and/or girlfriend on the other end of the telephone.	Use built-in intercoms or amplifiers on telephone or incorporate the use of a personal messaging program that allows Rafal to talk with friends/girlfriend through the computer.

Source: Compiled by Amy Mateer, OTS, Towson University.

therapy assistant may have the child hunt for treasure clues in different parts of the room and on different surfaces. While assembling the clues, the child is encouraged to maintain correct body alignment and place the clues near the midline of the body. The goal is for the child or adolescent to establish a useful habit of consistently utilizing correct posture throughout the day.

To effectively utilize a writing utensil, a child or adolescent also must **calibrate** the appropriate grip strength. The child or adolescent holds the writing utensil firmly enough to prevent slippage but not so tightly as to impede in-hand manipulation and movement. If a child or adolescent has difficulty exerting sufficient pressure to grip a utensil, the occupational therapy assistant may provide age appropriate activities to strengthen upper extremity muscles. For instance, the occupational therapy assistant may suggest that a preschooler play with sponges, turkey basters, and squirt guns during bath time or manipulate play dough into different shapes and objects. The occupational therapy assistant may suggest that an adolescent work on macramé craft projects or knead dough when baking. If client factors hinder the child or adolescent from increasing strength, the occupational therapy assistant may provide an adaptive device, such as a universal cuff or writing splint, that eliminates the need to grasp the utensil. Table 13.5■ gives further examples of appropriate interventions.

Community Mobility

Depending on the age, abilities, and environment, children and adolescents use a variety of different means to move around their communities. Younger children may use tricycles, scooters, and bicycles, while adolescents may use public transportation

■ **Table 13.5**
Grasp

OCCUPATION	OCCUPATIONAL CHALLENGES	INTERVENTIONS
Brandan, an 8-year-old who has a learning disability and is hypotonic, is responsible for unpacking/packing materials from his backpack at the beginning/end of the school day.	Unable to open and close book-bag to access materials and supplies.	Incorporate gross-motor exercises into classroom routine to facilitate tone in upper extremity prior to start of classroom work.
		Provide a loop tag to zipper pull on book bag or apply Velcro strips to open and close book bag.
Ossian, a 6-year-old who has Down syndrome, is working with class to complete art project at school.	Unable to hold regular paintbrush in right hand when painting at easel.	Provide Ossian with a paintbrush that has a built up handle to use when standing at easel, or instruct Ossian to use fingers to paint during art project.
	Has difficulty holding glitter in the palm of one hand as he sprinkles it on paper with the fingers of the other hand.	Place glitter into a shaker which will allow Ossian to use grasp with one hand and apply to the paper.
Sosanna, a 10-year-old who has cerebral palsy, needs to write in her daily word journal for English class.	Unable to hold pencil using a tripod grasp due to spasticity in her upper extremity.	Provide Sosanna with a custom-made pencil holder that allows for a spherical grasp on the device and insertion of the pencil into the device. If spasticity is severe, allow Sosanna to use either in-class computer or word processing system.
Jiang Li, a 12-year-old who has mild muscular dystrophy, needs to learn how to open the door to his home after being dropped off from the school bus.	Has difficulty opening the door using a key due to weakness in upper extremity.	With low-temp splinting material, attach an extension to the key that requires less force to open the lock. If finances are available, recommend installing a touch keypad opener.

Source: Compiled by Amy Mateer, OTS, Towson University.

or drive a car. Children and adolescents with motor performance difficulties may use a walker, wheelchair, or cane. Various options are available that enhance independent community mobility.

Wheelchairs

Some children and adolescents with motor difficulties use wheelchairs to participate in their daily occupations. The wheelchair should accommodate the child's or the adolescent's physical, environmental, and occupational needs. To assist with wheelchair selection, maintenance, and utilization, the occupational therapy assistant must understand the basic principles of wheelchair measurement and accessory selection, as well as be able to instruct the child or adolescent in the proper use of the chair.

Wheelchair Selection   Regardless of the type, the wheelchair should allow the child or adolescent to sit in a symmetrically aligned position with hips, knees, and ankles at approximately 90°. Proper chair seat surface, width, depth, and height promote alignment of the pelvis and trunk. Most pediatric wheelchair seats are a solid insert that allows equal distribution of weight over the thighs and buttocks and possible adjustments for later growth. Seat width is usually 1–2 inches wider than the measurement across the widest section of the child's or the adolescent's hips or thighs (see Figure 13.1a■). The seat depth needs to be 1-2 inches less than the measurement from the back of the buttock to the politeal fossa (See Figure 13.1b■) to eliminate the rubbing of the edge of the chair on the back of the legs. The height of the seat depends upon sitting balance and chosen means of propulsion. If the child or adolescent manually propels the chair, the seat back height needs to be under the scapular area to allow hyperextension of movement of the arm. As the seat height is lowered, the child or the adolescent needs more developed sitting balance. If the child or adolescent requires a power driven wheel chair, the back seat height is raised to a level to support the motor ability (Cook & Hussey, 2002). Since those who provide funding expect a wheelchair to fit a child for approximately 5 years, measurements must anticipate changes in body sizes. Some wheelchairs have adjustments that allow for growth. Often a customized seat or back insert is constructed for the wheelchair, and can be removed or altered as the child grows.

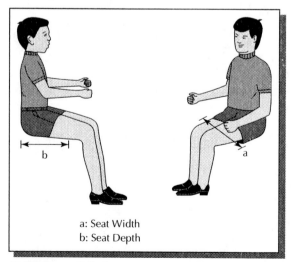

a: Seat Width
b: Seat Depth

■ **Figure 13.1**
(a) Seat width measurement; (b) seat depth measurement.

In addition to seat and back dimensions, the occupational therapist and occupational therapy assistant also must determine the overall height of the chair. In order for a younger child to transfer independently into and out of the chair, the occupational therapist and occupational therapy assistant may need to select a frame that is closer to the floor. A lower frame chair, however, is too low for a standard size table and is difficult for an adult to push. This decision, made in collaboration with the family and team members, must take into account the child's abilities and anticipate the child's environments, family preferences, and community setting.

Based upon performance skills, body function deficits, and anticipated environments, a child or adolescent uses either a manual or power wheelchair. Manual wheelchairs are usually lightweight. Accessory options include different types of leg rest, arms rest, seat cushion, seat belt, lapboard, and wheel size. Table 13.6■ illustrates how options are combined to customize a wheelchair.

Besides the feature mentioned for the manual chair, a means to operate the controls must be selected when customizing a power wheelchair. By examining the capabilities of the child or adolescent, the occupational therapist and the occupational therapy assistant may recommend the use of a particular body part or a combination of body parts and specific activation devices to operate the chair. Frequently, the occupational therapist and occupational therapy assistant recommend that children and adolescents use hand or head controls. A joystick is the most common hand switch for controlling the direction, speed, and turning of the power chair. The joystick is positioned at the center or side of the chair for optimal performance. The chair can be operated by head controls that consist of a pressure switch or motion detection device. The children and adolescents also may use mouth, foot, or shoulder movement to

■ **Table 13.6**
Manual Wheelchairs

OCCUPATION	OCCUPATIONAL CHALLENGES	ADAPTATIONS
SaQuan, a 5-year-old who has moderate spastic cerebral palsy, has out grown her stroller and needs a wheelchair to use at school.	Unable to sit independently, sliding out of her chair as lower extremity tone increases.	Secure the pelvis by installing a low seatbelt and carve the seat cushion to increase hip flexion.
	Unable to grip handrail to propel chair.	Install spokes on the handrails so SaQuan can push rather than grasp rim to propel the wheelchair.
Lisa, a 14-year-old who has spina bifida, wants her new chair to be easy to use in the community.	Due to low endurance, unable to propel wheelchair for long distances.	Choose a lightweight frame that requires less energy to propel.
	Has difficulty maneuvering her wheelchair in small spaces.	Choose smaller front wheels that provide a smaller turning radius and more maneuverability in small areas.
Jim, a 10-year-old with diplegic cerebral palsy, lives on a farm and needs his chair to handle a variety of outside terrains.	Has difficulty propelling his chair outside around the farm.	Recommend pneumatic caster wheels that will maneuver better on outside terrain.
Palmer, a 16-year-old with a spinal cord injury, would like to participate in wheelchair sports.	Often tips over his chair when playing sports.	Increase the camber on the wheels to improve the stability of the wheelchair base.
	His backrest and armrests interfere with UE movement during sports.	Investigate specific wheelchairs built for Palmer's chosen sport.

■ **Table 13.7**
Power Wheelchair

Occupation	Occupational Challenges	Adaptations
Antone, a 6-year-old with muscular dystrophy, wants to be able to play with his friends on the playground.	Unable to manually propel a wheelchair due to decreasing strength.	Select a child-sized power chair that sits Antone at the height of his peers.
Pam, an 18-year-old with a C3–4 spinal cord injury, needs to be able to sit in her chair for extended periods of time at her after-school job.	Unable to weight shift manually to relieve pressure on her buttocks. Unable to use hand or arms to operate joy stick.	Select tilt-in-space accessory that will allow Pam to eliminate pressure while still sitting in chair. Consider controls that can be activated by head or chin movement.
Manuel, a 12-year-old with spastic cerebral palsy, wants to be able to independently maneuver his wheelchair.	Unable to sit upright in chair without support. Although he can manipulate the joystick with his right arm, Manuel begins to slump to the right side which interferes with arm movement.	Provide lateral supports, seat belt, and adductor wedge. Reposition joystick closer to midline to encourage symmetrical posture and less slumping.

operate the wheelchair, if needed. Table 13.7■ illustrates various power wheelchair selections that enhance the child's or the adolescent's ability to successfully operate the chair.

Wheelchair Education   An occupational therapy assistant often will be responsible for instructing children or adolescent in wheelchair maneuverability and safety. In collaboration with the occupational therapist, the occupational therapy assistant identifies performance skills, performance patterns, and body functions deficits that hinder the child's or the adolescent's ability to safely maneuver in the community and address those issues. For instance, if a child or adolescent lacks upper body strength and endurance to manually propel the wheelchair, the occupational therapy assistant may introduce age appropriate strengthening activities. For a younger child this could be tossing weighted beanbags at a target, building structures with heavy blocks, or painting at an easel. The occupational therapy assistant might have the older child or adolescent participate in a basketball free throw shooting contest or work on a vertically suspended macramé project. If a child or adolescent has difficulty safely maneuvering the wheelchair in the classroom, the occupational therapy assistant might design an obstacle course to allow for practice opportunities. By grading the complexity of the obstacle course, the occupational therapy assistant could foster the development and mastery of different maneuverability strategies.

Mobility Devices
Although physical therapists often are responsible for the evaluation and initial training of mobility devices, occupational therapists and occupational therapy assistants reinforce the physical therapy instruction, ensure that the device is used safely, and incorporate the mobility device into other areas of occupation. The three categories of mobility devices children and adolescents commonly use are walkers, canes, and mobile standers.

Walkers   Children and adolescents may use **hand held walkers** and **support walkers** to assist in ambulation. In order to use a hand held walker, the child or adolescent must be able to assume a standing position while maintaining a grip on the walker handle. Hand held walkers come in different sizes and are adjusted for the individual child or adolescent. Two different types are available—an **anterior walker** which is placed in front and a **posterior walker** which is placed behind [Figure 13.2(a), (b)■]. The physical therapist usually determines which type of hand held walker is most appropriate for the child or adolescent. A support walker surrounds the body and supports body parts and weight [Figure 13.2(c)■].

A child or adolescent needs only to be able to move the lower extremities in a walking motion to propel the support walker. The walkers are wheeled; the larger the wheel, the more easily it maneuvers on different textured flooring and outdoors.

Canes   Children and adolescents whose occupations are challenged due to limited vision or motor difficulties use canes to assist in independent mobility. Children and adolescents with visual impairment may use a cane to maximize auditory and tactile information from the surrounding environment (Cook & Hussey, 2002). Specially trained mobility therapists often assume responsibility for the initial training; the occupational therapist or occupational therapy assistant incorporates these skills into intervention strategies when addressing other areas of occupation. The cane consists of three parts—the grip, the shaft, and the tip. The shaft and tip convey both auditory and tactile information which the child or adolescent either hears or feels through the grip. For instance, the child or adolescent can determine that a walkway is changing from concrete to grass, not only by the sound of the tap but also by the change in vibration sent up the cane handle. Since a high level of concentration is needed when interpreting this information, it is important not to distract the child or adolescent when learning to use the cane.

Children and adolescents with physical challenges also may use a cane during ambulation. As with other mobility devices, a physical therapist often provides the initial training; the occupational therapist and occupational therapy assistant incorporates safe usage of the cane into everyday activities, always adhering to safety precautions

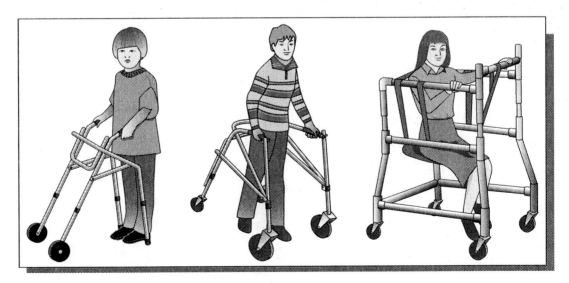

■ **Figure 13.2**
(a) Anterior hand held walker; (b) posterior hand-held walker; (c) support walker.

in its usage. Canes come in a variety of sizes and adjust to the height of the child. Children or adolescents use either a straight cane [Figure 13.3(a)■] or a quad cane [Figure 13-3(b)■], depending on the level of support needed.

A quad cane provides more support than a straight cane. If a child or an adolescent has difficulty grasping the cane handle, the occupational therapist or occupational therapy assistant may modify the cane grip.

Mobile Stander   Children and adolescent who are nonambulatory and who have the ability to push and maneuver large size wheels may use a mobile stander (Figure 13.4■) as an alternative to a wheelchair.

The standing position provides static weight bearing to the lower extremities while allowing the child or adolescent to maneuver around the environment. These devices often are used in a school based setting and can easily be positioned for participation in classroom activities. An occupational therapist or occupational therapy assistant working in school based practice may adapt the environment so that activities are accessible to mobile standers and other assistive devices such as prone standers, crutches, and paripodiums. They also may participate in the training of classroom teachers and aides in the proper positioning and safety issues related to these devices.

Riding Toys

Throughout their development, children and adolescents engage in activities that involve the use of riding toys. For the young child, this may include Big Wheels™, tricycles, or foot propelled riding toys. An older child or adolescent may use a bicycle, scooter, or skateboard. The occupational therapy assistant may need to adapt commercially available riding toys that children and adolescents have difficulty utilizing or may need to suggest an alternative adaptive piece of equipment. For instance, if a

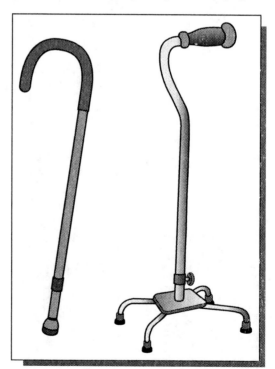

■ **Figure 13.3**
(a) Straight cane; (b) Quad cane.

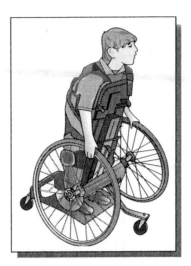

■ **Figure 13.4**
Mobile stander.

young child is unable to maintain balance and pedal a tricycle, the occupational therapy assistant may adapt the seat and pedals to provide added support. If a child is unable to use the legs to pedal a riding toy due to lower extremity bracing, the occupational therapy assistant may suggest an arm propelled riding toy (Figure 13.5■).

Table 13.8■ offers possible adaptation and alternative devices that enable children and adolescents to access riding toys during play.

Automobiles

Most adolescents delightedly anticipate when they are old enough to learn to drive. However, for the adolescent who is occupationally challenged due to sensory or motor limitation, obtaining a driver's license is not a routine occurrence. Although vehicle modification and adaptive driving programs are available, recent studies indicate that only 46 percent of students with disabilities have a driver's license compared to

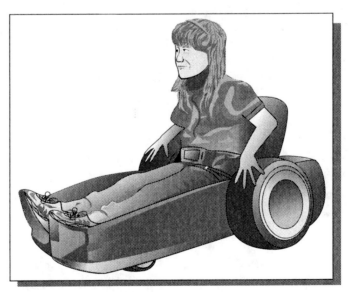

■ **Figure 13.5**
Child uses a caster cart in place of a tricycle.

■ **Table 13.8**
Riding Toys

OCCUPATION	OCCUPATIONAL CHALLENGES	ADAPTATIONS
Trey, a 6-year-old with developmental delays, wants to ride a Big Wheel™ with his brothers in the backyard.	Unable to sit upright unsupported on the seat.	Install side supports and seat belt to the original seat.
	Due to small stature, cannot reach the pedal or handle bars.	Attach blocks to the pedals and extend handle bars to decrease the distance.
Rylee, an 8-year-old with JRA wants to ride her bike in the town July 4th parade. The parade is three miles long, and she has filled the front basket with holiday decorations.	Unable to sustain grasp of handle bars for extended periods of time.	Increase circumference of handle bars to decrease stress on the hand joints during sustained grip.
	Does not want to use front basket to carry water bottles. Using a backpack increases stress on shoulder joints.	Assist Rylee in locating a new place to attach a water bottle, such as to side of frame. Install light weight saddle bags to back frame.
Alexander, a 12-year-old with Down syndrome, wants to complete a safety driver's course so that he can ride his bike on the street.	Has difficulty remembering the rules of the road when driving through the course.	Install picture reminders on handle bars for reference during the course.
	Has difficulty independently fastening his bike helmet.	Substitute an easier manipulated fastener for the originally one. Investigate that the new fastener meets safety standards.
Gee, a 3-year-old with autism, unsuccessfully attempts to propel a foot driven riding toy.	Unable to establish reciprocal foot motion to propel toy.	Assist Gee in moving his legs to propel, initiating the reciprocal movement from hip and knees.
	Cries when he wants to get off the toy.	Encourage Gee to use a gesture to indicate that he wants "off." Reward attempts with promptly assisting him off the toy.

88 percent of the typical teens in America (Vogtle, Kern & McCauley, 2002). The occupational therapy assistant may need to become an advocate for those adolescents with motor and sensory limitations to be able to access necessary resources to learn to drive.

Modifications to seating, driving systems, hand and foot controls, and steering controls can be installed on many automobiles.

- Power steering or power brakes reduce the physical effort to operate these systems.
- A left foot accelerator eliminates the need to lift and cross the legs if unable to access the foot controls with right foot.
- A right hand turn signal allows access to control when only right hand is available.
- Foot pedal extensions raise the height of the brake and accelerator pedals if unable to reach standard length.
- Hand controls that operate wipers, horn, turn signals, and light dimmer switch also can operate brake and accelerator.
- Steering wheels can be adapted by using spinner knobs, amputee ring, or tri-pin.
- Custom seating can improve sitting balance, align posture, and provide stability (Cook & Hussey, 2002).

Examples of other modifications can be found on such websites as www .adaptivedriving.com, www.infinitec.org, or www.aota.org. Although car modifications can be expensive, there are some funding sources available to families. Major car manufacturers provide reimbursements up to $1,000 on the cost of installing adaptations to new automobiles or leased vehicles. The Department of Vocational Rehabilitation and private charity groups often will offer financial assistance. Driver's education programs, provided within an academic setting or out patient service, also can be adapted for adolescents with occupational challenges.

Accessing Public Transportation

Depending on the community resources, children and adolescents may access public transportation. With the passage of American with Disabilities Act (ADA), municipalities are required to adapt public transportation vehicles or provide alternative systems for all individuals with disabilities. Some transportation companies have installed wheelchair lifts on all or some of their buses. Others have fitted their buses with pneumatic devices that lower the front end to curb height to allow easy access. A teenager who would like to take the bus to attend a baseball game with friends can use the wheelchair lift or the pneumatic feature to board the bus and secure his wheelchair safely during the travel. In those municipalities that have provided alternative systems, the adolescent needs to learn the phone number and the procedure for scheduling rides.

In addition to physical challenges, cognitive limitations may interfere with a child's or adolescent's ability to access public transportation. In order to use public transportation, a child or adolescent must know the transit routes; access the correct bus, subway, or train; determine the correct fare; recognize if an alternative money system is used; recognize the correct transportation stop; and activate a signaling device, if necessary. Table 13.9■ describes appropriate occupational therapy intervention strategies that may help a child or adolescent with cognitive or processing limitations to access public transportation.

Meal Preparation and Cleanup

The IADL of meal preparation and cleanup consists of different age appropriate tasks which are influenced by the child's and adolescent's abilities and family expectations. For instance, simple meal preparation of pouring milk into cereal or spreading peanut butter on bread can be accomplished by a 5-year-old (Allen & Marotz, 2007). However, if a family employs a cook or a child receives all meals at a homeless shelter, even though the child has the potential to perform these tasks, he will not develop the ability, since there is lack of opportunity or importance to develop the skills. Meal preparation and cleanup skill development in children and adolescents is dependent upon family expectations, opportunities, and cultural values.

Meal preparation and cleanup are multistep processes that involve many different activities. Regardless of the type of meal to be prepared, a child or adolescent must gather supplies, open and close any necessary containers, and manipulate required kitchen tools. Cleanup may include putting away supplies, washing and drying dishes, wiping off the countertop or table, and loading a dishwasher. For safety reasons, a young child needs adult supervision, but an adolescent may learn to operate kitchen appliances independently. Older children and adolescents may follow a written recipe, while young children may follow verbal directions from an adult or only prepare an uncooked meal such as a sandwich and a powdered drink. Other occupational therapy intervention strategies for each of these areas also might be utilized when working with a child or adolescent on food preparation and cleanup.

■ **Table 13.9**
Public Transportation

Occupation	Occupational Challenges	Interventions
Hannah, an 18-year-old who has a developmental disability, needs to learn how to take the bus to her new afternoon job at a local grocery store.	Unable to identify proper bus route from school to store on community bus schedule.	Acquire bus route map and work with Hannah to highlight route information from school to work. Take practice rides on the bus route, gradually decreasing how much assistance to give to Hannah. When she consistently demonstrates skill without prompts, shadow Hannah to make sure that she is independent.
	Unable to determine if she has proper amount of money for bus fare.	Instruct Hannah to prepare for work by setting the proper bus fare aside for each day of work. Instruct Hannah to place money in color coded envelopes for each day of the week. This visual cue will allow her to select an envelope each morning before going to school.
Brody, a 20-year-old who has a traumatic brain injury and decreased cognition, needs to take the subway into town for a work-training program.	Unable to remember directions and subway route from home to training program.	Construct wallet size cue cards that have pictures of route markers along the way for Brody to follow. Input directions and cues into a cellular phone or PDA, if accessible to Brody.
Rilla, a 4-year-old who has autism, travels with her mom into the city each morning. Rilla attends a full day developmental preschool program while her mom is at work.	Unable to process auditory stimulation in route to program.	Provide Rilla with a hand held listening device and personal headphones to use while in high frequency areas (subway, bus station).

Source: Compiled by Amy Mateer, OTS, Towson University.

Gathering Supplies

Depending on the reason for the difficulty, the occupational therapy assistant utilizes different intervention strategies to help the child or adolescent successfully gather needed food preparation supplies. For instance, if the challenge is due to limited ability to carry items to a work table, the occupational therapy assistant might instruct the child or adolescent to use a piece of adaptive equipment such as a utility cart to transport the needed items. If a child or adolescent has difficulty remembering what supplies are needed for the task, the occupational therapy assistant might help in the development of a checklist and provide opportunities for the child or adolescent to practice using checklists so that the skill becomes a useful habit. Additional intervention examples are listed in Table 13.10, on page 258.

Opening and Closing Containers.

During food preparation, numerous types of different containers must be opened and closed. For instance, when a child pours a glass of milk, he may need to manipulate a plastic screw-type milk lid or a cardboard spout opening. Each of these openings requires different motor and cognitive skills to successfully manipulate. For this reason, it is important for the occupational therapy assistant to investigate and observe what types of equipment are used within a given environment and modify the instructions or adaptations accordingly. Although providing practice in different contexts would encourage generalization, the occupational therapy assistant must remember to practice skills in the natural environment where the child or adolescent will frequently use them.

When selecting an appropriate intervention, the occupational therapy assistant keeps in mind the child's or adolescent's overarching occupation based goal and the performance skills or body function deficit that hinders full participation in this aspect of the IADL. For example, if the child or adolescent is unable to open a jar of peanut butter, what information in the occupational therapy evaluation explains the problem? If hand strength is inadequate to open the jar, can a program be designed to improve strength, or should the task be adapted so that it is within the child's or the adolescent's present abilities? Is the problem due to limitations in bilateral tasks? If so, can bilateral skills be facilitated, or will the task need to be adapted so that bilateral tasks are avoided? Are there any body function contraindications requiring the child or adolescent to learn to complete this task without stressing the finger joints or encouraging ulnar deviation of the wrist? Because of the complexity of IADL tasks, the occupational therapy assistant critically looks at the task and the child's or the adolescent's strengths and limitations to develop an optimal intervention. Refer to Table 13.10 for further intervention considerations.

Kitchen Tools Manipulation

There is a variety of different types of tools that a child or adolescent uses when preparing food. Depending upon the kitchen used, children and adolescents are exposed to an assortment of knives, peelers, can openers, ladles, measuring cups, and spatulas. With the introduction of universal design, tools with larger handles and nonslip grips are available commercially to assist the child or adolescent who has difficulty holding or calibrating the tool grip during usage. Regardless of the tool, however, safety is the most important aspect in tool usage. When selecting appropriate kitchen tools, it also is important to consider the size and strength of childrens' and adolescents' hands. Children or adolescents who are challenged due to limited vision often require tools that have Braille markings or safety guards during usage. Table 13.10 lists additional interventions that can be used for manipulation of kitchen tools.

Simple and Complex Meals

Before beginning cooking intervention with children or adolescents, the occupational therapy assistant considers the developmental age, cultural preferences, and complexity of the menu. When accessing the cooking activity, the occupational therapy assistant determines the complexity by considering the number and difficulty of required steps to complete the activity, as well as the required manipulation of cooking tools. The occupational therapy assistant grades the complexity based on the strengths and abilities of the child or adolescent. The child or adolescent should learn to prepare simple meals that only require assembly, such as making a sandwich or adding precut vegetables to a salad before attempting those that require cooking or manipulating kitchen tools. The occupational therapy assistant considers the child's or adolescent's developmental level before introducing a written recipe, using illustrations rather than written phrases, if necessary. The cooking activity that she chooses should be graded not only to ensure success but also provide an opportunity to improve the child's or adolescent's skills. Table 13.10 further illustrates how meal complexity is incorporated into an intervention session.

Cleanup

Cleanup is an important aspect of food preparation and the environment may need to be adapted for children or adolescents with special needs. Kitchens may need to be adapted so that work areas are accessible for wheelchairs. Adaptation to the hand grips of cleaning supplies or alternative equipment may be necessary. Table 13.10■ includes adaptations that you might need to make in this area.

Besides the physical aspect, cleanup also requires the child or the adolescent to recognize the necessity to perform the task and monitor that the task is completed correctly. For instance, an adolescent may know that dishes need to be washed after a meal but is unable to recognize when the dish is thoroughly washed. The occupational therapy assistant may need to teach a strategy whereby the adolescent visually checks all surfaces of the dish before rinsing off the soap. The occupational therapy assistant may need to provide visual and auditory cues until monitoring the task becomes a useful habit.

■ Table 13.10
Meal Preparation and Cleanup

OCCUPATION	OCCUPATIONAL CHALLENGES	INTERVENTIONS
Isabella, a 9-year-old who has ADHD, needs to assume responsibility for setting the table for dinner each night.	Unable to gather all dishes and utensils for meal without being distracted by external stimuli.	Place dishes and utensils in a designated area/same vicinity as one another within the kitchen.
	Unable to remember proper order for dishes and utensils on the dining table.	Provide a visual cue card that has a picture of a table setting for Isabella to follow when setting the table.
Jokin, a 13-year-old who has spina bifida, needs to prepare his lunch before leaving for school each morning.	Unable to reach all supplies and food within the pantry to prepare and organize his lunch for the day.	Arrange lunch items on a height appropriate shelf within the pantry and refrigerator to allow Jokin to navigate to and retrieve items using his walker.
Naavah, a 16-year-old who has mild mental retardation and muscular dystrophy, enjoys helping prepare dinner for the family.	Unable to follow multistep directions for preparing a side dish for dinner.	Construct single step cards for Naavah to use. Each card will have a picture of the ingredient and corresponding step.
	Unable to control utensils within mixing bowl when stirring batter or ingredients.	Instruct Naavah on how to use a hand held mixer when mixing ingredients together for meal.
Ade, an 11-year-old who has juvenile rheumatoid arthritis, is responsible for clearing the table and assisting with the dishes.	Unable to stand at sink for an extended period of time due to decreased endurance.	Instruct Ade to pace self during routine so that he does not get tired easily, and to sit on a stool at the kitchen sink to wash dishes.
	Unable to bend over to place dishes in bottom rack of dishwasher due to limited range of motion.	Create a buddy system with sibling or parent whereby Ade rinses the dish and his buddy loads the plate, bowl, or glass into the dishwasher.

Source: Compiled by Amy Mateer, OTS, Towson University.

Table 13.10 describes different strategies that might be used when working with a child or adolescent on meal preparation and cleanup. Notice that within the occupation, the child or adolescent may require multiple intervention strategies to more than one aspect of the IADL. It is important to incorporate these strategies in such as a way that assists the child adolescent to perform the skills and are also acceptable to the child, adolescent, and family members.

Personal Safety

Throughout their development, children and adolescents gradually assume more responsibility for personal safety. These safety skills often are learned initially within social situations and daily routines. For instance, when a family takes a walk to the park, a young child begins to learn safe street-crossing skills. When building a birdhouse with a grandparent, a child or adolescent learns to handle sharp tools correctly. In school, a child practices exiting the building when the fire alarm sounds and often attends age appropriate assemblies on stranger awareness, drug education, and the importance of seat belts. For children and adolescents with exceptional needs, however, incidental learning may not be sufficient.

An occupational therapist or occupational therapy assistant may provide adaptations to equipment or instruction so that the child and adolescent can successfully gain independence in age appropriate areas of personal safety. For instance, if a child or adolescent has processing limitations and does not understand the meaning of the colors, words, or crosswalk symbols, he may have difficulty learning safe street-crossing skills. The occupational therapy assistant may adapt age appropriate games and activities to incorporate the stop and go concepts of the colors, words, and symbols so that the child or adolescent develops these safety concepts. There are many other ways to incorporate and teach personal safety concepts to children and adolescents. Table 13.11■ illustrates some interventions used to enhance the child's or adolescent's independence in personal safety.

Shopping and Money Management

The occupations of shopping and money management are highly complex tasks that involve a variety of different activities. In order to shop for an item, the child or adolescent must recognize where to obtain the object, how to negotiate within the store, and how to pay for the item. This might require the child or adolescent to make a shopping list, maneuver a shopping cart safely, calculate the purchase price, or write a personal check. As with most IADL occupations, children and adolescents gradually acquire shopping and money management skills by initially imitating adults engaging in these occupations. Younger children will play store or accompany a parent on a shopping trip. Older children and adolescents begin shopping on their own for a few family groceries or personal items. Initially, younger children receive money for a purchase and are told to "wait for change" while older children or adolescents need to determine whether they have sufficient allowance or after-school job money saved to afford a purchase. Practice opportunities allow children and adolescents to develop useful habits that enable them to competently complete age appropriate shopping and money management activities.

When working with children and adolescents who are challenged due motor or processing performance limitations, the occupational therapy assistant may need to design interventions that improve participation in shopping and money management.

■ **Table 13.11**
Personal Safety

Occupation	Occupational Challenges	Adaptations
LeBron, a 9-year-old with Down syndrome and asthma, wants to participate in an after-school track program.	Unable to operate his inhaler due to lack of finger dexterity.	Teach LeBron to use a spacer or aerochamber.
	Unable to lace and tie his cleats.	Use backward chaining to teach LeBron shoe tying. Use Velcro™ fasteners.
Rebecca, a 12-year-old with fragile X syndrome, wants to go with her family on vacation, where they will be rafting.	Needs to wear a life jacket but dislikes friction from the texture of the vest.	Encourage Rebecca to wear a long-sleeved cotton or nylon shirt underneath vest to minimize discomfort.
	Unable to determine how to match vest straps and securely fasten them.	Color code straps. Mark spot where to fasten straps.
Shane, an 8-year-old with cerebral palsy, wants to maneuver her wheelchair in the school hallways and down ramps independently.	Does not remember to pause at intersections and often runs over other children when turning down a hallway.	Place stop signs at end of hallways. Incorporate signs into activities and games until she understands the meaning of the sign.
	Unable to control the speed down the ramp.	Teach Shane how to slow down her speed by holding the rim or gently applying her hand brakes.
Tamara, a 16-year-old with hand tremors, wants to complete an advanced cooking class at the youth center.	Unable to safely use kitchen knives.	Adapt the kitchen knives with hand/finger guards.
	Unable to retrieve items from oven without burning upper arms.	Teach Tamara to pull out oven rack before removing items. Use hot pad mitts that extend to elbows.

Source: Compiled by M. Poague, OTAS and T. Hayward, OTAS, Penn State University

The children and adolescents may need to improve impoverished habits or establish useful habits to successfully participate in these IADL occupations. In order to discuss specific strategies, the occupational therapy assistant considers how to provide age appropriate interventions to specific tasks such as preparation to go shopping, navigation within the store, and payment for purchases.

Preparations
There are many tasks that take place before a child or adolescent goes shopping and makes payment. To purchase a predetermined item, the child or adolescent must know what type of store or Internet site sells the object. To purchases multiple items, the child or adolescent may need to learn how to make a list to take to the store. If funds are limited, the child or adolescent must prioritize purchases and determine how to use available money. All of these tasks require multiple problem solving skills that may be difficult if the child or adolescent has limited processing skills.

Opportunities for children and adolescents to work on organizational skills to participate successfully in the occupation of shopping need to be age appropriate and meaningful. For example, an occupational therapy assistant working with an adolescent group to develop age appropriate shopping skills may plan a holiday party. During the planning meetings, the occupational therapy assistant might encourage the members to discuss any cultural diversity issues that would influence the choice of food or activities for the party. After the members choose a menu and activities, the occupational therapy assistant might guide them in making a shopping list by asking leading questions and encouraging discussion about the products they need to purchase. The occupational therapy assistant also might direct the group members to estimate and compare projected expenses with the party budget, then make financial decisions if projected items exceed the party budget. If needed, the occupational therapy assistant also helps the group recognize the appropriate stores to purchase items. By guiding the group members through this preparatory process rather than making all the decisions for them, the occupational therapy assistant allows the adolescents to develop useful habits for future shopping needs.

Store Navigation

In order to locate purchases and carry them to the checkout counter, a shopper must be able to navigate within a store. This can be a challenging task for an adolescent or child who has difficulties processing visual information. Children and adolescents with **topographical orientation** problems will have difficulty knowing how to navigate around a store and remember paths that lead to certain departments or exits; those with **depth perception** problems may struggle with judging distances when reaching for items or pushing the shopping basket through aisles and checkout. Those with **visual figure-ground perception** challenges may not be able to locate and select a particular item off a crowded shelf (Schneck, 2005).

As already discussed in Chapter 10, intervention can be directed toward the person through restoring or establishing the abilities, or toward the task and environment by utilizing adaptations. The occupational therapy assistant, working in collaboration with an occupational therapist, determines the focus of intervention based on the child's or adolescent's strengths and limitations in the areas of performance skills, performance patterns, activity demands, and body functions. Table 13.12■ illustrates a variety of therapeutic uses of age appropriate occupations and activities that address the person, activity, or environment.

Money Management

In order to complete any purchase transaction, some type of payment must take place. By the end of their teenage years, adolescents are expected to be able to pay by cash, write checks, and understand how to use credit cards. These skills require the ability to recognize and know the value of coins and bills and to complete math calculations. If a child or adolescent has limited vision or cognitive functions, the occupational therapy assistant may need to design interventions to increase their participation in money management skills. There are many intervention options to consider.

The occupational therapy assistant might instruct the child or adolescent with limited vision in compensatory techniques to recognize coins and bills. Since there are no tactile marking on bills, the occupational therapy assistant might instruct the child or adolescent to distinguish among them by folding each denomination is a unique way so that it can be recognizable. The occupational therapy assistant also might instruct the child or adolescent to feel distinct tactile markings and keep coins in separate compartments of a coin purse. In order to complete a check, an adolescent may learn to place a template over the check and write the correct information in a given area. Calculators with raised numbers or Braille marks can be used to complete necessary calculations.

■ **Table 13.12**
Shopping

OCCUPATION	OCCUPATIONAL CHALLENGES	ADAPTATIONS
Suzanne, a 9-year-old with ADHD, would like to purchase a birthday present for her grandmother.	Unable to decide what to buy or where to purchase the item.	Help Suzanne problem solve by making a list or calling her grandmother for a wish list. Prior to shopping, help Suzanne identify where she could locate the item in a large department store.
	Often wanders away from adults and gets lost in the store. Immediately starts to cry and is unable to ask a store attendant for help.	Carry an ID card which she can hand to store attendants. Establish a designated meeting place, if she wanders away. Role play shopping, emphasizing staying in line of sight of adult.
Manuel, a 16-year-old with spina bifida, wants to shop independently for his personal items.	Unable to reach items on shelves and racks while sitting in his wheelchair.	Instruct Manuel in the use of a long handled reacher.
	Has difficulty maneuvering his wheelchair without knocking over displays.	Set up an obstacle course for practice with stop/go techniques and wide angle turns.
Kim, a 12-year-old with autism, would like to help her mother grocery shop.	Unable to locate items in the grocery store. Wanders up and down the aisles aimlessly.	Using the same grocery store and a list with one category of items, practice shopping skills.
	Becomes anxious and upset when she is accidentally bumped by a cart or person passing her in the aisle.	Shop in nonpeak hours. Engage Kim in games that require close contact with others such as tag, Twister™.

Source: Compiled by T. Nero, OTAS, and T. Kelly, OTAS, Penn State University.

When a child or adolescent is having difficulty with money management due to limited cognitive functions, the occupational therapy assistant may need to break tasks down into manageable steps. Interventions may be structured to allow the child or adolescent to practice skills. Table 13.13■ further illustrates interventions that can be designed to practice these money handling and management tasks.

SUMMARY

As addressed in this chapter, IADL occupations require children and adolescents to perform tasks in multiple contexts. Before intervention strategies can be suggested, the occupational therapist or occupational therapy assistant must analyze both the occupation demands and the contexts where the IADL will be performed. This information can be used to develop occupation based strategies for intervention.

In order to provide effective IADL strategies, the occupational therapist and occupational therapy assistant must remember some key principles of intervention. Regardless of the area of occupation, these principles provide a foundation from which successful intervention can be designed.

■ **Table 13.13**
Money Management

OCCUPATION	OCCUPATIONAL CHALLENGES	ADAPTATIONS
Carlos, a 10-year-old with a learning disability, wants to be able to work in the school store.	Unable to give correct change back to a customer.	Teach Carlos to use a cash register that automatically determines the correct amount of change. Teach him to count back rather than subtract the amount.
Marissa, a 16-year-old with Down syndrome, would like to be able to purchase snacks in the vending machine at her after-school job.	Does not recognize values of coins and bills to make purchases.	Supply picture cue cards to remind her of the value coins and bills. Attach actual coins, construct flash card to use for practice.
	Does not automatically check for return change from the machine.	Place visual reminder in wallet or vending machine. Teach her a jingle to help her remember to check for change.
Jeff, a 14-year-old with bipolar disorder, would like to have a morning paper route to earn spending money.	Often oversleeps and is late completing his route.	Help him establish a routine and learn to set an alarm clock.
	Frequently makes mistakes on the route. When customers complain, gets angry and throws their paper into the bushes.	Develop a system to check himself throughout the route for accuracy. Role play situations that allow him to problem solve anger management and social interaction skills.

Source: Compiled by A. Fryer, OTAS, and S. Round, OTAS, Penn State University.

Before interventions can be introduced, the direction of the intervention must be decided. A decision must be made whether the intervention should be directed to the person, the task, the environment, or a combination of all three. The occupational therapist and occupational therapy assistant, in collaboration with the child, adolescent, or caretaker, make this decision based on the strengths and challenges of the individual, along with the identified occupation based outcome. The direction of intervention focuses all intervention decisions.

When an intervention is selected, it must be appropriate for the age and developmental level of the child or adolescent and also must be acceptable to the family's culture and beliefs. It is important to suggest and implement interventions that can fit easily into the existing daily routine and not be seen as an extra burden by family members and caretakers. It is important that the occupational therapist or occupational therapy assistant collaborate with the child, adolescent, and family members, and modify a strategy that is not acceptable to them. Everyone who will be involved in the intervention should be involved in the collaboration process in order to feel ownership for the success of the strategy.

Whenever possible, it is best to choose items or strategies that are available to the general public, rather than those that draw attention to the impairment and emphasize the disability. With the adoption of universal design principles, many commercially made items are available that can be adapted to meet special needs.

REVIEWING KEY POINTS

1. Define IADL. Give age appropriate examples for young children, school aged children, and adolescents.
2. Explain what is meant by directing the intervention to the person, activity, or environment.
3. Provide and justify four examples for modifying each of the following:
   - Communication device use
   - Community mobility
   - Pet care
   - Meal preparation and cleanup
   - Personal safety
   - Shopping

APPLYING KEY CONCEPTS

1. Choose an IADL that would be appropriate for a young child. List 10 possible adaptations that you could provide for this IADL. Remember to consider addressing the person, activity, and environment.
2. Using the same IADL, list 10 adaptations that you would make for an adolescent. Compare the differences and discuss the expanded contexts.

REFERENCES

American Occupational Therapy Association (2002). Occupational therapy practice framework: Domain and process. *American Journal of Occupational Therapy, 56*(6), 609–639.

Allen, E., & Marotz, L. (2007). *Developmental profiles: Pre-birth through twelve* (5th ed.). Clifton Park, NY: Thomson Delmar Learning.

Cook, A., & Hussey, S. (2002). *Assistive technologies: Principles and practice* (2nd ed.). St. Louis, MO: Mosby, Inc.

Schneck, C. (2005). Visual perception. In J. Case-Smith, *Occupational therapy for children* (5th ed.) (pp. 412–445). St. Louis, MO: Elsevier Mosby.

Vogtle, L.K., Kern, D., & McCauley, A. (2002). Differences in perception of social function between adolescents with and without disabilities. Abstract. *Developmental Medicine and Child Neurology,* Supp. 83, 16.

Chapter 14

Interventions for Education

Margaret J. Pendzick
and Dorothy L. Rockwell

Key Terms

Academic participation
Education
Environment
Establish
Figure-ground
Formal education participation
Form constancy
Inclusion
Individualized education program (IEP)
Least restrictive environment (LRE)
Mainstream
Maintain
Nonacademic participation
Person
Position in space

Prevent
Promote
Rehabilitation Act of 1974 (504)
Related service
Remediation
Restore
Scope of impact
Task
Transition plan
Transition process
Transition services
Transition team
Visual attention
Visual closure
Visual discrimination
Visual memory
Vocational preparation

Objectives

- Clarify the role of the occupational therapist and occupational therapy assistant in the intervention process for education.
- Explain intervention approaches that address children's and adolescents' educational needs and are developmentally and contextually relevant.
- Develop intervention plans to address education.

INTRODUCTION

This chapter describes occupation-based interventions that enable children and adolescents to participate in their **education** occupations. Education includes both **formal education participation** and informal education (AOTA, 2002).

SCHOOL BASED PRACTICE

Interventions that impact a child's or an adolescent's formal academic education take place primarily within a school setting. In order to understand how occupational therapy services are implemented within the educational system, it is necessary to review current special education policies. Occupational therapy services are mandated by federal laws and specific special education guidelines must be followed in order for students to qualify for services. Legislation frequently is revised and often reauthorized under a new title. Appendix D provides a historical listing of the federal laws pertaining to educational services to children and adolescents with special needs.

Initially passed by Congress as the *Education for All Handicapped Children Act* (PL94-142), special education programs currently are mandated under the *Individuals with Disability Education Improvement Act* (IDEA) and *No Child Left Behind Act* (NCLB). Federal guidelines mandate that all children (3–21 years) with disabilities are entitled to a free, appropriate education in the **least restrictive environment (LRE).** In accordance with the LRE mandate, students with disabilities must be educated whenever possible with their nondisabled peers. **Inclusion** describes a setting whereby students with disabilities are educated within a regular classroom. In order to meet individual needs, school systems must offer a continuum of services in the following settings:

- *Regular classroom:* The student with disabilities receives instruction from the regular classroom teacher. This inclusion placement often only requires modifications to regular education curriculum.

- *Regular classroom with consultation:* The regular education teacher provides instruction with consultation from special education teacher and other team members, as appropriate. This is an inclusion setting.

- *Regular classroom with supplementary instruction and services:* The student with disabilities receives all instruction in the regular education classroom with the special education teacher and other team members providing intervention within the classroom. This often is referred to as "push-in" services and is an inclusion setting.

- *Resource room:* Throughout the day, the student with disabilities leaves the regular classroom to receive instruction from a special education teacher or other team members in another room. This often is referred to as "pull-out" services and is a noninclusion setting.

- *Self-contained special education classroom:* Housed within a regular education building, the student with disabilities receives educational instruction from the special education teacher with other special education students. Within this noninclusion setting, the students with disabilities often are **mainstreamed** with regular education students for nonacademic instruction such as music, physical education, or art. They can be mainstreamed also for those academic subjects that they can complete at grade level.

- *Separate school:* This is a day program where students with disabilities attend a specially designed facility and receive all education and related services as indicated on the Individualized Education Program.
- *Residential school:* Specially trained staff, related service providers, and teachers provide education, related services, and 24 hour care (Heward, 2006).

Since occupational therapists and occupational therapy assistants may be required to provide intervention a variety of different education models within the educational setting, it is important to understand these different settings.

Under federal law, occupational therapy is considered a **related service** that supports the student's special education program. The occupational therapy process addresses the child's or the adolescent's role as a student. As discussed in Chapter 11, an **individualized education program (IEP)** is developed for each child or adolescent that qualifies for special education services. The IEP documents the required occupational therapy services, intervention goals, and objectives.

Student with disabilities who do not qualify for special education, may receive occupational therapy services through Section 504 of the **Rehabilitation Act of 1974 (504)**. Unlike an IEP, recommended services under a 504 pertain only to the student's current classroom placement and expire at the end of that school year. Consistent with Section 504, the occupational therapist and occupational therapy assistant can provide direct interventions to the student or make environmental accommodation (AOTA, 2004).

FORMAL EDUCATION PARTICIPATION

The Occupational Therapy Practice Framework (AOTA, 2002) defines formal education participation to include **academic participation**, **nonacademic participation**, and **vocational preparation**. This comprehensive definition emphasizes that full participation in formal education includes more than the ability to complete classroom based academic subjects. The occupational demands associated with education require the student to utilize performance skills and performance patterns within a variety of contextual situations within the school setting. Contextual situations include school convocations, athletic and arts programs, recess, extracurricular activities, and field trips. School settings include hallways, lunchrooms, libraries, auditoriums, gymnasiums, natatoriums, bathrooms, outdoor areas, school buses, and off-site learning environments. Importance is placed on how the student learns, interacts with peers, and navigates and uses resources in all of these situations and contexts. For instance, by middle school, students often are expected to use their lockers. To do so they must remember the combination, manipulate the lock and door, organize the placement of belongings into and out of the locker, and sustain balance while juggling books and coat. They also need to negotiate and interact appropriately with hallway crowds while remaining focused on the task and coping with distracting environmental noises and movement. Difficulty with these and other performance skills and patterns, and barriers within the environment, limit students' full academic participation.

Consideration also must be given to the **scope of impact** of particular performance skills, patterns, and habits on successful participation within various contexts. Some skills, patterns, and habits may be necessary for the completion of only a few tasks, while others may have a wider area of impact. For instance, a kindergartener who struggles with manipulating snaps may have difficulty only completing dressing tasks, whereas a kindergartener who has problems with processing skills and organizational patterns may have difficulty with a number of tasks. The kindergartener who struggles with snaps might use different fasteners that he maneuvers more easily, or may require some extra minutes during self-dressing. Since classroom materials and tasks do not usually involve manipulating snaps, his decreased snapping speed has limited impact on his school performance. In contrast, processing skills and organizational patterns may have a broader impact. For example, a kindergartener who has processing and organizational difficulties may be challenged throughout the school day in his effort to complete the beginning and end of school day routines, gather and return instructional materials, and clean up play areas. Because these processing difficulties affect a broader area of occupations and tasks, not a specific academic problem, they may be the central focus of occupational therapy intervention.

Occupation-Based Intervention

Occupation-based interventions designed to facilitate the ability of the children and adolescents to participate fully in their education are directed to the **person**, the **task**, and the **environment**. The specific intervention is based on the results of the occupational therapy evaluation and is selected in collaboration with the student, the family, and the teaching staff. As part of this process, the occupational therapist and occupational therapy assistant decide whether they can help the students achieve the desired outcomes most effectively by focusing on establishing or restoring a new skill or routine, adapting the task, modifying the environment, or attending to all three areas. When establishing or restoring a new skill or routine, the occupational therapist and occupational therapy assistant identify the student's underlying deficits and structure interventions to concentrate on these areas. An adaptive approach focuses on utilizing the student's present abilities to perform a task, often adapting the environment or the task to achieve the outcome. In best practice models, the occupational therapist and the occupational therapy assistant work collaboratively with other members of the educational team to provide such services in an efficient and effective manner.

Interventions Directed at the Person

Students with disabilities may experience limited participation in the formal educational process due to motor, processing, or communication difficulties or a combination of all three. Occupational therapy intervention often is included in the student's IEP to **remediate** or **restore** these difficulties or **prevent** them from occurring. Likewise, the occupational therapy intervention may focus on **promoting**, **establishing**, restoring, or **maintaining** the ability of the student to perform educationally related tasks. For instance, due to a medical condition, a student may have limited hand strength that interferes with his ability to hold a pencil for long periods of time and complete his schoolwork. The occupational therapist or occupational therapy assistant might design a program of occupation-based activities to remediate the strength of the weak hand muscles and restore the ability to grasp the pencil. The occupational therapy assistant might suggest that the student learn or establish new skills such as keyboarding or voice activated word processing to complete longer projects and restrict pencil tasks to shorter assignments. In another instance, the occupational therapist and occupational therapy assistant may provide interventions to promote useful routines that enable a student to complete educational tasks. For example, an occupational therapy assistant may help a high school student who has limited organizational skills to establish routines that he can use throughout the day to complete frequent tasks. If the school student is having trouble sustaining focus to task due to over or under stimulation, the occupational therapist might direct the occupational therapy assistant to incorporate sensory modulation principles to maintain the student's attention to task. As indicated in the IEP, the occupational therapist and occupational therapy assistant also might provide interventions to address the impoverished social skills of a grade school student who struggles to complete required group projects because of his inapt peer interactions. The student could join a social skills group led by the occupational therapy assistant to provide opportunities to establish cooperative level social skills needed for classroom work and prevent further social isolation.

Table 14.1■ provides additional examples of interventions that might be directed at students within a school setting. The table is divided into columns. The first column presents a brief description of the child or adolescent engaging in a school task. The second column lists the student's occupational challenges. Columns three and four provide interventions that might be utilized by an occupational therapy assistant.

Interventions Directed at the Task

Occupational therapy interventions also may be directed toward adapting the myriad of educational and daily life tasks in which students engage during the school day. Occupational therapists and occupational therapy assistants can make adaptations to academic and other educational activities, ADL and IADL school-related tasks, social participation tasks, and prevocational tasks. These adaptations enable students with disabilities to participate in their educational process and achieve success. Table 14.2■ gives examples of interventions directed to the task.

Interventions Directed to the Environment

Since student learning takes place within a variety of different school environments such as hallways, lunchrooms, classrooms, and playgrounds, occupational therapists and occupational therapy assistants also need to consider them as part of the intervention plan. School environments present unique characteristics that may assist or hinder a student's ability to participate. For instance, a crowded high school hallway at the beginning of the day may encourage social interaction for one student, while the loud noises may distract another student from organizing material for morning classes. A multilevel outdoor playground may allow some children to climb, jump, or explore but hinder other children from propelling their wheelchairs from one level to another. In order to increase student participation, the occupational therapist and occupational therapy assistant may need to alter or adapt the environment to fit the student's capacities (Hemmingsson & Borell, 2000). Table 14.3■ provides examples of how different environments can be adapted or altered to increase a student's participation in the educational process.

Interventions Directed Concurrently at the Person, Task, and Environment

When children and adolescents struggle with their education occupations, the occupational therapist and the occupational therapy assistant may decide that it is best to direct intervention concurrently at the person, task, and environment, rather than

■ **Table 14.1**
Interventions Directed to the Person

OCCUPATION	OCCUPATIONAL CHALLENGES	INTERVENTIONS	
Markel, a 4-year-old who has limited vision, attends a special needs preschool at a Head Start center.	Unable to serve himself at snack time.	Provide opportunities for Markel to practice pouring and scooping during water play and art activities.	During snack time, provide hand-over-hand instruction with verbal cues as he pours himself juice and scoops a serving of Jello.
Linda, a 6-year-old who has cerebral palsy, attends first grade in a regular education classroom in her neighborhood school.	Unable to isolate finger movements to use computer keyboard.	During free play, engage Linda in activities such as finger puppets, thumb print art, and pointing games that encourage isolated finger movements.	Provide Linda with a hand splint that isolates and supports one finger into extension.
Tricia, a 5-year-old, attends a developmental kindergarten class.	Has difficulty working independently. Quickly gets frustrated, cries, then damages or throws the project.	Teach Tricia how to use words to express her emotions; teach her strategies for asking for assistance from peers or aide.	Set up a buddy system for Tricia to work on early projects with a peer.
Geisha, a 9-year-old who has ADHD, attends fourth grade in a rural community.	Has difficulty participating in project level group activities due to distractions and frequently talking out of turn.	Model appropriate turn taking and provide feedback on social skills, while Geisha works in a group.	Assist Geisha in identifying distractions and developing habits to focus on task.
Lee, a 10-year-old, attends fifth grade in a resource room for children with behavioral difficulties.	Has difficulty managing stress and either runs out of the classroom or gets into fights with children.	Teach Lee stress management and relaxation techniques; teach verbal assertiveness skills to manage conflicts.	Assist Lee in identifying triggers that cause stress and physiological responses that are warning signs of stress.
Anthony, a 12-year-old who has Down syndrome, attends seventh grade in a special education classroom.	Unable to place items on lunch tray and carry to assigned table.	Throughout the day, provide opportunities for Anthony to carry items on trays. Allow him to experiment on how to place and carry items to different areas of the room.	Teach Anthony to follow the design on the premarked placemat to place items on the tray.
Tia, a 16-year-old who has JRA, attends eleventh grade at a large urban high school.	Unable to manipulate combination lock on school locker.	Encourage Tia to engage in hobbies that maintain finger and wrist movements such as macramé, jewelry making, and card playing.	Encourage Tia to problem solve her difficulty and choose a different locking system that she can more readily manipulate.

■ **Table 14.2**
Interventions Directed to the Task

Occupation	Occupational Challenges	Interventions	
Khadijah, a 7-year-old with a learning disability, attends a second grade classroom in a small, rural town.	Unable to complete worksheets that require cutting and pasting.	Provide Khadijah with precut materials.	Adapt the worksheet so that she can draw a line rather than cut and paste.
Bryce, a sixth grader with Down syndrome, attends a physical education class with a regular education classroom.	Unable to complete his dressing in the allotted time.	Eliminate one clothing item by allowing Bryce to wear his gym shirt to school.	Eliminate all fasteners by only wearing pullover shirts and pull on pants. Choose Velcro gym shoes.
Inderbir, a ninth grader with spastic cerebral palsy, is enrolled in a regular education history class.	Unable to raise his hand to answer a teacher's question.	Install a switch that Inderbir taps to turn on a light when he wants to answer.	Assign him a buddy who will raise his hand to alert the teacher.
Lottie, a 4-year-old with arthrogyposis, attends a Head Start preschool program.	Unable to extend her fingers in order to cut with scissors during art projects.	Provide Lottie with a pair of automatic opening scissors.	Alter the task so that Lottie can tear the paper rather than cut or precut items.
Reona, a 6-year-old with sensory modulation difficulties, attends a multi-aged kindergarten classroom.	Unable to tolerate sticky substances on fingers or hands.	Provide a glue stick rather than glue bottles.	Substitute painting with brushes rather than finger painting.

focus only on one area. For instance, in the scenario in Table 14.3, the occupational therapist and occupational therapy assistant also may teach Miles relaxation techniques to manage his anxiety, and provide a digital rather than a rotary dial lock. In the scenario about William, the occupational therapy assistant may model how to notice and count doorways, or hold onto the hallway railings rather than a schoolmate's hand. When working with a student who has processing, motor skill, and social skill difficulties to complete a group science project, the occupational therapist and occupational therapy assistant might:

- Teach turn taking and group communication skills
- Modify the sequence of steps
- Adapt the science equipment
- Rearrange the workstation
- Alter the background noise and visual stimuli

The occupational therapist and occupational therapy assistant consider the needs and capacities of the student, and the effectiveness and efficiency of the intervention strategies, when deciding whether to utilize one or several strategies. They also

■ **Table 14.3**
Interventions Directed to the Environment

OCCUPATION	OCCUPATIONAL CHALLENGE	INTERVENTION
Rhonda, a 16-year old, sophomore high school student who has diplegic cerebral palsy, walks with the assistance of bilateral canes.	Rhonda is unable to sit at the picnic bench seating with her friends.	Replace the lunch bench with chairs on one side of the table. If the bench is attached to the table, request that chairs be placed at the ends of the table.
Athea, a third grader who has autism, rides a school bus to her rural grade school.	Athea is very sensitive to noise. When riding the bus, she becomes agitated and starts to cry as more children board and the noise level increases.	Reserve a seat in the front row where noise level may be less. Place a headset and music at Athea's bus seat for her to use during the bus ride.
William, a kindergarten student with limited vision, attends a large urban neighborhood school.	When William arrives at school, he cannot find his classroom. He would like to be able to learn his way and not have to hold anyone's hand walking down the hallway.	Place tactile markings along the hallway that leads to William's classroom. Place talking picture frames outside key places that alert William to where he is.
Miles, a seventh grader with fragile X syndrome, who attends a large junior high school, needs to access his locker throughout the day.	Miles becomes anxious when standing close to others and cannot access his locker or manage the rotary combination lock.	Assign Miles a locker at the end of a hallway where he only has someone on one side. Allow Miles to access his locker before classes begin to change and when the hallways are less crowded.

consider the availability of other personnel to provide services such as an instructional aide, a mobility specialist, counselor, and speech and language pathologist.

Educational Activities and Tasks: Handwriting, Tool Usage, and Group Participation

Throughout the school day, children and adolescents engage in a variety of different tasks and activities that involve handwriting, tool usage, and group participation. Students write, use tools, and participate in groups during their science, language, and social studies classes, as well as, during industrial and creative art classes, and after-school club and athletic events. Writing, tool usage, and group participation require the integration of multiple performance skills, performance patterns, and habits. Students who struggle in these areas may benefit from occupational therapy intervention directed at improving needed skills, patterns, and habits, or at modifying the task and adapting the environment. Below are some interventions that might be used for handwriting, tool usage, and social skills.

Handwriting

One of the frequent reasons cited for a school based occupational therapy referral, handwriting often is a challenging task for children and adolescents with disabilities. Based upon the results of an occupational therapy evaluation, the age of the student, and the conceptual model chosen by the occupational therapist, intervention strategies focus on establishing underlying motor or processing skills, adapting the handwriting tasks or instruction, or preventing difficulties through prewriting activities. All of these approaches can be quite complex and may be used in conjunction with each other.

Prewriting skills. Since mandated federal laws include services for preschoolers with disabilities, occupational therapists and occupational therapy assistants often provide intervention strategies for preschoolers who demonstrate delays in prewriting skills. While young children are not expected to perform many printing tasks, most preschool curriculums include prewriting activities such as imitating and copying simple strokes and geometric shapes; printing first name, completing simple mazes, dot-to-dot, and coloring sheets; finger painting; and drawing with markers, crayons, or paint brushes. In this setting, the occupational therapy assistant, supervised by the occupational therapist, provides opportunities for the preschoolers to establish prewriting skills through age appropriate occupation-based activities, and provides consultation to the preschool teaching staff. In best practice models, the occupational therapist and occupational therapy assistant work in collaboration with the teaching staff and parents so that the child receives consistent instruction.

Based on the results of an occupational therapy evaluation and in consultation with educational team, the occupational therapist determines if motor or processing obstacles exist and whether intervention should focus on establishing new skills or adapting required tasks. The occupational therapist and occupational therapy assistant provide meaningful, age appropriate, and culturally sensitive interventions that address the identified problem. For example, if a preschooler has difficulties coloring within age appropriate lines and frequently abandons the project before completion, the teacher may refer the child for an occupational therapy evaluation. If the problem is due to inability to adjust the crayon in the hand, the occupational therapy assistant may provide in-hand manipulation activities so that the child can establish the skills. If hand strength hinders the coloring activity, the occupational therapy assistant may suggest that the teacher incorporate age appropriate strengthening activities, such as play dough or squeeze toys at the water table, into center stations. If visual processing difficulties interfere with the preschooler's ability to distinguish the outside line of the drawing from the background, the occupational therapy assistant may provide figure ground activities to help establish the skill or suggest raising the border around the primary figure.

Table 14.4■ provides additional examples of interventions that might be used in a preschool setting. The table is divided into columns. The first column presents a brief description of the preschooler engaging in a pre-writing task. The second column lists the preschooler's occupational challenges. Columns three and four provide interventions that might be utilized by an occupational therapy assistant or given as suggestions to classroom teaching staff.

Visual processing skills. Handwriting difficulties also may stem from processing problems. An occupational therapy evaluation that includes standardized, nonstandardized, and informal observational testing may detect visual perceptual skill deficits that hinder a student's ability to perform handwriting tasks. Occupational therapy intervention may focus on establishing the visual processing skills or minimize the task demands in order to increase student success in handwriting tasks. Chapter 10 provides a description of these processing skills.

■ **Table 14.4**
Interventions Directed to Prewriting Skills

Occupation	Occupational Challenges	Interventions	
Drylene, a 5-year-old preschooler with limited vision, attends a special needs preschool program.	Unable to draw shapes or letters due to lack of vision.	Use stencils and textured lines to provide shape and letter boundaries.	Using 3-D textured shapes and letters, play a memory game.
Noah, a 4-year-old preschooler with Down syndrome, attends a neighborhood day care.	Unable to exert enough pressure to make a mark on paper with crayon or marker.	Provide hand-over-hand assistance and verbal cues when Noah makes a mark.	Encourage Noah to push cookie cutters, beads, and fingers into play dough.
Sedrick, a 3-year-old preschooler with autistic-like tendencies, attends a Head Start program.	Refuses to participate in finger painting activities or other tactile experiences.	Provide deep pressure to palms of hands before beginning a tactile experience.	Increase tactile input on Sedrick's favorite toys. Gradually encourage him to engage in tactile activities.
Alisa, a 3-year-old preschooler with cerebral palsy, attends a developmental preschool program.	Has difficulty controlling crayons and markers because she does not extend her wrist spontaneously.	Using large handled ink stamps, facilitate active wrist extension by positioning paper to vertical plane.	Encourage Alisa to paint and draw in vertical plane to facilitate wrist extension.
Dante, a 5-year-old preschooler with developmental delays, attends a noncategorical developmental preschool program.	Unable to imitate or copy diagonal strokes and figures such as + and ×.	Using wands and streamers, assist Dante to make diagonal strokes and figures in the air.	Using toy cars, encourage Dante to follow a road composed of diagonal movements.
Vanessa, a 4-year-old preschooler with ADHD, attends a Head Start program.	Unable to make horizontal or vertical strokes due to difficulty sustaining attention to task.	Prior to prewriting activities, encourage Vanessa to modulate her sensory input by bouncing on a therapy ball or jumping on a minitramp.	Encourage stroke development by using multisensory experiences, such high textured finger paints and bright colored markers and crayons on nonglare paper.

- **Visual memory** helps the student to recall individual letter strokes. It also helps the student to speed up a copying task by remembering clusters of letters of words.

- **Visual attention** involves alertness during a writing task, and dividing focus between two tasks. Visual attention allows a student to return to a writing task when momentarily distracted by another student or required to attend to the teacher.

- **Visual discrimination** helps the student to detect differences and spatial relationships between letters and words. Visual discrimination includes the following skills:
  - **Form constancy** helps the student remember that a letter remains the same regardless of changes in size, font style, or background.

- **Visual closure** allows the student to identify a letter or word even though it may be partially erased on a blackboard or incompletely replicated on paper.
- **Figure ground** enables the student to locate the letters and words when presented on a distracting background or when written on a poorly erased blackboard.
- **Position in space** assists the student in recognizing the direction that a letter is turned, placement of a letter in relationship to the lines on paper, and distance between words in a sentence (Schneck, 2005).

After completing the evaluation, the occupational therapist may recommend that the occupational therapy assistant design age-appropriate interventions that focus on establishing or strengthening the student's underlying visual perceptual skills. These interventions provide opportunities to practice the specific visual perceptual skills and to establish new strategies to adapt for the visual processing difficulty. The occupational therapist also may request the occupational therapy assistant to adapt the handwriting task to decrease the visual perceptual demands. Students who are referred for an occupational therapy evaluation due to handwriting difficulties often are frustrated or disinterested in the writing process. Therefore, it is necessary to design creative intervention sessions that not only meet the desired outcomes but also actively engage the student and promote self-confidence in the task.

ALEX

Alex, a second grade student who is having difficulty completing his printing class assignments due to slow speed and illegibility, is referred for an occupational therapy assessment. An analysis of the evaluation results indicates that the Alex has difficulty remembering how to form letters and frequently needs to refer to the writing chart on his desk. When copying from the board, he does not read the sentence before beginning to copy and only remembers one letter at a time. He inconsistently forms letters, often adding strokes and squiggles to attempt to make the letter to look like the model. He frequently erases letters, which also decreases his printing speed and leaves smudges on his paper. The occupational therapist determines that Alex has difficulty with visual memory but has developed age appropriate visual discrimination skills that allow him to recognize when he has formed a letter poorly and needs to erase it. After sharing the results with the parents and the teacher, the IEP team adds occupational therapy service to Alex's current school IEP.

Occupational therapy intervention is provided in a variety of different ways. While meeting with parents and teachers, the occupational therapist and occupational therapy assistant explain the impact that the visual memory deficit has on his handwriting skills and suggests that the teacher and parents encourage Alex to engage in games and activities that promote his visual memory. The occupational therapy assistant provides a list of memory games and quick memory activities to use at home and at school.

In order to address the difficulty in correct letter formation, the occupational therapy assistant provides multisensory experiences to reinforce his letter formation memory. Keeping in mind that working on handwriting can seem boring, the occupational therapy assistant uses a variety of media such as shaving cream, gel pens, and colored chalk to work on specific letters and letter combinations. The occupational therapy assistant praises Alex's effort and encourages him to produce his best work during his classroom assignments.

After understanding Alex's difficulties, the teacher alters her instructional style to meet Alex's needs. Before initiating board-copying tasks, she reads aloud the sentence while one child points to each word in the sentences. She often changes the copying activity by providing each child with cut out letters or full words that the child arranges to copy the board sentences rather than printing them.

There are many different ways that visual perceptual skills impact handwriting skills. Table 14.5■ provides additional examples of intervention strategies that address visual perceptual difficulties.

Motor skills.   Along with processing skills, motor skills are a critical element in completing a handwriting task. Handwriting is influenced by the student's posture, shoulder, forearm, and wrist stabilization, in-hand manipulation skills, and bilateral coordination (Benbow, 1999). Evidence based research indicates that in-hand manipulation skills, which involve precise control of fingers and thumb, influence letter formation in handwriting more than the type of pencil grip utilized (Cornhill and Case-Smith, 1996; Rosenblum, Goldstand & Parush, 2006). Pencil grasp, which was discussed in Chapter 13, is often a well established habit by second grade and difficult to alter. Following best practice guidelines, it may be more appropriate to continue with rather than to alter a well established grasp pattern unless it causes pain in the hand or interferes with the writer's view of the completed print. Based upon evaluation results and clinical judgment, the occupational therapist decides whether to focus the intervention on restoring or establishing motor skills necessary for handwriting or adapting the handwriting task. Once the occupational therapist makes these determinations, the occupational therapy assistant can design age appropriate occupation-based interventions.

MIA

Mia, a third grade student who receives assistance from the learning support teacher, is referred for an occupational therapy evaluation due to teacher concerns of illegible handwriting and slow pace. During classroom observations the occupational therapy assistant notes that Mia often slumps over her desk, dangling her legs from her chair. Mia allows the paper or workbook to slide around her desk without stabilizing it with her nondominant hand. As the writing surface moves, she leaves stray pencil marks on the paper and does not form letters that are in proportion to lines and spaces. When erasing, she uses both hands to readjust the pencil, often dropping it on her desk. She often turns her wrist and forearm to align with the eraser end, and then uses her nondominant hand to assist with maintaining grip.

The analysis of the occupational therapy evaluation indicates that Mia has age appropriate visual perceptual skills. However, her upper extremity strength, in-hand manipulation skills, and bilateral coordination skills are not well developed and are interfering with her ability to control the pencil. In addition, Mia's basic sitting posture undermines good upper extremity control.

During a meeting with the parents, classroom teacher, and resource teacher, the occupational therapist explains the evaluation results. They collectively decide to add occupational therapy services to the IEP. The occupational therapist and parent discuss age appropriate out-of-school activities that would enhance Mia's overall upper body strength, ways to adapt her homework area so that she has better seated posture, and home activities that would encourage bilateral hand use.

■ **Table 14.5**
Intervention for Visual Processing Difficulties

Occupation	Occupational Challenges	Interventions	
		Establish or Restore	Adapt
Victoria, a 10-year-old fifth grader, needs to complete school writing assignments.	Victoria uses print rather than cursive to complete handwriting assignments. Since she moved in and out of different school districts, she did not receive instruction in cursive handwriting. Printing is illegible due to inconsistent placement of letters on lines and little spacing between words.	Increase Victoria's awareness of lines and space placement. Using ink stamps and stickers, complete pictures and projects that require precise placement of stamps or stickers on, under, and between designated lines.	Eliminate manuscript printing and provide Victoria with instruction in cursive handwriting. Involve Victoria in activities to learn computer keyboarding skills.
Tobias, a 6-year-old first grader, needs to complete his worksheets independently.	When given a worksheet, Tobias needs assistance to locate the correct space to print his name or answers due to figure-ground difficulties.	Provide Tobias opportunities to complete hidden picture games such as Where's Waldo?™ Grade the figure-ground activities so that Tobias is challenged but not frustrated.	Eliminate unnecessary information and decorations from worksheets. Before giving Tobias a worksheet, highlight where to print his name at the beginning of each answer line.
Gil, an 8-year-old third grader, needs to read and write in cursive.	Gil is having difficulty transitioning from printing to cursive handwriting. Due to a problem with form constancy, he does not associate the similarities of manuscript and cursive letters.	Provide opportunities for Gil to develop form constancy skills. Help him construct a collage of pictures that contain a certain shape. Explore the playground, hallway, or gymnasium looking for things that are of a certain shape.	Help Gil associate cursive letters with printed letters. Adapt games such as Go Fish™ or Memory!™ card so that he practices matching cursive and printed letters.
Janelle, a 7-year-old second grader, needs to copy lessons from the board.	Janelle is having difficulty copying from the board due to a problem with visual closure.	Encourage Janelle to engage in games that develop her visual closure skills. Provide a dot-to-dot or jigsaw puzzle and have her to try to guess what the picture is prior to completing the puzzle. Encourage Janelle to construct letters and words using a pegboard or a Light Bright toy. Have her trace the lines with her fingers and recite the letter or words.	Encourage the teacher to thoroughly erase marking off board before each use. Eliminate any glare on the board from natural light or overhead light fixtures.

As directed by the occupational therapist, the occupational therapy assistant addresses the IEP goals to improve handwriting legibility and handwriting speed within the classroom setting. She assists the teacher in adjusting the desk and chair so that Mia can place her feet flat on the floor and maintain better posture (Erhardt & Meade, 2005). The occupational therapy assistant engages Mia in activities to establish in-hand manipulation skills and bilateral coordination, and also adapts some classroom tasks to ensure immediate improvement. For instance, she instructs Mia to use a clipboard to help keep her papers in place. She also tacks visual reminders on Mia's desk to encourage her to use her nondominant hand as a helper. During indoor recess time, the occupational therapy assistant works with Mia and her peers to complete a hallway mural that requires them to stabilize stencils with their nondominant hand while tracing and coloring with their dominant hand. The occupational therapy assistant encourages upper extremity strengthening by positioning the mural paper so that Mia works with her extended arms at or above shoulder height. She fosters the development of Mia's in-hand manipulation skills by instructing all the students to use only their fingers to grasp and manipulate the pompoms and sequins available to finish the mural.

There is a variety of different ways that motor skills can be established or tasks can be adapted to enhance writing skills. Table 14.6■ gives additional intervention examples.

Adapting Handwriting Instruction or Tasks

Each school system selects a specific handwriting curriculum that suggests letter presentation sequence, student practice activities or workbooks, and a timeline transition from manuscript to cursive writing. Using the curriculum guide and stated benchmarks, individual teachers typically provide whole group instruction and practice sessions. Regardless of the curriculum chosen, adequate time and instruction must be provided in order for children to develop the skills and habits to successfully master the handwriting task.

For students who do not readily acquire handwriting skills through grade level workbook practice, instruction may need to be modified to reflect individual learning styles. Although occupational therapists and occupational therapy assistants are not responsible for classroom instruction, their ability to analyze tasks may assist the classroom teacher in altering the current curriculum or developing learning experiences to accommodate for those additional needs. For example, the occupational therapy assistant might recommend that the classroom teacher use raised or highlight-lined paper for those students who have difficulty with letter placement and spacing. The occupational therapy assistant also might suggest that the teacher reinforce letter placement when writing on the board by using different colored chalk for letters that drop below the baseline.

Handwriting tasks also may be altered to decrease the activity demands that hinder the student's performance. The occupational therapist and occupational therapy assistant may help teachers and administrators to understand specific client factors that require adaptations of given written tasks. For instance, in order to cause less stress on the joints, the occupational therapist and occupational therapy assistant may recommend that students with JRA write only key words rather than whole sentences. They also may recommend that children with motor difficulties circle rather than write out complete answers or use word processing prediction programs (Hadley-More et al., 2003).

Classroom Tools

Depending upon the grade level, students use a variety of different tools throughout the day within the school setting. Younger students often use scissors, paste,

■ **Table 14.6**
Interventions for Motor Difficulties

OCCUPATION	OCCUPATIONAL CHALLENGES	INTERVENTIONS	
		ESTABLISH OR RESTORE	ADAPT
Fatia, an 8-year-old second grader who has low muscle tone, receives learning support services within her regular education classroom.	She is unable to make firm strokes on the paper, making her handwriting very light and difficult to read. She holds the pencil high on the shaft with thumb and digits extended. Only her fingertips touch the pencil. Her wrist is flexed. She uses whole arm movements to control the pencil.	Provide carbon paper during writing activities. Instruct Fatia to press down hard enough to make a mark on the copy paper. Include Fatia in craft group activities that require her to use a tripod grasp, i.e., embossing greeting cards, scratch art bookmarks. Have Fatia and her classmates complete handwriting activities at the blackboard using small pieces of chalk. This encourages tripod grasp and active wrist extension.	Provide Fatia with soft leaded mechanical pencils rather than #2 pencils. This allows her to make a firmer mark on the paper without exerting more pressure. Place a pencil grip on the pencil to encourage Fatia to use a more mature grip. Position Fatia's paper on top of a slanted clipboard to encourage her to extend her wrist to write.
Troy, a 6-year-old who has JRA, attends a developmental kindergarten.	Troy is unable to maintain a grip on markers or crayon to prevent them from slipping out of his hand while moving across the paper. He completes a project very slowly, and often cries when he has trouble keeping up with his classmates.	Have Troy form the letter of the day using play dough. Have him use a plastic knife to cut the letter into pieces. Teach Troy work simplification techniques, such as eliminating unnecessary steps, to speed up his work. Encourage Troy to express his feeling of frustration verbally rather than crying.	Provide Troy with crayons and markers that have built up shafts. Adapt instructions so that less writing and coloring is required, i.e., circle, rather than color, the correct picture.
Sasha, a 10-year-old who has arthrogyposis, attends fifth grade.	Sasha is unable to make letters small enough for the fifth grade workbooks and paper. She doesn't like to draw attention to her handwriting difficulties so she often pretends that she doesn't know an answer, leaving the space blank.	Instruct Sasha to practice making letters within specific boundaries, gradually decreasing space for writing. With teacher permission, help Sasha develop abbreviations for frequently used words. Encourage Sasha to request a writing partner for lengthy writing assignments.	Instruct a classroom helper to adapt the workbook page to allow increased space for writing. Scan workbook pages into a word processing program that allows Sasha to complete work by typing in answers.

paintbrushes, and a variety of math manipulatives on a daily basis. In middle school, students may be introduced to pencil compasses, protractors, calculators, and rulers in math and may be required to use ink pens for written assignments. High school science classes often require students to use microscopes or scalpels in biology lab; Bunsen burners, test tubes, and flasks in chemistry lab; and manipulative apparatus in physics labs. Depending on the art, physical education, and music curriculums, all ages of students may be exposed to a variety of art tools and materials, musical instruments, or physical education equipment. Occupational therapists and occupational therapy assistants often help students establish performance skills and performance patterns required to properly use classroom tools or adapt a specific tool for easier use by the student.

ESTELLE

Estelle, a high school student who has motor challenges due to muscular dystrophy, has difficulty performing lab experiments in her chemistry class. Although she could be paired with a lab partner, Estelle would like to participate as much as possible in the experiments rather than be a passive observer or recorder of events. The occupational therapist interviews the chemistry teacher, observes the student in the chemistry setting, and assesses Estelle's motor strength and coordination. Based on the interview and the observations, the occupational therapist determines that the motor difficulties cannot be altered. The chemistry teacher provides a list of frequently required lab techniques and lab materials. The occupational therapy assistant adapts the classroom chemistry lab so that Estelle can participate more fully in experiments. At Estelle's lab station, test tube holders are provided, chemicals are placed in easy pour containers, and the work surface is lowered so that she can work from her wheelchair rather than balance on a lab stool. Estelle is encouraged to discuss her motor limitations with her lab partner and explain what techniques she can complete independently.

Numerous adaptations can be made to classroom tools to optimize a student's ability to fully participate in the educational process. Table 14.7■ provides additional intervention examples.

Social Skills and Group Participation

Within the American school systems, students primarily are educated in a group environment. The expected level of social skills and group participation are based on the child's chronological age and cultural norms. While in preschool and early primary grades, a student learns classroom rules such as raising one's hand before speaking in the group, walking in a line quietly when moving from one classroom to another, and taking one's turn to use classroom or playground equipment. Young children learn to share toys in a group; older students learn to work cooperatively in groups to accomplish learning goals, with or without teacher supervision. Classroom teachers encourage growth in social skills and group participation by designing group-learning experiences and establishing classroom routines and rules.

For many reasons, students may have difficulties fully participating in group activities or demonstrating appropriate social skills within the educational setting (Mancini & Coster, 2004). A student who sits in a wheelchair may lack the self-esteem to raise his hand and offer an answer within a class discussion. A student who is ADHD may not pick up the social cues to modulate his voice to the inside environment. A student who has been hospitalized for prolonged periods may have limited

■ **Table 14.7**
Interventions to Establish or Adapt Classroom Tool Use

Occupation	Occupational Challenges	Interventions	
		Establish or Restore	Adapt
Paul, a 5-year-old child with cerebral palsy, attends kindergarten in a small, rural community.	Paul is able to open but not close blades of scissors due to limited finger and thumb flexion. He does not spontaneously use his nondominant hand to hold the paper even though he has the necessary motor skills.	Encourage Paul to engage in bilateral tasks so that he establishes the consistent habit of using his nondominant hand as helper. Examples include building block structures that require him to use his nondominant hand to steady materials, and decorating greeting cards using stencils which require him to use his nondominant hand to stabilize the paper.	Instruct Paul in the use of adaptive easy open loop scissors that have one side attached to a base.
Kylie, a 12-year-old with low vision, is taking Algebra I. All of the students are expected to be able to use a calculator to set up and solve algebraic problems.	Kylie understands the math problem but is unable to use the calculator provided by the schools district due to its poor color contrast and small buttons.	Using a large cardboard model of the school calculator, assist Kylie in memorizing key placements and function key locations.	Provide Kylie with a calculator that meets the needs of the classroom teacher, can be programmed to operate in the same sequence of steps as the one used by her peers, and meets her low vision needs.
Kendall, a 10-year-old boy who sustained a closed head injury, sits at a classroom desk that requires him to raise the lip to retrieve school supplies.	Kendall is able to use his right UE for fine motor tasks but has severely limited ROM, grasp, and release in the left UE.	Provide the opportunity for Kendall to engage in bilateral activities and provide positioning for the left UE so that he does not sit all day with it in a retracted position.	Adapt his desk by attaching a horizontal storage area for books and workbooks to the outside of the right side of his desk. Provide a bag to fit over the armrest of his chair for other school tools. The classroom aide can assist to be sure the right books and tools are accessible in the morning and again in the afternoon if they will not all fit in the storage area.

experience interacting with peers and difficulty developing a rapport with classmates. An occupational therapist or occupational therapy assistant may provide interventions when limited interaction skills interfere with a student's ability to participate within the school environment.

CALVIN

Calvin, an 8-year-old third grader with ADHD, has difficulties interacting with his classmates during learning activities and recess. Although his impulsive behaviors are controlled by medication and behavioral interventions, Calvin does not demonstrate age appropriate social skills and is beginning to alienate his peers. He has difficulty working with a partner or in a small group, does not share art supplies, and interrupts others during discussions. During an annual review of the IEP, his grandparents, who are the legal guardians, and the classroom teacher request an occupational therapy evaluation for social interaction skills. The occupational therapist and occupational therapy assistant observe Calvin during a variety of different social situations; interview the teacher, grandparents, and child; and conduct a social skill inventory. Results of the evaluation indicate that Calvin frequently uses parallel level play skills while the rest of his peers prefer cooperative level of play. He does not pick up on the social cues from his peers and is unaware of his negative impact. His classmates indicate that they do not like to include him in playground games because he doesn't wait his turn and often walks away from the game before the end, resulting in a penalty for his side. As the results of the evaluation are discussed, the team decides to add occupational therapy services to Calvin's current IEP to address his delayed social interaction skills.

During the IEP meeting, the occupational therapist, classroom teacher, and the grandparents discuss ways to encourage the development of Calvin's social skills at home and at school. The grandparents agree to encourage Calvin to join in family group activities and provide Calvin with feedback on his behaviors. The classroom teacher and occupational therapist discuss strategies to improve Calvin's skills within the classroom. The classroom teacher decides to conduct class discussions with chairs in a circle and use a discussion baton to encourage all the children to look around the circle before sharing their comments. During indoor recess, the classroom teacher encourages the students to engage in board games with specific rules and turn taking requirements. She places Calvin with a group of students who are good social role models.

Calvin also joins a weekly Pals Group planned by the occupational therapy assistant to promote social skills. The occupational therapy assistant designs projects and organizes noncompetitive games that require the students to share materials and ideas, using socially acceptable behaviors. In the group, she helps the students learn how to ask for and provide direction, initiate conversations, respond to questions of others, and take turns talking. She provides opportunities for them to practice how to join in and exit from a group. She ends each session by asking the students to draw pictures of them being "good pals."

NONACADEMIC PARTICIPATION

Children and adolescents participate in a variety of different nonacademic learning experiences as they explore different interest areas. Young children often take swimming or tumbling lessons at the local recreation center or attend story time at the community library. School age children participate in drama lessons at the community theater, join the science club at the children's museum, or learn about their cultural backgrounds at ethnic programs. Adolescents often engage in modeling lessons at the local mall, take a driver's education course in the community, or attend youth leadership programs. Regardless of the interest, occupational therapists and occupational therapy assistants may need to provide intervention strategies to allow children and adolescents with disabilities to participate in programs of interest.

As with any other area of occupation, the need for intervention is determined by the analysis of an occupational therapy evaluation, in consultation with the child or adolescent, and parent or guardian, within the context of the activity. As each child and adolescent is unique, the interest areas are numerous with each intervention designed to the specific needs of the child or adolescent. Table 14.8■ gives examples of interventions used in informal educational activities. While reading the list, consider other possible interest areas and situations that may require occupational therapy intervention.

TRANSITION FROM HIGH SCHOOL

Every student who qualifies for an IEP is required to have a written plan for transition from high school. This is mandated by IDEA as a part of the IEP that is in place when the student reaches the age of 16 [δ614(d)(1)(A)(i)(VIII)]. Since most school districts schedule IEP meetings according to an established process, such as scheduling them alphabetically, it is important for the individuals responsible for the IEP to make note of the student's birthday and address transition issues in a timely manner. The IEP may be developed many months before the student reaches 16, but if it is in effect at that date, transition planning must be included in the written document. Transition planning is necessary to assist the student in making the change from daily life as a high school student to that of a college student, an employee, an apprentice, or other post school roles. The **transition plan** must address further vocational training, employment, higher education, or other post school occupations (Rockwell, 2006). These statistics show an alarming need for coordinated planning.

- 21 percent of people with a disability drop out of high school compared with 9 percent of those without a disability.

- 35 percent of people with a disability are employed full or part time compared with 78 percent of those without a disability.

- 26 percent of people with a disability live in poverty with an annual household income below $15,000, compared with 9 percent of those without a disability (NOD, 2004).

The reauthorization of IDEA in 2004 defines **transition services** stating they are a coordinated set of activities for a child with a disability that

- Is designed to be within a results oriented process, that is focused on improving the academic and functional achievement of the child with a disability to facilitate the child's movement from school to post school activities including: post secondary education, vocational education; integrated employment (including supported employment), continuing and adult education, adult services, independent living, or community participation

- Is based on the individual child's needs, taking into account the child's strengths, preferences, and interests.

■ **Table 14.8**
Interventions for Nonacademic Participation

Occupation	Occupational Challenges	Interventions
Analiese, a 15-year-old with cerebral palsy, wants to join the pompom squad at the high school.	Unable to hold pompom handles without dropping them during movement.	Modify handles for easier grip and attach Velcro straps to stay on during movement.
	Apprehensive about attempting a routine from a wheelchair.	Help Analiese analyze a current pompom routine and identify arm movements that she can accomplish from her wheelchair.
Raphael, a 6-year-old with autism and sensory modulation difficulties, wants to attend a zoo sponsored day camp.	Has difficulties transitioning from one activity to another.	Provide Raphael with a picture chart that shows the activities for the day. Several minutes prior to the transition, refer Raphael to the chart to anticipate the transition.
	Reacts negatively to his hand being held or being touched by strangers.	Rather than hold a partner's hand, have the children hold onto the knots of a knotted rope to stay with the group. When needed, use firm—not light—touch because it is less offensive.
Zach, a 10-year-old with ADHD, wants to join a karate program.	Easily distracted by other children. Has difficulty following instructions.	Suggest that instructor place Zach in the front row with no children to one side of him. Instruction should incorporate mirrored demonstrations.
	Attempts moves that are unsafe and beyond his ability due to impulsive behaviors.	Outside of class, have Zach make a list of karate moves with level of difficulty. Post list near his spot in class and instruct him to consult list prior to attempting a move.
Maria, a 16-year-old with ADHD, would like to take a driver's education course in the community.	When behind the wheel, Maria has difficulty dividing her attention between the watching the road and manipulating the car controls.	Suggest she attend a driver's school that includes car simulated driving where she can learn the controls without being in traffic. If not available, have Maria practice using turn signals and other needed controls without car in motion. Provide Maria extended practice so these skills become habit and not distracting for her.
	Maria has difficulty deciding when it is safe to pull out into traffic or when to change lanes.	While a passenger, have Maria practice decision making by verbalizing when it is safe to make the maneuver. Point out visual cues to assist in her decisions. Gradually decrease feedback to her decisions so that she begins to rely upon her own judgment.

- Includes instruction, related services, community experiences, the development of employment and other post-school adult living objectives and, when appropriate, acquisition of daily living skills and functional vocational evaluation. (IDEA, 2004)

The student and his parents or legal guardians are the core members of a transition team. The transition team is intended to be the *dream team* that helps the student set and achieve life goals. The makeup of the transition team is important to the development of an effective transition plan. In addition to the student and his parents or legal guardians it should include individuals from the school district such as teachers, therapists, and others who are familiar with the student, his abilities, and his needs. Occupational therapists and occupational therapy assistants included in transition teams do not need to provide school based services to participate. Occupational therapy practitioners in community based settings may participate on the team if their knowledge of the student contributes to the transition planning process. Family members also may have developed significant relationships with medically based occupational therapy practitioners over a long period of time and may wish to include them on the team. Representatives of community agencies who may assist the student in the transition process or following graduation also should be included. The student and his family may ask any other individual who knows the student well to participate in the transition planning process, such as a religious leader or youth organization leader. The team also may include current or potential employers. The goal of developing a transition team is to assemble a group of individuals who are invested in the success of the student and who know him and the community well enough to act in an advisory capacity. Parents and school personnel should plan ahead as they determine whom to include on the transition team. Parents and school personnel should invite the team members to the IEP meeting in a timely manner, and provide adequate information to them about the transition process so that they are prepared to discuss the plans of the student for his future. The written transition plan should:

- Consider the strengths and needs of the student
- Focus on both academic and functional achievements
- Outline the processes and services required to meet the student's goals
- Enable the student to meet employment goals and life style goals.

There are three steps in the **transition process**:

1. Determine the long term plans of the student for the future. This should include both short term and long term outcomes. Some students may know what they would like to do in their adult life. For other students, investigating possible options may be the starting place.
2. Develop a written plan to take the student from his present setting to the desired future life. The written plan should identify specific steps and specific individuals responsible for oversight of each step.
3. Implement the plan and review progress on an established schedule. Members of the team need to communicate with one another about progress toward established goals. This may be done at the IEP review or by another method determined by the team. Progress must be reported at subsequent formal IEP meetings. The transition plan is updated as necessary at each subsequent IEP meeting.

The transition plan must include specific goals for the student related to employment including any additional education and services required to meet these specific goals. In addition the transition plan should address domestic goals, leisure goals, and community goals (Case-Smith, 2005). The case study of Angela clarifies this process.

ANGELA

Angela, age 16, attends both mainstream and life skills classes in her high school located in a mid-sized community. As part of her life skills class she works two mornings a week in a local family owned restaurant where she fills the salad bar, rolls packets of napkins and silverware, and refills the condiment holders on each table. She has been successfully employed at this setting for several months. Angela enjoys her work. She hopes to be able to work at this restaurant following her graduation from high school and the owners have indicated their willingness to continue employing her. Angela's goal is to be a food server in addition to the work she already does. Angela would like to live in an apartment and to use public transportation for community mobility. In addition to working, Angela is active in a student-bowling league sponsored by the church her family attends. She enjoys bowling and would like to be part of an adult league when she finishes high school. One evening a month she also helps with a children's activity group sponsored by her church. She enjoys her interaction with the children. Angela's family supports her goals and believes they are realistic.

A transition team was developed at her last IEP. The following members were included:

- Angela and her parents
- The life skills classroom teacher

- The owner of the restaurant where Angela works
- Vocational rehabilitation counselor from a community agency
- Occupational therapy assistant employed by the school district
- Youth pastor from her church

The transition team addressed five goal areas when writing a transition plan for Angela's IEP.

- *Domestic:* Where does Angela hope to live and is it feasible in this community?
- *Employment:* What long term employment does Angela hope to have and is it possible in this community?
- *Education:* What further skills training or specific education program is needed to equip Angela for employment in her chosen career?
- *Leisure:* What does Angela enjoy doing in her free time? Are these activities that will meet her needs as an adult? Does Angela need to explore other leisure time opportunities?
- *Community:* What services and resources will Angela need as an independent adult? Are they available in this community? Does Angela have the skills to access them independently? (Wehman, 2006; Case-Smith, 2005)

The transition team assigns oversight responsibility for each specific goal that is written during the IEP meeting. The assignment of responsibility is based on the identified needs of the student and the expertise of the various team members. The occupational therapist and the occupational therapy assistant may be responsible for

- Evaluating current occupational performance capacity
- Directing the intervention in school or community settings
- Consulting with other service providers
- Managing the transition team

Table 14.9■ illustrates potential responsibilities that the occupational therapist and occupational therapy assistant may assume for Angela's transition plan. Rather than immediately addressing all of these areas, the occupational therapist and occu-

■ **Table 14.9**
Potential Responsibilities for Occupational Therapy

Area of Occupation	Occupational Goal	Occupational Therapy Transition Plan Responsibilities
Domestic	Angela wants to live in an apartment when she graduates from high school and is employed.	Evaluate ADL and IADL skills essential for apartment living. Provide direct intervention to develop needed skills.
Employment	Angela wants to be a food server at the family owned restaurant where she now works as part of her life skills class.	Consult with office of vocational rehabilitation to review a detailed job description of skills needed to be a food server. If no job description exists, complete an activity analysis of the essential functions of a food server. Provide essential functions information to the life skills teacher for inclusion in the classroom curriculum.
Education	Angela wants to be a successful food server.	Consult with the life skills teacher to determine the best method of providing training in essential functions of a food server. Provide direct intervention in the classroom setting or in the work setting to develop those skills.
Leisure	Angela wants to be a member of the adult bowling team. She also wants to continue working with the young children in their activities group. She has not identified any other leisure interests.	Administer an interest checklist to identify other leisure pursuits appropriate for Angela. Provide direct intervention to develop the skills needed for one individual leisure activity and one additional group activity.
Community	Angela wants to use public transportation for community mobility.	Evaluate Angela's current functional ability to use public transportation. Work within the community setting to develop or advance her ability to use public transportation.

pational therapy assistant may sequence them according to a timetable necessary for completion.

SUMMARY

When providing intervention in the school setting, occupational therapists and occupational therapy assistants adhere to federal legislative guidelines and address performance skills, patterns, and body functions as they relate to the child's or adolescent's role as a student. Occupational therapy services are provided under an IEP or a 504 plan; a transitional plan from school to work must be added to the IEP by age 16.

Age appropriate occupation-based interventions are designed and directed to impact the person, the task, or the environment, or a combination of the three. The occupational therapist and occupational therapy assistant work in collaboration with the teachers, aides, support staff, family members, and students. Occupational therapists and occupational therapy assistants frequently provide intervention to increase participation in educational tasks, ADL and IADL school-related tasks, and social activities. Collaborative consultation and individual or group interventions are directed toward establishing or restoring performance skills and patterns, creating routines, or modifying the tasks or the environments so that students with special needs can more fully participate in their education. The occupational therapist and occupational therapy assistant must be aware of the child's or the adolescent's physical, cognitive, and psychosocial needs and include these areas within the intervention services.

REVIEWING KEY POINTS

1. Define education as an occupation. Give examples of formal and informal education.
2. Explain the concept of least restricted environment (LRE).
3. Explain the difference between:

   "push-in" and "pull-out" service
   mainstream and inclusion
   IEP and 504 plan

4. Outline the federal laws affecting occupational therapy services within the educational setting.
5. Give examples of educational interventions directed to the person, to the task, or to the environment. Explain the rationale for directing these interventions to the person, the task, and the environment.
6. Discuss the impact of motor and processing skills on handwriting.
7. Identify and explain intervention strategies directed at handwriting tasks.
8. Identify and explain intervention strategies directed at improving tool usage.
9. Identify and explain intervention strategies directed at improving group participation.
10. Explain the purpose and the steps involved in a transition plan.
11. Identify possible roles for occupational therapists and occupational therapy assistants in the transition plan.
12. List the five goal areas of transition. Give an example for each goal.

APPLYING KEY CONCEPTS

1. Interview an occupational therapist or occupational therapy assistant who works within the school setting. Determine what frequent developmental challenges they address and intervention they provide. Ask about the demands of the setting in terms of paperwork, caseload, and additional duties. If possible, review an IEP and discuss the occupation-based goals and objectives.
2. Observe an occupational therapist or occupational therapy assistant working within a classroom setting. Compared to your understanding of clinic-based intervention, what is different? What is similar? What interaction do you observe among the teacher, students, and therapist?
3. Refer to Table 14.4 and reread the intervention strategies. Determine if the suggested interventions are directed to the person, the task, or the environment.

4. Refer to Table 14.9. Design a series of intervention sessions that would address several of Angela's transition goals.

REFERENCES

American Occupational Therapy Association (2002). Occupational therapy practice framework: Domain and process. *American Journal of Occupational Therapy, 56*(6), 609–639.

American Occupational Therapy Association (2004). Occupational therapy services in early intervention and school-based programs. *American Journal of Occupational Therapy, 58*(6), 681–685.

Benbow, M. (1999). *Fine motor development: Activities to develop hand skills in young children.* Columbus, OH: Zaner-Bloser, Inc.

Case-Smith, J. (2005). *Occupational therapy for children* (5th ed.). St. Louis, MO: Mosby, Inc.

Cornhill, H., & Case-Smith, J. (1996). Factors that relate to good and poor handwriting. *American Journal of Occupational Therapy, 50,* 723–730.

Erhardt, R., & Meade, V. (2005). Improving handwriting without teaching handwriting: The consultative clinical reasoning process. *Australian Occupational Therapy Journal, 52* (3), 199–210.

Hadley-More, D., et al. (2003). Facilitating written work using computer word processing and word prediction. *AJOT, 57* (2), 139–151.

Hemmingsson, H., & Borell, L. (2000). Accommodating needs and student environment fit in upper secondary schools for students with severe physical disabilities. *The Canadian Journal of Occupational Therapy, 67*(3), 162–175.

Heward, W. L. (2006). *Exceptional children: An introduction to special education* (8th ed.). Upper Saddle River, NJ: Pearson Prentice Hall.

Individuals with Disabilities Education Improvement Act of 2004. P. L. 108–446.

Mancini, M., & Coster, W. (2004). Functional predictors of school participation by children with disabilities. *Occupational Therapy International,* 11 (1), 12–25.

National Organization on Disability (2004). *2004 N.O.D./ Harris Survey Documents Trends Impacting 54 Million Americans.* Retrieved January 6, 2006, from http:// www.nod.org/index.cfm?fuseaction=page.viewPage& pageID=1430&nodeID=1&FeatureID=1422&redirected= 1&CFID=6327008&CFTOKEN=83972026.

Rosenblum, S., Goldstand, S., & Parush, C. (2006). Relationships among biomechanical ergonomic factors, handwriting product quality, handwriting efficiency, and computerized handwriting process measures in children with and without handwriting difficulties. *American Journal of Occupational Therapy, 60*(1), 28–39.

Rockwell, D. (2006). Transition services under IDEA: What is OT's role in the high school setting? *OT Practice, 11*(13), 15–17.

Schneck, C. (2005). Visual Perception. In J. Case-Smith. Occupational therapy for children (5th ed.) (pp. 412–445). St. Louis, MO: Elsevier Mosby.

Wehman, P. (2006). *Life beyond the classroom: Transition strategies for young people with disabilities* (4th ed.). Baltimore: Paul H. Brookes Publishing Co.

15

Interventions for Play, Leisure, and Social Participation

Janet V. DeLany

Key Terms

Associative group interactions
Attachment
Competitive play
Constructive play
Cooperative group interactions
Egocentric cooperative groups
Exploratory play
Fantasy play
Functional play
Games with rules
Gross motor play
Leisure occupations

Onlooker play
Parallel group interactions
Playfulness
Play occupations
Relational play
Rough-and-tumble play
Social competency
Social participation occupations
Social play
Solitary play
Symbolic play
Unoccupied play

Objectives

- Define play, leisure, and social participation occupations.
- Explain intervention approaches that address the play, leisure, and social participation needs of children and adolescents, and that are developmentally and contextually relevant.
- Clarify how the occupational therapist and occupational therapy assistant provide interventions to promote play, leisure, and social participation.
- Examine personal, environmental, and task related factors that occupational therapists and occupational therapy assistants consider when providing interventions to promote play, leisure, and social participation occupations.

INTRODUCTION

Chapter 1 reviewed working definitions for play, leisure, and social participation. **Play occupations** are those exploratory and participatory activities that provide pleasure or amusement, stimulate curiosity and creativity, or offer diversion. Play can be spontaneous, such as when jumping in a puddle after a rainstorm, or organized, such as when playing a game of basketball. Children and adolescents who demonstrate **playfulness** are internally motivated, feel internal control, and suspend reality when they play (Bundy, 1993). They are joyful, curious, creative, and totally absorbed in the play occupation (Knox, 1996). This playfulness can be seen in young children who take on the persona of superheroes while dressing up in pajamas and capes, or in elementary children who become explorers as they construct forts from old cardboard and lumber scraps. Viewed within occupational therapy literature as the primary occupation of children, play promotes physical, cognitive, linguistic, and social-emotional development (Bundy, 1992; Nevill-Jan, Fazio, Kennedy, & Snyder, 1997).

Leisure occupations also include exploratory and participatory activities. Because they are nonobligatory, they are done during discretionary time to satisfy an area of curiosity or interest, provide pleasure, or afford learning and creative opportunities. The distinction made between play and leisure often is related to age. Play is the term used more frequently to describe the freely chosen activities of children; leisure is the term used more frequently when referring to pleasurable, discretional use of time by older adolescents and adults (Christiansen, Baum, & Bass-Haugen, 2005; Parham & Fazio, 1997). Young children may be described as playing with dolls, clay, and trains; older adolescents may be viewed as pursuing leisure interests in doll collecting, ceramics, and miniature trains.

Social participation occupations involve interactions with family, friends, peers, and community members in organized patterns that are recognized by society (AOTA, 2002, nd; Mosey, 1996). Attending a family wedding, going to the ice cream store with friends, and participating in a community parade are examples of social participation activities. In contrast to play and leisure occupations that may be done alone or with others, social participation occupations involve interactions with other people. When successful, these interactions are characterized by a level of intimacy or connectedness among the people that reflect their cultural norms and roles (Christiansen, Baum, & Bass-Haugen, 2005).

Within the daily life of children and adolescents, the occupations of play, leisure, and social participation often overlap or become fused with one another. For example, a group of friends walking home from the bus stop swap football cards and then decide to spend time playing football in a vacant lot. One of the friends initially is reluctant to play, since his favorite game is soccer. However, because his friends encourage him to join the game, he does so. The friends agree to play again the next day, if the weather permits. Card swapping, playing an informal game, decision making about the way to spend leisure time, and socially participating with a group of friends all come together in this pick up game of football.

Social participation occupations, and play and leisure occupations, when done with others, requires **social competency**. Williamson and Dorman (2002) define social competency as the ability of the child or adolescent to:

- Discriminate the demands of the social setting
- Determine the verbal and nonverbal skills necessary for the situation
- Execute those skills in a fluid manner appropriate to the social norms

- Effectively perceive the reactions of others
- Adjust to this feedback (p. 4)

Children and adolescents learn to become socially competent by observing and modeling other socially competent people with whom they interact. They are able to integrate and apply cognitive and social skills to effectively regulate their behaviors, communicate, demonstrate prosocial behaviors, and make social decisions. They can greet, compliment and include others in the social situation; give and accept negative feedback; seek and offer information; negotiate conflicts; and appropriately terminate involvement in the social exchange (Williamson & Dorman, 2002). In the above pick up football scenario, the friends who are socially competent are able to figure out an activity that includes everyone. They can listen to and respect the viewpoints of all participants as they negotiate where and how to play the game. They give and provide feedback in a nonoffending manner so that they improve their level of play, fairly resolve debates over application of game rules, and smoothly terminate participation in the game. Throughout the game they maintain an appropriate balance between playfulness and competition.

Levels and Types of Play, Leisure, and Social Participation

Chapters 5, 6, 7, and 8 provided examples children and adolescents engaging in developmentally relevant play, leisure, and social participation occupations. Play, leisure, and social participation occupations can be categorized by the level of interaction with others and by the type of activity.

Level of Social Interaction

Initially, infants engage in **unoccupied play** behavior. They briefly watch others and the activities that occur in their environment, or they engage in body play and gross motor activities. As infants develop into toddlers, they become more aware of the presence of others and begin to watch how they play for longer periods of time. This is called **onlooker play** (Williamson & Dorman, 2002). The initial efforts of the toddlers to join the play are brief and basic. Thus, after watching their older siblings stack blocks or color with crayons for a few minutes, the toddlers simply may knock over the block structure or scribble on the drawings.

By age 2, children often spend time playing by themselves. This is called **solitary play**. In their zest to discover their world, they may bang on the kitchen pots, roll in the leaves, and dump out containers of household objects.

Between the ages of 2 and 3, children begin to engage in **parallel level groups**. This is the ability to play and to socialize alongside other children but not directly interact with them. For example, the children may play near one another in the same room, but each child explores different toys (see Figure 15.1■).

By 3½ years of age, children begin to borrow and share some toys and materials from those who are physically near them and who are engaged in similar activities. Through this process, the children begin to learn turn taking. This is called **associative group interaction**. For example, while in the sandbox, the children take turns with some of the sand toys, and move into and out of each other's digging spaces. Brief efforts to play with the same toy may occur (Cronin & Mandich, 2005).

By elementary school, children begin to participate in **egocentric cooperative group** interactions. That is, the children cooperate with one another because they realize that through this cooperation, their individual needs are met. This can be seen in a Little League baseball game where the children agree to take turns fielding the ball because this allows each of them to get a turn at bat. Around middle school, children and adolescents learn how to engage in cooperative groups. At this level, they can es-

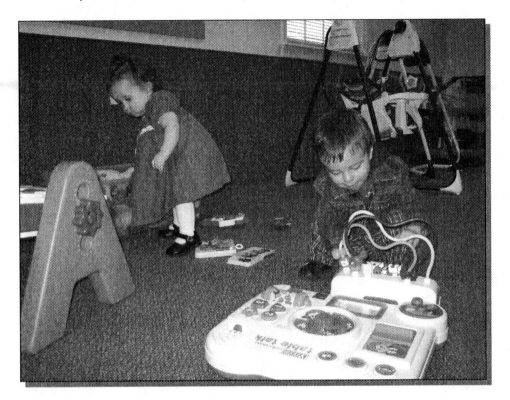

■ **Figure 15.1**
Parallel play.

tablish and abide by group rules, divide the workload, and assume roles to accomplish a common task. This is the time when children and adolescents become involved in extracurricular school activities and youth groups. The need to belong to the group and the sense of group identity are a central part of the play, leisure, or social activity (Vander Zanden, Crandell, & Crandell, 2003).

As children and adolescents develop, they do not lose their ability to engage in the earlier levels of social interaction. Typically, they expand the repertoire of the type and complexity of activities they perform at each of these levels of social interaction. Thus, the adolescent who is able to cooperate with his peers to play in a band may enjoy being an onlooker when watching a concert. As likely, the adolescent will use parallel group level skills to practice blowing his trumpet in a room with several other horn players, or will use associative level skills to share music scores with other musicians.

Types of Play, Leisure, and Social Participation Occupations

Infants engage in **social play** with their parents and caregivers through verbal, tactile, visual, kinesthetic, and affective means. As part of this social interaction, they coo and smile, whimper and cry. They visually examine and tactilely explore their parents and caregivers, increasing their body movements when they are excited, squirming when they are distressed, and snuggling peacefully when they are content. When these social interactions are positive, frequent, and predictable, they promote a sense of safety and freedom for the infant to explore the surrounding environment. **Attachment**, which is an enduring emotional bond, develops between the child and the parent or primary caregiver through these social interactions (Williamson & Dorman, 2002). During this same time period, infants begin to engage in **exploratory play** or sensorimotor play by

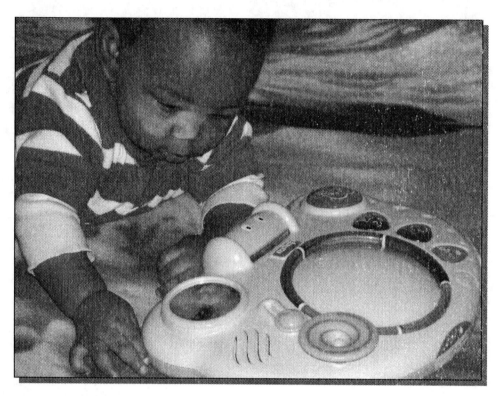

■ **Figure 15.2**
Sensorimotor play.

seeking and repeating activities that produce sensory and motor experiences (Case-Smith, 2005). They suck their fists, explore surfaces with their feet and hands, kick their legs, wave their arms, swat at mobiles, and experiment with the sound of their own voices (see Figure 15.2■).

Between the ages of 12 months and 18 months, children demonstrate **functional play** and **relational play.** Functional play is reality based; children use objects for the purpose for which they are designed. They may bring a cup or spoon to their mouth, or push a toy vacuum cleaner across the carpet. Functional play expands into relational play. In relational play, children combine a sequence of related actions such as putting a stuffed animal into a wagon and pulling it, or putting dishes into a cupboard (see Figure 15.3■).

During this same time, children spend significant time in **gross motor play** to explore spaces and textures of objects. They delight in full body movements that provide proprioceptive and vestibular input such as running, swinging, and spinning. They also enjoy tactile exploration such as water and sand play (Case-Smith, 2005).

As their expressive language and cognitive capacities develop, 2- and 3-year-old children expand upon their relational play to begin engaging in **symbolic play.** They use objects in novel ways and take on imaginary roles (Case-Smith, 2005; Feldman, 2004). For example, the paper cutout becomes a bird, or the child becomes the family dog. **Constructive play** emerges as children begin to draw, play with puzzles, and build simple block structures (see Figure 15.4■). Social play advances to include parallel and associative level interactions. Two- and 3-year-old children can play near others; some share materials and toys (see Figure 15.5■).

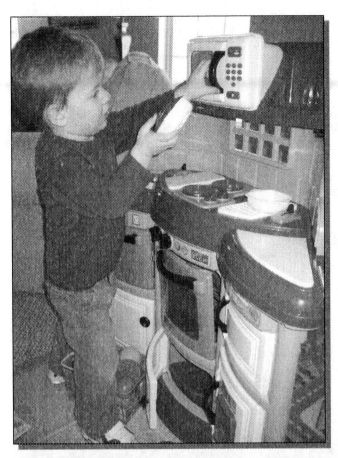

■ **Figure 15.3**
Relational play.

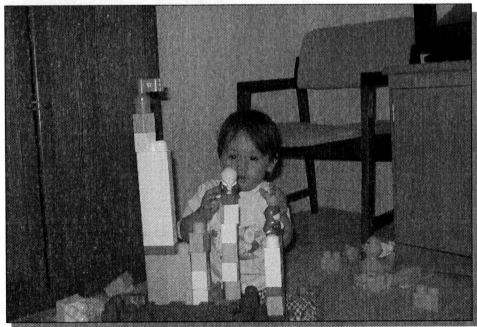

■ **Figure 15.4**
Constructing with blocks.

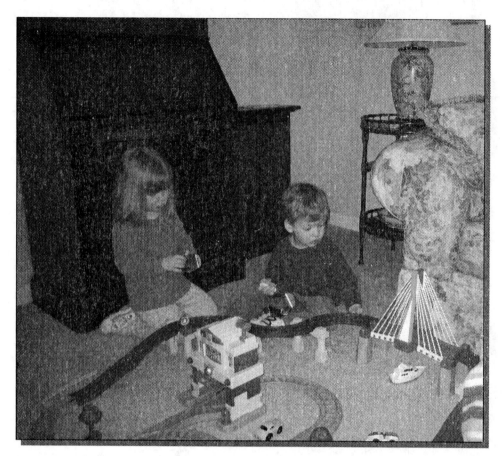

■ **Figure 15.5**
Children sharing a train set.

Between the ages of three and five years, symbolic play advances into **fantasy** or sociodramatic **play**. The blanket becomes the tent, and the stick becomes the fishing pole as the children embark on their imaginary camping trip. The toy jeep becomes a prop for imagined role of an auto mechanic (see Figure 15.6■). Gross motor play includes more **rough-and-tumble play**, such as climbing on playground equipment, sledding down hills, and rolling down sand dunes. Constructive play becomes more complex as the children experiment with stones, Legos®, interlocking puzzles, and art materials to build items. During this time, children begin participating in simple **games with rules** such as ring-around-the-rosie and duck-duck-goose (Case-Smith, 2005).

By 6 years of age children can play computer games and board games that require adherence to several rules. This may include the number and color sequence to follow, such as when playing a card game, and the pattern for moving game pieces forward and backward, such as when playing checkers. Most of the children are ready to participate in games requiring a mild level of competition and cooperation, as long as the emphasis is on participating rather than winning. While some cultures de-emphasize **competitive play**, others foster it by encouraging participation in organized sports programs. Those youth sports programs that are most successful for 6-year-olds have

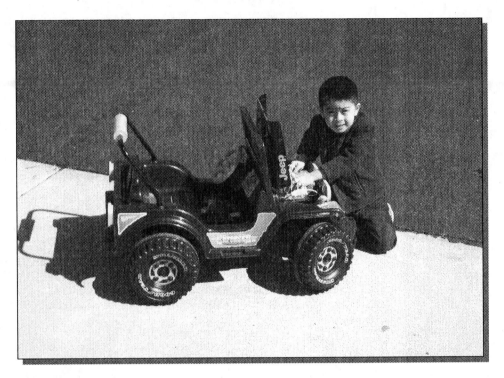

■ Figure 15.6
Fixing the Jeep.

established a system that allows all of the children to win frequently throughout the season.

The types of play interests that young children develop during the first 6 years of life serve as a foundation for the types of play, leisure, and social participation they enjoy as they grow older. For example, children who enjoy constructive play may become interested in designing complex models and making craft projects as they advance in their cognitive and physical skills. Fantasy and dramatic play may evolve into interests in music performance and theater. Exploratory play may emerge into leisure pursuits that involve hiking and orienteering. Children who receive pleasure from the vestibular and proprioceptive based gross motor play and who enjoy competition might remain actively involved in competitive sports programs. Simple board and computer games may evolve into more complex ones such as chess that require strategy, memory, forward planning of a series of moves, and prediction of the moves of others. Those who enjoy social play may develop an interest in organizing and attending social functions such as parties, festivals, and youth groups. Though there is no uniform system for clustering leisure pursuit, a few commonly cited categories include: arts, crafts, hobbies, cooking, woodworking, gardening, video gaming, outdoor recreation, sports, dance, and reading. Social participation can be clustered into community functions, religious functions, and family functions. Participation in family, school, religious, and community groups help children and adolescents expand their interests and advance their play, leisure, and social skills.

Influence of Context on Play, Leisure, and Social Participation

When providing interventions to address the play, leisure, and social participation occupations of children and adolescents, occupational therapists also must consider the contexts. As described in Chapter 1, these contexts include the physical, social, cultural, personal, spiritual, temporal, and virtual contexts. They influence what play, leisure, and social participation occupations are available to the children and adolescents, and how they engage in these occupations.

Physical Context

The physical context affects the exposure that children and adolescents have to various play, leisure, and social participation occupations, and to the materials for engaging in those occupations. Children and adolescents who live near the ocean have more opportunity to build sand castles, stroll along the beach, boogie board, deep sea fish, and ride dune buggies. Those who live near the mountains may spend more time playing in the stream, rock climbing, hiking, hunting, and camping. In contrast, those who live in the city may play sidewalk games such as hopscotch, step-ball, wire ball, and double-Dutch; wander through museums; and attend rock concerts and city fairs.

Social Context

The social context establishes behavioral norms that are to be followed during play, leisure, or social participation occupations. For example, in the social context of a birthday party for a peer, children and adolescents may play physical games, dance to music, and eat pizza. In the social context of a birthday party for a grandparent, children and adolescents may need to sit calmly and converse politely around the dinner table. In public places, they may be expected to maintain physical distance from strangers; at the neighborhood block party, they may be expected to speak with every adult they meet, and to use the adult's surname in the exchange.

Cultural Context

The culture context influences the form of play, leisure, and social participation occupations that are considered appropriate; for example, children from Amish families may play only with handmade, nonelectric toys. Native American children and adolescents may spend time doing beadwork and quillwork in preparation for ceremonial rituals. Male and female adolescents from Orthodox Jewish families swim and dance only with those of their own gender. Youth from Jamaican communities may learn to play steel drums as part of a band, while those youth from Mexican communities may learn to dance to Mariachi music (Arlon, 2004).

Personal Contexts

Age, gender, and socioeconomic status influence the level of supervision, and the types of materials available during play, leisure, and social participation activities. For instance, young children more commonly play in protected spaces under the supervision of older siblings or caregivers (see Figure 15.7■).

In contrast, adolescents frequently socialize in varied settings within their communities, out of view of the caregivers. Girls are more likely to have toys painted in pastel colors such pink, lavender, and yellow, and to be encouraged to participate in nurturing and fine detail activities. Boys are more likely to have toys painted in primary colors such as blue, red, and green, and to be encouraged to participate in ex-

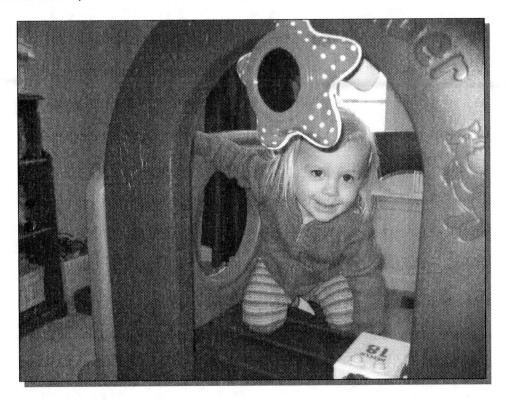

■ **Figure 15.7**
Playing in a protected space.

ploratory and large movement activities. Children and adolescents with limited fiscal resources are more apt to engage in cost-free play and leisure pursuits, whereas those with substantive fiscal resources are more apt to have costly toys and pursue costly interests. Some adolescents find part time employment to earn money to support their leisure interests. Because employment requires a time commitment, these adolescents may have to prioritize which of their leisure pursuits are most important to them.

Spiritual Context
The spiritual context influences the choice of materials that children and adolescents use when participating in play, leisure, and social participation activities. It also influences when they engage in those activities. Craft activities that involve valentines and Christmas ornaments reflect Christian beliefs, sand painting may reflect Navajo beliefs, and toys such as a dreidel reflect Jewish practices. Children and adolescents who are Jewish may need to reserve Friday nights and Saturdays to celebrate the Sabbath with their families and attend synagogue services. Those who are Muslims may need to arrange several times throughout the day to face east and respond to the call to prayer. Those who are members of the Christian faith may set aside time on Saturday or Sunday to attend church services.

Temporal Context
The temporal context includes internal and external time dimensions. These affect the frequency, duration, and time of day or season when children and adolescents participate in play, leisure, and social activities. Young children are more apt to play in short, frequent intervals throughout the morning and midafternoon. Elementary age children

are more likely to participate in play, leisure, and social activities for several hours in late afternoon on weekdays; adolescents may do so from late afternoon through late evening, depending on family and community curfews. Children and adolescents also may spend extended periods of time in a series of scheduled and spontaneous play, leisure, and social pursuits on Saturdays and Sundays, depending on other obligations and resources. Mild temperatures and prolonged periods of sunlight are conducive to outdoor activities. Extreme temperatures and shortened periods of sunlight often increase the amount of indoor activities.

Virtual Context

The virtual context, created by increased access to electronic media, has altered the time and space dimensions for engaging in play, leisure, and social occupations. Children and adolescents can play games through the Internet or communicate with one another almost instantaneously through instant messaging, text messaging, and emailing. These methods allow children and adolescents to suspend receiving and responding to the message, and to save their game moves until a more convenient time. Because these methods allow for real-time communication across multiple geographic places, children and adolescents can form and sustain personal relationships with people who live outside of their immediate locale.

Play, Leisure, and Social Participation Interventions

Play, leisure, and social participation occupations can be used as methods to achieve other goals or can be the outcome of intervention. As intervention methods, these occupations help to address problems children and adolescents may be experiencing in performance skills, performance patterns, body functions, or other areas of occupation. For example, after problem solving with the occupational therapist about the intervention plan, the occupational therapy assistants may have a young child play dress-up to learn dressing skills, or pretend to be a dentist to develop prehension skills necessary for oral hygiene tasks. The occupational therapy assistant may have an older child work on craft projects to develop visual motor skills, or have a high school student organize a group outing to refine problem solving and negotiation skills (see Figure 15.8■).

When planning such interventions, the occupational therapist and occupational therapy assistant consider the developmental appropriateness of the play, leisure, or social occupations, and the transferability of skills used during these occupations to problem areas being addressed.

When the ability to participate in play, leisure, and social activities is the outcome of intervention, occupational therapists and occupational therapy assistants focus on the skills, interests, playfulness, and social competency of the children and adolescents; environmental supports; and task modifications. For example, guided by the occupational therapist, the occupational therapy assistant might work with a young child to develop associative level play skills necessary for attending preschool, or with a middle school–age child to learn social competencies necessary to partake in youth programs. Collaborating with an adolescent as part of a transition plan, the occupational therapy assistant might address community leisure interests. As a consultant to a community recreation program, the occupational therapy assistant may consider accessibility of playground equipment and exercise paths. Common to planning for all of these interventions is the need for the occupational therapist and the occupational therapy assistant to consider the:

- Child's or adolescent's current levels of functioning
- Child's and adolescent's aspirations to participate in such in play, leisure, and social participation occupations

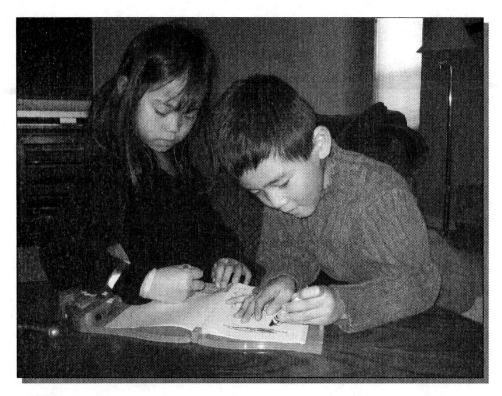

■ Figure 15.8
Developing visual motor skills.

- Tasks for participating in these occupations
- Context for participation in such occupations
- Occupational therapist's and the occupational therapy assistant's therapeutic interactions for promoting participation (Williamson & Dorman, 2002)

As described in Chapter 4, the occupational therapist assumes primary responsibility for all aspects of the intervention. The occupational therapy assistant assumes responsibility for implementing those aspects of the intervention delegated by the occupational therapist. To do so effectively requires the occupational therapist and the occupational therapy assistant to be knowledgeable about child and adolescent growth and development, the complexity and dimensions of play, leisure, and social participation occupations, and contextual influences. The interventions they devise may address person factors, the environment, or the task.

Interventions Directed at Person Factors
Performance Skills, Performance Patterns, and Body Functions
Through thoughtful planning and careful activity analysis, the occupational therapist and the occupational therapy assistant can use play, leisure, or social occupations to accomplish several goals. They can utilize play, leisure, and social participation activities to facilitate the development of a combination of physical, cognitive, social-emotional, and communication skills and patterns, or to help children and adolescents regain lost skills and patterns. They can upgrade the complexity of these occupations

to provide additional challenges as the child or adolescent becomes more competent. The following story of Jin demonstrates how the occupational therapy assistant uses the leisure occupation of card playing to address several rehabilitation goals.

JIN

Jin, an adolescent male, sustained a closed head injury as a result of a skiing accident. Jin now has difficulty with mental functions involving memory, judgment, problem solving, and self-control. He also has difficulty with movement functions involving fine motor control and bilateral integration. Using her ability to analyze activity demands, the occupational therapy assistant selects a card game that is of interest to Jin and addresses his performance problems. She chooses the card game War because it requires Jin to remember only a few rules and to wait only momentarily for his turn. She structures the game so that Jin picks up one card at a time from the pile and turns it face up. Next, she picks up a single card and places it face up on the table. Then she prompts Jin to identify the number or letter on each card and to determine which of the two cards is higher. Finally, she cues him to problem solve whether he or she won the round and should pick up the two cards. The combination of these strategies helps Jin to be successful in his efforts.

As Jin regains some mental and fine motor functions, the occupational therapy assistant upgrades the card game to Uno®. She now has him play with another person. Jin must communicate with the other person, hold the cards in his hands and focus on number and color sequences, and the rules for the number of cards to lie down or pick up. He must wait for his turn a bit longer, or skip his turn, if the cards indicate such an action.

As Jin continues to regain additional cognitive and motor functions, the occupational therapy assistant once again upgrades the card game to Casino. She structures the game so that he plays with a partner against another team. Now Jin must look at the cards in his hands and remember the plays made by his opponents to assess his potential to win tricks. This game requires higher level mental functions of memory, prediction, and judgment. It also requires fine motor and bilateral integration, the ability to wait while others plan their moves, and to organize his actions with those of his partner.

Prior to actually playing the occupation-based activity of cards, the occupational therapy assistant may engage Jin in both preparatory and purposeful activities. To improve pinch and bilateral integration, she may ask Jin to pick up poker chips and transfer them from his dominant to his non-dominant hand. She may have him practice drawing, discarding, and shuffling cards. If standard size cards are too difficult for him to manipulate, she may provide larger cards, and place the discard pile within easy reach at his midline. To address mental functions, the occupational therapy assistant may have Jin practice each step of the card game separately. She may have Jin read aloud written or pictorial cue cards that outline the basic rules of the game; use a timer to structure turn taking; and practice possible moves prior to playing the actual game to improve judgment. During these preparatory and purposeful activities, and the occupation-based card game, the occupational therapy assistant provides appropriate cues and feedback as needed for successful engagement in context.

Playfulness

Occupational therapists and occupational therapy assistants also may address the playfulness of children and adolescents through play. Children and adolescents who have little opportunity to engage in play because of traumatic life events or environmental deprivations may benefit from opportunities to develop playfulness. Curiosity, creativity, spontaneity, joyfulness, and a sense of internal control associated with playfulness may help children and adolescents to become flexible in their approaches for coping with other daily life demands (Knox, 2005; Morrison & Metzer, 2001). The following story of Shiva illustrates how occupational therapists and occupational therapy assistants may foster playfulness in a young child.

SHIVA

For the first two years of her life, Shiva lived in an orphanage. She spent most of her time in a crib because of understaffing of personnel available to care for more than her basic nutrition and clothing needs. Now adopted, Shiva attends an inclusionary preschool. As part of the intervention plan, the occupational therapist provides consultation to the classroom teacher and the parents regarding the development of play. The occupational therapy assistant works with Shiva in the classroom several times a week during creative playtime. Following the developmental sequence for play, he initially engages Shiva in social play and sensorimotor play. During this play, he models spontaneity, creativity, and pleasure, and lets Shiva take the lead as to those activities she enjoys. They make funny faces at one another, crawl through the sand piles, splash in the water, and roll on the pillows.

As Shiva initiates this type of play more frequently, the occupational therapy assistant introduces functional play and relational play. He encourages Shiva to play with bucket and shovel in the sand pile, use plastic pitcher to scoop up and pour the water, and line up the pillows in different sequences. Encouraging her development of gross motor play, the occupational therapy assistant prompts Shiva to carry buckets of sand from one pile to another, and to skip around the pillows. He includes another child in these activities to foster parallel level social skills.

Supporting Shiva as she continues to make progress, the occupational therapy assistant next introduces symbolic and constructive play. He adds dolls and animal figures, and models how to construct sand castles and water slides as play grounds for the toy people and animals. In an effort to promote associative level social skills, he then encourages Shiva to take turns sharing the space and the toys with two other children who are playing in the sand and water.

Throughout the sequence the occupational therapy assistant carefully observes Shiva's behaviors. He reports to the occupational therapist about the way Shiva moves her body, reacts to sensory input, and plans her play activities. He also reports about Shiva's play preferences, play patterns, emotional responses, and interactions with the other children. Using this information, the occupational therapist and occupational therapy assistant problem solve about the best approaches to promote Shiva's development, and to guard against over stimulation and adverse consequences.

Social Competence

Social competence is another area that occupational therapists and occupational therapy assistants address through play, leisure, and social participation occupations. Children and adolescents with problems in social competence have difficulty with:

- Age appropriate social and play behaviors
- Emotional and behavioral self-regulation
- Verbal and nonverbal communication exchanges
- Competent prosocial skills
- Prosocial skills and social decision making (Williamson & Dorman, 2002).

The following story of Alexi, a third grader, highlights some behaviors that children who have problems with social competence might exhibit.

ALEXI

Alexi's father requested an occupational therapy evaluation because of difficulties his son was having in getting along with other children his age. As directed by the occupational therapist, the occupational therapy assistant observed Alexi during the after school program. The occupational therapy assistant noted that Alexi tried to tell the other children what activities they were to do and how they were to do those activities. When the children rolled their eyes and stated that they wanted to choose their own activities, he told them that their ideas were stupid. As they started to walk away from him, he commanded them to do what he said. When the staff member confronted Alexi about these behaviors, he yelled at her then ran to another room. Later, the occupational therapy assistant observed Alexi at the preschool table, knocking over a block structure he just built, and mumbling that he can not do anything right. The occupational therapy assistant prepared a written report for the occupational therapist that outlined the observed behaviors.

The occupational therapist then met with Alexi's father and school personnel, who reported that he demonstrates similar behaviors when interacting with his cousins at family gatherings and with his peers during classroom activities. As a result, Alexi seldom gets invited to his cousins' or classmates' homes to play.

After analyzing the data, the occupational therapist meets with the occupational therapy assistant and Alexi's father to devise an intervention plan. They decide to use various teaching, modeling, coaching, and feedback techniques to help Alexi develop competent social skills. Table 15.1■ provides a list of intervention strategies that the occupational therapist and occupational therapy assistant may use to address Alexi's problems with social competence.

Interventions Directed at the Physical Environment

In addition to personal factors, it is important for occupational therapists and occupational therapy assistants to consider the physical environment when planning interventions to promote play, leisure, and social participation occupations. Children and adolescents react to the physical space that surrounds them. During interventions, occupational therapists and occupational therapy assistants can arrange these spaces to enable children and adolescents to constructively focus their physical, cognitive, and affective behaviors. Small spaces encourage sedentary play and leisure pursuits, whereas large spaces promote gross motor and rough and tumble play. Softly lighted environments with quiet colors, soothing sounds, and soft furniture have a calming affect. Brightly lighted environments, with vivid colors, multiple materials, and energizing sounds have an arousing affect. Using this information, occupational therapists and occupational therapy assistants might recommend using muted colors, fish tanks, waterfall sounds, and beanbag chairs in the library to promote quiet participation in storytelling and reading activities. To help children and adolescents with visual challenges to feel more secure, the occupational therapist and the occupational therapy assistant may suggest dividing large spaces into smaller ones that provide tactile and visual cues as the physical layout. To encourage movement for those children who are more sedentary or who are struggling with obesity, the occupational therapist and occupational therapy assistant may propose using vivid colors, fast paced music, and open spaces with exploratory enticing materials.

The temperature, smells, and number of people within the space also affect children's and adolescents' behaviors. What is an acceptable level of stimuli for one child or adolescent may over stimulate or under stimulate another, and thus affect the degree of successful engagement in the play, leisure, or social participation occupations.

■ **Table 15.1**
Intervention Strategies to Address Problems with Social Competence

AREA OF DIFFICULTY	INTERVENTION STRATEGY
Delay in social and play behaviors	Set up play activities with a few other children to encourage Alexi to interact successfully with his peers at the parallel and associative level. As he demonstrates prosocial skills at this level, advance to the egocentric cooperative level.
	Demonstrate and provide cues as to how to interact at the more advanced level.
	Place Alexi near another child who can model the next level of social interaction.
	Plan sequence of activities to include those that are familiar as well as novel, and contain tasks that are easy to accomplish as well as a few that are challenging to accomplish. As he feels safe with these activities, include more novel tasks.
Difficulty with self-regulation	Play "acting" games to teach Alexi how to monitor and adjust tone of voice, activity level, and emotional reactions.
	Teach Alexi how to calm himself by taking long, slow breaths, rocking slowly in a rocking chair, and rhythmically squeezing a squish toy, or slowly rubbing his arms and legs.
	Establish a cuing system to provide feedback to Alexi in a nonthreatening manner during the activity.
	Play "I saw something . . ." to practice attending to and interpreting nonverbal cues of others.
	Teach Alexi prediction and time management strategies for initiating, terminating, and transitioning between activities.
Difficulty communicating	Use puppets to rehearse how to initiate, continue, and switch a topic during conversation.
	Use language based board games to practice requesting, commenting, describing, clarifying, and turn taking skills.
	Have Alexi read poetry, songs, and short stories aloud to model story telling skills.
	Set up two-minute debates for Alexi to practice persuasion and compromise skills.
Limited prosocial skills	Have Alexi design greeting cards to practice greeting and complimenting others.
	Have Alexi role play skits from sit coms to give and receive feedback, and negotiate conflict.
	Have Alexi practice asking for and providing information to complete a scavenger hunt.
Limited social decision making skills	Using cut out pictures, have Alexi build a decision making tree to brainstorm ideas, consider consequences and impact of those ideas, implement ideas, and evaluate consequences of ideas.
	Have Alexi draw different versions of the same story to teach generation, selection, and evaluation of options.

■ Table 15.2
Physical Environments

PHYSICAL ENVIRONMENTAL SUPPORTS	PHYSICAL ENVIRONMENTAL FACTORS
Create a calming atmosphere	Provide soft lights, quiet colors, soothing sounds, soft furniture, and limited materials.
	Use head phones to reduce external noise, and sunglasses to reduce intensity of visual cues.
Create an arousing atmosphere	Provide bright lights, vivid colors, energizing sounds, and multiple materials.
Promote feelings of security and organization	Subdivide large spaces into smaller ones with boundaries; furnish with familiar objects.
	Establish a designated place for supplies and objects.
Promote physical activity	Play fast tempo music.
	Provide open spaces for movement; provide exploratory enticing materials.

Some children and adolescents perceive warm temperatures, lilac smells, and the presence of a few people as calming; they may perceive cool temperatures, citrus smells, and a crowd of people as invigorating. Other children and adolescents may become agitated by these same stimuli. A few children experience life threatening allergic reactions to some smells, such as those found in perfumes and fragrant-scented candles, shampoos, soaps, and lotions. Occupational therapists and occupational therapy assistants observe the responses of the children and adolescents carefully to various physical environments. Based on an analysis of this information, the occupational therapist and the occupational therapy assistant can determine the best match, and systematically modify the amount and types of physical stimuli in the environment. Through this modification, they can help the children and adolescents adjust their behaviors to participate successfully in their play, leisure, or social participation. Table 15.2■ summarizes key physical environmental factors.

Occupational therapists and occupational therapy assistants also need to consider safety features within these spaces. A number of safety practices apply to all children and adolescents, not just those who may be coping with additional physical, cognitive, and social emotional challenges. For example because of the potential of choking on or swallowing of small objects, young children and those who put objects into their mouths should not be given toys that are smaller than the size of their fists. Tables and counter tops should have nonbreakable surfaces and rounded edges. Painted surfaces should be lead and chip free. Plastic bags should be perforated. Work surfaces and supplies that are shared among several children and adolescents should be disinfected daily. Electric outlets should be covered, electric cords removed from traffic patterns, and sharp and hazardous materials stored in locked bins. Playground and gym equipment should be constructed from hard plastics and lumber, rather than metal. If constructed from lumber, care needs to be taken about the potential of splinters, particularly splinters from treated lumber that can cause allergic reactions. Playing surfaces should be covered with rubber mats, grass, sand, or other materials that can absorb the shock of falls. Depending on the type of contact sport, rough and tumble play, craft or cooking project, the children and adolescents should wear appropriate protective eye and head gear, body armor, mouth guards, ear plugs, and safety vests.

Occupational therapists and occupational therapy assistants need to pay additional attention to safety features when working with children and adolescents who have physical, cognitive, or social-emotional disabilities. Children and adolescents with physical disabilities may not have the strength, coordination, sensory acuity, or reaction time to adequately protect them from potential injury. Those with cognitive disabilities may have difficulty judging the safety risk and recalling safety procedures. Those with social emotional difficulties may struggle with self-control issues, or be at risk for self-abuse or suicide. Table 15.3■ summarizes key safety factors.

Occupational therapists and occupational therapy assistants also work to ensure that public spaces, such as playgrounds, parks, community centers, and schools are

■ **Table 15.3**
Safety Precautions

SAFETY CONCERN	SAFETY ACTION
Choking and swallowing hazard	Keep all objects small enough to be swallowed out of the reach of children who mouth objects.
	Keep medicine and toxic materials in child resistant containers and locked in cabinets.
	Keep curtain cords above head level.
Potential for collision and falls	Round the edges of table tops and other work surfaces.
	Replace glass table tops with wood or hard plastics.
	Install shatterproof windows.
	Construct railings that are at least three feet high, and have vertical slats that have a maximum of three inches between them on above ground walk surfaces.
	Install nonslip surfaces or nonslip safety strips, and nonglare lighting in traffic areas.
	Install safety precaution signs at intersections such as school hallways.
Ingestion of paint	Use lead free paint, sand and repaint chipped surfaces.
Spread of infections	Wipe all surfaces daily with a disinfectant.
	Wash hands between activities, before and after eating, and after toileting.
	Wear plastic gloves when touching body fluids.
Suffocation hazard	Perforate plastic bags large enough to cover the face and nose.
Electrocution hazard	Install GFCI protective outlets and cover outlets.
	Remove electric cords from traffic area.
Cutting hazard	Store all sharp tools in protective jackets and in locked cabinets.
Playground and gym hazards	Use hard plastic, splinter free lumber, and shock absorbing surfaces.
Sports and gross-motor play injuries	Wear appropriate protective gear such as helmets, kneepads, elbow pads, and shin guards.
Craft and hobby related injuries	Wear protective gear such as eye goggles, earplugs, safety gloves and aprons, and protective shoes.
	Remove jewelry, and secure loose clothing.

physically accessible for children and adolescents with disabilities. They may do this in an official capacity or as private citizens using their knowledge for the betterment of social conditions. As public or private school based employees, they may assess the safety and accessibility of playground equipment and communicate findings to appropriate individuals such as the building principal. In a consultant role to a sports equipment company, they may propose accessibility design modifications. Serving on a community committee, they may promote accessible theaters and restaurants. As constituent citizens, they may organize meetings with members of the state and federal government to discuss safety and usability issues at public parks. To do so requires occupational therapists and occupational therapy assistants to familiarize themselves with local and federal building codes that comply with Americans with Disabilities Act (ADA) guidelines. These include guidelines for entrances, exits, pathways, signage, work surface, bathrooms and water fountains, display and control boards, parking, communication, and transportation. Since most of these codes are based on adult bodies, modifications may be needed to accommodate child and adolescent bodies. Table 15.4■ provides some examples of how to modify environments to increase accessibility. Examples listed for one environment also may apply to other environments.

Examples of Interventions Directed at the Task

The occupational therapist and the occupational therapy assistant also may direct interventions at the task. Using their knowledge of both high- and low-tech modifications, they evaluate and grade activity demands to enable children and adolescents to engage in play, leisure, and social participation activities. Their interventions may focus on

- Modifying the tools, materials, or equipment
- Adjusting the sequence, number of steps, and time to complete the task
- Altering the physical, cognitive, or social emotional demands necessary to engage in the task
- Modifying the task so that it can be completed using alternative parts of the body (AOTA, 2002)

Modification to the Tools, Materials, or Equipment

Incorporating back supports, seat belts, and foot straps to the seat makes it possible for a young child with low muscle tone and muscle coordination difficulties to pump swings and gliders on the gym set. Adding Velcro® to a mitt and ball helps a child with deficits in fine motor control to play a game of catch. Using a T-ball stand helps a child who has difficulty visually tracking and quickly swinging at a thrown baseball, successfully bat the ball. Applicators made from smooth hard materials aids children and adolescents who are tactilely sensitive to complete arts and craft projects. A spring-loaded cast and rewind button on a fishing reel enable an adolescent with limited motor control to fish. A large print menu enables an adolescent with visual limitations to order food from a restaurant with friends.

Adjustments to the Sequence, Number of Steps, and Time

Eliminating backward movements and skipped turns enables a child with limited cognitive abilities or low frustration tolerance to participate in games such as Mother May I? Red Light-Green Light, and Chutes and Ladders®. Extending or eliminating the time requirement makes it easier for adolescents who have slower information

■ **Table 15.4**
Accessible Environments for Play, Leisure, and Social Participation

ENVIRONMENT	MODIFICATIONS TO INCREASE ACCESSIBILITY
Playground	Install table height water and sand tables. Build ramps for climbing structures. Install wheelchair accessible platform swings and mazes. Develop shaded play and rest areas. Build wheelchair tolerant basketball, tennis, shuffleboard, and volleyball courts.
National park	Build wheelchair accessible nature paths, fishing peers, and boat launches. Install guide ropes, rest areas, and signage along paths. Install emergency call boxes. Provide adapted sports rental equipment.
Amusement park	Install accessible changing rooms and bathrooms that allow a caregiver of either gender to provide needed assistance. Provide identification tags for caregivers to easily reunite with lost children or adolescent. Designate climate controlled rest areas for children and adolescents with special needs to attend to physical and medical needs. Design supportive seating on rides to accommodate children and adolescents with special needs.
Resorts	Design outriggers for adapted downhill and cross country skiing. Provide all-terrain wheelchairs for traversing sand and dirt surfaces. Install nonskid ramps or hydraulic lifts to enter and exit swimming pools. Provide full body flotation devices and shallow water areas for children and adolescents with special needs.
Place of worship Community center Theater	Design accessible seating at various locations throughout places of worship or theater. Install sound, lighting, and text messaging system to accommodate children and adolescents with limited vision and hearing.
Restaurant	Install wheelchair accessible tables in low traffic areas. Provide additional lighting and magnifying glasses for children and adolescents with limited vision. Provide picture versions of menus. Furnish adapted spoons, cups, plates, and eating utensils.
Shopping center	Design wide width shopping areas. Install motion sensitive doors and bathroom equipment. Install changing benches and assistance buttons in dressing rooms. Erect canopies over entrances. Install quiet play and reading areas.

processing rates to participate in decision making and memory recall games such as Charades®, Boggle®, or Trivial Pursuit®.

Alterations to the Physical, Cognitive, or Social Emotional Skills

Using a controller with a built up handle may make it easier for an older child with juvenile rheumatoid arthritis to play X-Box® games with his siblings. A touch access screen enables an adolescent who has difficulty isolating finger movements that are necessary to operate buttons on a small controller to play a computer game. Changing the rules of a game from those that reward the first person to succeed to those that reward the entire team for cooperating to complete the task, allows a child with low self-esteem to experience success. Going shopping at off peak hours and for short intervals helps an adolescent with self regulation problems better cope with environmental and social demands.

Completing the Task Using Alternative Body Movements

A riding toy with leg and arm propulsion mechanisms allows a child with limited strength to use all four limbs to propel forward. A cardholder enables the adolescent with hemiplegia to play a game of poker with friends. A plastic or wooden frame to hold fabrics provides the needed stability for that same adolescent to sew a needlecraft project with one hand. Paint brushes with mouth guards make it possible for children and adolescents with upper limb deficiencies or athetoid cerebral palsy to paint.

SUMMARY

Play occupations are those exploratory and participatory activities that provide pleasure and amusement, stimulate curiosity and creativity, or offer diversion and entertainment. Leisure occupations also include exploratory and participatory activities. Because they are nonobligatory, they are done during discretionary time to satisfy an area of curiosity or interest, provide pleasure, or afford learning and creative opportunities (Parham & Fazio, 1997). The distinction made between play and leisure often is related to age. Social participation occupations involve interactions with family, friends, peers, and community members in organized patterns that are recognized by society (AOTA, 2002; AOTA, nd; Mosey, 1996). Within the daily life of children and adolescents, play, leisure, and social participation occupations often overlap or become fused with one another. Children and adolescents need to be socially competent to engage in these occupations.

Play, leisure, and social participation occupations can be categorized by the level of interaction with others, and by the type of activity. The levels of interaction include solitary play, onlooker play, parallel, associative, egocentric cooperative, and cooperative. There are social, exploratory, functional, relational, symbolic, constructive, rough and tumble, gross motor, and rule bound types of play. Though there is no uniform system for clustering leisure pursuits, a few commonly cited categories include: arts, crafts, hobbies, cooking, woodworking, gardening, video gaming, outdoor recreation, and reading. Social participation activities can be grouped according to family, friend, religious, and community involvement. Children's and adolescents' level of growth and development, as well as the context in which they live, influence the level and type of play, leisure, and social participation occupations in which they engage.

Occupational therapists and occupational therapy assistants use play, leisure, and social participation occupations as methods to achieve other goals. They also target them as the outcome of intervention. Specifically, they use these occupations to address problems children and adolescents experience in performance skills, performance patterns, body functions, or other areas of occupation. Occupational therapists and occupational therapy assistants also design interventions to promote the ability of children and adolescents to engage in play, leisure, and social participation occupations. When engagement in these occupations is the outcome of intervention, occupational therapists and occupational therapy assistants focus on the skills, interests, playfulness, and social competency of the children and adolescents; environmental supports, and task modifications.

Whether as intervention method or as the outcome of intervention, occupational therapists and occupational therapy assistants need to have a solid understanding of child and adolescent growth and development; play, leisure, and social occupations; and the context influencing these occupations. They need to consider the child's or adolescent's current levels of functioning and their aspirations to participate in such in play, leisure, and social participation occupations. They also need to be able to analyze and adapt these occupations and the context for participation in such occupations. Finally, occupational therapists and occupational therapy assistants must assess their own ability to engage in therapeutic interactions that promote play, leisure, and social participation.

REVIEWING KEY POINTS

1. Define and distinguish among play, leisure, and social participation occupations.
2. Explain the different types of play.
3. Explain the different levels of social interaction.
4. Describe playfulness and its importance for participating in play, leisure, and social occupations.
5. Explain what is meant by social competence and why it is important in play, leisure, and social occupations.
6. Detail how context influences children's and adolescents' engagement in play, leisure, and social participation occupations.
7. Clarify how play, leisure, and social participation occupations can be methods to achieve an intervention goal or the goal of intervention.
8. Outline personal, environmental, and task related factors to consider when providing play, leisure, and social participation interventions.

APPLYING KEY CONCEPTS

1. Design a packet of handouts that parents and caregivers can use to create play centers for children ages 1 through 3.
   a. In these handouts, explain how the play centers promote different types of play and levels of social interaction.
   b. In these handouts, provide a list of suggestions that the parents and caregivers can use to modify the environment and task and thus enable children with special needs to participate.
2. Design a packet of handouts that parents and caregivers can use to create play centers for children ages 3 through 5.
   a. In these handouts, explain how the play centers promote different types of play and levels of social interaction.

  b. In these handouts, provide a list of suggestions that the parents and caregivers can use to modify the environment and tasks to enable children with special needs to participate.
3. Draft a plan to organize an after school program for children ages 6 through 12.
  a. Outline the type of play, leisure, and social participation activities available for the children. Provide a rationale for including these activities.
  b. Describe the context for each of these activities. Explain how these contexts influence the children's engagement in the activities. Explain how to modify these contexts for children with special needs.
  c. Describe safety features that should be incorporated for each of these activities. Outline additional safety features to consider for children with special needs.
4. Watch a video or a television show that depicts adolescents engaging in play, leisure, or social participation occupations. Describe those scenes where the adolescents are demonstrating social competency. Describe those scenes where the adolescents are having problems with social competence. Outline strategies for helping these adolescent to become socially competent.

REFERENCES

American Occupational Therapy Association (2002). Occupational therapy practice framework: Domain and process. *American Journal of Occupational Therapy, 56,* 609–639.

American Occupational Therapy Association (nd). Occupational therapy practice framework: Domain and process (2nd ed.). Draft.

Arlon, B. (Ed.) (2004). *How people live.* New York: DK Publishing.

Bundy, A. C. (1992, June). Play: The most important occupation of children. *Sensory Integration Special Interest Section Newsletter, 15* 1–2.

Bundy, A. (1993). Assessment of play and leisure. Delineation of the problem. *American Journal of Occupational Therapy, 47,* 217–222.

Case-Smith, J. (2005). *Occupational therapy for children* (5th ed.). St. Louis: Mosby.

Christiansen, C., Baum, C. M., & Bass-Haugen, J. (Eds.) (2005). *Occupational therapy: Performance, participation, and well-being* (3rd ed). Thorofare, NJ: SLACK.

Cronin, A., & Mandich, M. (2005). *Human development and performance throughout the lifespan.* Clifton Park, NY: Thomson Delmar Learning.

Feldman, R. (2004). *Child development* (3rd ed.). Upper Saddle, NJ: Pearson Prentice Hall.

Knox, S. (2005). Play. In J. Case-Smith (Ed.), *Occupational therapy for children* (5th ed., 571–586). St. Louis: Mosby.

Knox, S. (1996). Play and playfulness in preschool children. In R. Zemke and F. Clark (Eds.), *Occupational science: The evolving discipline* (pp. 81–88). Philadelphia: F. A. Davis.

Morrison, C., & Metzer, P. (2001). Play. In J. Case-Smith (Ed.), *Occupational therapy for children* (4th ed., 528–544). St. Louis: Mosby.

Neville-Jan, A., Fazio, L. S., Kennedy, B., & Snyder, C. (1997). Elementary to middle school transition: Using multicultural play activities to develop life skills. In L. D. Parham & L. S. Fazio (Eds.), *Play in occupational therapy for children* (pp. 35–51). St. Louis: Mosby.

Mosey, A. (1996). *Applied scientific inquiry in the health professions. An epistemological orientation* (2nd ed.). Bethesda, MD: American Occupational Therapy Association.

Parham, L. D., & Fazio, L. S. (Eds.) (1997). *Play in occupational therapy for children.* St. Louis: Mosby.

Vander Zanden, J. Crandell, T., & Crandell, C. (2003). *Human development* (7th ed. rev). Boston, MA: McGraw-Hill.

Williamson, G. G., & Dorman, W. (2002). *Promoting social competence.* San Antonio, TX: Therapy Skill Builders.

Chapter 16

Children and Youth with Intellectual and Developmental Disabilities

Margaret J. Pendzick and LuAnn Demi

Key Terms

Acquisition frame of reference
Adaptive behavior
American Association of Mental Retardation (AAMR)
Atlanto-axial joint
Developmental delay
Down syndrome
Extensive support
Family focused
Fetal alcohol syndrome (FAS)
Fragile X syndrome
Individualized education program (IEP)
Individualized family service plan (IFSP)

Intermittent support
ILEP system
Limited support
Mental retardation (MR)
Mild level of mental retardation
Moderate level of mental retardation
Pervasive support
Profound level of retardation
Radioulnar synostasis
Severe level of mental retardation
Vascular stenosis
Williams syndrome

Objectives

- Explain mental retardation (MR), fetal alcohol syndrome (FAS), Down syndrome, fragile X syndrome, and Williams syndrome.
- Examine how cognitive disabilities impact the daily occupations of children and adolescents within the context of their family and environment.

- Describe occupational therapy interventions to support the capacity of children and adolescents with cognitive disabilities to participate in their daily occupations.
- Examine how occupational therapists and occupational therapy assistants problem solve together during the intervention process.
- Describe how occupational therapists and occupational therapy assistants work with families and other professionals to provide services to children and adolescents with cognitive disabilities.

INTRODUCTION

This chapter contains an overview of **mental retardation (MR)** and several syndromes that include mental retardation—**Down syndrome, fetal alcohol syndrome (FAS), fragile X syndrome**, and **Williams syndrome**. The cognitive, physical, and social difficulties associated with mental retardation and those related conditions are discussed first. An examination of occupational therapy interventions to address the occupational challenges associated with mental retardation follows.

MENTAL RETARDATION

Mental retardation is characterized by substantial limitations in age appropriate intellectual functioning and **adaptive behavior** that originate before age 18 (AAMR, n.d.). Deficits in intellectual functioning for children and adolescents with mental retardation may include:

- Poor memory
- Slow learning rates
- Attention problems
- Difficulty generalizing skills and knowledge in new situations and different settings
- Difficulty knowing how to initiate and sequence tasks
- Difficulty with abstraction, judgment, categorization, and problem solving (Heward, 2006)

Deficits in adaptive behavior involve difficulty with performing those "conceptual, social, and practical skills that have been learned by people in order to function in their everyday lives" (Luckasson et al., 1992, p. 73). Making judgments on what to eat and wear, using words and gestures to communicate with peers, and manipulating various tools for play and school are adaptive behaviors. Because it is difficult to measure the cognitive capacity of children and adolescents with mental retardation, adaptive behavioral measurements rather than intelligence tests frequently are used (DSM-IV, 2000). On some measurement tools, such as the *Vineland Adaptive Behaviors Scales (Vineland-II)* (Sparrow, Cicchetti, & Balla, 2006) and the *Denver Developmental*

Screening Test (Denver II) (Frankenburg, Dodds, Archer, Shapiro, & Bresnick, 1992), adaptive behaviors are categorized according to self-help, fine motor manipulation, gross motor movements and mobility, and social communication.

How to define mental retardation has been debated and changed over time. Traditionally, the terms **mild**, **moderate**, **severe**, and **profound** have been used to classify the degree or level of intellectual impairment as measured by intelligence quotient (IQ) tests. Mild mental retardation represents an IQ range from approximately 55 to 70 and reflects the ability of children or adolescents to learn academic skills from the third to seventh grade level. Moderate mental retardation represents a range of approximately 40 to 55 on an IQ test and the ability to perform academic tasks at the second grade level. Children or adolescents who are classified as having severe mental retardation have an IQ range of approximately 25–40. These children and adolescents can learn to communicate basic ideas and perform self-care tasks. Profound mental retardation represents an IQ of below 25. Children and adolescents with this classification require extensive supports to live in the community (Behrman, Kliegman, & Jenson, 2004).

Recently, when considering the level of impairment of mental retardation, the focus has shifted from IQ test scores to the level of support and accommodations needed to function effectively in everyday settings (Thies & Travers, 2006). The **American Association of Mental Retardation (AAMR)** eliminated the mild, moderate, severe, and profound categories of mental retardation. Instead, the AAMR recognizes the importance of environment and the amount of support that a person needs for major life activities (Thies & Travers, 2006).

Although mental retardation impacts many aspects of the children's and adolescent's daily life, the environmental support can influence the degree of impact. Positive interactions within the environment enable the children and adolescents with mental retardation to become more independent, develop personal relationships, make societal contributions, and participate in school and the community (AAMR, 2004).

This focus on the importance of supports has created an alternative framework, called the ILEP system, for understanding the needs of children and adolescents with mental retardation. The **ILEP system** (as cited in Heward, 2006) defines four levels or intensities of support needed for the child and adolescent. These four levels are intermittent, limited, extensive, and pervasive. An interdisciplinary team assesses the intensity of support needed to improve functioning in school, home, community, and work environments (Heward). The AAMR (as cited in Heward) has defined these intensities of support:

- **Intermittent support** is support provided on an *as-needed basis*. It is short term and typically needed during life span transitions at home and school, such as the birth of a sibling, or enrollment in a new school.

- **Limited support** is more intensive than intermittent, but requires fewer staff members and less fiscal resources than the next level of support. Limited support is time bound and directed to the accomplishments of a specific objective. For instance, a child might need limited support for several months to participate in a Brownie or a Cub Scout troop. An adolescent might require limited support in the form of a job coach to transition from the school setting to the workplace.

- **Extensive support** implies regular or daily involvement with the individual in at least some environments, such as work or home. A classroom aide may provide daily assistance with using an alternative communication system, toileting, and dressing tasks.

- **Pervasive support** is constant support with high intensity. This support is provided across all environments for the child or adolescent and has a potentially life-sustaining nature. For example, this might involve professional support at school and home for all aspects of self-care, feeding, and health management (Heward, 2006).

The diagnosis of mental retardation usually is not given to a young child until a reliable intelligence test can be administered, which often is not until the child enters school. Initially, young children who demonstrate deficits in adaptive behaviors and delays in developmental milestones may be diagnosed as **developmentally delayed**. During this time, a variety of professionals may interact with the child to provide specialized interventions. As part of early intervention services, teachers, occupational therapists, occupational therapy assistants, physical therapists, and speech-language pathologists make important contributions to enhance the child's development.

Consistent with IDEA mandates, these early intervention services are **family focused** to compliment the strengths and wishes of each individual family. When the child reaches school age and receives a more precise diagnosis, intervention services may continue as part of the educational program. Chapter 11 describes early intervention services that are part of an **Individualized Family Service Plan (IFSP)** and educational related interventions that are part of an **Individualized Education Program (IEP)**.

Mental retardation also may be a characteristic of other health conditions such as Down syndrome, fetal alcohol syndrome, fragile X syndrome, and Williams syndrome. The following discussion explains each condition in more detail.

Down Syndrome

Down syndrome, also known as *trisomy 21*, is caused by one additional chromosome 21. Down syndrome is one of the most common causes of inherited mental retardation (Heward, 2006). It occurs approximately once in every 600–800 births and is characterized by a range of physical and mental problems (Behrman, Kliegman, & Jenson, 2004). The cause of the additional chromosomes is not completely understood. In some cases, the mother is a carrier. In other cases, neither parent has the abnormal number of chromosomes within the cell nuclei of the egg or sperm; the extra chromosome occurs spontaneously during cell division. The age of the mother greatly influences the incidence of Down syndrome. For mothers under the age of 20 the incidence of Down syndrome is approximately 1 in 200 births; for mothers 40 years and over the incidence of Down syndrome is about 1 in 40 (Reed, 2001).

Physical features that are common to most children and adolescents with Down syndrome are observable in the face. They include a broad or flat face, small nose, eyes which appear to slant upward with small folds at the inner corners of the eyelids, a small mouth which makes the tongue appear larger than normal, and ears that are abnormally shaped and located slightly lower on the head. Additionally, children and adolescents with Down syndrome have small hands and short fingers (Tocci, 2000).

Another common physical feature of Down syndrome is low muscle tone throughout the body. This also is apparent in the tongue. The low muscle tone results in tongue protrusion and causes speech articulation and eating difficulties (Tocci, 2000). Additionally, the low muscle tone in the rest of the body interferes with the typical developmental milestones of crawling, sitting, and walking, as well as the development of hand skills. These motor delays, coupled with communication and cognitive challenges, affect the development of play, self-care skills, and other occupations (Tocci). Not all children and adolescents with Down syndrome have all of these physical traits, but low muscle tone, upward slanted eyes, and small ears usually are present (Heward, 2006).

In addition, children and adolescents with Down syndrome also have a variety of other health problems including cardiovascular abnormalities, obesity, immune system inefficiency, respiratory complications, thyroid problems, gastrointestinal problems, and leukemia (Roizen, 2002). They also may have visual acuity problems that require correction.

A potentially dangerous problem of dislocation of the **atlanto-axial joint** exists for children or adolescents with Down syndrome. Instability of the first and second cervical vertebrae could result in spinal cord damage. Approximately 1 to 2 percent of children and adolescents with this instability develop an additional problem where the upper two vertebrae move apart from one another. This condition puts pressure on the nerves that travel through the spinal cord and can cause neck pain, constant contraction of neck muscles, and difficulty walking. Children and adolescents with this condition routinely receive X-rays of the neck starting at approximately age 5. If a problem is detected, an orthopedic doctor is contacted and fusion of the vertebrae may be necessary. Children and adolescents with this condition may not participate in any contact sports in school, and they may not do any other gymnastic activities that put strain on their necks, such as somersaults and trampoline exercises (Tocci, 2000).

Fetal Alcohol Syndrome

Fetal alcohol syndrome (FAS)—also known as alcohol related birth defect (ARBD)—is the leading preventable cause of mental retardation and the third leading cause of birth defects. It is estimated that FAS occurs in 1–2 per 1,000 live births worldwide and 1,200 births per year in the United States (Behrman, Kliegman, & Jenson, 2004). The cause of FAS is excessive alcohol use by a woman during pregnancy. The nature and extent of complications associated with FAS depends on the amount of alcohol consumed by the mother and the specific trimester during her pregnancy when alcohol abuse occurred. Excessive alcohol use by a woman during pregnancy damages organs and cells in the developing fetus, with the most sensitive organ being the brain (Thies & Travers, 2006). Because of this, prenatal alcohol exposure permanently compromises intellectual functioning and other body functions. The spectrum of damage ranges from clearly observable mental and physical limitations at birth, to subtle learning problems that are not detected until school age (Coles et al., 1991).

Three criteria are used to diagnose FAS in the presence of confirmed maternal alcohol use during pregnancy:

- Growth deficiency characterized by low birth weight, lack of weight gain over time, or disproportional low weight to height
- Central nervous system (CNS) problems, including small brain size at birth, structural brain abnormalities, impaired fine motor skills, neurosensory hearing loss, poor ambulation with a narrow base of support and decreased balance, poor eye–hand coordination, mental retardation, and other cognitive impairments
- Pattern of abnormal facial features such as a flat midface and thin upper lip (Thies & Travers, 2006).

The newborn with FAS is typically small for gestational age. As the child grows, craniofacial malformations, microcephaly, flat midface, thin upper lip, and differences in height, weight, and head circumference from typical children becomes more apparent. Minor joint and limb abnormalities include some restrictions of movement and altered palmar creases in the hands (Behrman, Kliegman, & Jenson, 2004).

Though the physical complications may be extensive, they usually are secondary to cognitive complications associated with FAS. Alcohol robs the brain of needed nutrients, resulting in diminished intellectual capacity and related central nervous system difficulties. Delayed development and mental deficiencies vary from borderline to severe, making FAS a common identifiable cause of mental retardation (Behrman, Kliegman, & Jenson, 2004).

In addition, children and adolescents who are exposed to excessive alcohol use prenatally have difficulty with psychosocial skills and prosocial behaviors (Thies & Travers, 2006). They and their parents may require intervention of mental health professionals. The children and adolescents may demonstrate inappropriate aggression, decreased attention span and ability to follow rules, increased impulsivity, distractibility, restlessness, reluctance to meet challenges, and poor social skills (Thies & Travers). The mother may continue to abuse alcohol, creating an unhealthy living environment for the child, and require substance abuse counseling and rehabilitation (Thies & Travers). The prognosis for children and adolescents born with FAS varies depending on the severity of the maternal alcoholism, and the impact it had on the child's various biological systems. Counseling the mother to eliminate alcohol intake after conception is the key to prevention (Behrman, Kliegman, & Jenson, 2004).

Fragile X Syndrome

Fragile X syndrome is a hereditary condition that causes learning problems and mental retardation in both male and female children and adolescents, although the condition is more common in males. The condition occurs in approximately 1 in 3,600 male births and 1 in 4,000–6,000 female births. Fragile X syndrome is the most common inherited form of mental retardation, the most common clinical form of mental retardation after Down syndrome, and the most common known cause of autism. Children and adolescents with fragile X syndrome often have language delays and characteristic facial features, including an elongated face, prominent jaw and forehead, and large prominent ears. Features also may include prolapse of the mitral valve, hyperextensive joints, and flat feet (Behrman, Kliegman & Jenson, 2004; National Fragile X Foundation, 2006).

The cause of fragile X syndrome is a repeat mutation of the X chromosome within the developing fetus' cell nuclei. This mutation interferes with normal production of a protein that is essential for normal brain functioning (Heward, 2006). Some infants are diagnosed with fragile X soon after birth, while others with subtle complications are not identified until they grow older and demonstrate delays in speech and language or ambulation (National Fragile X Foundation, 2006).

The extent of cognitive, behavioral, and language complications depends on the extent of the mutation of the X chromosome and the gender of the child. Thirty percent of females born with the full fragile X mutation have IQ scores of 85 or above, and 70 percent have IQ scores below 85 in the borderline or mild mental retardation range, requiring intermittent or limited support (National Fragile X Foundation, 2006). In contrast, males with fragile X syndrome are diagnosed at an earlier age than females and typically are more affected than females. Approximately 80 percent of males with fragile X are cognitively delayed, with 10–15 percent scoring in the borderline or mild mental retardation range and the remainder in the moderate or severe range, requiring extensive support (National Fragile X Foundation). Some males demonstrate a plateauing of intellectual abilities, followed by a decline in their IQ scores after puberty. Because fragile X is not a degenerative disease, possible explanations for this include neurological changes that slow learning, difficulty advancing from concrete thinking associated with childhood to abstract ways of learning associated with adolescents, and a decline in the overall rate of learning (National Fragile X Foundation).

Many children with fragile X syndrome display positive behavioral characteristics. They tend to be affectionate and have a positive sense of humor. However, they also struggle with a variety of behavioral challenges. Eighty to ninety percent of boys are impulsive and distractible. Ninety percent of boys also have sensory processing difficulties that include tactile defensiveness, oral motor defensiveness, and poor eye contact. They may flap their hands and chew their skin, clothing, or objects (National Fragile X Foundation, 2006). Girls show less hyperactivity than boys but are often inattentive to tasks (National Fragile X Foundation).

In addition, some children and adolescents with fragile X syndrome demonstrate persevering speech and self-talk. They tend to have more difficulty with social contacts, shyness, anxiety, and depression (National Fragile X Foundation, 2006).

Williams Syndrome

Williams syndrome (WS) is a rare genetic syndrome that affects approximately 1 in 20,000 births. It is only since 1993 that the condition was categorized as a genetic syndrome; prior to that, the etiology of Williams syndrome was a mystery and was hypothesized as being caused by maternal or teratologic factors (Pober, 2001). In 1993 genetic studies unveiled an abnormality on chromosome 7 of individuals with Williams syndrome. Missing is an elastin gene, an important protein source that contributes to the strength and elasticity of blood vessel walls and general connective tissue. The lack of this elastin protein in fetal development produces a variety of problems, including **vascular stenosis**, a condition where there is a narrowing of blood vessels. Cardiovascular disease occurs in approximately 80 percent of children and adolescents with Williams syndrome (Pober).

Other characteristics that are common in children and adolescents with Williams syndrome include:

- Mannerisms of excessive cheerfulness, happiness, and over friendliness
- Lack of reserve towards strangers
- Hyperactivity with attention and impulsivity problems
- Low tolerance for frustration and teasing
- Fear of loud sounds
- Pixie or elfin-like facial features (Heward, 2006).

Williams syndrome is a multisystem disorder that affects organ systems at birth and later in life. Accurate recognition and diagnosis of Williams syndrome is essential because of these potential medical complications and developmental implications. Many infants with Williams syndrome have difficulty coordinating sucking and swallowing; are irritable and colicky; have problems with gagging, choking, vomiting; and have difficulty transitioning to solid foods. Potential medical problems include aortic stenosis, blood vessel disease, stenosis of the pulmonary arteries, hypertension, hypercalcemia, ophthalmologic abnormalities, gastrointestinal abnormalities, renal anomalies, neurologic abnormalities, recurrent otitis media, and anxiety (Pober, 2001). Additionally, musculoskeletal abnormalities are common in children and adolescents with Williams syndrome. Most children and adolescents have impaired motor coordination and appear awkward in their movements. They display both gross and fine motor difficulties as well as balance problems (Semel & Rosner, 2003). Muscle tone shifts from being hypotonic during early childhood to being hypertonic in adolescents and adults (Semel & Rosner). As a result of the hypertonia, progressive joint limitations and contractures often develop, usually in the legs. Other musculoskeletal problems include lordosis, scoliosis, proximal muscle weakness, and **radioulnar synostosis**, which is fusion of the lower radius and ulna causing limitations in the child and adolescent's ability to rotate the lower arm and supinate the hand (Pober).

Children and adolescents diagnosed with Williams syndrome may have some degree of mental retardation, typically scoring within the mild range on an IQ test, and requiring intermittent support. Profound mental retardation that requires pervasive support is uncommon. IQ studies have shown that 5–20 percent of children and adolescents with Williams syndrome score in the low–average range (Pober, 2001). Mental retardation associated with Williams syndrome deviates from the traditional representation in other syndromes. Traditionally, mental retardation represents a uniform impairment in all domains of cognitive functioning, but in Williams syndrome the level fluctuates. The children and adolescents may perform in the average or near average range in some cognitive areas and have marked limitations in other areas (Crisco, Dobbs, & Mulhern, 1988; Pober, 2001). For this reason, reporting their full-scale IQ scores may be misleading if their particular strengths and weaknesses are not identified. Children and adolescents with Williams syndrome typically demonstrate intellectual strength in the areas of language and communication skills and long term memory for general information. They also successfully process meaningful information, such as remembering faces and interpreting illustrations. They struggle with visual-spatial skills, visual-motor integration, word retrieval skills, and fine motor skills. Additionally, some children and adolescents with Williams syndrome have short attention span (Semel & Rosner, 2003). Because they also are distractible, they may be diagnosed with attention deficit hyperactivity disorder (Pober). Given these variations in cognitive functions, children and adolescents with Williams syndrome perform some occupations at levels consistent with their chronological age, yet struggle to accomplish other age appropriate tasks (Pober).

INTERVENTIONS

Since mental retardation is a developmental disability that impacts all aspects of daily life, intervention involves the entire family with the focus and intensity of health, education, and community related services changing as the children and adolescents develop. Working in coordination with one another, health and educational professionals can provide integrated services to the children and their families through these stages of development.

Intervention often begins in infancy and early childhood with primary emphasis on family focused goals. Initially, physicians and nurses carefully monitor health related complications, coordinating medically relevant prevention and intervention efforts. They also provide well baby care to support the newborn's early growth and development. Early interventionists offer the families assistance in stimulating the infant's cognitive development. The occupational therapist works with the family and other children on daily life, social, and play related occupations. The speech-language pathologist addresses the communication needs of the infant, and in collaboration with the nurse and the occupational therapist, focuses on eating, feeding, and nutrition. The genetic counselor meets with the family to discuss the likelihood of other family members being carriers of or having the condition, while the physical therapist often provides intervention for postural and mobility issues.

As the children get older, health professionals continue to provide medically related intervention and prevention services. Within the school setting, intervention shifts focus from family issues to educationally related issues and later to vocational training and independent living skills training. Social-emotional skills are addressed to help the children and adolescents develop a sense of their own worth and the social competences they need to interact at school and the community with others. Community-based programs such as the Special Olympics offer opportunities for children and adolescents to compete and celebrate their talents at the local, state, and national levels.

Services for children and adolescents with mental retardation need to be individually tailored and to take into consideration the unique characteristics of specific diagnoses. For instance, some children with fragile X syndrome need only a very low intensity of stimulation to evoke a response. Thus, when providing interventions, it is important to modulate the amount of stimulation to foster an appropriate response level (Freund, 1994). Because children and adolescents with Williams syndrome often have heart related complications, joint limitations, and motor and balance problems that interfere with the acquisition of age appropriate skills, tasks and environments may need to be modified for them. Similarly, consideration needs to be given to coronary, pulmonary, autoimmune, and musculoskeletal complications that children and adolescents with Down syndrome have when determining the appropriate level and intensity of intervention.

Educational Interventions Strategies

Interventions for children and adolescents with mental retardation, often incorporate specific instructional strategies to promote learning. As introduced in Chapter 10, some of these strategies include teaching in context, backward chaining, grading the number of steps, providing pictorial cues of the sequence of steps, and offering hand-over-hand assistance. Table 16.1■ illustrates how some of the strategies can be utilized to promote learning.

In all of these examples, it is important that children and adolescents with mental retardation be given ample opportunities to practice new skills. By the very nature of the diagnosis, learning new skills quickly or out of context is difficult.

Occupational Therapy Intervention

Mental retardation negatively impacts the development of performance skills and performance patterns necessary for children and adolescents to engage in age appropriate occupations. Occupational therapists and occupational therapy assistants provide intervention to facilitate the development of these performance skills and performance patterns. They also consider strategies for adapting the environments and tasks to enable the children and adolescents to participate in developmentally appropriate occupations. Occupational therapy intervention can take place in the home, community, or school settings. Occupational therapists and occupational therapy assistants collaborate with the parent or primary caregiver and other professionals when providing occupational therapy intervention.

Coupled with an occupation based frame of reference, occupational therapists and occupational therapy assistants often use the **acquisition frame of reference** when

■ **Table 16.1**
Educational Strategies

OCCUPATIONAL CHALLENGE	INTERVENTION	STRATEGY
Brenna, an 8-year-old with Down syndrome, wants to tie her shoes independently.	Have Brenna consistently wear shoes that require tying. Have everyone agree upon an established shoe tying procedure.	Teach intervention in context of activity.
	Demonstrate tying Brenna's shoes and assist her in completing the last step of pulling knots tight. When she is successful with this step, assist her in next-to-last step of making the loop knots. Continue introducing the new steps until she ties her shoes independently.	Backward chaining
Levi, a 16-year-old with fragile X syndrome, has been selected as junior manager for the high school football team. He must learn to wash the team uniforms.	Set up baskets in locker room so that each team member sorts own dirty laundry. Use premeasured detergent and limit washer setting options.	Simplify activity.
	Instruct Levi in the laundry routine. Post step-by-step picture instructions over the washer.	Provide visual cues.
Fiana, a 10-year-old with FAS, wants to use a knife independently during mealtime.	Select an easily cut menu item such as pancakes or waffles. Place utensils in Fiana's hands and grasp her hands. Provide cutting motion.	Hand-over-hand assistance
	As she begins to initiate and complete movement, calibrate grip of her hands. Gradually increase the demands of the cutting tasks by changing texture.	Grade amount of intervention needed.

working with children or adolescents with mental retardation. Since this frame of reference emphasizes multiple repetitions during skill acquisition, it allows the sufficient practice needed to learn new skills.

During the occupational therapy evaluation and intervention process, the occupational therapist and occupational therapy assistant systematically consider the child's or adolescent's cognitive, physical, perceptual, psychosocial, and emotional capacities, the demands of the task that needs to be performed, and the context for performing the task. The aim is to determine the correct fit between the tasks, the environment, and the child's or adolescent's capability to perform the task.

Interventions are individualized to reflect the child's or adolescent's particular learning ability, based on the severity of mental retardation and level of needed support. Occupational therapy intervention for the child and adolescent with mild and moderate mental retardation requiring intermittent or limited support might include establishing performance skills and patterns through various play, work, ADL, and leisure occupations, using various skill acquisition and cognitive learning techniques (Heward, 2006). For example, an occupational therapy assistant might use skill acquisition strategies to teach an adolescent with mild mental retardation how to organize inventory into categories when stacking shelves as part of an after school job experience. The occupational therapy assistant might use cognitive learning techniques to help a younger child learn how to sequence the steps of craft projects she wants to make during an after school activity club. To help children and adolescents with moderate mental retardation learn ADL and IADL occupations, the occupational therapy assistant might consider backward chaining strategies or task simplification approaches. When working with children and adolescents with severe or profound mental retardation who need extensive or pervasive intervention, the occupational therapy assistant may focus on implementing positioning techniques to enhance feeding and self-care; adapting toys, tools, and communication systems to enable the child and adolescent to play and learn; and training family members and caregivers in proper techniques and body mechanics for care giving tasks. The following case studies of Anya and Tyler further illustrate occupational therapy intervention.

Case Studies Applying Interventions

ANYA

Anya is a 10-year-old sixth grader with severe mental retardation and limited vision. She requires extensive support. She recently transferred to Good Hope Middle School due to a new foster care placement. Anya has a working vocabulary of five words (juice, cookie, no, eat, puppy) and is beginning to use a communication board. Because she uses a gross grasp pattern, she has difficulty manipulating small items. Since her IEP is current, the Good Hope Middle School administrators and teacher accept the annual goals recommended by her previous school (see Figure 16.1■) and place her in a self-contained special education classroom. The foster

parents, classroom special education teacher, school administrator, speech-language pathologist, and occupational therapist meet to discuss implementation of the annual goals. Since Mr. Marino, the special education teacher, has minimal experience with students who are visually challenged, he requests occupational therapy assistance to help implement the IEP goals. The IEP team decides to add weekly occupational therapy services to Anya's IEP. They agree that occupational therapy should include consultation and direct services, as needed, to achieve the objectives. Mr. Marino indicates that he would like to first address the self-feeding goals.

---

1. With set-up to increase visual contrast and verbal cues for food location, Anya will feed herself a school lunch.
   1a. Anya will scoop and successfully bring spoon to her mouth, 8/10 attempts.
   1b. Anya will drink from cup without spilling, 4/5 attempts.
   1c. Anya will stab with fork and bring food to mouth, 4/5 attempts.
   1d. Anya will hold sandwich and other finger foods and bring them to her mouth, 4/5 attempts.
2. Anya will use adaptive switches independently throughout her school day.
   1b. Anya will use wall level switches to turn room lights on/off and open doors independently, when requested.
   2b. Anya will use enlarged switches to turn on/off audio recorder and simple toys independently, as needed.
   2c. Anya will use computer touch screen during educational activities independently, as requested.
3. Anya will use her communication board to indicate her wants and needs.
   3a. Using her communication board, Anya will express her food and drink preferences during snack time, 4/5 times.

(continued)

■ **Figure 16.1**
Anya's IEP goals.

3b. Using her communication board, Anya will indicate hygiene and dressing needs, 4/5 times.

3c. Using her communication board, Anya will express her choice of activities, given several options, 4/5 times.

4. Under supervision, Anya will complete basic school required hygiene.

4a. Given verbal reminders, Anya will wash her hands before eating and after toileting, 4/5 attempts.

4b. Given verbal reminders, Anya will wipe her mouth and hands with a napkin when eating, as needed, 4/5 attempts.

4c. Anya will complete toileting tasks, 4/5 attempts.

■ **Figure 16.1 (cont.)**

The occupational therapist and the occupational therapy assistant discuss intervention strategies to assist Anya in self-feeding. The occupational therapy assistant meets with Anya and classroom staff during lunch and brings a variety of different adaptive feeding devices to try. The occupational therapy assistant prepares a list of low vision suggestions (see Figure 16.2■) to increase the contrast between the food and eating surface. He demonstrates hand-over-hand assistance for using utensils and bringing the cup to the mouth. He also suggests food selections (see Figure 16.3■) that would be easier for Anya to handle. He answers the teacher's and teacher aide's questions and arranges to return next week to review Anya's progress.

The teacher also indicates that his next concern is identifying appropriate switches for Anya to use. Taking into consideration Anya's limited vision, the occupational therapy assistant chooses large, brightly colored switches that require a variety of different hand movements to operate. In order to try out different switches, the occupational therapy assistant adapts an audio player for switch usage. The teacher and occupational therapy assistant initially provide hand-over-hand assistance to help Anya activate the switch to play the music. Through trial and error, the occupational

The following suggestions may help Anya be more successful in self-feeding:

- Position Anya under bright, concentrated light to provide her the best opportunity to see her food.
- Place only the necessary items on the table during feeding. Avoid unnecessary items, clutter, and tablecloths with patterns on the table, to eliminate distractions.
- Use high contrast colors such as white or yellow on black, or vice versa when setting the table for Anya's meal. Use a solid color plate or bowl, cup or glass, and dinnerware, preferably white, on a dark colored placemat. Avoid the use of clear glass or plastic dinnerware.
- Use a solid color napkin in a contrasting color from the placemat.
- Use a plate guard or plate with a lip, along with a nonslip mat under the plate, to increase Anya's success when self-feeding. Place all meal items in the same location at each meal for consistency and increased success for Anya. For instance, always place the napkin on the left side of the bowl, the cup at the top right edge of the bowl, and so on.
- If a food item matches the color of the plate or bowl, place the food item in a contrasting-color dish for the meal.

■ **Figure 16.2**
Low vision suggestions.

The following suggestions may help Anya be more successful in self-feeding:

- Provide Anya opportunities where the food will stick to the spoon, such as mashed potatoes, pudding, yogurt, and applesauce. This success will reward her for each effort.
- Initially provide Anya with foods that are easy to stab and then gradually increase the difficulty. For instance, start with lightly browned French fries, soft cooked vegetables, or pieces of French toast. Make sure that all pieces are bite sized until a knife is introduced.
- Initially provide a small amount of thickened liquid into her drinking cup. Gradually increase the amount and decrease the thickness of the liquid as she is successful bringing it to her mouth without spilling.

■ **Figure 16.3**
Food selection suggestions.

therapy assistant assists the teacher in determining an appropriate switch and optimum placement. With this decision completed, the occupational therapy assistant further assists the classroom teaching staff in adapting objects with the chosen switches.

Tyler

Tyler was born with Down syndrome. As an infant, the family received occupational therapy through an early intervention program in their home. The occupational therapist worked with the family on feeding, positioning techniques, and facilitating motor and play skills. Occupational therapy services were discontinued when Tyler was 2 years old, as he was able to participate in age appropriate occupations and the family members were able to make any needed modifications independently. At time of discharge, Tyler was part of a toddler play group at the local YMCA and attended various community preschool activities with his 4-year-old sister, Victoria. When Tyler was 4, his mother became employed full time outside the home and needed full time day services for him. Though Tyler qualified for enrollment in the developmental half-day preschool program in the local school district, his parents wanted one setting for the whole day. Thus, they chose to enroll Tyler in a community daycare center and obtain any needed therapy services through a pediatric home health agency.

The following three vignettes describe occupational therapy intervention services provided to Tyler and his family as he started daycare, when he entered third grade, and when he transitioned into junior high school.

TYLER AT THE DAYCARE

Tyler is an energetic 4-year-old child with Down syndrome, who attends a community center daycare. His older sister, Victoria, joins him at the community center for an after-school program. Their father picks up both children on the way home from work.

Since Tyler is the only child in his class with special needs, the preschool teacher meets with the parents numerous times to discuss how to address his needs within her classroom. In collaboration with Tyler's developmental pediatrician, the parents decide that occupational therapy services can help to support Tyler's participation in the daycare setting activities. They selected a home health agency that specializes in pediatrics to provide consultative services at the daycare setting for a short period of time.

The occupational therapist meets with the parents and conducts an assessment of Tyler within the home setting. The occupational therapist administers the *Peabody Developmental Motor Scales—2* (Folio & Fewell, 2002) that is a standardized test of fine and gross motor skills, and the *Hawaii Early Learning Profile (HELP) Preschool Checklist* (Vort Corp., 1995), a curriculum based assessment to measure self-help skills that may be needed within the daycare setting. Evaluation results indicate that Tyler has difficulty with occupations that require hand manipulation and balance skills, such as picking up small objects off a tabletop or ascending or descending stairs independently. Although he generally is following typical development, he often performs tasks at a 3-year-old rather than 4-year-old level. When presented with a new task, Tyler needs physical prompts or hand-over-hand assistance.

Prior to the first session at the preschool, the occupational therapist interviews the preschool teacher about her concerns and description of the classroom routines and schedule. Figure 16.4■ describes a summary of the conversation.

Teacher Interview Summary

The preschool classroom follows a High-Scope curriculum. Activities are grouped around a central theme and each child, with teacher assistance, determines a schedule of activities. The day starts off with free play, often in the outside play area. All the children participate in the morning circle time and then complete a variety of different art, science, and play activities based on the chosen schedule. Snack, lunch, and naptime are included in the daily schedule.

The preschool teacher states that she primarily teaches through frequent verbal instructions. Her verbal directions are simple, and clear. The preschool teacher and aide make sure that they have the child's attention before giving instructions.

The preschool teacher reports that Tyler is a very energetic and friendly child. He gets along with all the children in the classroom and is very respectful of the teaching staff. He quickly alters his behaviors when corrected. She notices that Tyler has difficulty with his self-care. He can take off his coat and hat but does not put anything on independently. He can pull up on a zipper, which is engaged, but not pull apart snaps or buttons. He only self-feeds finger food and seems to get frustrated when offered a spoon. He frequently knocks over his glass during snack and meals and is unable to pour from the child sized pitcher.

Although Tyler politely listens to instructions, the preschool teacher indicates that he doesn't learn new things easily. Tyler often becomes frustrated during repeated verbal instructions; the teaching staff often completes the activity if he starts to get upset. During table top activities, he always chooses the same toys. He needs to be encouraged to try new toys, and often needs a demonstration. When the children are building with blocks, he only slides his block around making car noises and does not attempt to build. When given play dough, he just breaks it apart into small pieces and then puts it back into the container. He is unable to open or close scissors and usually tries to avoid that activity. He likes to finger paint and to join in the songs during circle time.

Although he likes to run around the playground, he has difficulty playing with and on the different equipment. He is unable to pedal a tricycle and uses his feet to scoot around the play area. He needs assistance to climb up the slide but enjoys sliding down independently. He has difficulty throwing or catching balls but likes to chase and run after them.

The preschool teacher would like Tyler to participate fully in all the activities with his peers. She identifies two skills that she would like Tyler to learn this year. First, she would like Tyler to improve his play skills so that the he freely explores new toys and activities. Second, she would like Tyler to be less dependent on adults and more independent in the classroom setting.

■ Figure 16.4
Summary of interview.

The occupational therapist concludes that Tyler's daycare teacher would like him to participate fully in the activities but she is unaware of Tyler's learning style and how to make changes within the classroom environment. Selecting the Ecology of Human Performance (Dunn, Brown, & McGuigan, 1994), as an occupation based model to guide interventions and the acquisition frame of reference (Royeen & Duncan, 1999) to aid in skill development, the occupational therapist discusses the results with the occupational therapy assistant. Together they attend a meeting with the teacher to discuss ways to modify the daycare environment so that Tyler is more independent. The occupational therapy assistant works with Tyler to introduce play skills, using acquisition strategies and hand-over-hand techniques that the teacher can incorporate into her interactions with Tyler. The occupational therapy assistant joins Tyler in the daycare setting. She attempts to expand his play skills and demonstrates teaching techniques to the classroom staff. As Tyler chooses to join the play dough activities and reverts to crumbing the clay into small pieces, the occupational therapy assistant helps him roll and squeeze the dough into to different shapes. She demonstrates the use of the rolling pin, cooking cutters, and other toys, giving hand-over-hand assistance for Tyler to complete the task.

During five consultative sessions, the occupational therapist and the occupational therapy assistant provide practical suggestions to increase Tyler's independence and modify the setting. They discuss how to break down tasks to simple steps, to incorporate physical cues with verbal instructions, and to provide multiple opportunities within the day for skill practice. The occupational therapy assistant models the intervention strategy while the occupational therapist provides an explanation to the daycare teacher. At the end of this intervention period, the daycare teacher demonstrates knowledge of Tyler's learning needs and ability to adapt demands and activities within the classroom setting.

Tyler continues at the daycare until he begins kindergarten in the local public school system at age 5 and switches to after school care. Since the kindergarten follows a routine similar to the daycare classroom, Tyler transitions easily to the program. As part of an IEP, he receives learning support for reading and math within his regular education kindergarten classroom. As was the parent's preference, Tyler continues to be included in a regular education classroom for first and second grade.

TYLER'S TRANSITION INTO THIRD GRADE

During a second grade annual IEP review meeting, Tyler's teachers and parents discuss his transition into third grade. His parents elect to have Tyler continue in an inclusion setting and prefer to limit one-on-one aide assistance. His classroom teacher expresses concerns over his ability to meet the increased independence demands of third grade. Typical third graders are expected to be independent in nonacademic areas such as school ADLs, lunchroom routine, and organization of books and supplies. The learning support teacher feels that Tyler still has many difficulties in these areas, even though she has tried to address them. The IEP team decides to request occupational therapy to assess these anticipated demands and Tyler's present ability to meet those demands.

After meeting with the third grade teaching team, the occupational therapist devises a list of grade expectations. She requests the occupational therapy assistant to observe Tyler throughout the school day to determine his current status in these areas. Table 16.2■ summarizes his observations.

■ **Table 16.2**
3rd Grade Expectations

| IDENTIFIED SKILLS | INDEPENDENT | | COMMENTS |
	Yes	No	
Personal Items			
Tie shoes		X	Requires adult assistance. Parents often buy nontie shoes
Put on and take off jacket independently and manipulate all clothing fasteners		X	Engages and zips front opening zipper. Requires assistance to snap jeans.
Store and retrieve all personal items in storage unit		X	Requires verbal reminders to store personal items and assistance to find and retrieve personal items.
Blow nose with tissue and dispose in trash bin	X		Not used that day, but teacher indicates he is independent.
Sharpen pencil	X		Electric sharpener in all classrooms.
Obtain permission for and uses toileting facilities independently.		X	Consistently asks for permission but needs assistance in redressing, if wearing jeans.
Lunchroom Routine			
Sign in for lunch ticket		X	Needs verbal reminder to complete this task at beginning of day.
Retrieve lunch line items		X	Forgets to retrieve all items.
Carry tray	X		Able to carry all items without tipping.
Open all containers		X	Needs assistance opening milk cartons. Independently opens utensil packaging and food covers.
Dispose of trash	X		Disposes in correct bins.
Classroom Routine			
Locate correct books/folders		X	Requires assistance to find correct book and supplies.
Waits his turn in line or in the classroom	X		Consistent behavior
Raises hand for assistance and before speaking	X		Consistent behavior
Finds and gathers needed supplies for the task		X	Able to locate one but not two items. He may find his reading textbook, but not find the workbook or pencil that he needs. Often classmates help him.
Put homework in correct bins		n/a	Not part of second grade routine

■ **Table 16.2**
3rd Grade Expectations (cont.)

| | INDEPENDENT | | |
IDENTIFIED SKILLS	Yes	No	COMMENTS
Return books to library weekly		n/a	Not part of second grade routine
Listens to and follows group instructions.		X	Attentively listens but does not follow through on multistep verbal directions. Has difficulty performing nonroutine instructions.
Navigates independently between classroom and other school areas	X		At present time, he is independent. When he enters third grade, however, his classroom will be in a different wing from the K–2 section and may need assistance.
Remains focused and works independently at desk for 15 minutes.	X		If task is within his skill level, he is able to complete. If not, he will look around the room or seek out teacher.
Remain focused and works with a group for 15 minutes.	X		Has good social skills and works cooperatively with work members on tasks.

After gathering and reviewing all the observations and comment sheets, the occupational therapist prepares a summary report for the IEP team. At the meeting, they discuss Tyler's current status and how skills could be addressed in preparation for third grade transition. Recognizing that Tyler requires multiple opportunities to learn new skills, occupational therapy services are added to the IEP to provide consultative and individual services for the remainder of the school year.

As part of these services, the occupational therapy assistant develops a systematic procedure to teach Tyler how to tie his shoes and fasten his trousers. The parents and teachers reinforce these procedures in the home and at school. The classroom teacher volunteers to alter her classroom routine to allow all the students the opportunity to develop the required third grade routine of placing assigned homework in specific bins and individually returning library books. The occupational therapy assistant develops a color coding and peer buddy system to help Tyler learn these new routines. In addition, the occupational therapy assistant works with Tyler on organizational skills and lunchroom skills.

Tyler in Junior High School

After a successful transition into third grade, Tyler does not require school based occupational therapy services until he enters junior high school and the IEP includes job related life skills. At the parents' request, a transition team is established when Tyler turns 13. Although IDEA legislation does not mandate school-to-work transition goals until age 16, the parents request that the IEP team begin to address these vocational areas before Tyler enters high school.

TYLER'S TRANSITION TO 8TH GRADE

As the end of the school year, Tyler's parents, teachers, and school administrator meet to review the annual IEP goals and make additions and changes for the next school year. Since the parents would like to discuss school-to-work transitional goals, the parents ask the occupational therapist to attend the meeting.

The team discusses the eighth grade optional courses and available out-of-class experiences. At home, Tyler shows an interest in cooking and slowly is learning some basic cooking skills. The owners of a local family restaurant indicate that they would consider Tyler for further employment and the parent feel that this is a feasible work option.

To help prepare him for this type of employment, the team feels that Tyler would benefit from including two new experiences in his educational program. They consider enrolling Tyler in the eighth grade family and consumer science class but express concerns about his ability to work in this traditionally large class, particularly during the weekly cooking session. The parents report that at home Tyler has difficulty safely using a variety of different kitchen equipment. Also, the IEP team members consider involving Tyler in the school store but are not sure what type of task he can perform successfully. The parents express their appreciation that everyone wants Tyler to experience success but they also would like him to be challenged to learn new skills as the year progresses.

The occupational therapist suggests that she conduct task analyses, which would allow the learning support teacher to better choose an entry level position for Tyler. She also indicates that she can provide consultative services throughout the school year to adapt any future work duties. Concerning the family and consumer science course, the occupational therapist suggests that the occupational therapy assistant coteach with the class teacher on the one day per week the students actually cook. The teacher assigns Tyler and two to three other students to the occupational therapy assistant's group, where she can provide individualized instruction and modify tasks as needed. The IEP team agrees with the occupational therapist's suggestions and adds these additional services for the following school year.

SUMMARY

Mental retardation often is due to genetic and chromosomal abnormalities, teratogens, infections, and environmental and nutritional deprivation. It can occur independently or as part of a syndrome such as Down syndrome, fragile X syndrome, Williams syndrome and fetal alcohol syndrome. The level of mental retardation can be defined in two different ways. Based on IQ and adaptive behavior testing, the terms mild, moderate, severe, and profound are used. The ILEP system describes four levels based on amount of support needed.

Occupational therapists and occupational therapy assistants provide occupation based interventions in the areas of ADL, IADL, play, leisure, education, and work to children and adolescents with mental retardation based on individual strengths and challenges. An acquisition approach often is combined with an occupation based model of practice to ensure that intervention includes adequate repetition, grading of skills, and consultation to immediate caregivers. Occupational therapists and occupational therapy assistants often adapt the task or environment to reflect the functional ability of the child or adolescent with mental retardation.

REVIEWING KEY POINTS

1. Explain what is meant by adaptive behaviors.
2. Explain the difference between mild, moderate, severe, and profound levels of mental retardation.
3. Describe the ILEP system's four levels of support.
4. Describe the following chromosomal causes of mental retardation: Down syndrome, fragile X syndrome, and Williams syndrome.
5. Explain the potential danger of dislocation of the atlanto-axial joint, as often seen in children or adolescents with Down syndrome.
6. Describe the importance of monitoring the stimulation level when working with a child or adolescent with fragile X syndrome.
7. List five occupations that might be difficult for a child or adolescent with Williams syndrome to perform. Explain your answer.
8. Describe fetal alcohol syndrome.

APPLYING KEY CONCEPTS

1. Consider Anya's case study. If you were the school based occupational therapy assistant providing intervention, what suggestions would you make for addressing the basic hygiene IEP goals?
2. Investigate different types of communication board. What system would you recommend for Anya? Justify your answer.
3. Consider Tyler's case study. Assuming the role as the occupational therapy assistant, how would you design interventions to address his needs in the lunchroom?
4. With a group of students, role play the occupational therapy assistant leading a small cooking group for adolescents who need limited support, and for adolescents who need intermittent support because of cognitive challenges.
   a. Choose a menu item that requires the use of at least two different cooking tools. Demonstrate how you would instruct the group.
   b. Choose a menu item that requires the use of the stovetop or oven. Demonstrate how you would instruct the students with special emphasis on safety.
5. Watch a video about the Special Olympics. Analyze how the coaches adapt the athletic events, the equipment, and the instructions to provide the right level of challenge for the Olympians.

REFERENCES

American Association on Mental Retardation (n.d.). *Mental retardation fact sheet*. Retrieved January 29, 2004 from *http://www.aamr.org/Policies/faq_mental_retardation.html*.

American Psychiatric Association. (2000). *Diagnostic and Statistical manual of mental disorders* (4th ed.rev.). Washington, DC: Author.

Behrman, R., Kliegman, R., & Jenson, H. (2004). *Nelson textbook of pediatrics* (17th ed). Philadelphia: Saunders.

Coles, C., Brown, B. T., Smith, I. E., Platzman, K. A., Erickson, S., & Falek, A. (1991). Effects of prenatal alcohol exposure at school age. *Neurotoxicology and Teratology, 13*, 357–367.

Crisco, J. J., Dobbs, J. M., & Mulhern, R. K. (1988). Cognitive processing of children with Williams syndrome. *Dev Med Child Neurol, 30*, 650–656.

Dunn, W., Brown, C., & McGuigan, A. (1994). The ecology of human performance: A framework for considering the effect of context. *American Journal of Occupational Therapy, 48*, 595–607.

Freund, L. (1994). Diagnostic and developmental issues for young children with fragile X syndrome. *Infants and young children, 6*(3), 34–45.

Frankenburg, W. K., Dodds, J., Archer, P., Shapiro, H., & Bresnick, B. (1992). *Denver Developmental Screening*

Tool (2nd ed). Denver, CO: Denver Developmental Materials.

Folio, M. R., & Fewell, R. R. (2002). *Peabody Developmental Motor Scales* (2nd ed). Denver: Pro Ed.

Heward, W. (2006). *Exceptional children: An introduction to special education* (8th ed). Upper Saddle River, NJ: Pearson Prentice Hall.

Luckasson, R., Coulter, D. L., Polloway, E. A., Reiss, S., Schalock, R. L., Snell, M. E., Spitalnik, D. N., Stark, E. A. (1992). *Mental retardation: Definition, classification, and systems of support* (9th ed.). Washington, DC: American Association of Mental Retardation.

National Fragile X Foundation (2006). *The NFXF.* Retrieved August 11, 2006, from http://www.fragilex.org.

Pober, B. (2001). Williams Syndrome. In A. Capute & P. Accardo, *Developmental disabilities in infancy and childhood* (2nd ed). *Volume II: The spectrum of developmental disabilities* (pp. 271–279). Baltimore: Paul H. Brookes Publishing Co.

Reed, K. (2001). *Quick reference to occupational therapy* (2nd ed). Gaithersburg, MD: Aspen Publications.

Royeen, C., & Duncan, M. (1999). Acquisition frame of reference. In P. Kramer & J. Hinojosa (Eds), *Frames of reference for pediatric occupational therapy* (2nd ed). Philadelphia: Lippincott Williams & Wilkins.

Roizen, N. J. (2002). Down syndrome. In M.L. Batshaw (Ed.), *Children with disabilities.* Baltimore: Brookes.

Sparrow, S., Cicchetti, D. V., & Balla, D. A. (2006). *Vineland Adaptive Behavior Scales* (2nd ed). Upper Saddle River, NJ: Pearson Assessments.

Semel, E., & Rosner, S. (2003). *Understanding Williams syndrome: Behavior patterns and interventions.* Mahwah, NJ: Lawrence Erlbaum Associates.

Thies, K., & Travers, J. (2006). *Handbook of human development for health care professionals.* Sudbury, MA: Jones and Bartlett.

Tocci, S. (2000). *Down syndrome.* Danbury, CT: Franklin Watts.

Vort Corporation (1995). *HELP for preschoolers: Assessment and curriculum guide.* Palo Alto, CA: Author.

Chapter 17

Children and Adolescents with Psychosocial, Emotional, and Behavioral Challenges

Janet V. DeLany

Key Terms

Anorexia
Anxiety disorders
Behavioral related disorders
Bipolar disorder
Bulimia
Conduct disorder
Cyclothymic disorder
Delusions
DSM-IV
Eating disorders
Emotional and behavioral disorder
Exacerbation
Hallucinations
Manic

Oppositional defiant disorder
Positive Behavioral Interventions and Supports system
Posttraumatic stress disorder
Psychotic symptoms
Reactive attachment disorder
Relational aggression
Schizophrenia
Separation anxiety disorder
Social competency
Social skills training
State of arousal
Substance abuse
Substance dependence
Violence prevention programs

Objectives

- Explain the psychosocial, emotional, and behavioral challenges negatively affecting the occupational performance of children and adolescents.
- Examine how these challenges impact the daily occupations of children and adolescents within the context of the family, school, and community environments.

- Describe occupational therapy interventions to support the capacity of children and adolescents with these challenges to participate in their daily occupations.
- Examine how occupational therapists and occupational therapy assistants work together during the intervention process.
- Describe how occupational therapist and occupational therapy assistants work with families and other professionals to provide services to children and adolescents with these challenges.

INTRODUCTION

Children and adolescents often address psychosocial, emotional, and behavioral issues as part of their typical growth and development. This chapter focuses on those challenges that are more complex and that are listed in *Diagnostic and statistical manual of mental disorder: DSM-IV-TR* (APA, 2000), or included under the classification of **emotional and behavioral disorders** (EBD) within *Individuals with Disabilities Education Improvement Act* (IDEIA) guidelines (2004). This chapter also addresses the secondary challenges that arise for those children and adolescents coping with other physical, cognitive, social, or learning difficulties. Vignettes throughout the chapter highlight occupational therapy services for children and adolescents coping with these challenges at various points in their occupational development.

A survey conducted by the National Institute of Child Health and Human Development (2005) found that 5 percent of parents believe that their children—an estimated 2.7 million children—have severe emotional or behavioral difficulties that interfere with their ability to learn, participate in family life, and form friendships, though only 65 percent of these receive services from the medical or educational community to address their emotional and behavioral concerns. It is estimated that 1 in 10 of the 73 million children and adolescents in the United States have a severe emotional disturbance, though only 20 percent of them receive professional interventions to address their complex needs (House, 2002; U.S. Department of Health and Human Services [DHHS] 2000). Similarly, between 6 and 8 percent of school children between the ages of 3 and 21 receive special education and related services because of their emotional and behavioral difficulties (U.S. Department of Education, 2003, 2005), though frequently these services are inadequate because of funding constraints, lack of well trained professionals and sustainable programs, and limited interagency collaboration and support networks (Federal Interagency Coordinating Council, 2002, as cited in Jackson and Arbesman, 2006; Koyanagi & Semansky, 2003)

The psychosocial, emotional, and behavioral challenges that children and adolescents experience may stem from environmental and personal factors that are acute or chronic in duration. These factors include: biological and genetic predispositions, failure of caretakers to bond and form attachments, parental and child depression, inadequate parenting, child abuse and neglect, sexual abuse, substance abuse, poverty, and personal or community trauma and violence. They also may stem from rejection by or bullying from peers, and feelings of loneliness and alienation (Center for Mental Health in Schools, 2003). The more chronic these factors, the more likely they will have long term consequences that continue to negatively affect children and adolescents into their adulthood. Fifty-eight percent of the youth with EBD who graduate from high school and 78 percent of the youth with EBD who do not graduate from high school are incarcerated within five years (U.S. Department of Education, 2000 as cited in Schultz, 2003). Their cognitive and behavioral problems, such as difficulty with impulse control, predicting the consequences of actions, reading social cues, and learning from experience, increase their risk of getting into difficulty with the law. Conversely, 33.4 percent of incarcerated youth as compared to 10 percent within the school population have a disability, including a learning disability or an emotional or behavioral disorder, which qualifies them for special education and related services under *IDEA* guidelines (Segal, 2006).

The U.S. Department of Health and Human Services has established a series of goals to address "the burden of suffering experienced by children with mental health needs and their families [that] has created a health crisis in this country" (2000, p. 1). These goals are as follows:

1. Promote public awareness of children's mental health issues and reduce the stigma associated with mental illness.
2. Continue to develop, disseminate, and implement scientifically proven prevention and treatment services in the field of children's mental health.
3. Improve the assessment and recognition of mental health needs in children.
4. Eliminate racial/ethnic and socioeconomic disparities in access to mental health care.
5. Improve the infrastructure for children's mental health services, including support for scientifically proven interventions across professions.
6. Increase access to and coordination of quality mental health care services.
7. Train frontline providers to recognize and manage mental health issues, and educate mental health providers in scientifically proven prevention and treatment services.
8. Monitor the access to and coordination of quality mental health care services (DHHS, 2000, p. 4).

DSM-IV CATEGORIES OF PSYCHOSOCIAL AND EMOTIONAL CONDITIONS

Within DSM-IV, psychosocial and emotional diagnoses are clustered into several categories: Some of these include **behavioral related disorders**, psychotic disorders, mood disorders, substance related disorders, **anxiety disorders**, **eating disorders**, and adjustment disorders (First, Frances, & Pincus, 2002). Below is a description of some of those diagnoses. Psychiatrists and psychologists gather data from personal histories, family histories, mental status examinations, laboratory tests, and observations of the children and adolescents over time to make the appropriate differential diagnosis and initiate intervention. Occupational therapists and occupational therapy assistants address how these disorders interfere with the ability of the children and adolescents to successfully participate in their daily life occupations at school, home, and the community.

Behavioral Related Disorders

Conduct Disorder

Children and adolescents who exhibit **conduct disorder** frequently violate major rules regarding expected behaviors and respect for the basic rights of others. Considered antisocial, they may repeatedly display acts of violence against people and animals, destroy or steal property, or serious violate societal rules (First et al., 2002; House, 2002).

Oppositional Defiant Disorder

Children and adolescents diagnosed as having **oppositional defiant disorder** demonstrate a persistent pattern of negativistic, hostile, and defiant behaviors that lasts at least six months, that is inconsistent with their developmental age, and interferes with their social, academic, and occupational tasks. Considered less serious a diagnosis than conduct disorder, children and adolescents with oppositional defiant disorder often lose their temper, argue with adults, and openly defy adults' requests or rules. They deliberately annoy and place blame on other people for their own mistakes and negative behaviors (House, 2002; Reid & Wise, 1995).

Anxiety Related Disorders

Separation Anxiety Disorder

Children and adolescents struggling with **separation anxiety disorder** display excessive anxiety about separating from their primary caregiver or other person with whom they are emotionally attached. Their level of anxiety is beyond that which is expected for their developmental age. They also may display severe anxiety about leaving those places, such as their homes, which make them feel secure. The symptoms last for at least four weeks, and cause a significant level of distress (House, 2002; Reid & Wise, 1995).

Posttraumatic Stress Disorder

Posttraumatic stress disorder can occur when the child or adolescent experiences a significant trauma such as war, kidnapping, community violence, personal violence, or family death, resulting in sustained and significant anxiety. The anxiety lasts for a minimum of one month, during which time the child or adolescent re-experiences the trauma, remains hypervigilant, and may avoid stimuli related to the trauma (First et al., 2002; House, 2002).

Reactive Attachment Disorder of Infancy or Early Childhood

Reactive attachment disorder of infancy or early childhood affects young children who received grossly inadequate or harmful care from their primary caregivers. These children have severe difficulty with personal relationships in most social and interpersonal contexts. They may have difficulty initiating and responding to social interactions in an age appropriate manner, be hypervigilant or extremely ambivalent, or be nondiscriminant and nonselective in their attachment to others (First et al., 2002; House, 2002).

Substance Related Disorders

Substance Dependence

Substance dependence results from intentional or unintentional exposure to toxic substances over a sustained period of time. Children and adolescents can misuse amphetamines, caffeine, cocaine, hallucinogens, cannabis, opiates, sedatives, alcohol, nicotine, and inhalants. Dependency results when they continue to use these substances in spite of adverse consequences, such as health complications, and educational, social, and occupational impairments. They may develop a tolerance for the toxic substance and experience withdrawal symptoms when they try to discontinue or reduce the usage. Substance dependence can occur in combination with other mental health challenges stemming from depression, impulse control difficulties, abuse, and learning difficulties (First et al., 2002).

Substance Abuse

Children and adolescents are considered to have a **substance abuse** problem when they exhibit maladaptive behaviors as a result of substance use. However, unlike those who have a substance dependence problem, those with a substance abuse problem do not have a history of tolerance and withdrawal reactions or a pattern of compulsive usage (First et al., 2002).

Eating Disorders

Anorexia Nervosa

Anorexia involves excessive loss of weight or failure to gain appropriate weight because of distorted body image and fear of gaining weight. Though occurring most commonly in adolescent girls, boys and girls as young as 10 years of age may struggle with anorexia nervosa. In spite of being hungry, they severely restrict caloric intake and may engage in prolonged and frequent exercise. They also may be depressed and suicidal. Youth in art and sports activities, such as ballet, gymnastics, wrestling, and competitive horse racing, where weight control is considered essential, are at increased risk (House, 2002).

Bulimia

Concerned with body weight and shape, youth struggling with **bulimia** over eat, binging on high calorie foods. To maintain their desired weight, they then purge their bodies by vomiting or using laxatives and diuretics. They also may starve themselves for an extended period of time. As result of purging, they disrupt the balance of their electrolytes and may suffer sudden coronary arrest. Youth coping with bulimia may become self-injurious, depressed, and suicidal (House, 2002).

Psychotic Disorder

Schizophrenia

Though more likely to occur in young adulthood, **schizophrenia** can develop in childhood and adolescence. Schizophrenia is marked by periods of exacerbation and remission. During periods of **exacerbation**, or the active phase of schizophrenia, children and adolescents may experience **psychotic symptoms** including delusions, hallucinations, disorganized speech and behaviors, or disturbances in affect and thought. A **delusion** is a severe misperception in thinking about what is real despite clear evidence to refute it; a **hallucination** is a visual, auditory, olfactory, gustatory, or tactile perception of a sensory experience that does not exist. The psychotic symptoms last over a month, with some persisting for more than six months. During the exacerbation phase, children and adolescents function below the highest social and cognitive level they previously achieved. Types of schizophrenia include paranoid type, disorganized type, catatonic type, undifferentiated type, and residual type (First et al., 2002; House, 2002).

Mood Disorders

Major Depressive Episode

Children and adolescents experiencing a major depressive episode demonstrate depressed and irritable moods that last for a minimum of two weeks. They no longer show pleasure in tasks they previously enjoyed, and may lose weight or fail to gain expected developmental weight. Young children may demonstrate agitation and restlessness, and complain of somatic discomforts. In contrast, adolescents may act out, misuse substances, and have difficulty with academic tasks (House, 2002).

Bipolar Disorders

There are three types of **bipolar disorder** that affect children and adolescents: type I, type II, and cyclothymic. Though rare, children and adolescents with bipolar I disorder have a current or past history of at least one full-blown episode of manic behaviors. Children and adolescents with bipolar II disorder have had a least one major depressive and one hypomanic (mild manic) episode. Those with **cyclothymic disorder** have had numerous depressive and hypomanic over a period of a year or longer. While **manic**, the children and adolescents may be highly distractible and hypersexual. They may demonstrate a flight of ideas, unstable mood swings, aggressive behaviors, and irritability. When depressed, they are sad, oversleep, over or under eat, and have difficulty completing school and home tasks. Ninety percent of the children and adolescents diagnosed with bipolar disorder have a history of attention deficit and hyperactivity disorder [ADHD] (First et al., 2002; House, 2002).

IDEA CLASSIFICATION OF BEHAVIORAL AND EMOTIONAL DISTURBANCES

As outlined IDEA (2004), schools are to provide positive and proactive behavioral interventions and supports for children and adolescents with disabilities whose behaviors interfere with their learning or the learning of others (Jackson & Arbesman, 2006). In addition, schools are to determine which children and adolescents with behavioral and emotional problems qualify for special education and related services under the Behavioral and Emotional Disturbance (EBD) classification of IDEA (2004). To receive services under this classification, children and adolescents must exhibit one or more of the following characteristics over a long period of time. These characteristics must adversely affect the student's ability to learn. These characteristics include:

- An inability to learn that cannot be explained by intellectual, sensory, or health factors
- An inability to build or maintain satisfactory interpersonal relationships with peers and teachers
- Inappropriate types of behavior or feelings under normal circumstances
- A general, pervasive mood of unhappiness or depression
- A tendency to develop physical symptoms or fears associated with personal or school problems (NICHCY, 2002, p. 1).

Overlap occurs between the DSM-IV diagnoses and school based IDEA classifications. Children and adolescents with diagnoses of behavioral, anxiety, psychotic, and mood related disorders under DSM-IV may qualify for services under the EBD category of IDEA. Children and adolescents with substance and eating disorders as categorized by DSM-IV may receive IDEA educational and related service support under the *other health conditions* classification. In addition, depending upon the school district's interpretation of what is meant by educationally relevant, some students may receive support to address emotional, behavioral, and psychological challenges stemming from other physical, learning, and cognitive classifications identified in IDEA. Some school districts narrowly define the words *educationally relevant* to mean that only children and adolescents who are failing academically are eligible for special education and related services. Other school districts broadly define the words and apply them to children and youth who are struggling with, but not necessarily failing some aspect of school life. The 2004 amendment to IDEA (P.L. 108-446) also permits schools to provide proactive early intervening services for children and adolescents in the general education system who have learning and behavioral difficulties, but who do not require special education services and a formal Individual Education Program (Jackson & Arbesman, 2006). Care must be taken to consider whether the learning and behavioral patterns reflect the children's and adolescents' cultural background and social context, or their cognitive capacities and developmental age, so that they are not inappropriately targeted as having learning and behavioral difficulties (DHHS, 2000).

OCCUPATIONAL THERAPY INTERVENTIONS

Children and adolescents with a **DSM-IV** diagnosis or who fit within the bounds of IDEA guidelines may be referred for occupational therapy services. As likely, children and adolescents with psychosocial and emotional difficulties, though initially referred for occupational therapy services for a different reason, also may receive occupational therapy interventions to address their psychosocial, emotional, and behavioral challenges. The children and adolescents may receive occupational therapy services within the home, school, and community settings. When their symptoms are severe, the children and adolescents may need to receive more intensive services within the hospital, a residential treatment center, or juvenile system. Occupational therapists and occupational therapy assistants often collaborate with the primary caregiver and other professionals when providing interventions to address these psychosocial, emotional, and behavioral challenges. Depending on the practice setting, these other professionals may include child and adolescent psychiatrists, developmental pediatricians, clinical and school psychologists, counselors, educators, school and psychiatric nurses, dietitians, and qualified mental health providers.

To provide services, the occupational therapist establishes and oversees a plan to evaluate, provide interventions, and measure intervention outcomes that address the children's and adolescents' ability to participate in their daily life occupations. The occupational therapist selects an occupational based model and reviews evidence based research related to the psychosocial, emotional, and behavioral challenges to guide this plan. Supervised by the occupation therapist, the occupational therapy assistant contributes to designing and carrying out the evaluation, intervention, and outcome (AOTA, 2004).

During the evaluation process, the occupational therapist and the occupational therapy assistant develop an occupational profile of the children and adolescents and gather data to analyze performance capacities. The occupational profile helps the occupational therapist and the occupational therapy assistant understand the

- Background, occupational history, and occupational goals of the children and adolescents
- Reasons for the occupational therapy request
- Occupational strengths and challenges of the children and adolescents
- Context supporting or blocking the children or adolescents' occupational performance (AOTA, 2002)

Information gathered through observations, interviews, and assessments allows the occupational therapist to analyze and make judgments about the children's or adolescents' psychosocial, emotional, and behavioral challenges, and the effect of these challenges on their occupational performance. Working with children and adolescents, their primary caregivers, and other members of the professional team, the occupational therapist and occupational therapy assistant then develop and carryout an intervention plan to promote occupational performance. Depending on the specific behavioral, psychosocial, or emotional challenges, the intervention may focus on establishing or restoring the children's and adolescents' performance skills and patterns, modifying the context and the tasks, and promoting healthy coping patterns and lifestyles. Intervention strategies may incorporate various play and leisure occupations, expressive arts occupations, social skill training, behavioral management techniques, skill acquisition approaches, biofeedback techniques, stress management techniques, cognitive learning techniques, and role playing. Outcome measures help to determine the effectiveness of the interventions (Jackson & Arbesman, 2006). The following school, community, residential, and hospital based scenarios illustrate occupational therapy services for children and adolescents whose psychosocial, emotional, and behavioral challenges interfere with their ability to effectively participate in their daily life occupations.

School-Based Program

As part of a grant funded project, the occupational therapist and occupational therapy assistant work with a team of professionals to design and implement a three-year project for elementary age children who are struggling with behavioral issues in the school setting. The children have a history of aggressive and disruptive classroom behaviors. Some of them have been formally diagnosed with oppositional defiant behavior, bipolar disorder, reactive attachment disorder, and conduct disorder.

In addition to the occupational therapist and the occupational therapy assistant, the team includes a psychologist, a nurse, a social worker, and a teacher. Each member contributes particular knowledge and skills. The psychologist offers expertise about cognitive and emotional development. The nurse assumes responsibility for managing the anticonvulsant, antidepressant, and antipsychotic medication that some of the children take to help control their behaviors. The social worker serves as a liaison between the home and school, and helps to identify additional community resources for the families. The teacher focuses on the academic needs of the children. The occupational therapist and occupational therapy assistant bring particular knowledge about the capacities and needs of the children to participate in their daily life occupations.

The immediate objectives of the program are to promote behavioral self-control, emotional self-regulation, social problem solving skills, and academic success for these students (Conduct Problems Prevention Research Group, 2002). The long term goal of the program is to reduce the likelihood of chronic academic difficulties, peer rejection, and confrontations with teachers that these students will experience during elementary school and chronic delinquency, and antisocial and criminal activities they may experience as adolescents (Conduct Problems Prevention Research Group, 2002).

Prior to initiating intervention programs, the team members conduct a series of evaluations of the children's academic, social, and emotional capacities. As part of the evaluation, the occupational therapist and occupational therapy assistant interview the parents and teachers regarding the children's patterns when performing daily life occupations at school and at home. They observe the children in the classroom, at recess, and during lunch regarding their group interaction, conflict resolution, and negotiation skills. The also record the context and the tasks that trigger disruptive and aggressive behaviors.

Social Enrichment Group

In collaboration with the psychologist, the occupational therapist and occupational therapy assistant conduct biweekly social enrichment groups for the children. They run one group for students in kindergarten through second grade, one for students in third and fourth grade, and one for students in fifth and sixth grade. They include peer buddies in each of these groups to serve as models and to foster potential friendships outside of the group sessions.

Each session begins with an activity during which the children share a picture, object, or drawing about what they do well or about what makes them feel positive about themselves. Then, after listening to a story or watching a video clip, the children identify examples of prosocial behaviors and effective strategies for managing feelings. Next, they identify examples of negative behaviors and ineffective strategies for managing feelings. For each of the examples the children then consider how the characters felt, what the characters thought, and why the characters behaved the way they did. For those examples where the characters displayed negative behaviors or ineffective management of feelings, the children identify two other options that may have been more successful. Then the children role play the altered version of the story or video clip, to practice the more successful options. Next, the children engage in play, art, and social activities that allow them to practice the prosocial problem solving skills, behavioral management, and emotional regulation skills they previously discussed.

Using their combined knowledge about occupations, and physical, cognitive, and emotional development, the occupational therapist, the occupational therapy assistant, and the psychologist carefully grade these activities to provide an appropriate amount of challenge and structure for the children. As the children engage in these activities, the psychologist, occupational therapist, and occupational therapy assistant take photographs of the children. Using the photograph as props, they conclude the sessions with a brief group discussion about what the children did, how they felt, and how they managed their behaviors during the activity.

Education

The psychologist, occupational therapist, and occupational therapy assistant also collaborate with the classroom teacher to foster the learning of the children. The psychologist establishes a behavioral management program with clear rules and expectations to promote prosocial behaviors and to extinguish negative ones. Based on the data collected from observations and interviews during the initial evaluation, the occupational therapist and the occupational therapy assistant recommend modifications to the classroom environment, routine, and seating arrangements to minimize factors that trigger the aggressive and disruptive behaviors. They recommend:

- Posting and discussing the classroom schedule daily
- Posting and reviewing classroom rules of conduct
- Dividing the classroom into clearly distinguishable work and social activity areas

- Creating quiet, independent working areas for the children
- Sandwiching the difficult part of a task between two easier parts of a task
- Interspersing structured academic tasks with physical movement
- Placing the at-risk children in small groups with peer buddies who can provide assistance and a calm working environment
- Establishing a signal system that the children and teacher can use to cue one another that the situation is becoming overwhelming
- Creating "safety areas," such as the nurse's or psychologist's office, where the children can obtain passes from the teacher to visit so that they can remove themselves from classroom situations that are becoming overwhelming

With the classroom teacher, they develop strategies for dividing worksheets into smaller units and for providing more immediate feedback on completed work to foster a sense of accomplishment and success.

Community-Based Domestic Violence Program

The occupational therapist and occupational therapy assistant work at a domestic violence program that provides crisis support, counseling services, and long term shelter. As defined by the Office for Victims of Crime, domestic violence is "coercive behavior designed to exert power and control over a person in an intimate relationship through the use of intimidating, threatening, harmful, or harassing behavior" (2002, ¶ 8). In addition to providing services for the adults who are survivors of domestic violence, the occupational therapist and occupational therapy assistant provide services for the children and adolescents who witnessed the domestic violence. Some of these children and adolescents also have been physical or emotionally abuse or neglected. Most of the children have difficulties calming themselves, going to sleep, engaging in play, and participating in social activities. Some demonstrate developmental delays and eating problems (Javaherian, Underwood & DeLany, 2007). The older youth are experiencing academic difficulties. They are anxious, and fluctuate between being belligerent and withdrawn.

In collaboration with the other staff and volunteers at the domestic violence center, the occupational therapist and occupational therapy assistant provide programs for the children, adolescents, and their families. Some of the programs include play, social participation activities, self-care, and educational support programs for the children and adolescents, and parenting strategies for the adults. Guided by the Person-Environment-Occupational Performance Model, the occupational therapist and occupational therapy assistant consider the capacities and needs of the children, youth, and their families, the influence of the environment on these capacities and needs, and the resultant occupational engagement.

Play and Social Participation

To facilitate the play and social participation capacities of the children and youth, the occupational therapist and occupational therapy assistant make a number of environmental adjustments. They subdivide the large community room into smaller areas with furniture, carpet remnants, and room dividers to absorb noise. They designate specific areas for exploratory, art, music, scientific, and constructive activities, board games, and gross motor movement activities. To provide structure to the day, the occupational therapist and occupational therapy assistant post time schedules for various activities and incorporate quiet time for study and rest. They make head-phones available to use with musical and other noisemaking equipment to reduce the number of competing sounds, and arrange a quiet area with soft sitting pillows and beanbag chairs where the children can read or calm themselves. To develop a sense of personal space, they help each child and adolescent design a storage bin that contains supplies for his or her exclusive use. To help the older children and adolescents deal with their anxiety, the occupational therapist and occupational therapy assistant offer yoga and meditation classes, and provide guidance on how to establish healthy sleep and eating patterns.

To address the social interaction level of each child and adolescent, the occupa-tional therapist and occupational therapy assistant conduct training sessions for the parents and volunteers about how to adapt the activities to be consistent with the chil-dren's and adolescents' parallel, associative, or cooperative levels of play. The occupa-tional therapy assistant also creates a reference book of ideas regarding how to adapt various activities to foster parallel, associative, or cooperative levels of interaction.

The occupational therapist and occupational therapy assistant conduct formal as-sessments of those children and adolescents who appear to be struggling with social participation. In collaboration with the social worker and the psychologist who work at the center, the occupational therapist and occupational therapy assistant use the Transdisciplinary Play-Based Assessment (Linder, 1993) for the younger children. They use the Children's Assessment of Participation and Enjoyment [CAPE] (King et al., 2004) and the Child Occupational Self-Assessment [COSA] (Keller et al., 2005) for the older children and adolescents. The Transdisciplinary Play Assessment provides in-formation about young children's cognitive, social-emotional, sensorimotor, and com-munication and language capacities. The COSA and the CAPE provide information about what the youth do with their time, where and with whom they perform these activities, and their level of satisfaction with their activity options. Based on this in-formation, the occupational therapist and occupational therapy assistant implement play based interventions for the younger children and social competency programs for the older children.

Education

To help those children and adolescents who are struggling academically, the occupa-tional therapist and occupational therapy assistant implement the Academic Inter-vention Monitoring System (AIMS)®. On the AIMS Student Intervention Form, the children and adolescents indicate their capacity and interest in setting expectations for learning and achievement, their motivators for accomplishing academic tasks, and their ability to self-monitor and evaluate their academic progress (Elliott, Di Perna, & Shapiro, 2001). With permission from the youth and their parents, the occupational therapist contacts the school to discuss the learning difficulties and to develop inter-vention strategies. At the domestic violence center, the occupational therapist and the occupational therapy assistant works with these children and adolescents to:

- Establish a daily study routine
- Design study areas that promote concentration
- Develop a system for studying that involves formulating a question about the materials prior to reading them, taking notes on and drawing graphic represen-tations of the reviewed materials
- Expand the length of time they can concentrate on work
- Develop time estimation skills

- Plan schedules for completing assignments
- Set goals for tasks to accomplish and
- Establish a reward system for achieving study goals (Elliott, Di Perna, & Shapiro, 2001)

Parents

In addition to working directly with the children, the occupational therapist and the occupational therapy assistant run parent–child groups. The purpose of these groups is to (1) promote nurturing interactions between the parent and the child, and (2) develop the parents' ability to use positive parenting skills. The occupational therapist and occupational therapy assistant conduct three different groups, one for parents with infants and toddlers, one for parents with elementary age children, and one for parents with adolescents. Parents who have children of different ages choose those groups that are important to them.

During the first part of the session, the child and parent listen to a story or CD, or watch a video clip that addresses and aspect of human relationships and expression of feelings. They then participate in a short discussion period about how the story, CD, or video clip relates to their interactions and feelings. Next, the parent and child play or socialize in dyads with one another, using developmentally appropriate toys, games, crafts, and building projects. The occupational therapist and occupational therapy assistant take photographs of the parent–child interactions. After the parent and child share a healthy snack with one another, the children move to a separate room where they participate in gross motor activities and games. The parents then meet with one another to reflect on the experiences they just had with their children. Using the photographs to trigger conversation, the parents discuss the verbal and nonverbal interactions they had with their children, their feelings about these interactions, their perceptions of what was successful, and what was not successful. Validating for the parents that their role is to be older, wiser, stronger, and more gentle then their children, the occupational therapist and occupational therapy assistant conclude the session with a conversation about nurturing and positive parenting strategies.

Residential Wilderness Program

The occupational therapist and the occupational therapy assistant work at a residential wilderness program for male youth who range in age from 12 to 16 years. The youth are sent to the program by the juvenile probation system, usually for a period of six months. Most of the youth have a history of school expulsion, petty crime, and misdemeanors. Some have experienced abuse, neglect, and personal or community trauma and violence. A number struggle with learning disabilities, impulse control, hyperactivity and short attention span. Some have difficulty reading social cues and predicting the consequences of actions.

The wilderness program has an established code of conduct and clearly defined behavioral management system. The youth earn privileges for socially appropriate actions and lose privileges for unacceptable behaviors. During the week, the youth attend school for 6½ hours a day, complete assigned chores, attend group therapy sessions, and engage in supervised recreational activities. On weekends, they participate in wilderness exploration programs to develop self-reliance, group trust, peer collaboration, and physical and emotional competence. Those who successfully remain in the program for 6 months go on a 2-week wilderness excursion. Those who do not abide by the program's code of conduct are sent to more regimented programs by the juvenile probation system.

As members of the interdisciplinary team, the occupational therapist and occupational therapy assistant collaborate with other professionals to design and implement interventions for the youth. The occupational therapist and occupational therapy assistant provide consultative services and direct interventions for the academic, therapeutic, and wilderness aspects of the program.

Academic Programs

The occupational therapy and occupational therapy assistant consult with the classroom teachers and the residential program staff who supervise evening study hours regarding environmental adaptations to promote learning. Because a number of the youth are distractible and have short attention spans, the occupational therapist and occupational therapy assistant help the teachers and staff erect designated work areas and study cubicles with supply bins that reduce visual and auditory distractions, and provide clear clues about the tasks to accomplish. They outline a daily study schedule that intersperses short breaks between 20 and 30 minute periods of focused concentration. During the breaks, they have the youth do yoga-type stretches and deep pressure movement activities. After reviewing educational reports and observing the youths' academic performance, the occupational therapist and occupational therapy assistant help the teachers and the staff redesign the visual layout of the worksheets and instructional guides to reduce the amount of clutter and to direct the youth's attention to the essential elements.

Group Therapy Sessions

Because studies have indicated that young offenders have a narrow range of healthy leisure occupations (Farnworth, 2000), the occupational therapist and the occupational therapy assistant collaborate with the recreational therapist to design a leisure exploration group. As part of this group, the youth participate in a sampling of athletic, art, and recreational occupations and learn about safe places in their community where they can participate in such occupations. They develop charts to compare how they actually spend their time with how they would like to spend their time when they are in their home communities. They then examine supports and barriers to participation in these occupations within their community.

Because a number of the youth struggle with impulse control and monitoring their internal readiness to participate in the various activities, the occupational therapist and occupational therapy assistant also run an eight-week Alert Program for Self-Regulation® (Williams & Shellenberger, 1996).

In this group, they help the youth to understand the relationship between their internal state of readiness, or **state of arousal**, and their over or under reactive behaviors when performing various daily occupations. Adhering to the guidelines outlined in the Alert Program, the occupational therapist and the occupational therapy assistant divide the activities for the eight weeks into three stages. During the first stage, the youth learn about and become attuned to their specific patterns and states of arousal. During the second stage, the youth experiment with various sensory and motor approaches to reduce or increase their level of arousal. During third stage, the youth learn to control their level of arousal to match that necessary for optimal performance of their daily occupations. As part of the eight-week program, each student completes a series of How Fast Does Your Engine Run?® worksheets to help them focus on their states of arousal and develop oral, motor, tactile, visual, auditory, and movement-related strategies to regulate them (Williams & Shellenberger, 1996).

Wilderness Activities

Staff members who are knowledgeable about outdoor recreational programs run the wilderness activities. The weekend activities include hiking, kayaking, whitewater rafting, rock climbing, and overnight survival camps. The two-week programs involve driving cross-country wagon trains and sailing schooners. Because the goals of the wilderness program are to foster self-reliance, group trust, peer collaboration, and physical and emotional competence, resources are kept at a minimum. The occupational therapist and occupational therapy assistant provide consultative services regarding how to adapt the equipment and the activities to provide an appropriate amount of cognitive, physical, and social-emotional challenge for each of the youth. Based on analysis of the youth's language processing and cognitive capacities during various academic group activities, the occupational therapist and occupational therapy assistant make recommendations as to how to give written and verbal instructions, and sequence the steps of the tasks. They suggest ways to provide physical guidance and adapt the equipment for those youth who are less coordinated or struggle with dyspraxia. Concerned with fostering group collaboration, they propose strategies for how to organize the youth into parallel, associative, or cooperative level groups, depending on their capacity to work with others. Finally, sensitive to the linkage between the youth's capacity to manage their behaviors and ability to regulate their state of arousal, the occupational therapist and occupational therapy assistant outline strategies for adjusting the amount of sensory stimuli during each of the activities.

Hospital-Based Inpatient Program

The occupational therapist and the occupational therapy assistant work with a group of health professionals to provide services to adolescents with eating disorders. The other health professionals include physicians, psychologists, nurses, psychiatrists, nutritionists, and social workers. For those adolescents at risk for dying because of starvation and metabolic and coronary complications, nutrition and stabilization of their medical conditions are of primary concern. Suicide precautions are put in place for those at risk for self-injurious behaviors. Behavioral management techniques are use to help the adolescents regain a healthy amount of weight. Services also focus on providing education regarding healthy eating and sleep patterns, developing a positive body image, and fostering healthy perspectives about one's self-concept, self-esteem, feelings, and attitudes. Counseling services are provided to the entire family to address family issues and to minimize the chances of relapse when the adolescents return home (Yager et al., 2004).

As part of these inpatient intervention services, the occupational therapist and occupational therapy assistant focus on helping the adolescents establish a healthy balance of daily life activities. Because it provides a method for considering the adolescents' sense of personal control and choice, interests, habits, and performance skills, the occupational therapist and occupational therapy assistant use the Model of Human Occupation to guide their critical reasoning and service delivery. They have the adolescents complete the Canadian Occupational Performance Measure to establish interventions goals that are important to the adolescents, and to learn what daily life occupations are most challenging for them (Law et al., 1998). The occupational therapist and occupational therapy assistant also have the adolescents complete the Occupational History Interview II (Kielhofner, 2004), and the Pediatric Interest Profile (Henry, 2000) to gain a sense of what occupations and leisure activities are important to them.

Based on the data collected from these assessments, the occupational therapist and occupational therapy assistant organize a series of occupation based group sessions for the adolescents throughout the day. Because the adolescents revealed that they spent most of their time thinking about food and ways to control their weight, the occupational therapist and occupational therapy assistant conduct a leisure group to encourage the adolescents to explore alternate interests that promote a sense of positive accomplishment and that do not involve excessive energy consumption. They offer yoga and meditation classes to help the adolescents learn relaxation techniques and to develop positive approaches for developing a sense of control over their bodies. The occupational therapist and occupational therapy assistant also offer a creative expression group. In this group, the adolescents work with fabric arts to explore their creativity, and make projects that reflect their sense of self. As part of the creative expressions group, the adolescents also write stories or poem to help them learn how to put their feelings and thoughts into words. Working with the psychologist, the occupational therapist and occupational therapy assistant help the adolescents explore the meaning of their stories and poems. Because the adolescents shared that they struggle with food preparation activities, the occupational therapist and occupational therapy assistant organize a cooking group. In the group, the adolescents learn how to plan healthy meals, and practice becoming comfortable with touching and preparing foods. To measure the effectiveness of their programs, the occupational therapist and occupational therapy assistant again have the adolescents complete the COPM and the Pediatric Interest Profile, and provide writing samples about positive and negative days. The occupational therapist then compares the results from the initial assessment with those at the time of discharge from the hospital.

VIOLENCE PREVENTION PROGRAMS

In addition to providing interventions focused on individual children and adolescents, occupational therapists and occupational therapy assistants may work as members of school or community teams to design and implement programs to prevent violence at the systems level. These **violence prevention programs** focus on helping the students to master five core competences: self-awareness, social awareness, self-management, relationship skills, and responsible decision making (Collaborative for Academic, Social, and Emotional Learning, as cited in Jackson & Arbesman, 2006, p. 71). Such prevention programs may include the implementation of: **Positive Behavioral Interventions and Supports system** (PBS), social skills training within the school curriculum, and activity based programs that foster social competency (Jackson & Arbesman, 2006).

PBS is a system designed to promote socially appropriate behaviors within the school or community program using positive instead of punitive approaches. School and community teams that implement a PBS system do not adhere to a zero-based tolerance policy that results in suspension or expulsion regardless of the severity of the infraction, Rather, they consider the reason behind the problem behavior, the context influencing the behavior, interventions consistent with the behavior and the desired outcomes, and the implementation of outcomes acceptable to the student, the family, and the members of the school or community (Jackson & Arbesman, 2006). As members of school or community teams, occupational therapists and occupational therapy assistants bring their understanding of the influence of environments and occupational demands on performance, their knowledge of activity demands, and their sensitivity to the health conditions and learning capacities of children and adolescents, to establish developmentally and contextually appropriate PBS systems.

Working in concert with the teachers, occupational therapists and occupational therapy assistants also devise strategies for incorporating **social skills training** within the daily routine of the classroom to reduce violence and other disruptive behaviors. In the community, they work with youth coordinators to integrate social skills training into the scheduled recreational and service activities. Through the social skills training program, students learn how to effectively listen to and communicate with their peers and teachers, manage their behaviors, take turns, compromise, problem solve, and resolve conflicts. Simulations and role playing allow students to practice social problem solving strategies in small groups. Teaching social skills clarifies school and community expectations regarding acceptable behaviors (Jackson & Arbesman, 2006).

Occupational therapists and occupational therapy assistants also offer occupation-based programs that promote **social competency**, particularly for at risk students. Within the school system, occupational therapists and occupational therapy assistants may offer such programs as part of activity classes during or after the school day. In the community, they can offer the programs as part of wellness initiatives. Occupation based social competency programs emphasize direct and incidental learning about social interactions within the context of play and leisure occupations. These programs help children and adolescents develop generalizable capacities for engaging in and sustaining social interactions with others in a variety of situations (Williamson & Dorman, 2002). The following scenario describes how an occupational therapist and occupational therapy assistant work together to offer violence prevention programs.

The middle school principal and staff are concerned about the increase in incidents of **relational aggression** occurring among the seventh grade girls. Relational aggression is a form of bullying used more frequently by girls than by boys to hurt one another. It involves the use of name-calling, rumors, gossip, printed and verbal insults, and shunning rather than physical violence to cause emotional and social pain. Incidents of relational aggression can be very subtle and couched within apparently nonoffending statements, or can be very blatant and direct. One girl usually is the **aggressor**, while another girl usually is the **victim**. In addition, there often are **bystanders**, that is, girls who observe the act of relational aggression, and either try to stop, encourage, or ignore it (Dellasega & Nixon, 2003). Currently, the principal and staff have observed or heard about incidents of relational aggression that occur during school arrival and departures, in the cafeteria and locker rooms, and through phone text messages and instant messaging on the computers. They have noted an increase in the number of girls crying, sitting by themselves, and being absent from school. The principal and staff are concerned that if they do not address the issue, the relational aggression might escalate to physical violence, as has occurred in other schools.

As a member of the school violence prevention team, the occupational therapist proposes that she and the occupational therapy assistant develop a social competency program that focuses on reducing relational aggression. Given administrative approval, the occupational therapist conducts a review of literature regarding effective strategies to address relational aggression (Dellasega & Nixon, 2003) and discusses with the occupational therapy assistant how to incorporate these strategies into the social competency program. The occupational therapist selects the Person-Environment-Occupational Performance Model as the theoretical framework to guide her thinking about the needs of the girls, and the influence of the physical and social context on their behavior. She also uses the model to guide the developmental of the intervention plan and the outcome measures used to determine the effectiveness of the program for improving the occupational performance of the girls in social situations (see Chapter 2 for a description of that model).

The occupational therapist next approaches the language arts teacher, who also is a member of the violence prevention team. They discuss the feasibility of using the literature the girls are reading as the basis for activities for the social competency programs. They draft a schedule whereby all of the seventh grade girls rotate in small groups through the program. Each girl participates in the program for a series of eight sessions, to coincide with the activity period on the girls' course schedules. During the sessions the girls learn about relational aggression, gain insight into the reasons why others act the way they do, and practice prosocial communication strategies. The girls then create skits from the various stories they have read during their literature class that depict incidence of relational aggression. Each girl role plays being a victim, an aggressor, and a bystander, and journals about her feelings when she assumed each of the roles. The girls then problem solve how to rewrite the script to depict positive assertive communication and interaction skills. Again, through role playing, they learn how to deflect the relational aggression, constructively resolve conflicts, and develop alternative outlets to express feelings. They identify safe places and activities to reduce the risk of relational aggression, and develop behavioral contracts to stop the aggression against girls who are being victimized.

The occupational therapy assistant coleads each of the group sessions with the occupational therapist. The occupational therapy assistant also helps with collecting outcome data. At the beginning of each session, she has the girls anonymously report the number of relational aggressive incidences in which they were the aggressor, bystander, or victim, and the number of relational aggressive incidents they stopped during the past 24 hours. In addition, the occupational therapy assistant collates data from school administrators and counselors regarding the number of reported incidents of relational aggression each week. The occupational therapist uses this data, along with other measures of social competency and exit interviews, to measure program outcomes.

SUMMARY

Children and adolescents often address psychosocial, emotional, and behavioral issues as part of their typical growth and development. Those with more complex psychosocial, emotional, and behavioral challenges may be diagnosed as having a condition listed in *Diagnostic and statistical manual of mental disorder: DSM-IV-TR* (APA, 2000), or included under the classification of emotional and behavioral disorders (EBD) within Individuals with Disabilities Education Improvement Act (IDEIA) guidelines (2004). It is estimated that 1 in 10 of the 73 million children and adolescents in the United States have a severe emotional disturbance (House, 2002; U.S. Department of Health and Human Services [DHHS], 2000). Similarly, between 6 and 8 percent of school children between the ages of 3 and 21 receive special education and related services because of their emotional and behavioral difficulties (U.S. Department of Education, 2003).

The psychosocial, emotional, and behavioral challenges that children and adolescents experience may stem from environmental and personal factors that are acute or chronic in duration. These factors include: biological and genetic predispositions, failure of caretakers to bond and form attachments, parental and child depression, inadequate parenting, child abuse and neglect, sexual abuse, substance abuse, poverty, and personal or community trauma and violence. They also may stem from rejection by or bullying from peers, and feelings of loneliness and alienation (Center for Mental Health in Schools, 2003). The more chronic these factors, the more likely they will have long term consequences that continue to negatively affect children and adolescents into their adulthood.

The DSM-IV categorizes conditions according to behavioral problems, psychotic disorders, mood disorders, substance-related disorders, anxiety disorders, eating disorders, and adjustment disorders (First, Frances, & Pincus, 2002). Overlap occurs between the DSM-IV diagnoses and school based IDEA classifications. Children and adolescents with diagnoses of behavioral, anxiety, psychotic, and mood related disorders under DSM-IV may qualify for services under the *emotional and behavioral disturbance* (EBD) category of IDEA. Children and adolescents with substance and eating disorders, as categorized by DSM-IV, may receive IDEA educational and related service support under the *other health conditions* classification. In addition, depending upon the school district's interpretation of what is meant by educationally relevant, some students may receive support to address emotional, behavioral, and psychological challenges stemming from other physical, learning, and cognitive classifications identified in IDEA. Care must be taken to consider whether the learning and behavioral patterns reflect the children's and adolescents' cultural background and social context so that they are not inappropriately targeted as having learning and behavioral difficulties (DHHS, 2000).

Children and adolescents with a DSM-IV diagnosis or who fit within the bounds of IDEA guidelines may be referred for occupational therapy services. As likely, children and adolescents with psychosocial and emotional difficulties, though initially referred for occupational therapy services for a different reason, also may receive occupational therapy interventions to address their psychosocial, emotional, and behavioral challenges. The children and adolescents may receive occupational therapy services within the home, school, and community settings. When their symptoms are severe, the children and adolescents may need to receive more intensive services within the hospital, a residential treatment center, or juvenile system. When providing such services, the occupational therapist and occupational therapy assistant often work with a team of health and educational professionals including psychiatrists, physicians, nurses, teachers, counselors, social workers, psychologists, and genetic counselors.

REVIEWING KEY POINTS

1. Describe the incidence of children and youth in the United States with severe behavioral and emotional difficulties.
2. Explain the factors contributing to these behavioral and emotional difficulties.
3. Explain the relationship between youth with disabilities and those who are incarcerated.
4. Explain the relationship between DSM-IV classifications and IDEA classifications related to psychosocial, behavioral, and emotional challenges
5. Describe each of the following conditions:

Anorexia	Anxiety disorders
Behavioral related disorders	Bipolar disorder
Bulimia	Conduct disorder
Cyclothymic disorder	Eating disorders

Emotional and behavioral disorder	Oppositional defiant disorder
Posttraumatic stress syndrome	Reactive attachment disorder
Relational aggression	Schizophrenia
Separation anxiety disorder	Substance abuse
Substance dependence	

6. Describe the current IDEA guidelines for providing services in the school system to children with behavioral and emotional challenges.
7. Describe the roles and responsibilities of the occupational therapist and the occupational therapy assistant when providing services to children and youth with behavioral, emotional, and psychosocial challenges.
8. Identify other health and educational professionals who also provide services to children and youth with behavioral, emotional, and psychosocial challenges. Describe their roles and responsibilities.
9. List evaluation tools that occupational therapists and occupational therapy assistants might use when evaluating children and youth with behavioral, emotional, and psychosocial challenges.
10. Describe the Alert Program.
11. Describe strategies for adapting the classroom environment to support the learning needs of children and adolescents with behavioral, emotional, and psychosocial challenges.
12. List five challenges that make it difficult for elementary children with behavioral and emotional difficulties to participate in their daily life occupations.
13. List five strategies that occupational therapists and occupational therapy assistants can use to help children with behavioral and emotional difficulties successfully engage in their daily life occupations.
14. List five challenges that make it difficult for children and youth coping with domestic violence to participate in their daily life occupations.
15. List five strategies that occupational therapists and occupational therapy assistants can use to help children and youth coping with domestic violence successfully engage in their daily life occupations.
16. List five challenges that make it difficult for youth with eating disorders to participate in their daily life occupations.
17. List five strategies that occupational therapists and occupational therapy assistants can use to help youth with eating disorders successfully engage in their daily life occupations.
18. List five challenges that make it difficult for adjudicated youth to participate in their daily life occupations.
19. List five strategies that occupational therapists and occupational therapy assistants can use to help adjudicated youth successfully engage in their daily life occupations.
20. Describe the Positive Behavioral Interventions and Supports system and how occupational therapists and occupational therapy assistants can contribute to violence prevention programs.
21. Explain relational aggression and outline a program that occupational therapists and occupational therapy assistants can implement to reduce relational aggression.

APPLYING KEY CONCEPTS

1. Review the school based case study about elementary age children struggling with behavioral and emotional control issues.
   a. For each of the age groups, select three stories or videos to promote discussion about behavioral management and emotional regulation. Justify your selections.

     b. For each of the age groups, design three activities to help the children practice behavioral management and emotional regulation. Explain how these activities can be used to achieve your objectives.

2. Volunteer time at a shelter for homeless families or families recovering from domestic violence.
     a. Organize play and leisure groups for the children.
     b. Keep a journal of your experiences. In the journal reflect on your feelings and behavior toward the children. Describe how the children use materials and space. Record and reflect about the verbal and nonverbal patterns they use when interacting with one another. Consider the obvious and the underlying messages they are conveying and the reasons for those messages.

3. Interview an adolescent coping with an eating disorder or view a tape about adolescents discussing their eating disorders. Consider how the adolescents describe their daily life occupations and how they engage in those occupations. Consider more positive ways for the adolescents to participate in those daily life occupations as well as additional occupations to promote health.

4. Arrange a class trip to visit a juvenile detention center or a residential program for adjudicated youth.
     a. Assess the environment. Consider how it structures the occupations in which the youth at the center or the residential program engage. Consider how these occupations prepare the youth to return to their home communities.
     b. Design an occupation based program that occupational therapists and occupational therapy assistants could provide at the center or residential program. Outline the objective for that program. List the supports and barriers for implementing such a program. List resources that would be needed. Outline safety precautions that must be established.

5. Read *Girl wars* (Dellasega & Nixon, 2003).
     a. Describe an incident of relational aggression you experienced in middle school and high school.
     b. Consider how you (1) contributed to the relational aggression; (2) were the victim in the situation; and (3) stopped the situation from escalating.
     c. With peers, role play how to guide a group of middle school and high school to: (1) respond to acts of relational aggression; and (2) stop them.

REFERENCES

American Occupational Therapy Association (2002). Occupational therapy practice framework: Domain and process. *American Journal of Occupational Therapy, 56*(6), 609–639.

American Occupational Therapy Association (2004). Guidelines for supervision, roles, and responsibilities during the delivery of occupational therapy services. *American Journal of Occupational Therapy, 58* (November/December).

American Psychiatric Association (2000). *Diagnostic and statistical manual of mental disorder: DSM-IV-TR.* Washington, DC: American Psychiatric Association, http://alias.libriaries.psu.edu/eresources/STATREP>.

Center for Mental Health in Schools (2003). *An introductory packet on social and interpersonal problems related to school age youth.* Los Angeles: University of California. Available online at http://smhp.psych.ucla.edu.

Committee on Education and the Workforce (2005). *Individuals with Disabilities Education Act: A Guide to Frequently Asked Questions.* Retrieved April 20, 2006 from http://edworkforce.house.gov/issues/109th/education/idea/ideafaq.pdf.

Conduct Problems Prevention Research Group (2002). Evaluation of the first three years of Fast Track prevention trial with children at high risk for adolescent conduct problems. *Journal of Abnormal Child Psychology, 30*(1),19–35.

Dellasega, C., & Nixon, C. (2003). *Girl wars.* New York: Fireside.

Elliott, S., DiPerna, J., & Shapiro, E. (2001). *Academic Intervention Monitoring System: Guidebook.* San Antonio, TX: Harcourt Assessment.

Farnworth, L. (2000). Time use and leisure occupations of young offenders. *American Journal of Occupational Therapy,* 54(3), 315–324.

First, M., Frances, A., & Pincus, H. (2002). *DSM-IV-TR: Handbook of differential diagnosis.* Washington, DC: American Psychiatric Publishing.

House, A. (2002). *DSM-IV diagnosis in the schools.* New York: Guilford Press.

Javaherian, H., Underwood, R., & DeLany, J. (2007). Domestic violence statement. *American Journal of Occupational Therapy, 61,* November/December.

Individuals with Disabilities Education Improvement Act of 2004, Pub. L. 108–446.

Jackson, L., & Arbesman, M. (2006). *Occupational therapy practice guidelines for children with behavioral and psychosocial needs.* Bethesda, MD: AOTA Press.

Henry, A. (2000). *Pediatric Interest Profile.* San Antonio, TX: Harcourt.

Keller, J., Kafkes, A., Basu, S., Federico, J., Kielhofner, G. (2005). *Child Occupational Self Assessment* (Version 2.1). Chicago: MOHO clearinghouse.

Kielhofner, G., Mallinson, T., Crawford, C., Nowak, M., Rigby, M., Henry, A., & Walens, D. (2004). *Occupational Performance History Interview II* (version 2.1). Chicago: MOHO Clearinghouse.

King, G., Law, M., King, S., Hurley, P., Hanna, S., Kertoy, M., Rosenbaum, P., & Young, N. (2004). *Children's Assessment of Participation and Enjoyment (CAPE) and Preferences for Activities of Children (PAC).* San Antonio, TX: Harcourt Assessment.

Kramer, J. (2002). *Children and youth self-report assessments: Evidence to support best practice in OT.* Chicago: MOHO Clearinghouse.

Koyanagi, C., & Semansky, R. (2003). *No one's priority. The plight of children with severe mental disorders in Medicaid systems.* Washington, DC: Brazelton Center for Mental Health Law.

Law, M., Baptiste, S., Carswell, A., McColl, M.A., Polatajko, H., & Pollock, N. (1998). *The Canadian Occupational Performance Measure* (3rd ed.). Toronto: CAOT, from http://www.caot.ca.

Linder, T. (1993). *Transdisciplinary Play-Based Assessment* (rev.). Baltimore, MD: Brookes.

National Center on Education, Disability, and Juvenile Justice. (2005, February). *EDJJ Notes, 4*(1).

National Institute of Child Health and Human Development Federal Interagency Forum on Child and Family Statistics (2005). *America's children: Key national indicators of well-being, 2005.* Washington, DC: Retrieved May 2, 2006 from http://nichd.nih.gov/new/releases/americas_children05_bg_parents.cfm.

National Dissemination Center for Children with Disabilities (NICHCY; 2002). *General information about disabilities: Disabilities that qualify infants, toddlers, children, and youth for services under the IDEA.* Retrieved April 20, 2006 from http://www.nichcy.org/pubs/genresc/gr3.htm.

Office for Victims of Crime. (2002). National Victim Assistance Academy: Foundations in victimology and victims' rights and services. Chapter 9: Domestic Violence. Retrieved June 8, 2006 from http://www.ojp.gov/ovc/assist/nvaa2002/chapter9.html.

Reid, W., & Wise, M. (1995). *DSM-IV training guide.* New York: Brunner Mazel.

Schultz, S. (2003). Psychosocial occupational therapy in schools. *OT Practice, 8*(16), CE1–8.

Segal, A. (2006). *IDEA and the juvenile justice system: A fact sheet* National Evaluation and Technical Assistance Center. Retrieved April 20, 2006 from http://www.neglected-delinquent.org/nd/resources/spotlight/spotlight200503f.asp

U.S. Department of Education (2003). *Twenty-fifth annual report to Congress on the implementation of the Individuals with Disabilities Education Act.* Washington, DC:Author.

U.S. Department of Education, Office of Special Education Programs, Data Analysis System (DANS) (2005). *Report of children with disabilities receiving special education under Part B of the Individuals with Disabilities Education Act.* Washington, DC: Author.

U. S. Department of Health and Human Services (2000). *Conference on children's mental health issues: A national action agenda. A report of the Surgeon General.* Bethesda, MD: National Institute of Mental Health. Retrieved May 9, 2006 from http://wwwsurgeongeneral.gov/cmh/default.htm.

Williams, M. S., & Shellenberger, S. (1996). *How fast does your engine run? A leader's guide to the alert program for self-regulation.* Albuquerque, NM: Therapy Works.

Williamson, G., & Dorman, W. (2002). *Promoting social competence.* San Antonio, TX: Therapy Skill Builders.

Yager, J., Anderson, A., Devlin, M., Egger, H., Herzo, D., Mitchell, J., Powers, P., Yates., & Zerbe, K. (2004). Practice guideline for the treatment of patients with eating disorders. In American Psychiatric Association, *Practice guidelines for the treatment of psychiatric disorders: Compendium 2004* (pp. 675–744). Arlington, VA: Author.

Chapter 18

Children and Adolescents with Orthopedic and Muscular Conditions

Margaret J. Pendzick and LuAnn Demi

Key Terms

Arthrogryposis multiplex congenita
Asymmetrical pattern
Biomechanical techniques
Body powered prosthesis
Cable
Cock-up splint
Congenital limb deficiency
Cosmetic hand
Energy conservation
Exacerbation
Externally powered prosthesis
Functional prosthesis
Harness
Hook
Joint protection techniques
Juvenile rheumatoid arthritis (JRA)
Longitudinal
Micrognathia
Myoelectric hand
Nonsteroidal anti-inflammatory drugs (NSAIDs)

Pauciarticular JRA
Passive prosthesis
Phocomelia
Polyarticular JRA
Prosthesis
Prosthetist
Pulmonary hypoplasia
Resting pan splint
Rheumatologist
Socket
Splinting
Still's disease
Systemic onset JRA
Terminal device
Transverse
Transverse complete forearm deficiency
Transverse complete humeral deficiency
Ulnar deviation
Ulnar deviation splint
Wrist unit

Objectives

- Explain the orthopedic and muscular conditions of arthrogryposis multiplex congenita, congenital limb deficiency, and juvenile rheumatoid arthritis (JRA).
- Examine how orthopedic and muscular conditions impact the daily occupations of children and adolescents within the context of their family and environment.
- Describe occupational therapy interventions to support the capacity of children and adolescents with orthopedic and muscular conditions to participate in their daily occupations.
- Examine how occupational therapists and occupational therapy assistants problem solve together during the intervention process.
- Describe how occupational therapists and occupational therapy assistants work with families and other professionals to provide services to children and adolescents with orthopedic and muscular disabilities.

INTRODUCTION

This chapter contains an overview of three orthopedic and muscular conditions that affect children and adolescents. These conditions are: **arthrogryposis multiplex congenita**, **congenital limb deficiencies**, and **juvenile rheumatoid arthritis (JRA)**. This chapter then examines how various professionals address the health care and educational needs of these children and adolescents, and how occupational therapists and occupational therapy assistants address the occupational performance challenges confronting them. Vignettes highlight occupational therapy's focus on the developmentally appropriate adaptive techniques and environmental modifications to enable these children and adolescents to participate fully in their daily life occupations.

ARTHROGRYPOSIS MULTIPLEX CONGENITA

Arthrogryposis multiplex congenita, often simply called arthrogryposis, is a general category of conditions that involves congenital contractures in two or more of the joints and sometimes affects other body systems (Cassidy & Allanson, 2005). Approximately 1 in 3,000 infants are born with arthrogryposis multiplex congenita. Though variability exists among the body systems affected, typically, the contractures and limitations in joint movement are nonprogressive (Cassidy & Allanson; Cassidy & Petty, 2005).

There are three classifications or groups of arthrogryposis: involvement of limbs only, involvement of limbs and body systems that exclude the central nervous system, and limb involvement with severe central nervous system dysfunction (Cassidy & Allanson, 2005). Two-thirds of children and adolescents with arthrogryposis have contractures and movement restrictions in multiple joints in all four extremities and multiple joints, while the other one-third of the children and adolescents are affected predominantly in the lower limbs (Morrissy & Weinstein, 2006). Those children and adolescents with upper extremity involvement typically have shoulders that are adducted and internally rotated, elbows that are extended, wrists that are severely flexed with ulnar deviation, and fingers that are flexed and clutching the thumb. Those children and adolescents with lower extremity involvement have flexed, abducted, and externally rotated hips, extended knees, and club feet. The distal portion of their legs is more severely affected, and the contractures are more rigid. These children and adolescents also may have hips that are unilaterally or bilaterally dislocated (Morrissy & Weinstein).

Arthrogryposis is caused by decreased intrauterine movement stemming from factors associated with the fetus or the mother. Those associated with the fetus include structural anomalies of the central nervous system and peripheral nerves, muscular abnormalities, and connective tissue disorders. Those associated with the mother include insufficient uterine space due to multiple births or a uterine fibroid, maternal illnesses such as myotonic dystrophy, myasthenia gravis, infections and metabolic imbalances, medication use during pregnancy, including misoprostol, curare, and muscle relaxants, and injuries in the first trimester (Cassidy & Allanson, 2005). A decrease in or lack of movement can be diagnosed prenatally by ultrasound that can detect fixed contractions, clubfoot, and thin ribs in a developing fetus (Cassidy & Allanson).

A fetus typically begins to move around at 8 or 9 weeks gestation and continues moving throughout pregnancy. The earlier in fetal development that decreased movement occurs, the more severe and immobilizing the contractures (Cassidy & Allanson, 2005).

Lack of movement in utero can cause many different problems. It can retard bone growth and predispose the infant to osteoporosis. Many infants with arthrogryposis experience fractures at birth, and up to 10 percent have a fracture within the first week of life (Cassidy & Allanson, 2005). Since lack of fetal movement hinders the normal stretching of the umbilical cord, these infants may experience respiratory problems during labor (Cassidy & Allanson). They also may be born with an immature intestinal tract secondary to lack of fetal swallowing in utero and **pulmonary hypoplasia**, a condition where the lungs are atrophied or underdeveloped. Infants born with severe pulmonary hypoplasia often have difficulty being weaned off the respirator and may require a permanent tracheostomy and ventilation. The bone retardation and lack of movement also may cause craniofacial abnormalities including **micrognathia**, an unusually small jaw, cleft palate, underdeveloped maxilla, prominent nose bridge, and depressed tip of nose (Cassidy & Allanson).

The ability of children and adolescents with arthrogryposis to engage in their daily occupations is affected by the type and severity of their musculoskeletal condition. As infants, they may experience feeding problems because of decreased musculature and lack of maturation of intestinal muscle coordination. Limitations in jaw movements and the size of the mouth also may interfere with their feeding and dental care. As the infants grow, they may develop an aversion to solids and require speech-language therapy, occupational therapy, and nursing interventions to aid in developing swallowing habits (Cassidy & Allanson, 2005). Though their level of intelligence typically is within the average to above average range, these children may experience language delays because of these early oral motor difficulties. It is important that these early speech problems are not misinterpreted as mental retardation (Morrissy & Weintein, 2006).

Joints that are fixed or contracted and spinal problems that may include stiffness, weakness, kyphosis, and scoliosis also interfere with the abilities of these children and adolescents to participate in other self-care skills, school-related tasks, and play activities. For example, at home they may have difficulty reaching for and manipulating grooming and hygiene supplies, and household materials. At school, they may struggle to manipulate various prewriting and writing materials, access school supplies, and navigate playground equipment (Cassidy & Allanson, 2005). Children and adolescents with compromised pulmonary systems may not have sufficient stamina and endurance to ride bicycles, join in running games, or engage in more organized sports and activities such as soccer, swimming, cheerleading, or marching band. Since hips commonly are dislocated, older adolescents frequently experience osteoarthritis (Cassidy & Alanson) and need to avoid high impact sports.

Vision problems may include cataracts, retinal changes, macular abnormalities, or scarring. Auditory problems can result from chronic otitis media and fluid in the middle ear if the children remain in a horizontal position for extended periods of time. Deafness can occur due to ossicle fusion or neural dysfunction (Cassidy & Allanson, 2005). These visual and auditory deficits present additional complications for the children and adolescents as they attempt to develop the skills needed to perform their daily occupations and to engage in organized sporting or community events, and school and work-related tasks.

Multiteam Approach

Interventions for children and adolescents with arthrogryposis involve a variety of team members and strategies. Regular orthopedic exams are required to monitor the effects of the condition (Cassidy & Allanson, 2005). Physicians, ophthamologists, and respiratory therapists address issues specific to osteoporosis, dislocations, visual deficits, and pulmonary deficits. Physical therapists concentrate on facilitating the highest level of ambulation and joint mobility possible (Cassidy & Allanson).

The occupational therapist and occupational therapy assistant provide occupation-based interventions directed at increasing the children's and adolescents' ability to participate in age appropriate tasks. Working in collaboration with the children, the adolescents, and their families, they actively problem solve how to adapt tasks and the environment to minimize barriers that interfere with occupational performance. They also may incorporate **biomechanical techniques** such as stretching, positioning, and proper joint alignment into the occupation-based interventions to increase active joint range and independent occupational performance.

In the school setting, the occupational therapist and the occupational therapy assistant partner with the teacher to determine what adaptive equipment and task modifications to incorporate into the daily school routine. They monitor the academic needs of the children or adolescents as they progress through school. For example, as the demand for independent written work increases, the occupational therapist and the occupational therapy assistant may recommend specific computer software that will enable older children to complete the written tasks in a timely manner (Cassidy & Allanson, 2005). They also may consider specialized seating, workstations, keyboards, or other technology to enable the children and adolescents to complete their academic tasks (Reed, 2001).

As adolescents prepare to transition from high school, the occupational therapist and occupational therapy assistant may work with the transition team to help identify independent living arrangements and workplace or postsecondary education accommodations. Environmental modifications may be warranted in the home, school, and worksite to accommodate a wheelchair, limited upper and lower extremity use, and energy conservation needs (Reed, 2001). Since children and adolescents with arthrogryposis often recognize their limitations, special attention needs to be made to build their sense of self-worth and self-esteem throughout all stages of their development (Reed). The following vignette of Levi further illustrates occupational therapy intervention.

Occupational Therapy Services: A Case Study

Levi

Levi, an 8-year-old third grader with arthogryposis, is a new student at Hilltop Elementary School. Until this year, Levi was home schooled by his mother. He is at grade level for all his academic subjects but was placed on an IEP for classroom accommodations necessary for his health impairment. The classroom teacher and parents request an occupational therapy evaluation due to Levi's difficulty performing specific ADL and school related tasks. The parents and teacher are concerned that Levi's self-esteem is being affected by his inability to function in the school setting independently. He requires assistance in toileting since he is unable to manipulate the front zipper on his pants and/or manage his clothing when using the urinal. He becomes frustrated during art activities when projects require cutting, as he is unable to manipulate scissors. He has difficulty making a firm pencil mark on the paper and completing written work. Although Levi uses a voice activated word processing program to complete assignments, the teacher and parents would like Levi to be able to complete minimal writing tasks in a manner similar to his peers. The only solution they have found was allowing Levi to use markers, but Levi feels that is babyish.

After discussing the need for the evaluation with the parents and teacher, the occupational therapist and occupational therapy assistant plan the assessment. Recognizing that Levi will need to problem solve solutions and generalize those solutions to maximize his occupational performance within the context of the school, the occupational therapist chooses to use the Person-Environment-Occupational Performance Model (Christiansen & Baum, 1997; Baum & Christiansen, 2005) to guide her evaluation. Besides requesting the occupational therapy assistant to observe Levi during toileting, she decides to include observations during lunch and recess to ascertain if any potential problems exist in those environments. She assesses Levi's functional hand, arm, and mobility skills. Levi completes the Activity Scales for Kids (ASK) (Young, n.d.) so that he can self-report the effects of the musculoskeletal disorder on ADL, play, and mobility. The parents and teacher provide information through the School Functional Assessment (SFA) (Coster, Denney, Haltiwanger, & Haley, 1998).

The occupational therapist compares the SFA and ASK standardized test results, informal functional motor assessment, and environmental observation report. She notes that Levi's limited hand function—no active thumb movement, 15 degrees active digit flexion, no extension—hinders his ability to grasp and manipulate objects. Although elbow and shoulder movement are adequate to perform dressing and grooming skills, Levi experiences difficulty removing items above shoulder height or throwing an overhand ball with force. Although he has full lower extremity movement, his difficulty grading movements results in a jerky gait pattern that interferes with carrying items and performing toileting tasks.

The observations recorded by the occupational therapy assistant and the teacher's SFA responses indicate that Levi is having difficulty interacting socially with his peers. In order to participate fully in informal recess games, Levi requires modifications to the sports equipment or playground area. The teacher reports that Levi participates well with others on teacher-assigned group tasks.

The occupational therapist completes her evaluation report (Figure 18.1■) and shares the findings with the parents and teacher. After adding occupational therapy as a related service to Levi's current IEP, the parents, classroom teacher, and the occupational therapist further discuss Levi's social skills. Since Levi enjoys reading, the classroom teacher suggests that she encourage Levi to join the Reading Buddy program, where third grade students are paired with first graders for a weekly library program. The classroom teacher agrees to identify some leadership role that Levi can assume in the classroom, which should help boost his confidence. The parents indicate that Levi has expressed interest in joining Cub

Levi, an 8-year-old third grader at Hilltop Elementary School, was referred for an occupational therapy evaluation by his classroom teacher, Mrs. Peters, and his parents. Mrs. Peters reports that Levi's academic skills are at grade level but he requires accommodations in the classroom due to his musculoskeletal developmental disability. From kindergarten through third grade, Levi was home schooled, requiring fewer accommodations in that setting. Current major concerns include Levi's dependence in dressing during toileting, inability to use scissors during art class, and difficulty making a firm stroke with his pencil on paper. He independently uses a voice activated computer software program for written work. Although he used thick markers to print short answers in the home setting, Levi currently refuses the accommodation stating that it makes him "look like a baby."

The occupational therapy evaluation is a synthesis of the following assessment tools: functional assessment of motor skills, School Functional Assessment (SFA) completed by the parents and classroom teacher, Activity Scales for Kids (ASK) completed by Levi, and observations during toileting, lunch, and recess. Test results are as follows:

Functional Motor Skills: Due to Levi's medical condition, his hand function is limited by no active thumb movement and little active movement of his fingers, resulting in a weak and inefficient grasp pattern. He requires adaptations to manipulate objects such as zipper tabs, scissors, and cafeteria eating utensils. Although Levi's elbow and shoulder movements are adequate for dressing and grooming skills, he experiences difficulty removing items from above shoulder height or throwing an overhand ball with force. He independently ambulates but his gait is jerky, having difficulty maintaining his balance when he bends over. These motor patterns interfere with his ability to maintain his balance during toileting and keep his tray steady when walking. Without accommodations, he is unable to join his peers during playground ball games.

Self-Help Skills: For the majority of self-help skills, Levi is independent, often spontaneously incorporating adaptive techniques. Due to Levi's difficulty manipulating fasteners, his parents primarily select clothing that require minimal or no fasteners. Elastic waist pull down pants, however, interfere with his ability to maintain balance during toileting. When Levi wears front zipper pants, he requires assistance to manipulate the fastener. When the zipper is opened, Levi has difficulty maintaining the wide base stance needed to keep his pants from falling to the floor. This creates a soiling problem when using the urinal.

Levi is experiencing some difficulties in the lunchroom setting. He is unable to grasp the cafeteria supplied disposable sporks so he chooses finger foods or sandwiches. He usually avoids carton packaged drinks, choosing to stop at the water fountain after lunch. After eating, he has difficulty carrying his tray to the cleanup area. The empty containers slide around the tray as he walks, frequently requiring him to stop and attempt to pick up dropped trash. Doing so requires him to set the tray down before reaching for the floor.

Social Skills: Although Levi works well in a classroom cooperative group project, he cannot identify any specific friends at school. On the playground, he watches group games from the sidelines and does not initiate any conversations with other children. He does not join a specific lunchroom group but seems to choose a free seat closest to the cafeteria lunch line.

Summary: Since his physical limitations cannot be altered, Levi requires modifications and adaptation to increase his successful participation in multiple contexts. Levi needs to learn strategies that will help him succeed in school and increase opportunities to interact socially with his peers.

Recommendations: Levi would benefit from the addition of occupational therapy services to his current IEP. Occupational therapy should address needed adaptations and modification and help Levi acquire age appropriate social competencies.

■ **Figure 18.1**
Levi's occupational therapy evaluation.

Scouts but they are apprehensive about his participation. If Levi joins Cub Scouts, the occupational therapist offers to meet with the leader to help adapt the program to meet Levi's needs. The occupational therapist suggests that the classroom teacher help Levi identify some classroom buddies who he could join at lunchtime and at recess. The occupational therapy assistant offers to work with the adaptive PE teacher to introduce some adapted games during recess. ■

CONGENITAL LIMB DEFICIENCY

Although limb deficiencies occur rarely in children, they primarily are caused by congenital problems stemming from errors in the genetic control of limb development, disruption of the developing arterial supply, and intrauterine amputation from amniotic bands (Morrissy & Weinstein, 2006). Because the development of a limb is complex and requires the precise interaction of a large number of genes, the opportunity for errors in this system is great (Morrissy & Weinstein).

Classifications and Types of Anomalies

Congenital anomalies are classified as **transverse**, where the defect extends across the entire limb, or **longitudinal**, where only the pre- or postaxial portion is affected (Morrissy & Weinstein, 2006). Table 18.1■ describes specific upper extremity anomalies.

The term **phocomelia** refers to the condition where the distal portion of the extremities attaches directly to a proximal part of the body. For instance, the child or adolescent's hand or portion of a hand attaches directly to the shoulder or a residual arm stump. The hand may or may not be functional. Children and adolescents with a nonfunctional hand or little arm length often learn to use their feet and body strength to complete self-care skills (Morrissy & Weinstein, 2006).

Transverse complete humeral deficiency refers to a unilateral above-elbow amputation, and **transverse complete forearm deficiency** refers to a congenital below-elbow amputation. The below-elbow amputation is the most common of all the upper extremity anomalies and occurs more often in the left arm (Morrissy & Weinstein, 2006). Families who have an infant with a congenital limb deficiency have the option to wait and see how the infant develops and learns with the existing limb deficiency, or to choose to have the infant fitted with a prosthesis. Families generally choose to treat their infant with a prosthesis (Olson & DeRuyter, 2002).

Multiteam Approach

A multidisciplinary team approach is important from a very early age to address the child's limitations caused by a congenital limb deficiency. Physicians and surgeons are involved initially if any surgical intervention is required prior to prosthesis assessment. A **prosthetist** is important to the children and adolescents throughout their growth and development to evaluate and fit the most appropriate type of prosthesis, routinely service it, and recognize the need for a new one. The skilled prosthetist ensures that the highest functional need of the children and adolescents are met through prosthetic intervention or, if appropriate, through no intervention at all (Morrissy & Weinstein, 2006). When the children and adolescents are in school, the teacher becomes a part of the multidisciplinary team that aids the child in the proper use of the prosthesis, especially when the children and adolescents receive a new prosthesis or

■ **Table 18.1**
Upper Extremity Anomalies

TRANSVERSE CONGENITAL ANOMALIES	
TYPE	DEFINITION
Amelia	Absence of a limb
Hemimelia	Absence of forearm and hand
Partial hemimelia	Part of forearm is present
Acheiria	Absence of the hand
Complete adactlia	Absence of the five digits and metacarpal bones
Complete phalange	Absence of one or more phalanges from all five digits
LONGITUDINAL CONGENITAL ANOMALIES	
TYPE	DEFINITION
Complete paraxial hemimelia	Complete absence of a forearm element and corresponding portion of the hand
Incomplete paraxial hemimelia	Partial absence of a forearm element and corresponding portion of the hand
Partial adactylia	Absence of one to four digits and metacarpal bones
Partial phalange	Absence of one or more phalanges from one to four digits

Source: Morrissy & Weinstein, 2006.

have school related requirements where specific prosthetic training is necessary (Case-Smith, 2005).

Prosthesis: An Overview

A **prosthesis** is an artificial part that is fabricated to substitute for a missing body part. The purpose of an upper extremity prosthesis is to provide the child or adolescent with a hand to use and to position the hand so that it can be used effectively (Morrissy & Weinstein, 2006).

There are different types of upper extremity prostheses used by children and adolescents. Prosthetic devices are recommended and selected based on the level of limb amputation and the preferences of the child, adolescent, and caregivers (Pendleton & Schultz-Krohn, 2006).

The higher the level of amputation, the greater the functional loss of the arm, and the greater the need for a more complex prosthesis and more extensive training. For instance, those children and adolescents who are missing part of the humerus and all structures below have only shoulder movements of extension, flexion, abduction, and adduction available. In order to gain full use of the extremity, the prosthesis must be capable of elbow, wrist, and grasp movement. In contrast, children and adolescents who are missing the wrist and below also can flex and extend their elbows and supinate and pronate their forearms. Thus, they need a prosthesis that is capable of performing wrist and hand actions. The fewer the number of actions that the prosthesis needs to control, the easier it is for the child and adolescent to learn to operate it.

The child's social, cognitive, and emotional development affects the level and type of orthotic intervention. If a child or adolescent requires a prosthetic device to independently perform self-care, play, or school related tasks, the least noticeable and least cumbersome prosthetic device should be utilized (Olson & DeRuyter, 2002).

Types of Prostheses

Depending on the need of the device, a prosthesis is either passive or functional. A **passive prosthesis** has no moveable parts and often is used to provide postural balance or to assist the functional limb. The infant is given a lightweight, passive limb between 4 and 6 months of age in order to become comfortable with it. It is in this developmental age range that a child typically brings hands to midline while supine, props up on elbows in prone, and then props up on extended arms in sitting and rolling over. Introducing the passive hand at this time attempts to aid in the development of central cortical pathways for bimanual dexterity (Morrissy & Weinstein, 2006). A **functional prosthesis** has the capability of grasping and holding objects. It may be body powered or externally powered (Pendleton & Schultz-Krohn, 2006).

Body Powered Prosthesis.   The **body powered prosthesis** has five components (see Figure 18.2■):

* The **socket** [Figure (a)] fits snugly over the residual limb and is the fundamental component to which the other parts of the prosthesis are attached.

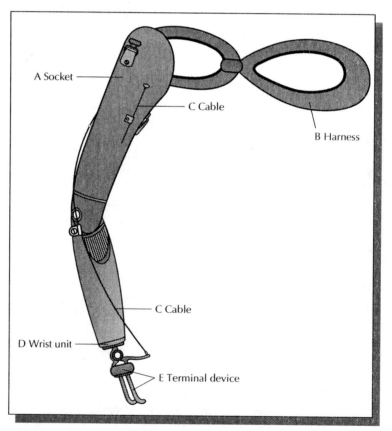

■ **Figure 18.2**
Components of a body powered prosthesis.

- The **harness**, (b), is commonly a figure-8 system that is worn across the back and shoulders or around the chest. It fastens to the socket to secure the prosthesis.
- The stainless-steel **cable**, (c), attaches to the harness at one end and to the functional component of the prosthesis at the other. Specific body movements by the child or adolescent can create tension on the cable and operate the prosthesis.
- The **wrist unit**, (d), serves to pronate and supinate the terminal device, rotating and repositioning it for various functional needs.
- The **terminal device**, (e), functions to grasp and hold objects. The child or adolescent can choose between two styles of terminal devices, the **hook** and the **cosmetic hand**. The hook has greater grip and tension than the hand; different types of hooks are available for various activities. The hand looks more natural and can function to push, pull, and stabilize objects (Pendleton & Schultz-Krohn, 2006).

When initially placing the prosthesis on the child, the prosthetist often immobilizes or "fixes" it at the elbows to make it easier for the child to learn how to operate it.

Externally Powered Prosthesis.   An **externally powered prosthesis** utilizes a **myoelectric hand**. An electrode is placed on the surface of the skin and picks up electromyographic (EMG) signals to operate an electric hand. A child younger than 2 years of age is fitted with a one site system. The child learns to voluntarily contract a muscle to open the hand. When the muscle relaxes, the hand automatically closes. Children as young as 3 to 3 1/2 years often can learn to operate a more complex two site system. The EMG signal of the flexors is used to close the hand and the EMG signal of the extensors is used to open the hand (Morrissy & Weinstein, 2006).

Occupational Therapy Intervention

The occupational therapist and occupational therapy assistant provide occupation-based intervention directed at the specific needs of the child or adolescent with a congenital limb deficiency. Intervention for children and adolescents is developmentally structured, beginning with bilateral self-care and play activities and progressing to school related activities and more skill intensive self-care tasks. Children and adolescents with congenital limb deficiencies are taught age appropriate ADL, IADL, and play skills both with and without the prosthesis.

Depending on the type of prosthesis chosen, the occupational therapist may focus on helping the child or adolescent to learn the subtle body movements to activate the body powered prosthesis or to isolate the muscle contraction to fire the electrodes in the externally powered prosthesis. In order to effectively provide this instruction, an occupational therapy assistant must obtain additional training beyond entry level competency in the field.

Self-concept and self-esteem are addressed with the children and adolescents as they attempt to incorporate the prosthesis into their body image, or decide to accept their body image with a congenital limb deficiency. The children and adolescents are supported in age appropriate social play and interaction experiences. They are encouraged to incorporate their affected extremity, with or without a prosthesis, into all aspects of life and to set realistic goals. They are provided with information and resources to develop skill mastery in chosen occupations of interest (Meier & Atkins, 2004). The case study of Travis further illustrates occupational intervention.

Travis

Travis, a 3-year-old with a congenital limb deficiency, attends the local school district's developmental preschool program. Travis recently has been fitted with a left upper extremity below elbow prosthesis. Currently, the cable is nonoperative but Travis is encouraged to use the terminal device to actively assist with his right hand movements. The occupational therapy assistant works with Travis in a small group setting within the preschool classroom.

The occupational therapy assistant prepares for the weekly preschool session by choosing activities that require bilateral hand skills and allow Travis multiple opportunities to place objects into the terminal device. The occupational therapy assistant suggests that the preschool teacher include musical instruments during circle time. Triangles, cymbals, and rhythm sticks are used that require bilateral hand usage. The occupational therapy assistant plans a craft project that requires Travis to hold the paper plate with his terminal device while snipping fringe to make the lion's mane, and while applying glue and glitter to decorate the lion's face.

Following the preschool session, the occupational therapy assistant meets with the preschool teacher to answer any questions she may have about the prosthesis. They develop a list of possible ways to incorporate Travis' use of the prosthesis into existing preschool activities. Figure 18.3■ lists some examples. ■

- After donning his jacket, encourage Travis to use his terminal device to hold the bottom of his coat taut while engaging the zipper.
- When gathering supplies, encourage Travis to place lightweight objects into his terminal device and carry them to the table.
- Encourage Travis to play with insert puzzles on a tabletop rather than on the rug. Have him steady the formboard with his prosthesis while inserting the puzzle piece with his right hand.
- Challenge Travis to attempt to do a task with his prosthesis and hand at the same time such as holding two cookie cutters and inserting them into play dough, or holding a paintbrush in both his hand and prosthesis to paint a picture at the easel.
- Play catch with a large playground ball, which requires Travis to use both arms.

■ **Figure 18.3**
Suggestions to incorporate the prosthesis into everyday activities.

JUVENILE RHEUMATOID ARTHRITIS

Juvenile rheumatoid arthritis (JRA) is a condition that affects between 57 and 113 per 100,000 children under the age of 16. The specific cause of JRA is unknown; some possible causes include infection, trauma, and autoimmunity in conjunction with a genetic predisposition for arthritis (Morrissy & Weinstein, 2006).

JRA is diagnosed when inflammation of the peripheral joints is chronic and begins before the age of 16, although any joint may be involved. Symptoms of limited range of motion, tenderness or pain in motion, and heat must be present for a minimum of six weeks with no known cause or diagnosis (Brown, 2002). In addition to muscle weakness and joint deformity, children and adolescents with JRA may experience symptoms of growth difficulties, fever, eye inflammation, fatigue, and abnormalities of the heart, liver, and spleen (Brown).

The term JRA is an umbrella term for three forms of childhood arthritis, each having a different pattern and prognosis (Dunkin, 2002). The first is **systemic onset JRA**, also called **Still's disease**. This type of arthritis affects many body systems, often beginning with a fever and chills that appear on and off for weeks. The child or adolescent also may develop a rash on the thighs and chest, and have joint inflammation, enlarged lymph nodes, anemia, and inflammation of the liver and heart and surrounding tissues (Dunkin).

Polyarticular JRA involves more than four joints. The joints affected are typically symmetrical, meaning if a joint on the left side is affected, the same joint on the right side will be affected. With this form of JRA, the small joints of the hands, the knees, ankles, hips, and feet commonly are affected.

The third type of JRA, **pauciarticular JRA**, generally affects four or fewer joints in an **asymmetrical pattern**, meaning if a joint on the left side is affected, it typically is not affected on the right side. The joints most commonly involved are the knees, elbows, wrist, and ankles (Dunkin, 2002).

Although symptoms of JRA may be controlled with medication, the child or adolescent still may experience periods of **exacerbation**, or flareup, of their symptoms as the disease activity fluctuates (Brown, 2002). Many drugs are available to treat JRA and often two or more must be used simultaneously in order to achieve disease control (Morrissy & Weinstein, 2006). **Nonsteroidal anti-inflammatory drugs (NSAIDs)** typically are the initial therapeutic intervention used because they provide both analgesia and an anti-inflammatory effect. In the United States, the most commonly used NSAID for children and adolescents with arthritis is naproxen, although other drugs, which fall into the NSAID category, include ibuprofen, and aspirin (Morrissy & Weinstein). Though NSAIDs are generally safe and well tolerated in most children, the medications may cause gastric upset with accompanying reduced general health and well-being in the child or adolescent (Brown, 2002). Other medications used to treat JRA include corticosteroid injections to provide rapid control for severe arthritis and methotrexate, an immune system medication, which is given in a weekly dosage either orally or subcutaneously (Morrissy & Weinstein).

The impact of JRA on a child or adolescent's occupations depends on the age of onset and extent and severity of involvement. Functional skill acquisition and performance needed for play, mobility and ambulation, and self-care are affected by the progression of the child or adolescent's arthritis during the developing years (Brown, 2002). A child or adolescent with debilitating symptoms and multiple joint involvements may struggle with restricted mobility and require assistance or modifications in a variety of occupations (Brown). A toddler may have difficulty achieving developmental skills associated with self-care, especially dressing, because of problems moving arms and legs into a shirt or pants or maintaining a grasp to pull up pants or straightening a shirt on their body. School aged children and adolescents with JRA may have limitations in more physically demanding tasks such as walking long distances or engaging in sports (Brown). It is important to assess their interests and help to make appropriate matches for sports or activities that aren't as demanding on the joints, such as swimming, horseback riding, or certain forms of low-impact dance. These children and adolescents also may have trouble completing ADL, IADL, school related activities, and play activities that require refined wrist or hand involvement or where specific joint limitations exist. Adolescents may have additional limitations when required to write long essay answers on school exams or to work at a part time job which places stress on their joints (Brown).

Interdisciplinary Team Approach

An interdisciplinary team approach is needed to address the various needs of a child and adolescent with JRA. A pediatric **rheumatologist** is a specialist in providing non-surgical treatment to children with rheumatic disease, such as JRA. This specialist provides comprehensive care to the child or adolescent, as well as the family members. The rheumatologist serves as a consultant to the child's or adolescent's primary care physician to discuss treatment plans and medications. An orthopedist may be consulted to assess joint and bone integrity and determine if there are any surgical needs. The child or adolescent with JRA also will benefit from intervention by a physical therapist who provides stretching of the lower extremities and gait training, if needed.

Occupational Therapy Intervention

The goal of occupational therapy for children and adolescents with JRA is to help them learn techniques and strategies to engage in occupations as independently as possible with limited pain and chance of exacerbation. Occupational therapists and occupational therapy assistants use a combination of **joint protection** and **energy conservation** techniques, instruction, exercise, **splinting**, and environmental adaptations to enable children and adolescents to engage in daily occupations.

Joint Protection Techniques

Children and adolescents are instructed to protect their joints and prevent excessive force on joints during occupations (see Table 18.2■). These techniques need to be

■ **Table 18.2**
Joint Protection Techniques

Joint Protection Technique	Example
Use large joints for heavy work.	Carry items in a backpack, over the shoulders or in a wheeled bag, rather than in a bag by the handle.
	Use the forearms and palms of hands rather than fingers to help support a lunch tray, textbook, or other heavy item being carried from one place to another.
Avoid holding any joint in a static position.	When coloring or writing over an extended period of time, take frequent breaks.
	When required to sit for long periods of time, change body positions frequently, getting up to stretch or walk around the area.
Maintain good joint alignment.	Choose a chair that allows feet to rest comfortably on the floor.
	When rising from a seated position, avoid leaning to either side.
	When seated, select a desk height that allows the forearms to rest comfortably.
	Avoid activities that require tight squeezing, pinching, or twisting motion. Instead, use the palm of the hand to turn doorknobs and open lids on containers. Use built up grips on pencils.
Respect pain.	Be aware of personal limits and stop or modify any activity before pain occurs. If pain occurs, discontinue the movement pattern.

Source: Trombly, C. A., & Radomski, M. (Eds.) (2007). *Occupational therapy for physical dysfunction* (6th ed.). Baltimore, MD: Williams & Wilkins.

incorporated into the child's or adolescent's routine so that they become useful habits for preventing further joint damage (Harris, 2001).

Energy Conservation Techniques

Fatigue is a frequent symptom of JRA and can affect the child's or the adolescent's ability to participate in age appropriate occupations. The occupational therapist or the occupational therapy assistant instructs the child or adolescents in energy conservation techniques which help to pace the effort needed to perform a task and avoid excessive fatigue. Table 18.3■ lists common energy conservation techniques with examples applicable to children and adolescents. It is important for a child or adolescent to minimize fatigue that may contribute to an exacerbation of the condition (Harris, 2001).

Exercise

Exercise promotes general health and fitness and should be encouraged for all children and adolescents with JRA as part of a healthy lifestyle. Exercise keeps the muscles and joints functioning as normally as possible by maintaining or improving range of motion, maintaining muscle strength, and preventing disuse atrophy (Pendleton & Schultz-Krohn, 2006). Physical exercise, particularly minimal weight bearing activities such as swimming, water aerobics, and horseback riding, strengthens muscles and increases endurance without adding stress to the joints. Exercise improves posture, overall strength, and flexibility (Harris, 2001). Since chronic pain and fatigue may be present, it is important to individualize exercise suggestions to take into account personal preferences, needs, and tolerances (Pendleton & Schultz-Krohn).

Splinting

Splints are external devices that are applied to a body part for support, to provide immobilization, to correct or prevent deformity, or to provide assistance with movement

■ Table 18.3
Energy Conservation Techniques

ENERGY CONSERVATION PRINCIPLE	EXAMPLE
Minimize effort to complete a task.	Keep toys in smaller containers that are easier to lift.
	Use faucets and door handles with levers rather than twist knobs.
Break down tasks to smaller components.	When completing a large task, such as cleaning the bedroom, divide the job into individual tasks; take rest breaks between individual tasks. Alternate the easy and difficult tasks. Take at least a 10 minute break each hour.
Plan ahead.	When beginning a task, gather all of the supplies at once and avoid unnecessary walking. Allow sufficient time to minimize the need to rush.
Sit whenever possible.	Regardless of the activity, consider ways to sit rather than stand for at least a portion of the time.
Use good body mechanics.	Incorporate good posture into the activity. Keep the back straight and the knees bent when lifting an item from the floor.
	Use a reacher for out of reach items. Push or pull an item rather than carry it. Slide items across a desk, table, or counter rather than pick them up. Use a wheeled book bag or rolled cart to transport items.

Source: Trombly, C. A., & Radomski, M. (Eds.) (2007). *Occupational therapy for physical dysfunction* (6th ed.). Baltimore, MD: Williams & Wilkins.

of the body part (Sladyk & Ryan, 2005). Splints can be custom made by creating a pattern, heating the splinting material, and draping and molding the material on the extremity. Splints also can be ordered already precut in common patterns and be adjusted on the child or adolescent for proper fit (Sladyk & Ryan, 2005).

The fundamental goal of splinting with JRA is to maximize function (Pendleton & Schultz-Krohn, 2006). Often children or adolescents keep their joints bent for long periods of time, such as when sleeping, which causes increased stiffening of the joints. A static splint, or splint with no moving parts, rests and protects a joint or extremity to allow healing, reduce pain, or prevent contractures (Sladyk & Ryan, 2005). A child or adolescent with JRA may benefit from wearing a **resting pan splint** [Figure 18.4(a)■] at night to help keep joints straight, especially the wrist and hand, knee, and ankle, and to aid in preventing night pain and morning stiffness (Cooke, 2004). In cases where the child or adolescent requires additional stability of the wrist during occupational engagement, a wrist splint, called a **cock-up splint** [Figure 18.4(b)■], may be used to provide the necessary support at the wrist, while allowing functional use of the hand. **Ulnar deviation**, or drifting of the metacarpalphalangeal joints toward the small finger, may be a symptom of JRA. If this condition occurs, an **ulnar deviation splint** [Figure 18.4(c)■] may be used to provide improved stability and alignment of the MP joints. This splint, however, can impede functional hand use (Pendleton & Schultz-Krohn, 2006).

Although splinting may be a major part of occupational therapy intervention, it is important to understand that splinting is just one of a multitude of events and experiences for the child and their family (Schroder, Crabtree & Lyall-Watson, 2002). Parents report that their children's cooperation with a splinting regime is essential and that when their children are younger they more easily comply with the program, since they cannot remove the splints. However, as the children grow older, they often remove the splints when they are unsupervised. Wearing the splint can become uncomfortable and make the children feel as if they stand out and are different from others their age. The quality of the therapeutic relationship with the child or adolescent, as well as the parent who is responsible for supervising and following through with the splinting regime, has a strong impact on compliance with splinting. The occupational therapist and occupational therapy assistant who take time to communicate a caring attitude, answer questions, and address personal needs will be more likely to see positive attitudes toward splinting in the child and adolescent with JRA and in their family (Schroder, Crabtree & Lyall-Watson).

Environmental Adaptations

The occupational therapist and the occupational therapy assistant also educate the child, adolescent, family members, and teachers about needed environmental adaptations in the home and at school. The family may need to make modifications in the home so the child or adolescent can navigate easily and independently and have the

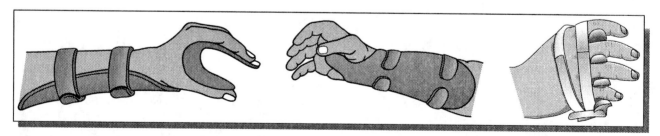

■ Figure 18.4

(a) Resting pan splint; (b) cock-up splint, and (c) ulnar deviation splint.

ability to perform daily occupations with ease and independence. For instance, doorways may need to be widened or nonslip flooring installed to accommodate a child or adolescent with JRA and mobility limitations. Doorknobs and knob type faucets in showers and sinks should be replaced with levers that do not require grasping and turning. Grab bars and nonskid mats in the shower may be necessary for safety. Lowering closets racks and raising or lowering electrical outlets and light switches in the child's or adolescent's bedroom may provide easier access (Arthritis Foundation, 2006).

Additionally, the occupational therapist and the occupational therapy assistant can discuss environmental adaptations that need to be considered by the teacher in the school environment. The child or adolescent may need built up handles on pencils, crayons, scissors, and other manipulatives required for a specific class. The child or adolescent may benefit from a seating evaluation that suggests proper ergonomic positions and alternative seating arrangements to break up long periods of sitting in one position. The occupational therapy assistant might need to assess the different school environments and make suggestions. For example, adaptations may be necessary for the child or adolescent to operate classroom computers, turn handles on faucets or commodes, carry lunch trays through the cafeteria, or manipulate a school locker. Further discussion of occupational therapy interventions are presented in the case study of Alisha.

Alisha

During a routine appointment with her rheumatologist, Alisha, a 14-year-old high school freshman with JRA, informs her doctor that she would like to participate in high school extra-curricular activities and the sports program. Although the doctor explains the importance of avoiding high impact activities and incorporating energy conservation and joint protection techniques during activities, the doctor is uncertain that Alisha understands how to make sensible activity choices. Dr. Angular refers Alisha to the occupational therapy department to help her choose activities that would be compatible with her chronic condition.

After reviewing the referral and medical chart, the occupational therapist requests the occupational therapy assistant to meet with Alisha to review the principles of energy conservation and work simplification, and to analyze sports and activities. Prior to the session, the occupational therapy assistant gathers departmental handouts, modifying the information so that language and examples are pertinent to a high school freshman. She requests that Alisha bring a list of available high school sports and activities and rank them in order of interest.

During the intervention session, the occupational therapy assistant begins by educating Alisha on work simplification, energy conservation, and joint protection techniques. Together they discuss the activities and sports that interest Alisha. The occupational therapy assistant helps her to analyze her chosen activities, often helping her make choices that are more compatible with her chronic condition. For instance, when Alisha indicates an interest in gymnastics, the occupational therapy assistant helps her identify events such as floor exercises or balance beam that would be less stressful on her joints than vaulting or uneven bars. When Alisha indicates that she would like to join the cross-country team but the distance running causes her increased pain, the occupational therapy assistant suggests that she consider volunteering to be a team manager or timer. Alisha also indicates that she likes to work on the school newspaper but often finds the increased typing causes joint pain. The occupational therapy assistant suggests that Alisha use a voice-activated word processing program or a word predictor program that would decrease the number of keyboarding strokes needed to compose her article. The occupational therapy assistant suggests that Alisha join the hospital sponsored adolescent wellness group that focuses on lifetime sports and activities that are compatible with chronic illnesses. She also provides Alisha with information on the Arthritis Foundation aquatic and exercise programs. The occupational therapy assistant documents the intervention session in the medical chart (Figure 18.5■). ■

S: "I would like to join sports and activities at school."
O: 14-year-old female with JRA was referred for occupational therapy consultation to assist adolescent in selection of sports and leisure activities that would not aggravate chronic condition. Reviewed and provided handouts on joint protection, energy conservation, work simplification, and low vs. high impact activities. Initially assisted adolescent in analyzing available high school sports and activities but as session progressed, adolescent was able to complete analysis independently. Also, provided information on programs provided through the hospital and arthritis foundation.
A: Adolescent demonstrated ability to independently analyze activities based on principles presented.
P: No further follow-up required, at this time. Adolescent and parent were advised to contact OT clinic if any questions arise.

■ **Figure 18.5**
Medical chart documentation.

SUMMARY

Three musculoskeletal conditions that often require occupational therapy intervention are arthrogryposis, congenital limb deficiency, and juvenile rheumatoid arthritis. Arthrogryposis, which is caused by decreased movement of the fetus, results in multiple contractures and loss of active range of motion requiring modification to tasks. An upper extremity congenital limb deficiency may require a child or adolescent to learn to operate a prosthesis. Children and adolescents with juvenile rheumatoid arthritis frequently require occupational therapy services to provide joint protection and energy conservation instruction, upper extremity splinting, or modification to tasks during exacerbation of the condition.

Occupational therapist and occupational therapy assistants who work with children and adolescents with orthopedic and musculoskeletal conditions must consider the medical diagnosis and the impact that it has on the ability of children or adolescents to participate in age appropriate occupations. Occupational therapy intervention addresses both the physical and social aspect of the condition.

Many times occupational therapy interventions directed toward adapting or modifying the task or environment will enable better performance and allow success. To provide effective services, the occupational therapist and the occupational therapy assistant work with the child and adolescent and the entire team, which often includes family members, medical providers, and educators.

REVIEWING KEY POINTS

1. Define arthrogryposis, congenital limb deficiency, and juvenile rheumatoid arthritis.
2. Briefly explain how arthrogryposis interferes with a child's or adolescent's ability to perform an age appropriate task.
3. Compare and contrast the following types of prostheses: body powered and externally powered prosthesis, functional and passive prosthesis.
4. Discuss the difference between the following types of terminal devices: hook, myoelectrical hand, and cosmetic hand.
5. Explain the importance of the wrist unit on a prosthesis.

6. Explain the importance of joint protection and energy conservation techniques, particularly for children and adolescents with JRA. Give examples of how to incorporate these principles into a child's or adolescent's daily occupations.
7. Explain the purpose of the following types of splints for children and adolescents with JRA: resting pan, cock up, and ulnar deviation.

APPLYING KEY CONCEPTS

1. Reread Levi's case study. Make a list of five functional tasks that he is unable to complete independently. Develop an intervention plan that adapts or modifies the task or environment. Keep in mind that Levi does not like to look or act different than other children in his classroom.
2. Discuss the possible causes for Levi's difficulties making friends. Develop an intervention plan to help Levi develop his social competency skills.
3. Consider the case study of Travis. What additional interventions may work? Develop other preschool activities that would encourage bilateral hand and prosthetic use.
4. Consider the impact that JRA has on Alisha's occupations as a teenager. List five additional tasks that Alisha might find challenging. List ways she can complete these tasks while adhering to joint protection and energy conservation principles.

REFERENCES

Arthritis Foundation. *Home life: 10 simple household solutions.* Retrieved 9/9/2006. http://www.Arthritis.org/resources/home_life/solutions.asp

Baum, C. M., & Christiansen, C. (2005). Person-environment-occupational performance: An occupation-based framework for practice. In C. Christiansen, C. Baum, & J. Bass-Haugen (Eds.), *Occupational therapy: Performance, participation, and well-being.* Thorofare, NJ: SLACK.

Brown, G. T. (2002). Functional assessment tools for paediatric clients with juvenile chronic arthritis: An update and review for occupational therapists. *Scandinavian Journal of Occupational Therapy, 9*(1), 23–34.

Case-Smith, J. (2005). *Occupational therapy for children* (5th ed.). St. Louis: Mosby.

Cassidy, J., & Petty, R. (2005). *Textbook of pediatric rheumatology* (5th ed.). Philadelphia: W. B. Saunders.

Cassidy, S., & Allanson, J. (2005). *Management of genetic syndromes* (2nd ed.). Hoboken: John Wiley & Sons.

Christiansen, C., & Baum, C. M. (Eds.). (1997). *Occupational therapy: Enabling function and well-being* (2nd ed.). Thorofare, NJ: SLACK.

Cooke, K. (2004). Splinting joints with juvenile rheumatoid arthritis. *Healthwise.* Retrieved August 12, 2006, http://www.yahoo.com/topic/rheumatoidarthritis/resources/article/healthwise/hw100907.

Coster, W., Denney, T., Haltiwanger, J., & Haley, S. (1998). *School Functional Assessment (SFA).* San Antonio, TX: The Psychological Corporation.

Dunkin, M. A. (2002). Arthritis 101: Juvenile rheumatoid arthritis. *Arthritis Today, 6*/28/2002.

Harris, E. D. Jr. (2001). Clinical features of rheumatoid arthritis. In S. Ruddy et al. (Eds.), *Kelley's textbook of rheumatology* (6th ed.), vol. 2. Philadelphia: Saunders.

Meier, R., & Atkins, D. (2004). *Functional restoration of adults and children with upper extremity amputation.* New York: Demos Medical Publishing, Inc.

Morrissy, R., & Weinstein, S. (2006). *Lovell and Winter's pediatric orthopaedics* (6th ed.). Philadelphia: Lippincott, Williams & Wilkins.

Olson, D., & DeRuyter, F. (2002). *Clinician's guide to assistive technology.* St. Louis: Mosby.

Pendleton, H. M., & Schultz-Krohn, W. (2006). *Pedretti's occupational therapy practice skills for physical dysfunction* (6th ed). St. Louis: Mosby.

Reed, K. (2001). *Quick reference guide to occupational therapy* (2nd ed.). Gaithersburg, MD: Aspen Publications.

Schroder, N., Crabtree, M., & Lyall-Watson, S. (2002). The effectiveness of splinting as perceived by the parents of children with juvenile idiopathic arthritis. *British Journal of Occupational Therapy, 65*(2), 75–80.

Sladyk, K., & Ryan, S. (2005). *Ryan's occupational therapy assistant: Principles, practice issues, and techniques* (4th ed). Thorofare, NJ: SLACK.

Trombly, C. A., Radomski, M. (Eds.). (2007). *Occupational therapy for physical dysfunction* (6th ed.). Baltimore, MD: Williams & Wilkins.

Young, N. L. (n.d.) *The Activities Scale for Kids manual.* Toronto: The Hospital for Sick Children.

Chapter 19

Children and Adolescents with Neural Tube Defects

Dorothy L. Rockwell

Key Terms

Alpha-fetoprotein (AFP)
Anencephaly
Arnold Chiari malformation
Flaccid paralysis
Hydrocephalus
Incontinent
Kyphosis
Level of lesion
Lordosis
Meningocele

Myelomeningocele
Neural tube defect
Orthosis
Orthotics
Scoliosis
Shunt
Spina bifida
Spina bifida occulta
Tethered cord

Objectives

- Explain the group of birth defects known as neural tube defects.
- Examine the impact of myelomeningocele on the occupations of children and adolescents.
- Describe occupational therapy interventions to support the capacity of children and adolescents with myelomeningocele to participate in their daily occupations.
- Examine how occupational therapists and occupational therapy assistants problem solve together during the intervention process.
- Describe how occupational therapists and occupational therapy assistants work with families and other professionals to provide services to children and adolescents with myelomeningocele.

INTRODUCTION

This chapter contains an overview of the most common neural tube defects followed by an extensive discussion of myelomeningocele, or spina bifida, and its impact on the occupations of children and adolescents. It then discusses appropriate occupational therapy interventions for various age levels of children and adolescents with spina bifida in a variety of practice settings.

NEURAL TUBE DEFECTS: AN OVERVIEW

Types of Neural Tube Defects

The term **neural tube defect** refers to a group of birth defects which occur during the first 30 days of embryonic development. During the first days of embryonic development the layer of cells that become the central nervous system folds onto itself and becomes a closed tube. A neural tube defect results when the developing tube fails to close correctly. The spectrum of neural tube defects ranges from spina bifida occulta to anencephaly. Each is described briefly below (Sandler, 1997).

The cause of neural tube defects is unknown. However, current research shows that having an intake of 0.4 mgs of the B vitamin folic acid before conception decreases the incidence of neural tube defects by 70 percent (March of Dimes, 2006). Prenatal screening for neural tube defects is accomplished by a simple blood test that looks for elevated levels of **alpha-fetoprotein (AFP)** in the mother's blood stream. AFP is a type of antigen or protein present in the developing fetus. An AFP screening at 13 weeks of pregnancy is part of routine prenatal care in many countries, including the United States (Sandler, 1997). An elevated AFP result is followed by ultrasound to determine if a neural tube defect is present. If the defect exists, the pregnant woman is advised of the condition and the medical options available to her and the fetus. The incidence of neural tube defects in the United States is 1 per 1,000 live births (March of Dimes).

The least problematic form of neural tube defect is **spina bifida occulta**. The term spina bifida means cleft spine; the term occulta means hidden. In spina bifida occulta there is an opening in the bones that form the spinal column. There is no mark on the skin to show what has happened to the bones and there is no damage to the spinal cord (see Figure 19.1■). There may be a small hairy patch on the back at the level of the defect. It is estimated that 3 to 5 percent of people who have spina bifida occulta are never diagnosed unless they have another reason to have their spine x-rayed (NICHCY, 2006).

The next level of involvement is **meningocele.** In this condition, the meninges or covering around the spinal cord are pushed out through the opening in the spine and through an opening in the skin. At birth, a balloon like sac is noted on the back (see Figure 19.2■). Surgical closure of the defect and repair of the spine is required to prevent infection or damage to the spinal cord. When this is complete, the child should have normal sensory and motor function of the spinal cord (Sandler, 1997).

The most severe neural tube defect which always results in infant death is **anencephaly.** In this defect the majority of the brain, skull, and skin fail to form, exposing the brain stem. These children usually are stillborn or die shortly after birth (NINDS, 2006).

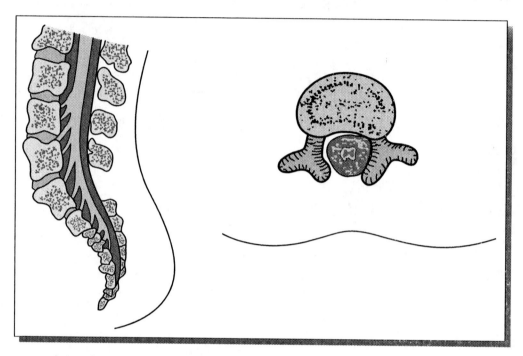

■ **Figure 19.1**
Spina bifida occulta.

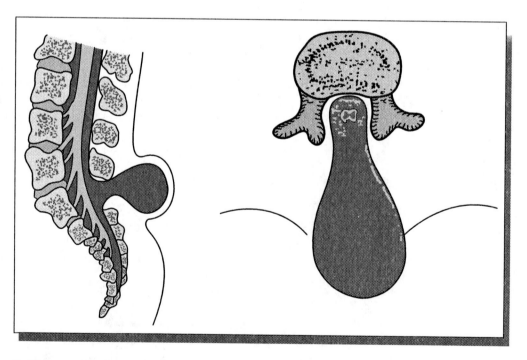

■ **Figure 19.2**
Meningocele.

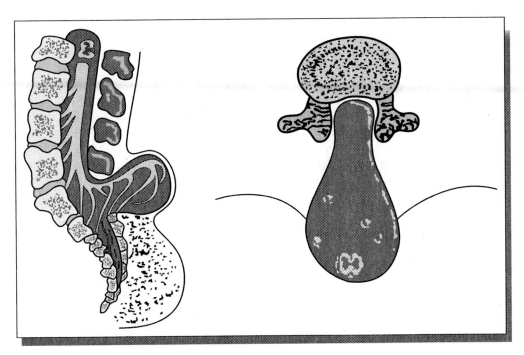

■ **Figure 19.3**
Myelomeningocele.

Myelomeningocele is the most common and the second most severe type of neural tube defect. Ninety-four percent of all neural tube defects are of this type. Infants born with myelomeningocele survive. A myelomeningocele may be present at any place along the spine, from the cervical to the lumbar areas, with 80 percent occurring in the lumbar and sacral areas of the spinal column (NICHCY, 2006). Medical professionals who work frequently with children with myelomeningocele use the shorthand phrase **level of the lesion** to discuss where the defect occurs and to understand the functional implications of the defect. In myelomeningocele, the meninges, deformed spinal cord, and cerebral spinal fluid are seen in prenatal ultrasound scans and are visible as a sac on the child's back at the time of birth (see Figure 19.3■). Once the child is born, surgical closure of the back generally is completed within 24 to 48 hours as long as the child is medically stable. This prevents possible systemic infection from entering the body through the opening (Sandler, 1997).

The spinal cord, including both motor and sensory nerves below the level of the lesion, almost always is damaged and nonfunctional. While the surgical repair of the back prevents infection and restores the integrity of the spinal column, it can not restore spinal cord function. Thus, the child has sensory and motor quadriplegia or sensory and motor paraplegia of the flaccid paralysis type depending upon where the lesion occurs along the spinal column. Quadriplegia means that all four extremities are involved, while paraplegia means the lower extremities are involved. **Flaccid paralysis** means there is no underlying muscle tone present in the muscle groups affected (Sandler, 1997). This is in contrast to a child with spastic quadriplegia, such as a child with cerebral palsy, who has high muscle tone in the muscles affected. Limbs affected by flaccid paralysis are at risk for dislocation and fracture if they are not properly protected during positioning and movement. The muscles and tendons are not able to keep the bones in alignment (Sandler).

Occupational therapists and the occupational therapy assistants need to be familiar with the functional implications of spinal cord injury and the muscle groups that are affected at each level when planning the interventions for children and adolescents with myelomeningocele. Though both sensory and motor functions are lost beginning at the level of the lesion, slight motor, sensory, and functional differences may occur between the right and left sides of the children's body. Table 19.1■ illustrates the motor function and functional implications of the different levels of myelomeningocele. Young children with flaccid paralysis have difficulty moving in the environment to engage in their daily living, play, and exploratory occupations. Thus, they may experience delays in their development. In addition, spina bifida compromises the amount of sensory information these children feel as they move their bodies, and as they touch and are touched by people and objects, limiting an important way to learn about the environment.

Though **spina bifida** is not the correct medical term, it is used commonly to describe the myelomeningocele level of neural tube defect. The Spina Bifida Association of America promotes this word usage in its publications (Spina Bifida Association of America, 2007). In the intervention portion of this chapter, the term spina bifida refers to children and adolescents with the myelomeningocele form of neural tube defect.

Related Medical Complications

In addition to the deformed spinal cord and spinal column 90 percent of children with spina bifida also have **hydrocephalus** (NICHCY, 2006). The brain contains four ven-

■ **Table 19.1**
Functional Expectations of Levels of Spina Bifida

LEVEL OF LESION	MOTOR FUNCTIONS PRESENT	FUNCTIONAL IMPLICATIONS
C8–T1	Has full use of upper extremities. Has poor or absent trunk control. Is incontinent in bowel and bladder functions.	Needs assistive technology for mobility; needs thoracic, hip, knee, and ankle orthotic for body alignment and ambulation
T4–T6	Has increased trunk control because long muscles of the back are active. Is incontinent of bowel and bladder functions.	Ambulates short distances using thoracic, hip, knee and ankle orthosis
T9–T12	Has improved trunk control because of active abdominal muscles. Is incontinent of bowel and bladder functions.	Ambulates longer distances using thoracic, hip, knee, and ankle orthosis
L2–L3	Has good trunk control. Can flex hips, and abduct and extend knees. Is incontinent of bowel and bladder.	Needs knee, ankle foot orthosis. Uses a wheelchair for energy conservation
L4, L5	Can flex hips and extend knees. Has weak knee flexion. Is incontinent of bowel and bladder functions.	Needs ankle and foot orthosis
Sacral	Has limited ankle control. May have some bowel and bladder control.	May need ankle and foot orthosis

Rothstein, Roy, & Wolf, 2005.

tricles connected by channels through which the cerebrospinal fluid (CSF) flows. The CSF passes into cisterns at the base of the brain. It then is absorbed into the bloodstream. When something prevents the fluid from passing from ventricle to ventricle or from being absorbed into the bloodstream, it builds up in the ventricle. This increases the size of the ventricle and compresses the tissue of the brain against the bones of the skull, resulting in damage of the brain tissue. Prolonged pressure causes irreparable brain damage (Sandler, 1997).

Untreated hydrocephalus causes the head circumference to enlarge or the fontanelles to bulge. Ultrasound scans of the head help to determine if hydrocephalus is present and if a **shunt** is needed. A shunt is a thin, flexible tube with a one way valve and reservoir. One end is inserted into a ventricle through a small hole in the skull. The remaining length of tubing then is threaded under the skin and inserted into the abdominal cavity or the atrium of the heart where the fluid drains (see Figure 19.4■). The reservoir can be pressed through the skin to test if it is working. It also holds a small amount of CSF. A needle can be inserted into the reservoir to check the CSF for infections. If hydrocephalus is detected at birth, the neurosurgeon inserts a shunt following closure of the open area on the back as soon as it is medically possible (Sandler, 1997).

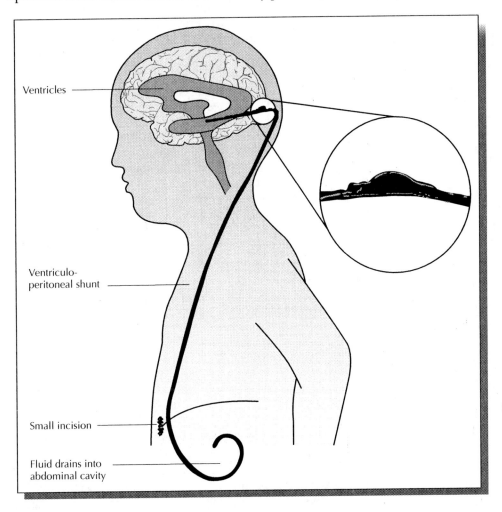

Ventricles

Ventriculo-
peritoneal shunt

Small incision

Fluid drains into
abdominal cavity

■ **Figure 19.4**
A shunt.

The **Arnold Chiari malformation**, or the Chiari malformation, is an associated condition present in almost all children with spina bifida (Batshaw, 1997). It is a downward displacement of a portion of the brain into the neck through the foramen magnum, an opening in the base of the skull through which the spinal cord passes. The Arnold Chiari malformation can cause life threatening breathing problems in the infant, feeding and swallowing difficulties, and upper extremity weakness or spasticity. Treatment requires surgical replacement of the tissue into the cranium. Permanent damage can be averted if the malformation is corrected when it is detected (Batshaw, 1997).

Another frequently occurring problem confronting children with myelomeningocele is the **tethered cord** syndrome. The spinal cord becomes trapped or tethered on the deformed bony tissue of the spinal column or on the scars formed as a result of the surgical repair of the original spina bifida. Because of this tethering or entrapment, the spinal cord does not move freely within the spinal column when the body flexes and extends. This causes the spinal cord to become stretched and can result in additional, permanent damage. Children with spina bifida who begin to experience changes in the sensory or motor functions of the lower extremities or changes in bowel and bladder habits may have a tethered cord. Surgical release of the cord can prevent permanent damage; affected functions will resume as healing takes place (National Institute of Neurological Disorders and Stroke, 2006).

Children and adolescents with spina bifida also may develop spinal deformities as a result of their neural tube defect, resulting in improper bony growth. Spinal deformity secondary to flaccid paralysis or improper positioning over a prolonged period of time may occur. One common spinal deformity is **scoliosis**. Scoliosis is present in 80 percent of children with thoracic level lesions, 50 percent of those with mid-lumbar level lesions, and 20 percent of those with low-lumbar lesions (Sandler, 1997). With scoliosis, the spine curves in an S shape and can cause uneven pressure on the ischium, the bones upon which an individual sits. Because of the scoliosis, the internal organs may become compressed and pushed out of their proper position as the body collapses upon itself. A child with scoliosis may have decreased respiratory capacity and be at risk for pneumonia. The deformity can cause difficulty with mobility, decreased voice production, and impaired bowel and bladder function. It also can restrict upper extremity function because it puts the trunk in a compromised position that limits full range of motion. Early detection and proper intervention by the orthopedist is critical in addressing potential spinal deformity. Treatment of scoliosis may require surgery to align the bones of the spine and hold them in alignment, or may involve wearing a body brace for a specified period of time to apply external pressure to the bones and guide them into alignment.

Other spinal deformities found in children with spina bifida are **kyphosis** and **lordosis**. Kyphosis is characterized by a rounding of the back into a forward curving posture. Lordosis is characterized by an inward curving of the lower back, sometimes called a sway back. Similar to scoliosis, lordosis and kyphosis can compromise the functions of internal organs and interfere with body movements (Lutkenhoff, 1999). (See Figures 19.5■ and 19.6■.)

Finally, children with spina bifida are at risk for developing osteoporosis. The bones of the child with spina bifida may become brittle and osteoporotic secondary to flaccid paralysis. In flaccid paralysis the muscles do not exert any pull on the bone and there is no active weight bearing. As a result, they may fracture easily (Lutkenhoff, 1999).

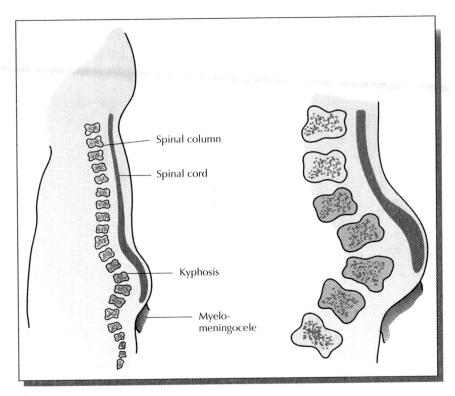

■ Figure 19.5
Scoliosis and kyphosis, lateral view.

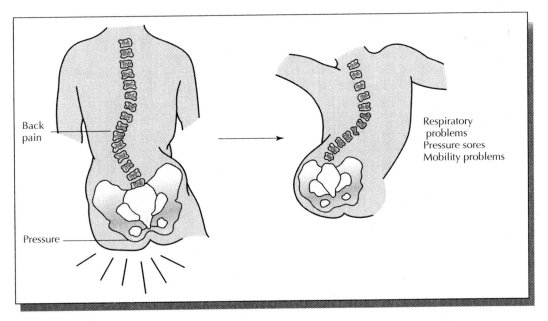

■ Figure 19.6
Scoliosis and kyphosis, posterior view.

IMPACT OF SPINA BIFIDA ON BODY FUNCTIONS

Spina bifida negatively affects movement related, sensory, genitourinary, reproductive functions, and mental functions (AOTA, 2002). Consequently, children and adolescents with spina bifida cope with multiple performance challenges that can limit their participation in their daily life activities.

Movement Related Functions

Depending on the level of lesion, young children with spina bifida may not acquire developmentally typical motor skills such as rolling over, coming to a sitting position, getting into a quadruped position, crawling, and coming to stand followed by cruising and walking. Providing external supports for their flaccid leg muscles and flaccid or decreased trunk muscles assists the children and adolescents in achieving and maintaining functional positions such as sitting or standing, and in accessing their environment. External supports worn on the body are called **orthotics**. The level of lesion and the resultant paralysis determines the type of orthotics needed. Some children and adolescents need orthotics that provide support for the entire body from the trunk to

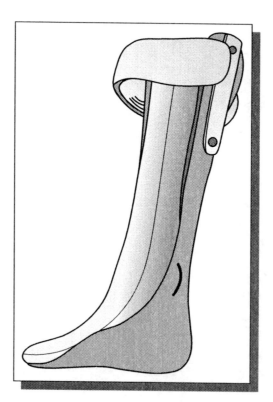

■ **Figure 19.7**
Ankle-foot orthosis.

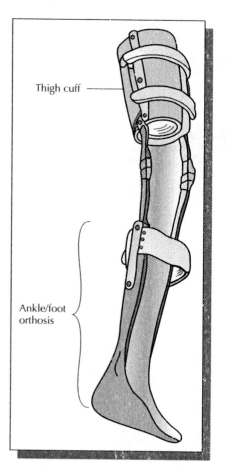

Thigh cuff

Ankle/foot
orthosis

■ **Figure 19.8**
Knee-ankle-foot orthosis with
thigh cuff.

the toes; others need support only for the ankle and foot. Orthotists, medical professionals skilled in the design and fabrication of orthotics, fit them to the child's or adolescent's body. Properly fitting orthotics provide enough support for the children and adolescents to sit independently and to maintain or be placed in a standing position (Lutkenhoff, 1999; Sandler, 1997).

Orthotics are named for the body parts they support and generally are spoken of by their initials. An AFO is an ankle-foot **orthosis;** a KAFO is a knee-ankle-foot orthosis; and a HKAFO is a hip-knee-ankle-foot orthosis. The HKAFO usually has an attachment which provides support to the trunk. This trunk support may be a thermoplastic support molded to fit the trunk of the child and provide maximum support, or it may be a sturdy fabric which closes with Velcro fasteners over the abdomen. Various orthotics are illustrated in Figures 19.7■, 19.8■, and 19.9■.

External orthotic supports allow children and adolescents to bear weight through their lower extremities. Lower extremity weight bearing contributes to bone development and may prevent the development of osteoporosis. Orthotics provide protection for the hip, knee, and ankle joints by keeping them in good alignment; the orthotics

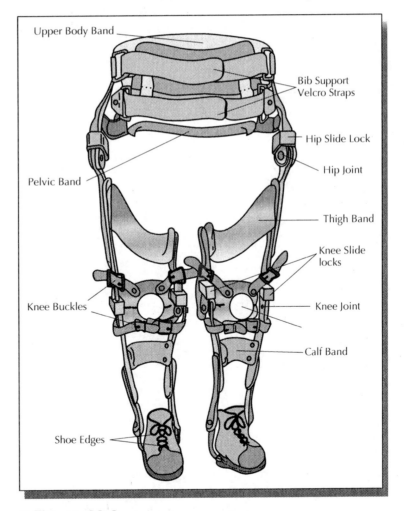

■ **Figure 19.9**
Hip-knee-ankle-foot orthosis with pelvic band and thoracic support.

also cushion the bones of the lower extremities, thereby decreasing the chance for fractures. Proper positioning prevents contracture and facilitates mobility, which allows the children to explore and develop mastery over their environments. Through this movement, children and adolescents learn about their own bodies and how they interact with objects in the environment. In addition, through physically exploring the environment, the children and adolescents refine their visual perceptual abilities.

When providing interventions, it is important for occupational therapists and occupational therapy assistants to know how the orthosis functions, how to correctly position the children and the adolescents in their orthosis, and how to check for pressure areas following its wear. A schedule of times is developed to help the children and adolescents develop wearing tolerance. Those children and adolescents who have the capacity to do so are taught how to don and doff their orthosis, and to inspect the skin under the orthosis for signs of pressure or redness when it is removed. Exact guidelines for donning and doffing the orthosis and for developing wearing tolerance may be established by the orthopedist or by the orthotist. The occupational therapist and occupational therapy assistant involved in donning and doffing new orthotics need to be familiar with the wearing times and report any problems to the appropriate professional.

Orthotic devices may be used either alone or in conjunction with a belly board, stander, crutches, or a wheelchair to enable children and adolescents to become mobile. Children can explore their environment safely while lying prone on a belly board. To accommodate the difference in their body sizes, there are belly boards designed for infants and young children, and belly boards designed for older children. A belly board is a flat, padded board with wheels that extends from the child's upper chest to the ankles (see Figure 19.10■). The child uses his upper extremities to propel the belly board. A strap fastened over the back prevents the child from accidentally rolling off the board. A variety of standing devices is available to enable the children and adolescents to stand independently, freeing their arms and hands for environmental ac-

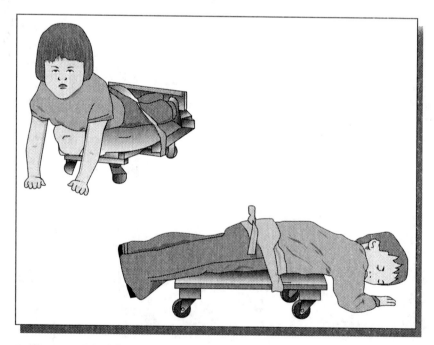

■ **Figure 19.10**
Belly board.

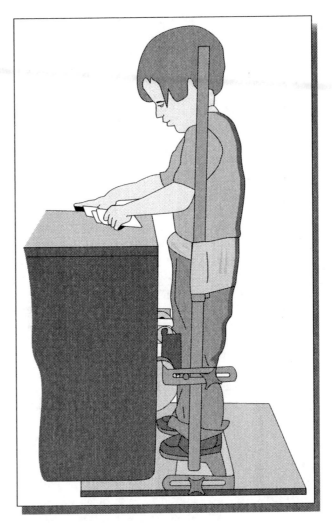

■ Figure 19.11
Prone stander or parapodium.

cess. There are prone standers (see Figure 19.11■) and wheelchairs that convert to a standing position. Straps attached to the standing devices provide support to the trunk, hips, upper and lower legs, and feet, as needed. Standing devices can be used in the classroom or in the home settings as an alternative to sitting (Lutkenhoff, 1999; Sandler, 1997).

Children and adolescents may be taught to ambulate using crutches or walkers. The physical therapist works with the orthopedic specialist to determine the best method of independent ambulation. Regardless of the level of lesion, many children and adolescents elect to use a wheelchair for mobility over long distances to conserve energy or to transport materials in the school setting. Using crutches limits their ability to transport anything else with their hands while standing or walking. While a backpack may be used to transport lightweight objects, doing so requires adjustments to the gait pattern. The physical therapist explores options with the child or adolescent who wants to use one. Older adolescents often elect to use a wheelchair exclusively for mobility because the weight of their orthosis makes independent ambulation too difficult. Regardless of the method of mobility, children and adolescents use their orthosis to maintain proper body positioning, stand, and transfer (Lutkenhoff, 1999).

Many children with spina bifida are overweight due to inactivity. Because the additional weight makes transfers and mobility more difficult, it is important for children and adolescents to be involved in leisure time activities that allow for appropriate physical exercise without risking fractures. The occupational therapist or occupational therapy assistant can work with the children, the adolescents, and their families to identify active leisure pursuits available within the community such as swimming, conditioning training, and recreational walking. Many children and adolescents are able to participate in the Special Olympics and organized competitive wheelchair sports. Children and adolescents also can attend camps, such as those sponsored by the Spina Bifida Association of America, which provide opportunity for the development of lifelong leisure skills and friendships (Sandler, 1997).

Sensory Functions

Children and adolescents with spina bifida do not have sensory function below the level of their lesion. Because the sensations of touch, pressure, pain, temperature, and body position are affected, these children and adolescents need to learn to visually monitor their lower body position and to protect their lower extremities from potentially dangerous insults to the skin. They need to inspect their skin as part of their everyday activities of daily living. Full length mirrors and hand held mirrors that have flexible, tube handles are useful for checking all body surfaces.

Genitourinary and Reproductive Functions

The majority of children and adolescents with spina bifida are **incontinent** in their bowel and bladder functions. Only 15 percent of children with low sacral level lesions have bowel and bladder control without the use of medication or other intervention. All other children and adolescents will require specific intervention for bowel and bladder control. The urologist is the specialist who determines the specific program for each child. The goal of bowel and bladder management is to prevent bladder infections and to achieve controlled continence by the time other children learn bowel and bladder control. This means the child learns to time when and how to empty the bowel and bladder to avoid accidental wetting or soiling. Management of bladder control may include medication to increase bladder tone and the ability of the bladder to hold and release urine, timed emptying of the bladder by catheterization or by pressure on the bladder, and dietary control of liquid intake. Management of bowel control includes scheduled times when the child sits on the toilet, dietary management, and the use of stool softeners. Most children with spina bifida can achieve bowel and bladder control at the age when other nondisabled children achieve control, facilitating social integration (Sandler, 1997).

Adolescents with spina bifida experience the body changes associated with puberty in the same way as other adolescents. However, there is documentation associated with the early onset of puberty in children with spina bifida. This early onset of puberty is called precocious puberty. It may bring premature sexual development and cause the growth plates of the bones to mature, limiting full growth (Sandler, 1997). The occupational therapist and the occupational therapy assistant can collaborate with the family and the educational staff to provide developmentally appropriate education about these body changes, and about body image and sexuality.

Mental Functions

The cognitive abilities of children and adolescents with spina bifida range from severely mentally retarded to gifted, but most commonly are average to below average. The children and adolescents tend to score higher on verbal than on motor skills on standardized tests (Sandler, 1997). Regardless of their basic cognitive level, most children and adolescents with spina bifida have some learning and visual perceptual difficulties (Porr & Rainville, 1999). Learning strategies that emphasize verbal skills tap into these language strengths. Chapter 22 describes additional interventions useful for children and adolescents with spina bifida who demonstrate learning difficulties and perceptual deficits.

THE ROLE OF THE OCCUPATIONAL THERAPIST AND OCCUPATIONAL THERAPY ASSISTANT IN THE INTERVENTION PROCESS

Because spina bifida affects multiple body functions, it can compromise the ability of these children and adolescents to participate fully in their daily life occupations throughout their life. As part of the occupational therapy process, the occupational therapist and occupational therapy assistant consider how to adapt the occupations and the task demands, promote performance skills and useful performance patterns, and modify the context to facilitate the ability of the children and adolescents to participate in occupations important to them. Interventions are provided at different times, in a variety of practice settings, and on multiple occasions as the children grow and develop from infancy through adulthood. In their provision of services, the occupational therapist and the occupational therapy assistant work collaboratively with the family and many other health care and educational professionals, such as nurses, urologists, orthopedists, orthotists, learning specialists, counselors, and physical therapists. They must have a thorough working knowledge of the anatomy and physiology of spinal cord, and the impact of spinal cord injury on body structures and body functions to provide competent services. They also must have a solid understanding of child and adolescent growth and development, and family cultures to provide services that are age appropriate and socially relevant. The following case studies outline occupational therapy services that may be offered to children and adolescents with spina bifida at varying points in their development.

Kelli

Kelli is 5 years of age and lives with her aunt, grandmother, and cousins. She attends the prekindergarten inclusion class offered by her school district. Kelli has a T7 level of spina bifida and hydrocephalus controlled by a ventriculo-peritoneal shunt. She has full range of motion and intact sensation in her upper extremities. All muscle groups controlling her arms and hands are fully functional. Her lower extremities have no sensation or tone. Her trunk is weak because only the muscles of her upper chest are active. Her lower abdominal muscles and back extensors are not active. When placed in a sitting position with her legs out in front of her she collapses forward unless she uses at least one arm to keep her trunk upright. Kelli tends to lean on her left arm, as she prefers to use her right hand for most one-handed activities. This limits her opportunities to experiment with activities that develop bilateral upper extremity coordination.

Kelli requires full bracing to sit with an erect back, to stand, and to facilitate mobility. Her bracing includes a thoraco-lumbar-sacral orthotic, also called a body jacket, attached to long leg braces with a positioning device for the foot. There are locking joints at the hips and knees which can be unlocked to allow for movement but which can be locked in extension for standing or walking. Kelli uses a belly board, also called a prone scooter, to move around the house and in her classroom. She also uses a manual wheelchair for traveling long distances and for seated positioning at a table. Kelli is learning to ambulate with cuff crutches. She is fearful of movement experiences other than moving herself on her belly board or in her wheelchair.

As part of her Individualized Education Program, the occupational therapist administers the Peabody Developmental Motor Scales (Folio, 2000) and the Developmental Test of Visual Motor Integration (Hammil, Pearson, & Voress, 1998). On these standardized assessments, Kelli scores within the 3.5 year range of development. Like many other children her age with a high level of spina bifida, Kelli demonstrates delays in performing academic, self-care, and play occupations that involve fine motor coordination and visual perception. Her fear

of movement also limits her participation in these occupations. For example, she has difficulty cutting with scissors, coloring, completing puzzles and craft projects, manipulating food and storage containers, and managing school bag and jacket fasteners. Because she is hesitant about leaning forward to retrieve objects that are not within her immediate grasp, she does not spontaneously participate in ball playing activities or games that require her to reach across the table. She also is afraid to reach forward to wash her hands or assist with toileting care.

In collaboration with the teacher, the occupational therapist and the occupational therapy assistant work with Kelli in the classroom to promote her participation in school related academic, self-care, and play occupations. They specifically focus on facilitating the development of visual motor, visual perceptual, fine motor skills, and adaptive movement patterns necessary for her to participate in her school related occupations. In addition, they work with the teacher and the administrators to adapt the tasks and environment to support Kelli's inclusion in school life.

To guide the occupational therapy intervention, the occupational therapist and the occupational therapy assistant draft a series of goals and objectives (see Figure 19.12■). Prior to implementing the plan, they meet with the other members of the IEP team and Kelli's aunt and grandmother to modify and finalize the draft.

The occupational therapist and the occupational therapy assistant select the Person-Environment-Occupation model (Law et al., 1996) to guide their clinical reasoning as they design and implement the intervention. Consistent with this model, they direct their interventions toward facilitating the development of Kelli's motor and perceptual skills as well as toward adapting the task and the environment to maximize Kelli's engagement in her academic, self-care, and play occupations. Consistent with the model, most of the interventions take place in the natural environment of the school classroom, bathroom, cafeteria, and play areas. Occasionally, when Kelli needs a private or distraction reduced environment to practice, the occupational therapist or occupational therapy assistant works with her in the occupational therapy room which is in a mobile unit outside the main building. Table 19.2■ illustrates examples of using the PEO model to implement Kelli's occupational therapy program.

As requested by the occupational therapist, the occupational therapy assistant completes an analysis of various classroom activities and discusses Kelli's ability to use school tools and manipulate objects with the classroom teacher. Jointly they decide which activities Kelli should be encouraged to try to complete independently, and which activities should be modified for her. They also determine how to implement a Best Buddy system within the classroom. The occupational therapy assistant evaluates the workspace, and adjusts the height of the table to accommodate the wheelchair and provide a secure working surface. The occupational therapist then suggests ways the teacher may include activities in the classroom that promote the development of the radial side of the hand while stabilizing with the ulnar two fingers. This is the pattern needed for both cutting and the successful control of writing tools. The teacher and the occupational therapy assistant create several activity stations in the classroom that contain fine motor manipulatives that all of the students can use. They construct

- An art station with small scraps of paper, materials, wooden sticks, tape, scissors, and glue for creating collages
- A food preparation station with containers, clay, tongs, and cookie cutters
- A building station with construction toys, marbles, and marble run designs

1. Kelli will use school tools selected by her teacher to complete activities within the classroom independently.
   a. Kelli will control alignment and manipulation of scissors to cut out basic shapes within 1/2" of the line 4/5 times.
   b. Kelli will use art and craft supplies to color and paint within a target area staying within 1/2" of the outside margin 4/5 times.
   c. Kelli will retrieve desk supplies, including stapler, tape dispenser, and glue stick, to fasten objects together 4/5 times.
   d. Kelli will align puzzle pieces to independently complete 10-piece interlocking puzzles that are 2 inches or smaller in size.
2. Kelli will open and close food and school supply containers, independently.
   a. Kelli will open and close food containers including milk carton and snack boxes independently without spillage 4/5 times.
   b. Kelli will open the packet containing utensils for eating and drinking 4/5 times.
   c. Kelli will open and close school supply containers, including crayon boxes, paint bottles, art supply bags, and construction toy bins, independently 4/5 times.
3. Kelli will manipulate the fasteners on her school bag and upper body clothing independently.
   a. Kelli will manipulate the zipper and buckle on her school bag independently 4/5 times.
   b. Kelli will manipulate the zipper and large size buttons on her jacket and shirts independently 4/5 times.
4. Kelli will perform self-care activities and participate in play activities with her peers.
   a. Kelli will wash her hands independently while maintaining balance at the sink using adaptive strategies.
   b. Kelli will retrieve materials that are 2 or more feet beyond the center of her body using adaptive strategies to maintain her balance.
   c. Kelli will use adaptive equipment to reach for materials that are more than 2 feet beyond the center of her body.

■ **Figure 19.12**
Kelli's IEP goals.

■ **Table 19.2**
Intervention Strategies Using the PEO Model

	INTERVENTIONS TO DEVELOP SKILLS	INTERVENTION TO COMPENSATE FOR LIMITED SKILLS
Person	Provide activities to develop the use of the radial side of the hand: pinching bits of play dough, pushing in and pulling out large plastic pegs, tearing paper into small pieces to complete a mosaic picture.	Use double loop scissors to pattern the cutting process. Position Kelli in wheelchair or in a freedom stander that provides trunk support and place objects on a slant board to promote upper extremity function.
Environment	Seat Kelli at table next to peers who model classroom performance expectations. Work with Kelli in the natural environment associated with the task.	Provide additional time for Kelli to complete the task in a distraction reduced workspace. Install extended handles on faucets and doors. Arrange for a Best Buddy system to assist Kelli with completing difficult tasks.
Occupation	Upgrade the complexity of the cutting task and the containers to open as Kelli gains more skill.	Provide Kelli with precut materials and easy open containers. Substitute Velcro for clothing fasteners.

All of the stations contain patterns and designs that the students can copy when arranging their art, cooking, or building projects. All of the stations also have smocks for the students to use to protect their clothing. The smocks have various types and sizes of fasteners. There is a sink in the classroom where the students are expected to wash and dry their hands after participating in each of the activity stations to help maintain cleanliness and control the spread of germs. The occupational therapy assistant joins Kelli at these play stations, grading the activities to promote Kelli's fine motor, visual motor, perceptual, and balance skills. After this, the occupational therapy assistant works with Kelli in the classroom, bathroom, and cafeteria to promote her use of school tools and supplies in their natural context. ■

Brooke

Brooke is a 10-year-old. He attends fifth grade and is an excellent student. He has a T12–L1 level of lesion and hydrocephalus controlled by a ventriculo-atrial shunt. He has full range of motion, strength, and sensation in his upper extremities. He has good trunk control and active hip flexion, but no sensation below the waist. Brooke uses a knee-ankle-foot orthosis (KAFO) and ambulates using cuff crutches and a four point gait pattern. He uses a wheelchair for long distance mobility and for speed, and to conserve energy. He is incontinent of bowel and bladder but, until recently, remained dry and avoided soiling accidents by following a program established by the urologist and physiatrist. The program included intermittent catheterization for bladder management and dietary routine with regular toileting for bowel emptying. Recently, however, Brooke began to have soiling and wetting accidents at school despite following the established routine. He complained that he was getting tired walking at school and was having headaches. Brooke's parents recognized these as possible signs of a tethered cord and called his primary care physician. Brooke was admitted to Children's Hospital and scheduled for a surgical release of the tethered cord.

Following the surgery he was referred to occupational therapy for evaluation and intervention to develop strategies for sustaining his health and participation in age appropriate activities and occupations. The occupational therapist administered the Functional Independence Measure (FIMs), the Canadian Occupational Performance Measure (COPM), and the Pediatric Activities Card Sort (PACS). The FIMS provided an objective measurement of Brook's self care and mobility skills. The COPM enabled the occupational therapist to identify Brooke's and his parents' concerns about skin care, bladder management, weight control, and participation in community activities. The PACS provided a means for Brooke to self-rate his frequency of participation in personal care, school/productivity, hobbies/social, and sports occupations. Based on the data gathered from these measurement tools, Brooke and his parents identified a desire for Brooke to learn to complete his bladder care independently and to assume responsibility for daily skin inspection, so that he could have more ownership of his body functions and more privacy in regard to toileting functions. In addition, Brooke and his parents identified that they wanted to find community sports and fitness programs where Brooke could socialize and help manage his weight. (See Figure 19.13■.)

1. Brooke will complete self-catheterization at bedside and in the bathroom successfully 4/4 times.
   a. Brooke will list and gather the materials needed for self-catheterization.
   b. Brooke will list the steps needed to maintain a clean field during self-catheterization.
   c. Brooke will demonstrate the ability to handle the catheter, wash his hands and body parts, and complete the catheterization.
2. Brooke will complete skin inspection successfully 4/4 times.
   a. Brooke will identify the areas of his body that need to be inspected daily.
   b. Brooke will develop a checklist for use in daily skin inspection.
   c. Brooke will gather the necessary supplies and demonstrate the ability to inspect his body for skin integrity, using the checklist.

■ **Figure 19.13**
Brooke's Goals.

3. Brooke will participate in community sports and fitness programs.
   a. Brooke will describe the importance of maintaining health through participation in community fitness and sports programs.
   b. Brooke will identify three sports and fitness programs that interest him.
   c. Brooke will locate and enroll in a weekly community sports and fitness program.

■ **Figure 19.13**
Brooke's Goals (cont.)

The occupational therapist and the occupational therapy assistant collaborate with Brooke and his parents to develop the intervention plan. They schedule Brooke for five days of occupational therapy services and choose a biomechanical model to guide their teaching of self-catheterization and skin inspection skills. During the first intervention session the occupational therapy assistant interviews Brooke to determine his familiarity with self-catheterization and skin inspection procedures. Together they design a chart for Brooke to use to monitor his catheterization times and the results of his skin inspection. The occupational therapy assistant provides a long handled mirror for use in inspecting his back side. Since Brooke likes to draw, the occupational therapy assistant provides supplies for Brooke to create a chart with an outline of his body from the waist down. He includes arrows pointing to areas over bony prominences where he must carefully check his skin. Together the occupational therapy assistant and Brooke create a table to record the frequency and the results of the skin inspection. They conclude the session with a creating a poster of sports and fitness activities that interest Brooke.

Over the next four days Brooke learns to use the mirror and inspect his skin successfully. He marks the chart appropriately. He also learns how to self-catheter. Supplies are brought from home by his parents because he already is familiar with them. The occupational therapy assistant helps Brooke to develop a checklist of supplies, steps for maintaining a clean field, and a timetable where he can indicate when he completed his self-catheterization. The occupational therapy assistant provides verbal cues and encouragement as Brooke attempts the procedure for the first time. Brooke repeats the process multiple times at bedside and in the bathroom, until he develops the necessary competency. In addition, the occupational therapy assistant helps Brooke to use the Internet to investigate sports and fitness programs for children within the community. The occupational therapy assistant meets with the parents and Brooke to discuss the success of his program and to provide copies of his charts for use at home. The occupational therapy assistant also provides a detailed description of community fitness and sports programs that are of interest to Brooke and that accommodate his physical challenges. With their approval, the occupational therapy assistant helps Brooke to enroll in one of these programs online. Brooke is discharged from occupational therapy services at the end of five days. The occupational therapy intervention is documented using the SOAP format (see Figure 19.14■). ■

S: Brooke states, "I am so glad that I learned how to do this by myself. I did not know it would be so easy. It is time I did this now that I am getting older. I am also glad that I will join a sports program."
O: Brooke was seen daily to develop the ability to independently complete self-catheterization and skin inspection. He initially was seen bedside. A skin inspection mirror, catheter, sterile gloves, cleansing wipes, and lubricant were provided. Brooke was instructed in the use of the inspection mirror and in the process of self-catheterization. He learned to follow a skin inspection routine and to self-catheter at bedside. Once Brooke was able to ambulate, he learned to perform self-catheterization and skin inspection in the bathroom. Brooke also learned to use charts to track the daily completion and monitor the results of his skin inspection and self-catheterization activities. In addition, Brooke identified and enrolled in a community sports and fitness program to help manage his weight and increase opportunities for social participation in the community.
A: Brooke is able to complete self-catheterization and skin inspection at bedside and in the bathroom independently. Brooke is able to inspect his skin for integrity independently. He has enrolled in a community fitness and sports program to help with weight management. Brooke has met all goals for intervention.
P: Brooke will follow established program upon discharge. No additional intervention is indicated.

■ **Figure 19.14**
Discharge Summary.

Alex

Alex is a 17-year-old boy with an L4–5 level of lesion. He uses molded ankle foot orthoses (AFO) for support wearing them in a variety of shoes, including sneakers and boots. He uses cuff crutches for additional support, ambulating quickly with a swing through gait pattern. For long distance mobility he elects to use a sports style wheelchair. It provides speed and ease of carrying his backpack and other personal items. Alex is in the academic track at his high school and plans to attend college to become a math teacher. He hopes to combine teaching and coaching, since he is an accomplished athlete. He is a weight lifter and participates in organized wheelchair basketball in the community. Alex has an IEP in place which provides accommodations that allow him to leave class three minutes before the period ends to avoid the congestion of the hallways. His IEP also permits him to use the building elevator when moving from floor to floor. Because Alex is 17, his annual IEP includes a transition plan. Alex's family included the occupational therapist and the occupational therapy assistant from the Children's Hospital spina bifida clinic on his team. The spina bifida clinic is an outpatient service which coordinates appointment schedules with numerous professionals on one day. During his a clinic appointment there, he routinely was seen by the urologist, orthopedist, physiatrist, physical therapist, occupational therapist, occupational therapy assistant, social worker, dietician, and orthotist. The occupational therapist and the occupational therapy assistant have known Alex for the past six years, having followed him at clinic appointments and most recently during a brief hospitalization for the treatment of a pressure sore on his right heel. Their long term relationship with Alex and his family and community contacts make them effective members of the transition team.

The transition plan is a required element of an IEP when a student reaches the age of 16. Alex's last IEP included the development of his transition team and the establishment of initial goals for career exploration. At the current IEP meeting, his team members include Alex, his family, his math teacher, the guidance counselor, the school psychologist, the basketball coach, and the occupational therapist and occupational therapy assistant from Children's Hospital. Alex and his family review the progress toward their goals for him following graduation from high school. These goals include attending college, getting a job, living independently, and continuing to participate in organized sports. Two goals are written which address his ability to access the services he needs within the community and his ability to access the campus of State University, where he plans to enroll next year. The occupational therapist and occupational therapy assistant assume responsibility for these education and community related accessibility goals (see Figure 19.15■).

The occupational therapist and the occupational therapy assistant select the PEO model to guide their clinical reasoning and intervention approaches. They choose this model because it helps them to concurrently focus on Alex's capabilities and needs, the environmental supports and press, and occupation based opportunities and barriers. As part of the intervention to identify and access transportation systems, Alex and the occupational therapy assistant develop a comprehensive list of community resources which may be used by a college student. Together they find bus schedules and maps from the transit authority which are available online and print them. Alex locates the phone numbers of alternative transportation carriers to use when there is no appropriate bus route. Using these, he works with the occupational therapy assistant to develop a plan for accessing three services he has listed. Alex and the occupational therapy assistant then leave the school and put his plan into practice. They revise the plan after identifying any environmental challenges they had not anticipated. Finally, Alex creates sample daily activity schedules requiring varying needs for the use of public transportation on a daily basis.

To assist Alex with independently negotiating the campus of State University, the occupational therapy assistant implements a similar intervention plan. The occupational therapy assistant works with Alex to access an online campus map and descriptions of the different buildings. They then develop a list of the buildings Alex wants to access. Alex and the occupational therapy assistant next use public transportation to travel to and determine the accessibility of the campus. Alex uses both his wheelchair and his crutches for mobility, evaluating the effectiveness of each in different situations. Finally, they establish the location of classes he plans to take and create a daily plan for mobility using the information he gathered while on campus. ■

1. Alex will utilize public transportation independently to access desired community services.
   a. Alex will develop a list of community services needed by college students.
   b. Alex will identify the bus routes and timetables needed to access six desired community services.
   c. Alex will identify alternate carriers to access community services if there is no bus route available.
   d. Alex will utilize public transportation to access a desired service.
2. Alex will navigate independently through the campus of State University.
   a. Alex will use a map to identify the best route to take from location to location on the campus.
   b. Alex will establish time frames and identify transportation options to move from one location to another.
   c. Alex will travel on campus using the routes and transportation options he identified.

■ **Figure 19.15**
Transition Goals for Alex.

SUMMARY

Children and adolescents with spina bifida confront numerous performance challenges. Their needs are multifaceted and include issues related to positioning for function and mobility, mastering self-dressing and bracing, developing appropriate leisure activities, and managing learning disabilities within the classroom. Spina bifida affects the ability of the children and adolescents to engage in their community and home occupations. In addition to these more obvious concerns, spina bifida also influences how these children and adolescents develop their sense of identity and competency. To address these changing concerns, children with spina bifida may require the services of an occupational therapist and an occupational therapy assistant from birth through young adult life in a variety of settings, including hospitals, rehabilitation centers, home based early intervention, and school based occupational therapy. The focus of occupational therapy interventions is to support the participation of the children and adolescents in the occupations that are important to them, so that they can live healthy and meaningful lives. Thorough knowledge of the spinal cord, spinal cord injuries, and of the skeletal, muscular, genitourinary, learning, and sensory processing functions affected by spina bifida is essential for providing competent services. With this knowledge of body functions, occupational therapists and occupational therapy assistants can provide interventions that promote the performance skills and performance patterns of the children and adolescents, and adapt the activities and context to support full inclusion and participation in daily life.

REVIEWING KEY POINTS

1. Explain what is meant by neural tube defect and what can be done to reduce the risk of neural tube defects.
2. Describe the differences among spina bifida occulta, myelomeningocele, meningocele, and anencephaly.

3. Distinguish between flaccid paralysis and flaccid quadriplegia resulting from myelomengingocele.
4. Clarify what is meant by Chiari malformation, and the complications associated with it.
5. Explain hydrocephalus and describe how it is managed.
6. Explain what is meant by tethered cord and the warning signs of a tethered cord. Outline procedures for managing a tethered cord.
7. Outline the motor and sensory functions that a child or adolescent with spina bifida has at each of the following levels: C8–T1, T4–T6, T9–T12, L2–L3, L4–L5, and sacral.
8. Describe how a person with spina bifida is at risk for orthopedic complications. Identify interventions to minimize the orthopedic complications. Clarify the difference among scoliosis, kyphosis, lordosis, and osteoporosis.
9. Clarify the purpose of orthotics and the management of orthotics for children and adolescents with spina bifida.
10. Identify sensory complications resulting from spina bifida and discuss the impact of those sensory complications on occupational performance; outline occupational therapy interventions to address these issues.
11. Explain the learning complications affecting a number of children with spina bifida and outline occupational therapy interventions to address these issues.
12. Describe the areas of intervention occupational therapists and occupational therapy assistants consider for children and adolescents with spina bifida.

APPLYING KEY CONCEPTS

1. Identify 10 strategies for adapting the home environment to accommodate dressing, toileting, and transportation activities for a 4-year-old child with spina bifida at the T4–T6 level.
2. Identify 10 strategies for adapting the community activities to accommodate social and play activities of a 7-year-old child with spina bifida at the T9–T12 level.
3. Identify 10 strategies for adapting the school environment and activities to accommodate a middle school child with spina bifida at the L3–4 level.
4. Identify 10 strategies for adapting the school environment to accommodate an adolescent with spina bifida at the L4–L5 and the sacral levels.
5. Search the Internet for resources and support groups for children and adolescents with spina bifida. Describe the services available, and services that should be added.
6. Speak with the disability coordinator at your university. Describe resources on campus to support full participation of a student with spina bifida in the life of the university. Identify barriers on campus to full participation.

REFERENCES

American Occupational Therapy Association (2002). Occupational therapy practice framework: Domain and process. *American Journal of Occupational Therapy, 56*(6), 609–639.

Batshaw, M. (1997). *Children with disabilities* (4th ed.). Baltimore, MD: Brookes Publishing.

Folio, R., & Fewell, R. (2000). *Peabody development motor scales–2.* Austin, TX: Pro-Ed.

Hammill, D., Pearson, N. A., & Voress, J. K. (1998). *Developmental test of visual perception (DVPT–2).* Austin, TX: ProEd.

Law, M., Cooper, B, Strong, S., Steward, D., Rigby, R., & Letts, L. (1996). The person-environment-occupational model: A transactive approach to occupational performance. *Canadian Journal of Occupational Therapy, 63,* 9–23.

Lutkenhoff, M., (Ed.) (1999). *Children with spina bifida: A parent's guide*. Bethesda, MD: Woodbine House.

March of Dimes (2006). *Birth defects and genetics: Spina bifida*. Retrieved May 25, 2006 from http://www.marchofdimes.com/printableArticles/4439_1224.asp.

National Dissemination Center for Children with Disabilities (NICHCY; 2004). *Spina bifida fact sheet*. Retrieved March 22, 2006 from http://www.nichcy.org/pubs/factshe/fs12txm.htm.

National Institute of Neurological Disorders and Stroke (NINDS; 2006). *NINDS anencephaly information page*. Retrieved March 22, 2006 from http://www.ninds.nih.gov/disorders/anencephaly.htm.

National Institute of Neurological Disorders and Stroke (NINDS; 2005). *Tethered spinal cord syndrome information page*. Retrieved December 7, 2005 from http://www.ninds.nih.gov/disorders/tethered_cord/tethered_cord_pr.htm.

Porr, S., & Rainville, E. (1999). *Pediatric therapy: A systems approach*. Philadelphia: F. A. Davis.

Reed, K. (2001*). Quick reference to occupational therapy*. (2nd ed.). Gaithersburg, MD: Aspen Publishers.

Rothstein, J., Roy, S., & Wolf, S. (2005). *The rehabilitation specialist's handbook* (3rd ed.). Philadelphia: F. A. Davis.

Sandler, A. (1997). *Living with spina bifida: A guide for families and professionals*. Chapel Hill, NC: University of North Carolina Press.

Spina Bifida Association of America (2007). What is spina bifida? Retrieved March 28, 2007 from http://www.spaa.org.

Chapter 20

Children and Adolescents with Neurological Challenges: Cerebral Palsy

Barbara B. Demchick
and Margaret J. Pendzick

Key Terms

Acquired cerebral palsy
Alternative and augmentative
   communication (AAC)
Ankle-foot orthosis (AFO)
Asphyxia
Ataxic cerebral palsy
Athetoid cerebral palsy
Biomechanical
Central nervous system lesion
Cerebral palsy
Compensatory
Constraint-induced movement
   therapy (CI therapy)
Contracture
Cytomeglovirus (CMV)
Diplegia
Feedback
Flaccid
Hemiparesis
Hemiplegia
Hyperbilirubinemia
Hypertonic

Hypotonic
Itinerant
Mild cerebral palsy
Moderate cerebral palsy
Muscle tone
Neurodevelopmental treatment
   (NDT)
Osteoporosis
Paresis
Plegia
Quadriparesis
Quadriplegia
Related service
Rubella
Selective dorsal rhizotomy
Severe cerebral palsy
Shaping
Spastic cerebral palsy
Tendon release
Tendon transfer
Thumb loop splint
Toxoplasmosis

Objectives

- Explain cerebral palsy.
- Examine how cerebral palsy impacts the daily occupations of children and adolescents within the context of their family and environment.
- Describe occupational therapy interventions to support the capacity of children and adolescents with cerebral palsy to participate in their daily occupations.
- Examine how the occupational therapist and the occupational therapy assistant problem solve together in the intervention process.
- Describe how occupational therapists and occupational therapy assistants work with other professionals to provide services to children and adolescents with cerebral palsy.

INTRODUCTION

This chapter describes the types and causes of **cerebral palsy** that affect the health and development of children and adolescents. It provides a brief overview of medical, physical therapy, and speech and language interventions to address the motor, sensory, and communication challenges associated with cerebral palsy. Occupational therapy interventions to support the occupational needs of children and adolescents with cerebral palsy and their families are examined in detail. Five vignettes illustrate occupational therapy services available to children and adolescents with cerebral palsy at various stages in their development.

CEREBRAL PALSY

Cerebral palsy (CP) refers to a heterogeneous group of conditions that affects a person's ability to move, and to maintain posture and balance (March of Dimes, 2004). It is due to a nonprogressive lesion in the developing brain, which usually occurs before or during birth. Because the lesion affects the brain, it is called a **central nervous system lesion**. A diagnosis of cerebral palsy also may be given to children injured in early infancy and often is referred to as **acquired cerebral palsy**.

Although the central nervous system lesion is nonprogressive, the resulting disabilities can change with time. This occurs because the lesion impacts a body and nervous system that still is growing and maturing (Stamer, 2000). For example, a young child initially may use crutches to perform functional mobility tasks but after an adolescent growth spurt, may require a wheelchair to perform the same tasks. The incidence of cerebral palsy is estimated to be 1–2 per 1,000 live births.

Children and adolescents with cerebral palsy have damage to parts of the brain that control **muscle tone**. Muscle tone is the amount of resistance to movement in a muscle. Typical muscle tone allows movement against gravity while maintaining stability within the joint. The term **hypertonic** describes increased muscle tone that often restricts full range of motion within the joints. The term **hypotonic** describes decreased muscle tone that often results in inability to stabilize against gravity or in floppiness. The specific location of the brain lesion affects the location and the quality of movement (Stanley, Blair, & Alberman, 2000).

Atypical muscle tone also causes children and adolescents with cerebral palsy to develop secondary musculoskeletal impairments. Lack of active movement causes muscles to become atrophied and weak, and joints to develop **contractures.** A contracture is tightness of the muscles, ligaments, and tendons that hinders joint movement. **Osteoporosis**, which is decreased bone density, may develop due to disuse and non–weight bearing joints. These secondary problems can influence the ability of children and adolescents with cerebral palsy to develop and perform age appropriate occupations (Shumway-Cook & Woollacott, 2006).

Cognitive deficits, speech and language deficits, seizures, and sensory deficits frequently occur in cerebral palsy (Pellegrino, 2002). Delays in cognitive development and seizures are seen in at least 50 percent of children and adolescents with cerebral palsy. Sensory deficits include problems in the visual system, including impaired vision, limited eye movements, and eye muscle weakness. Approximately 40 to 50 percent of children with cerebral palsy have some visual deficits and require glasses or low vision or visual perception training. Twenty-five percent of youngsters with cerebral palsy have auditory deficits as well (Stanley et al., 2000).

Additionally, feeding problems, such as difficulty swallowing, chewing, or biting, result from atypical movement, posture, and tone of the muscles of the face, tongue, upper extremities, and trunk. These feeding problems affect not only the occupational performance of the child, but that of the whole family, as eating is often a shared family occupation.

CLASSIFICATION

Cerebral palsy is classified according to the type of muscle tone and resultant motor impairment, and the parts of the body most affected (Stanley, Blair, & Alberman, 2000). Given wide differences in degrees of severity and involvement, each child and adolescent with cerebral palsy must be considered as an individual with unique abilities and challenges.

Types of Muscle Tone

About 70–80 percent of children and adolescents with cerebral palsy have the spastic type (March of Dimes, 2004). **Spastic cerebral palsy** is caused by damage to the motor cortex of the brain and results in increased muscle tone (Rogers, 2005) or hypertonicity. Because their muscles are stiff, children and adolescents with spastic cerebral palsy have difficulty isolating specific movements. Young children with spastic cerebral palsy often have low tone in the postural muscles of the head, neck, and trunk, and spastic tone in their arms and legs. As they grow, these children develop spastic tone in their postural muscles as well.

Approximately 10–20 percent of youngsters with cerebral palsy have the athetoid type (March of Dimes, 2004). Athetosis typically is caused by damage to the brain in the region of the basal ganglia (Rogers, 2005). Children and adolescents with **athetoid cerebral palsy** typically have fluctuating muscle tone. Often they appear to have slow, writing movements that they cannot control. Alternately, their movements may be rapid and jerky. Children and adolescents with athetosis often have great difficulty learning to control their bodies and make precise movements.

About 5–10 percent of children and adolescents with cerebral palsy have the **ataxic** type (March of Dimes, 2004). This results from damage to the cerebellar region of the brain, and causes balance and coordination difficulties (Rogers, 2005). Children with ataxia often walk with an unsteady gait with their feet far apart, and have difficulty with motions that require precise coordination. Their muscle tone generally is classified as low to typical, although as they grow, they may experience increased tightness in the flexor muscles of the lower extremities.

Some people use the term mixed cerebral palsy when more than one type of cerebral palsy is present in the same individual. The most common mixed pattern is spasticity combined with athetoid movements.

Although hypotonia is not a classification of cerebral palsy, some infants initially have markedly low or **flaccid** muscle tone. However, as they grow, these children are likely to develop characteristics of spastic, athetoid, or ataxic cerebral palsy.

No matter what the classification of muscle tone, most babies and young children with cerebral palsy demonstrate an abnormal quality of extensor muscle activity (Bly, 1983). There is an abnormal quality to their movement detectable after birth, with extension not balanced by flexion.

Distribution and Intensity of Motor Impairment

Cerebral palsy also is classified according to the distribution of the motor impairment and intensity of involvement. Athetoid and ataxic cerebral palsy usually affects the whole body; spastic cerebral palsy affects different parts of the body with varying degrees of intensity. The terms mild, moderate, and severe are used to describe the intensity of involvement. Children or adolescents with **mild cerebral palsy** typically display increased postural tone when they become excited or when they exert effort to perform a task. In spite of this increased postural tone, usually they can complete the task. Children and adolescents with **moderate cerebral palsy** often use primitive or abnormal movement patterns to complete a task, though their muscle tone during rest is nearer to typical. Children and adolescents with **severe cerebral palsy** have limited or no voluntary movements due to continuous atypical tone and obligatory primitive reflexes.

Spastic cerebral palsy also can be classified according to the degree of weakness or paralysis and the number of parts affected. The following terms are used to denote these distinctions. The suffix **plegia,** placed after the root word, describes a muscle paralysis while **paresis** describes a muscle weakness. However, this distinction is not consistently made in describing cerebral palsy.

- **Hemiplegia** or **hemiparesis**: Involvement of extremities on one side of the body
- **Quadriplegia** or **quadriparesis**: Involvement of all four extremities
- **Diplegia**: Involvement of primarily lower extremities, although there frequently is mild upper extremity involvement.

Based on the complexity of the classification of cerebral palsy, a diagnosis of cerebral palsy itself gives very little information about the occupational functioning of the child. A child with mild cerebral palsy may have mild coordination difficulties using one of her hands, and may otherwise be indistinguishable from the other children in class, whereas another child with severe cerebral palsy may need total care.

EARLY SIGNS AND SYMPTOMS

Early diagnosis of cerebral palsy is important to secure the services that the child and family may need to optimize the child's development (Rogers, 2005). For this reason, all heathcare providers must be alert to indicators that might suggest that a possible problem exists. Though the following are by no means conclusive indicators of cerebral palsy, they do warrant further evaluation and referral to the pediatrician.

In the first few months of life, a baby demonstrating the following movement patterns should be evaluated: limited random movements, a strong persistent startle reflex, poor development of head control, extreme irritability, difficulty feeding, or stiff or floppy muscle tone relative to other babies. In the middle of the first year, additional signs and symptoms which may indicate the presence of cerebral palsy include turning over by flipping the body as a unit, assuming unusual or asymmetrical positions when lying on the back, fisting of the hand or hands, and avoiding or fussing when in the prone position.

Signs and symptoms that may be seen in the latter part of the first year include poor trunk control, poor balance skills, and limited protective responses, that is, limited ability to reach out with a hand to keep from falling. These may result in the baby having difficulty maintaining sitting, crawling, creeping, kneeling, and standing positions. Additionally, difficulty developing fine grasp patterns that involve the thumb and index finger may be indicative of motor dysfunction.

CAUSES OF CEREBRAL PALSY

Cerebral palsy results from a number of factors that cause trauma to the brain. These include hemorrhages, asphyxia, jaundice, infections, toxins, maternal–infant blood incompatibility, and disease.

Premature babies that weigh less than 3 1/2 pounds are up to 30 times more likely to develop cerebral palsy than full term babies. The lower their birth weight, the greater is their likelihood of suffering from a brain hemorrhage, which can damage delicate brain tissue (March of Dimes, 2004). Since the survival rate of these extremely small premature infants is increasing with advancing technology, this particular cause of cerebral palsy is on the rise.

Infections in the mother during pregnancy can a cause cerebral palsy. These infections include **rubella** or German measles, **cytomegalovirus** (CMV), a usually mild infection, and **toxoplasmosis**, a usually mild parasitic infection. Reproductive and urinary tract infections and exposure to environmental toxins increase the chances of premature delivery and cerebral palsy. Insufficient oxygen reaching the fetus, as occurs when the placenta is not functioning correctly, or tears away from the uterus before delivery, also can cause cerebral palsy. Babies born with brain malformations, and with some genetic conditions and birth defects are at increased risk for cerebral palsy as well (March of Dimes, 2004).

Blood diseases are a less common cause of cerebral palsy. Rh disease, an incompatibility between the blood of a mother and her fetus, can cause jaundice and brain damage, resulting in cerebral palsy. This disease is preventable by giving a mother with Rh negative blood an injection of Rh immune globulin around the 28th week of pregnancy and again after the birth of a baby who has Rh positive blood. Blood clotting disorders in the mother or the baby also may increase the risk of cerebral palsy (March of Dimes, 2004).

Until recently, **asphyxia** during labor and delivery was believed to be the cause of most cases of cerebral palsy. While deprivation of oxygen during labor and delivery is a cause of cerebral palsy, the incidence of asphyxia has decreased in recent years (Pellegrino, 2002). It now is believed that asphyxia causes fewer than 10 percent of cases of cerebral palsy. Similarly, severe jaundice, or **hyperbilirubinemia**, which is a yellowing of the skin due to the buildup of a pigment called bilirubin in the blood, can pose a risk of brain damage to the developing infant, resulting in cerebral palsy. However, this cause of cerebral palsy also appears to be on the decline.

INTERVENTION

Intervention for children and adolescents with cerebral palsy involves a variety of team members. Physicians, surgeons, physical therapists, speech and language pathologists, educators, and occupational therapy practitioners work in collaboration with the children, adolescents, and parents to provide services that enhance medical, social, and educational needs. The occupational therapist and occupational therapy assistant need to have an understanding of the types of interventions that are performed by medical professionals to be able to meet the child's needs most effectively.

Medical and Surgical Intervention

Physicians may prescribe oral medications to reduce muscle tone in youngsters with spasticity. Examples of such medications include baclofen, diazepam, and detrolene. These may reduce spasticity and improve comfort in children for short periods. These medications have side effects such as drowsiness and drooling, which may limit their usefulness (Pellegrino, 2002). A child also may need to take oral medications for other problems associated with cerebral palsy, such as anticonvulsant drugs to control seizures.

Implanted medication pumps also are used for children with spasticity. A physician inserts a catheter into the skin of the abdomen, and routes the catheter into the lumbar area of the spine, where medication can be delivered directly into the spinal cord. Baclofen is the primary medication delivered in this manner. Smaller doses of medication can be administered this way than by mouth, which may limit the side effects; however, mechanical failures and infection do occur (Pellegino, 2002). Another medical intervention is a nerve block. Botulism toxin (Botox) injected in small quantities by a physician has been shown to reduce spasticity for up to six months without serious side effects.

Surgical interventions are used frequently with children and adolescents with cerebral palsy. Although cerebral palsy is considered to be nonprogressive, atypical muscle tone and movement patterns may cause the development of contractures and deformities over time. This may limit function as the child or adolescent matures. For this reason, surgery may be performed to reduce contractures that have resulted from atypical muscle tone. A **tendon release**, which is lengthening of a muscle, is the most common orthopedic procedure. Another common orthopedic procedure is a **tendon transfer**, which moves the point of attachment of a tendon on a bone. Other surgeries include corrections for hip dislocations and scoliosis, both which may be seen in children and adolescents with hypertonia and asymmetric posturing. Because of atypical tone, sometimes procedures need to be repeated as the child ages (Menkes, 2001).

A neurosurgical technique called a **selective dorsal rhizotomy** is performed less frequently. In this procedure, the doctor identifies and cuts some of the nerve fibers that are contributing most to spasticity. This procedure is recommended for children and adolescents with significant lower extremity spasticity without fixed deformities (Park & Owen, 1992).

Physical Therapy and Speech and Language Therapy Intervention

Physical therapists focus on enhancing motor skills and preventing the development of contractures. Sometimes braces, splints, and casts are used along with physical therapy to help prevent contractures and to increase function. Physical therapists also prescribe appropriate mobility aids for children and adolescents with cerebral palsy, such as wheelchairs and walkers, often with input from occupational therapy practitioners.

Children and adolescents with cerebral palsy may have speech and language deficits, both in expressing themselves and in understanding language. Limitations in communication skills may be a source of stress and frustration for the child and family, and may negatively influence socialization. Therefore, it is essential that the speech and language pathologist works with these youngsters to foster communication skills. Use of **alternative and augmentative communication (AAC)**, or communication that does not require speech, can be individualized to the unique needs of the child, and may be important to the development of communication skills in children with significant oral motor involvement. Often, the occupational therapist and occupational therapy assistant work collaboratively with the speech pathologists to determine the most appropriate devices and the best way for the child to activate them (Doster & Politano, 1996).

Feeding problems are associated with the abnormalities in muscle tone that affect children and adolescents with cerebral palsy. Sucking, chewing, and swallowing may be difficult to initiate or control; hypersensitivity or hyposensitivity to touch in and around the mouth complicates oral motor responsiveness. These difficulties make feeding stressful for families, especially when they increase the risk of choking and aspiration (Morris & Klein, 2000). Special positioning and feeding techniques may be required, and the child's diet may need to be adjusted. This is often a collaborative effort between occupational therapy and speech pathology.

Constraint Induced Movement Therapy

Constraint-induced movement therapy (CI therapy) is a new intervention approach that is utilized by both occupational and physical therapists. Originally developed as a protocol for adults with hemiplegia due to cardiovascular accidents (CVA) (Taub et al., 1993), research studies have begun addressing the use of constraint-induced movement therapy (CI Therapy) for children and adolescents with hemiplegia due to cerebral palsy (Charles, 2001). Traditionally, rehabilitative intervention focuses on increasing independence by introducing and emphasizing compensatory strategies for the noninvolved upper extremity (Charles & Gordon, 2005). CI therapy, however, focuses on increasing the voluntary usage of the involved hemiplegic side of the body (Charles, 2001) by restraining the noninvolved side. Rationale for CI therapy is based on central nervous system plasticity and the assumption that a person with hemiplegia learns not to attempt tasks with the involved extremity, since it is more efficient to accomplish the task one handed with the noninvolved extremity (Charles, 2001; Bonnier, 2006).

Although a specific protocol has not been developed for children and adolescents, current research studies (Taub, Ramey, DeLuca & Echols, 2004; Willis, Morello, Davie, et al., 2002) use splints, mitts, plaster casts, and bivalve casts to restrain the noninvolved side. For various numbers of days, children and adolescents participate in approximately six hours of structured intervention directed toward increasing the use of the involved side while the noninvolved side is retrained. Depending on the research study design, repetition, **shaping**, and **feedback** are provided throughout the session in varying degrees of intensity (Charles & Gordon, 2005; Gordon, Charles, & Wolf, 2005). Shaping involves breaking down a task and working on small increments, increasing complexity and speed as improvement occurs with practice. With each attempt, the children and adolescents are given feedback on how well they execute the desired motor movement.

During the intense intervention sessions, children and adolescents can become frustrated by attempting tasks with only their involved extremity. Family members report that it is difficult to watch the child or adolescent struggle with tasks and often are tempted to discontinue the treatment protocol (Glover, Mateer, Yoell, & Speed, 2002). Some studies allow the constraint to be removed for short periods of time at the request of the child or adolescent. Researchers Charles and Gordon (2005) reflect that CI therapy's success is due to the intense practice rather than the noninvolved arm restraint and speculate whether a protocol for children and adolescents can be developed that would provide the practice without the restraint.

At this time, constraint-induced movement therapy is still experimental. Preliminary research reports gains in upper extremity movement, but these studies often are limited in value due to lack of consistent protocols and lack of testing over large populations with control groups (Crocker, Mackay-Lyons & McDonnell, 1997; Fetters, Figueiredo, Keane-Miller, et al., 2004; Charles & Gordon, 2005). Future research is needed before CI therapy becomes an acceptable intervention strategy for children and adolescents with hemiplegic cerebral palsy (Hart, 2005; Hoare, 2004). Occupational therapists and occupational therapy assistants should continue to monitor research on this topic, being aware of new trends but adhering to best practice intervention principles.

Occupational Therapy Intervention

To provide appropriate intervention, the occupational therapist, with assistance from the occupational therapy assistant, evaluates the physical, sensory, cognitive, and social emotional capacities of the children and adolescents, the tasks they need to complete, and the environments in which they perform these tasks. Because cerebral palsy results from a central nervous system lesion that affects the children's and adolescents' ability to move, and to maintain posture and balance (March of Dimes, 2004), particular knowledge about central nervous system functions and motor control theory is essential during this evaluation process. Based on the results of the evaluation, the occupational therapist and occupational therapy assistant focus on skill development, and on environmental tasks and adaptations that promote the ability of the children and adolescents to participate in their daily life occupations at home, at school, and in the community. Using a variety of activities and approaches, they enhance the ability of children and adolescents to engage in ADL, IADL, education, work, play, leisure, and social participation occupations with their families, friends, and peers. In many cases, the occupational therapist and the occupational therapy assistant focus on helping the child or the adolescent to develop performance skills and performance patterns to complete these occupations independently, or with assistance. When the children and adolescents are severely involved physically and cognitively, the focus of the interventions may be on making caretaking tasks easier for the parent or caregiver.

Similarly, many children and adolescents with cerebral palsy and their families benefit from modifications to the environment or the tasks. Restructuring the physical and social environments minimizes barriers and enhances access to daily life occupations. For example, rearranging the placement and type of furniture can facilitate movement and social interaction. Positioning devices, such as customized seating systems, wheelchairs, and standers allow a child with abnormal posture to sit or stand appropriately. Computer based and adapted toys, educational materials, and communication devices permit children and adolescents with limited manipulation skills to participate in age appropriate play, education, and leisure activities. Chapters 13 and 15 of this text provide more detailed information about environmental and task adaptation.

There are various occupation based practice models and non–occupation based frames of reference that occupational therapists and occupational therapy assistants use to guide their critical thinking and intervention approaches when working with children and adolescents with cerebral palsy. Depending on the child's or adolescent's occupational profile and occupational challenges, the occupational therapist determines which ones are most appropriate to use. For example, when selecting the Person-Environment-Occupational (PEO) model (Law et al., 1996), the occupational therapist considers the skills of the child or adolescent, the environment in which a task is being performed, and the occupations, or tasks and activities being performed. The PEO model suggests that a person's occupational performance is a result of a dynamic interaction among the person, environment, and occupation (Law et al., 1996). Therefore, when working with children and adolescents with cerebral palsy, the PEO model can be used to identify factors in the person, environment, and occupation that facilitate or hinder performance. Occupational therapy intervention then can focus on facilitating change in any of these components. Other occupation-based practice models include the Ecology of Human Performance (EHP) (Dunn, Brown, & McGuigan, 1994), Person-Environment-Occupational Performance (PEOP) (Christiansen, Baum, & Bass-Haugen, 2005), Occupational Adaptation (OA) (Schkade & Schultz, 1992), and Model of Human Occupation (MOHO) (Kielhofner et al., 2002). All are discussed in Chapter 2 of this text. The person, the environment, and the occupation are emphasized in all of these models. Non–occupation based frames of references such as those described below can be used in conjunction with PEO or other occupation based practice models, to guide intervention approaches for children and adolescents with cerebral palsy.

Neurodevelopmental treatment (NDT) is an intervention approach used by occupational therapy practitioners and physical therapists when working with children with cerebral palsy. The NDT approach primarily addresses person aspects of the PEO model, although NDT principles do recognize the importance of the environment. A child with cerebral palsy has atypical muscle tone and movement patterns. These cause the child or adolescent to develop alternate ways of accomplishing movement goals, which may lead to the development of contractures and deformities over time (Bly, 1983). An occupational therapist or occupational therapy assistant applying NDT principles manually handles a child in the context of an activity to facilitate postural control. At the same time, through the placement of their hands, the occupational therapist and occupational therapy assistant attempt to limit abnormal patterns that could result in muscular and skeletal deformities (Howle, 2002). Using NDT principles allows the occupational therapist and the occupational therapy assistant to help the child actively participate in purposeful activities and occupations using appropriate movement patterns.

The **biomechanical** approach is used when a child or adolescent with cerebral palsy cannot maintain postural control on his or her own. It provides guidance about what artificial supports to use to substitute for the lack of postural control, and how to position the body to perform activities and occupations more efficiently (Colangelo, 1999). Because gravity affects the movements of children and adolescents with moderate to severe involvement, they frequently develop tightness in the upper extremity flexor muscles and lower extremity extensor muscles. The use of splints, bracing, and adaptive seating reduces the demands of gravity on the child by providing external control. Once proximal control is provided through these external devices, the child can focus on the environment. With the added external postural control, the child is better able to free the hands to interact with the environment, thereby enhancing occupational performance.

Occupational therapists and occupational therapy assistants use principles from both the neurodevelopmental and biomechanical approaches in order to position children and adolescents to maximize performance in daily life and school related activities. Sometimes, the occupational therapy practitioner encourages the child to actively assume certain positions to maximize fine motor skills and play. With more involved youngsters, the occupational therapy practitioner places or holds the child in certain positions to optimize performance. A specialized chair, wheelchair, prone stander, and other pieces of equipment can be used to hold the child in the desired position. Ideally, the occupational therapy practitioner should position the child as symmetrically as possible. However, in some older children with fixed deformities, symmetry may not be possible. To promote symmetry in sitting, hips should be flexed to 90 degrees, knees should be bent, and feet should be flat. Positioning improves postural stability for daily tasks such as feeding and toileting (Nelson, 2001). Additionally, optimal sitting is important for the performance of school related occupations.

Another approach to occupational therapy intervention with children and adolescents with cerebral palsy is called the **compensatory** model of practice. This model emphasizes adapting the manner in which the task is performed, the demands of the task, and the physical and social environment to minimize the limitations of the child or adolescent and to enhance occupational performance (Law, Missiuna, Pollock, & Stewart, 2005). For example, typical children usually pick up small objects using a pincer grasp between the thumb and index finger. Because this grasp pattern is difficult for most children or adolescents with cerebral palsy, they may learn to grasp objects using their thumb, index, and middle fingers. Also, handwriting may be cumbersome and time consuming for some children and adolescents with cerebral palsy. A typing program or a system that uses dictation or word prediction may enhance school performance. By using compensatory approaches, children and adolescents can increase their participation in a variety of occupations. This not only enhances the children's and adolescent's ability to perform activities, but also builds opportunity for social interaction and fosters self-esteem.

Due to the nature of the condition, a child or adolescent with cerebral palsy faces many unique challenges. The following four vignettes demonstrate different interventions occupational therapists and occupational therapy assistant utilize to encourage full participation in age appropriate occupations.

Occupational Therapy Intervention: Case Studies

Tim

Tim is a 4-year, 4-month-old youngster with right hemiparesis. He attends a prekindergarten program five mornings per week at the Harding Elementary School. Tim has been evaluated by the school-based occupational therapist. Tim scored age appropriately on the Beery-Buktenic Developmental Test of Visual-Motor Integration (2005). He was able to copy vertical, horizontal, and diagonal lines, and a circle and square on that evaluation. The occupational therapist reported that during the evaluation, Tim performed age appropriately in fine motor adaptive tasks except those requiring the refined use of both upper extremities such as bead stringing. Tim's teacher reported that he is performing successfully in the classroom. He even is managing to perform some though not all of his dressing activities. Based on formal testing and classroom performance, the occupational therapist has concluded that Tim does not qualify for services based on a 504 plan, as his hemiparesis does not limit performance in self care activities. She provides consultation to the teacher regarding strategies to facilitate independence in self care.

Tim's mother, however, remains concerned because, in spite of his successful performance, he does not use his right hand and leg routinely to complete activities. She rarely sees him use this hand and leg. Although she realizes that he is able to do what he needs to do, she worries that he will not use them to the fullest extent possible. For this reason, she had Tim evaluated by the community hospital occupational therapy outpatient department. The following describes his outpatient therapy.

As a result of the evaluation (Figure 20.1■), the outpatient occupational therapist recommends that Tim receive outpatient services to enhance his incorporation of the right side of his body into his daily activities. In collaboration with the occupational therapist, the occupational therapy assistant provides occupational therapy services to Tim. The occupational therapist and occupational therapy assistant establish the following goals for Tim, in conjunction with his mother. Since his mother's major concern is with Tim's ability to use his hand and leg in the course of his day, they focus on self care and play tasks.

Goal 1. Tim will perform fine motor activities while bearing weight on both sides of his body.

   Objective 1a. Tim will sit straight, bearing weight on both hips when playing while seated at the table.

   Objective 1b. When performing self-care tasks in standing, Tim will bear weight evenly on both legs.

Goal 2. Tim will incorporate his right hand into daily activities.

   Objective 2a. Tim will pick up and stabilize toys and household objects with his right hand while manipulating them with his left hand.

   Objective 2b. Tim will pull his pants down and up when he needs to with minimal assistance.

In conjunction with the occupational therapist, the occupational therapy assistant begins by fitting Tim with a prefabricated neoprene **thumb loop splint** (Figure 20.2■). This splint inhibits spasticity of the hand. This is an example of a biomechanical intervention that incorporates neurodevelopmental principles. Similar to the NDT handling technique, the splint inhibits spasticity by applying pressure.

The occupational therapy assistant carefully monitors Tim's splint wearing time, looking carefully at his skin to be sure it is not getting red. The occupational therapy assistant puts stickers of Tim's favorite cartoon character on his splint to aid in Tim's acceptance of the splint and his desire to wear it. Tim gradually builds up splint wearing time. The occupational therapy assistant discusses Tim's splint wearing schedule with his mother, and explains that the splint should be removed during rest periods. Before sending the splint home for Tim to wear there, the occupational therapy assistant makes sure that Tim is using it effectively during therapy sessions to enhance use of the right hand.

During therapy, the occupational therapy assistant has Tim sit at a small table, as he does at school. The occupational therapy assistant seats Tim on a wooden chair of the correct size and seat depth, and makes sure that he sits close to the table, with his elbows resting on the table surface. This helps Tim to sit symmetrically, with his hips, knees, and ankles at 90 degrees of flexion to incorporate his involved right hand as he plays. As alternatives, Tim sometimes sits on a bolster chair at an appropriate sized table, or kneels at a low table. These positions foster equal weight distribution and inhibition of spasticity, thereby enhancing upper extremity function. The occupational therapy assistant plays games with Tim that encourage weight bearing on Tim's right hand, also to inhibit spasticity. He does not wear his splint when doing these weight bearing activities.

Tim is an ambulatory 4-year-old male with a diagnosis of right spastic hemiparesis. His mother has requested an occupational therapy evaluation at this time due to concerns about his difficulty routinely incorporating his right hand and leg into self-care and play activities.

Tim's muscle tone is moderately increased throughout his right upper and lower extremities, the upper more than the lower. Tim walks and runs, leading with the left leg. He stands, taking weight on his left leg more than his right. Tim wears a right ankle foot orthosis to reduce spasticity in his right foot and to improve his standing position. When sitting, Tim is asymmetrical, taking more weight on his left hip than his right. His left arm is forward and his right is retracted. He needs encouragement to bring his right arm forward or to incorporate it into play. Tim demonstrates active range of motion (AROM) that is within normal limits in his uninvolved left upper extremity. AROM is decreased in his involved right upper extremity, particularly in shoulder flexion, abduction, external rotation, and elbow extension, forearm supination, and wrist extension. Passive range of motion is within normal limits, however. Sensation is grossly intact to light touch and temperature throughout his right upper extremity. Sensation, including stereognosis is intact throughout his uninvolved left upper extremity. Visual fields appear to be intact.

On his own, Tim holds an object against his body by adducting his right arm, after placing it with the left. He manipulates the held object with his uninvolved left hand. He employs mature grasp patterns, such as a superior pincer grasp with his left hand. He is able to control the movements of his left hand to release and stack more than 10 one-inch blocks. In contrast, Tim makes little effort to grasp with his involved right hand. When he does attempt to grasp, he tends to keep his right thumb in the palm of his hand in cortical thumb position. However, when the occupational therapist applies NDT handling techniques to his thenar eminence, he is able to open the hand, and actively grasp with a palmar pattern, inconsistently incorporating the thumb. He pulls objects placed in or held in his right hand out with his left. He can not voluntarily release objects with his right hand. He engages in age appropriate adaptive play when the task does not require the use of both hands, as per his mother's report and that of the school occupational therapist.

In activities of daily living, Tim needs moderate assistance to put on or take off his jacket, as well as to put on or take off his shirt. He also needs moderate assistance to pull down his pants for toileting, although he does manage his zipper, using a zipper pull. He needs maximum assistance to put on shoes and his ankle foot orthosis, although he can remove them with minimal to moderate assistance.

Visual perceptual motor tasks were tested by his school occupational therapist, so they were not examined at this time.

It is recommended that Tim receive outpatient occupational therapy twice per week to increase right upper extremity active range of motion, to facilitate the development of active grasp and voluntary release in the involved right hand, and to foster incorporation of the right arm and leg into play and self care skills.

■ **Figure 20.1**
Community hospital occupational therapy evaluation.

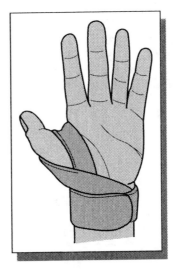

■ **Figure 20.2**
Thumb loop splint.

1. As an alternate play position, have Tim play while "standing" on his knees. Tim can color on a piece of paper taped to the wall. He can support the paper with his right hand.
2. When Tim is playing with toy cars, encourage him to crawl along the floor. He can hold the car with either hand.
3. Instruct Tim to put his right arm or leg into his shirt or pants before the left and remove the left one first. Encourage him to pull his pants up and down with both hands.
4. Position Tim at the kitchen table for play or mealtimes on a booster seat, so that he is sitting upright and bearing weight equally on both sides. Be sure he is tucked in close to the table.
5. Encourage Tim to use his right hand to hold a toy and his left to manipulate it. For instance, he should hold his puzzle down with his right hand and place pieces with his left hand.

■ Figure 20.3
Tim's home program.

During therapy sessions, the occupational therapy assistant initially encourages Tim to push and carry large toys such as cars and beach balls, with both hands. After several sessions, Tim begins to hold larger toys and objects spontaneously in his right hand, such as a formboard or bank, while placing the smaller objects such as puzzle pieces or pennies into them with his uninvolved left hand. He then gradually advances toward completing more difficult two handed activities such as bead stringing and scissors cutting. The occupational therapy assistant also encourages Tim to relax his grasp with his right hand so he can begin intentionally to release an object.

Also, the occupational therapy assistant encourages Tim to incorporate his involved hand into self-care tasks. He begins to hold his cup with his right hand and pour juice with assistance. He tries to hold his pants with both hands when he needs to pull them down for toileting. Once he gets better at this task, the occupational therapy assistant encourages his mother to have him wear pull on sweat pants, which are easier to move up and down. The occupational therapy assistant works with Tim on putting on his jacket, instructing him to push his right arm in the sleeve first.

In addition, the occupational therapy assistant provides Tim's mother with a home program of activities. She incorporates them into her daily activities with Tim. However, the occupational therapy assistant is careful to make sure that she doesn't give Tim's mother a list of extra things to do with her son, but rather tasks that she can easily fit into existing routines (Figure 20.3■). This is consistent with family centered principles. ■

Michael

Michael, a 3½-year-old with severe spastic quadriplegic cerebral palsy, attends a full day developmental preschool class at Beaver Elementary, a rural school district. The noncategorical class consists of eight preschoolers, one preschool teacher, and a teacher's aide. The other seven preschoolers have various degrees of speech and language delays but their motor skills are within a typical range. Seventh and eighth grade student volunteers assist the preschoolers during the all school lunch and recess; children in other grades participate in buddy programs, often reading stories, playing games, or assisting in craft activities.

Michael lives with his parents and two older brothers on a dairy farm. He has a dog, Spike, who Michael likes to pat when sidelying on the floor. His favorite foods are chocolate pudding and French fries, and he likes to watch cartoons with his brothers.

Michael has increased tone in all extremities; flexor tone dominates in his hand, causing a fisted hand position. Although he is dependent in all areas of self-care, with hand-over-hand support, he can bat at an object at shoulder height and bring his hands to his mouth. He is alert and interested in people and things in his environment. Even though Michael is too young for formal testing, the school psychologist speculates that his cognitive abilities are within the severe to moderate range of mental retardation. He vocalizes pleasure and displeasure, making a variety of sounds. When excited, he often extends his arms in a synergistic pattern, hyperextends his neck, and fully opens his jaw. Drooling increases when his neck is hyperextended. He has a customized highback manual wheelchair that he uses at school.

Consistent with IDEA, the county developmental disabilities board provides the federally mandated services of occupational therapy, physical therapy, and speech and language services to the children and adolescents throughout the district. Because of the small number of students requiring intervention at any one school, the occupational therapist and occupational therapy assistant travel among the schools providing **itinerant** services. At Beaver Elementary, they train the classroom staff how to position Michael for optimal school performance. They also address feeding and play, and work with speech and language pathologists on communication systems. Throughout the school year, the occupational therapy assistant provides ongoing staff training and direct services to Michael on a weekly basis.

The following are the IEP goals that the occupational therapist and occupational therapy assistant address while working with Michael.

Goal 1: By the end of the school year, Michael will assist in self-feeding.

Objective 1a: With hand-over-hand assistance, Michael will bring an adaptive spoon to his mouth, 3/5 attempts.

Objective 1b: With hand-over-hand assistance, Michael will hold his milk carton while attempting to drink through a straw, 2/5 attempts.

Objective 1c: With hand-over hand assistance, Michael will scoop pureed or soft food with his spoon, 4/5 attempts.

Goal 2: By the end of the school year, Michael actively will engage in play activities, 3/5 days.

Objective 2a: With assistance, Michael will play with an adaptive toy by pressing an adaptive switch, 2/5 times.

Objective 2b: With assistance, Michael will initiate interactive play by pushing a toy towards another person, 3/5 times.

Objective 2c: Michael will bat at a toy that is placed within reach and at his shoulder height independently, 4/5 times.

Goal 3: Michael will operate his scanning communication board through the use of an adaptive switch.

Objective 3a: With hand-over-hand support, Michael will choose between two picture options on his communication board by pressing a switch, 3/5 times.

Objective 3b: With minimal physical assistance, Michael will use his communication board to choose between four pictures to express his wants, 4/5 times.

Objective 3c: With verbal cueing, Michael will use his communication board to choose between four symbols to express his wants, 4/5 times.

Due to Michael's severe atypical postural tone and the necessity to adapt the classroom environment to his needs, the occupational therapist chooses the Ecology of Human Performance (Dunn, Brown, & McGuigan, 1994) and Neurodevelopmental Treatment (NDT) (Schoen & Anderson, 1999) to guide intervention decisions. Applying this practice model and frame of reference, the occupational therapy assistant pays close attention to the contextual demands and adapts the environment to enhance Michael's occupational performance. As directed by the occupational therapist, the occupational therapy assistant focuses on how he positions and handles Michael to maximize Michael's motor control.

He emphasizes symmetrical body alignment and positions toys and objects below Michael's eye level to discourage neck hyperextension. He demonstrates how different body positions influence Michael's ability to swallow properly, emphasizing ways to decrease Michael's tendency to drool. He suggests alternatives to wheelchair sitting such as prone lying over a wedge, sidelying on the floor, supported sitting in a beanbag chair, or supported standing in a prone stander. The occupational therapy assistant shows the classroom staff how to adjust the beanbag chair so that Michael's back and neck have full support while his hips and knees are flexed to 90 degrees. Before placing Michael into the stander, he demonstrates how to adjust the moveable pads and supports that hold the child into place. While placing Michael into the prone stander, the occupational therapy assistant emphasizes the importance of correct placement and tightness of straps at midchest, buttock, and knees.

He also demonstrates how to gently guide Michael's extremities movements by focusing on key points of control at the trunk, hip, shoulder, knee, elbow, and wrist rather than pulling and yanking them. When donning Michael's coat, the occupational therapy assistant supports the arm at the shoulder and elbow while moving it forward into the sleeve. If Michael's muscles are extremely tight, he suggests first gently ranging the extremity before attempting dressing or position Michael in sidelying to decrease the tightness.

When Michael hyperextends his trunk or legs, the occupational therapy assistant shows the classroom staff how to gently flex the trunk or legs to decrease the extension. When in a seated position, the occupational therapy assistant decreases Michael's hyperextension by placing one hand on the sternum while using the other hand and arm to gently cradle the shoulder girdle into flexion. Since Michael's position will be varied throughout the day, the occupational therapy assistant demonstrates how to use the pelvis, hips, and knees as lower extremity key points of control to obtain the necessary body adjustments. When Michael is lying supine, the occupational therapy assistant places his hands on the pelvic bone and gently flexes the hips. In sidelying, he places a support behind the head, trunk, and hips, making sure the neck is slightly flexed to discourage hyperextention. He writes down his suggestions and leaves a handout (Figure 20.4■) with the classroom teacher and aide.

- When positioning Michael over a wedge, try to keep his entire body aligned symmetrically.
- When placing him into a chair, make sure his hips and knees are flexed at 90 degrees and rest against the back of the chair.
- Support his feet and head in midline position when he is seated. Don't allow his feet to dangle or his head to flop backwards.
- If his muscles are tight, try to gently move the joints within his limited range. Starting with the joints closest to the midline of the body, use slow rotary movements, and gentle pressure. Do not pull or jerk on the joints or force movement.
- When placing his arms or legs into clothing, support him at the shoulders or hip and guide the extremity through the opening. Do not pull on the arms or legs.
- Try to place all items at or below Michael's eye level. Talk to Michael at or below his eye level so that he does not have to tilt his head.
- Try a variety of different positions throughout the day. If the children are playing on the floor, Michael may be able to join them by being placed in sidelying, prone over a wedge, or in a bean bag chair.

If you have any questions or problems positioning Michael, please don't hesitate to contact the occupational therapist or occupational therapy assistant!

■ **Figure 20.4**
Suggestions for positioning and handling.

The occupational therapy assistant and the classroom aide work together on Michael's self-feeding goals. During classroom snack time, he tries different adaptive spoons with various shaped and sized handle grips to determine which would be the easiest for Michael to grasp. He also determines the best placement for the milk carton so that Michael grasps it without excessive postural tone. He models how to assist Michael in a hand-over-hand approach, initially placing his hand directly over Michael's hand and giving assistance to Michael as he guides but not forces the spoon to Michael's mouth. He explains that he constantly adjusts the amount of assistance so that Michael is performing as much of the tasks as possible with each movement and completes the grasp and movement pattern. The occupational therapy assistant allows the classroom aide to practice the handling technique while he gives verbal feedback and encouragement. He emphasizes keeping Michael's overall posture erect and symmetrical and his chin slightly flexed to facilitate a more controlled swallow.

The classroom teacher, aide, occupational therapist, and occupational therapy assistant also discuss ways to adapt the classroom to Michael's needs. They rearrange the furniture to accommodate the wheelchair and move visual materials at or below Michael's eye level. They replace carpet squares with bean bag chairs for circle time and place the shelf and coat hook in Michael's cubby at a height visually accessible when sitting in his wheelchair.

The speech and language pathologist and the occupational therapy assistant work collaboratively with Michael and the classroom staff. Together they establish ways to introduce Michael to the communication device. The speech and language pathologist selects the device that meets Michael's cognitive and language needs while the occupational therapy assistant determines what adaptations will be necessary for Michael to activate the system. Choices are graded by the number of selections given and the visual display. First, real objects, then pictures, and finally symbols are used to represent choices. ■

Minnie

Minnie, a 5-year-old kindergarten student at Bayside Elementary School, has been referred for an occupational therapy evaluation. Even though she has a diagnosis of mild ataxic cerebral palsy, Minnie requires no special education services; therefore, she is referred for an occupational therapy evaluation on a Section 504.

Minnie is an energetic child who likes to tell "knock-knock" jokes and play on her swing set. She is an only child; she lives with her parents and grandmother and has many friends in her neighborhood. Her mother compensates for her ataxia by choosing clothing with minimal fasteners, providing seating with firm base of support, and encouraging chores that she can complete successfully. Minnie enjoys attending the library story hour with her grandmother, grocery shopping with her mom, and roughhousing with her dad.

Although she can participate fully in classroom activities academically, Mrs. Augustus, the kindergarten teacher, notices that Minnie is very awkward using the classroom manipulatives, often knocking over her math counters, breaking crayons and pencils when she colors or draws, and dropping items on the floor. Minnie prefers not to cut, often asking her tablemates to complete any cutting projects for her. Sometimes, she unsuccessfully attempts to tear rather than cut out an item. Quickly becoming upset, Minnie often needs a hug from Mrs. Augustus in the middle of an activity.

Mrs. Augustus worries that Minnie is getting frustrated with classroom tasks and schedules a parent-teacher conference to discuss her concerns. Minnie's parents notice that she is not excited about attending kindergarten even though she enjoyed her preschool experience. Her parents often find crumpled up, half completed projects in her backpack; Minnie refers to these as her "mistakes." Both her parents and teacher are concerned that Minnie is getting a "negative attitude," and wonder if accommodations are needed in the classroom. The occupational therapist meets with the parents and teacher and agrees that an occupational therapy assessment for classroom modification is needed.

Realizing Minnie's coordination problems are due to the ataxia and will require modifications of both the task and the environment, the occupational therapist chooses to structure her evaluation based on the Person-Environment-Occupational Performance Model (Christiansen, Baum-Haugen, 2007). The occupational therapy assistant completes observations (Table 20.1■), emphasizing how the environment assists or inhibits Minnie's participation.

■ Table 20.1
Classroom Observations

Occupations Observed	Performance Skills and Performance Patterns Observed	Performance Context
Math Lesson The children take turns passing and removing a handful of teddy bear counters from the bag.	Minnie takes the bag from a student. As she is removing the counters, she drops three on the floor. She passes the bag to the next student before retrieving the counters off the floor.	Four students are seated around each child-sized table in the kindergarten room. A container of crayons is in the middle of the table.
They place the counters on the table, separating them into four groups by color.	Minnie keeps dropping the teddy bears out of her hand while she is separating them; as a result, they fall into the wrong pile or fall on the floor. After picking up four counters off the floor, she looks around the room and kicks the remaining fallen counters away from her table. Although she was the second child to remove counters, she is the last to complete her piles.	Each child has a large piece of paper with a printed grid. A drawstring bag containing light weight plastic teddy bear counters is placed in the middle of the table.
After counting each color group of teddy bear counters, they color that same number of squares on the paper.	Minnie chooses the correct crayons and begins to color. She has difficulty staying within the lines of the grid. As she colors, she breaks one of the crayons. One of her classmates starts complaining about broken crayons at their table.	

■ **Table 20.1**
Classroom Observations (cont.)

OCCUPATIONS OBSERVED	PERFORMANCE SKILLS AND PERFORMANCE PATTERNS OBSERVED	PERFORMANCE CONTEXT
Art Project Each child draws in the facial features, glues on eyes, cuts and applies yarn hair. They cut out magazine pictures of things they like. They use the pompoms, pictures, crayons, and glitter to decorate the cutouts.	Minnie sits on a stool but uses her hand to brace herself when reaching toward the middle of the table to secure supplies. She draws facial feature of nose and mouth. She has difficulty maintaining grasp of the scissors to cut the yarn. She asks her friend to cut some yarn that she can use for hair. Quickly Minnie locates her magazine pictures. Her cutting is choppy. She often lops off parts of the picture. She unsuccessfully tries to tear the paper, then crumples up mistakes and pushes pictures to the side. She successfully cuts out and glues one picture to the cardboard. She uses glitter and pompoms to decorate. Minnie's area is messier than those of her peers.	Six children are seated on stools around each high table in the art room. Child-sized blunt scissors, glitter, glue bottles, crayons, yarn, magazine, glitter, and google eyes are in the middle of each table. Each child has a large cardboard cutout person.
Reading Lesson Each child stands up, one at a time, selects the correct picture and places it within a lettered square on the flannel board. The child then returns to the original place on the floor.	As Minnie stands up from floor, she turns in place and uses her hands to push up to standing. She bumps the children at her side and behind her. Minnie correctly selects her picture and places it on the board. The teacher adjusts the picture so that it fits into the square. Minnie returns to her seat, bumping other children as she sits on the floor.	Children sit crosslegged on carpet squares in a double semicircle. The teacher sits on a chair with flannel board to her side. Small laminated pictures are arranged on the floor in front of the students.

Using the *Canadian Occupational Performance Measure* (COPM; Law et al., 1998), the occupational therapist interviews the parents, kindergarten teacher, and Minnie in order to define school expectations and ascertain occupation based goals. The occupational therapist administers the Peabody Developmental Motor Scales (PDMS-2) (Folio & Fewell, 2002) to observe Minnie's motor skills.

At the followup meeting, the occupational therapist explains how Minnie's difficulty with balance and coordination interferes with her school tasks. The ataxic muscle tone makes it difficult for Minnie to precisely control her arm and finger movements, to carefully set objects down on a surface, to avoid bumping over object, or to use school supplies. To complete age appropriate motor tasks, Minnie uses a wider base of support to compensate for her balance difficulties; she needs more space to transition from sitting on the floor to standing, and

foot support when seated in a chair. The occupational therapist shares a list of classroom and task modifications (Figure 20.5■) and the occupational therapy assistant arranges to work with the teacher on making the modifications.

The kindergarten teacher, parent, and occupational therapy assistant collaborate to develop activities that will boost Minnie's self-esteem and provide positive school experiences. Minnie's parents share ways that they encourage Minnie's independence at home. The classroom teacher and occupational therapy assistant plan activities that will teach all the children respect for individual performance differences and way to offer assistance to each other. The teacher and aide identify leadership opportunities for Minnie within the kindergarten class. The classroom teacher monitors Minnie's participation and contacts the occupational therapist if future modifications are needed. ■

Kindergarten Room and Tasks

- To eliminate bumping into other children, substitute chairs for carpet squares in the reading circle.
- To eliminate reaching across the table, have two rather than four children share supplies.
- To keep coloring within a given space, use wikki sticks or colored glue to make a border around the color space.

Art Room and Tasks

- For better balance, allow children the option to work at lower tables where feet can rest on the floor.
- To minimize frustration, offer the option to use precut supplies to all children.
- On projects that require extensive cutting, allow children the option to work with a buddy.

Supplies

- To decrease breakage, provide chubby crayons, or place regular width crayons into holders.
- In order to eliminate opening scissors too wide and dropping out of her hand, place a rubber band around handles to decrease the opening.
- Substitute heavier weighted counters such as colored pebbles.
- If using light weight counters, place Velcro on the bottom of the counters and have a strip on desk for placement.

■ **Figure 20.5**
Environmental and task modifications to support Minnie's participation at school.

Rosetta

Rosetta, a 9-year-old child with mild spastic hemiplegia cerebral palsy and visual limitations, is a new fourth grade student at Oakland Elementary School. Daughter of migrant workers, Rosetta currently lives with her grandmother, who is employed as a nurse's aide in the local hospital. Rosetta, the youngest of six children, enjoys music and animals, expressing desires to be either a veterinarian or a rock star. Rosetta and her grandmother live in a large apartment complex within walking distance to her school. Rosetta attends the local community center after school program, where she participates in activities and receives tutoring in math and reading. She is a member of the organized singing group and likes to join spontaneous dance activities.

Since staying with her grandmother, Rosetta is followed medically by the children's hospital cerebral palsy clinic. She recently was fitted for an **ankle-foot orthosis (AFO)** due to her foot drop. She uses her hemiplegic side as an active assist to her dominant right side. She wears prescription lenses but her vision is still limited. Rosetta completes her own self-care and helps around the house. Since her grandmother is concerned about the vision and hemiplegia interfering with Rosetta's schoolwork, the clinic social worker explains the school referral process.

Due to frequent relocations, Rosetta has limited experience in an organized school setting. Although she converses in English, her primary language is Spanish and she receives English as a second language (ESL) services daily. The grandmother and teachers complete the referral process for a multidisciplinary team assessment to determine eligibility for services under IDEA. The team assessment includes cognitive and achievement testing, vision-specialist consultation, a physical therapy evaluation, and an occupational therapy evaluation.

After choosing the Person-Environment-Occupation Model (Law et al., 1996), the occupational therapist decides to include observations, teacher interviews, and the Canadian Occupational Performance Measure (COPM; Law, et al. 1998) in his evaluation. He interviews the classroom and ESL teacher, who indicate that Rosetta gets along well with her classmates and participates in class discussions. Except for shoe tying, Rosetta is independent in ADLs. Since keyboarding is taught in the fourth grade, the classroom teacher is unsure how Rosetta will access the computer with only one hand. After talking with the teachers, the occupational therapist concludes that although Rosetta has motor involvement due to the cerebral palsy, her visual limitations have a stronger impact on her ability to participate in the school setting.

The occupational therapist completes the COPM with Rosetta and the classroom teacher. Both the teacher and student agree that Rosetta needs to independently don and fasten her AFO and high top shoes, and independently operate a school computer. They also agree that it is important to adapt playground games so Rosetta can play with her peers.

The occupational therapy assistant completes observations of Rosetta in the cafeteria, the computer lab, and the playground. In the cafeteria, Rosetta completes the lunch line routine and primarily chooses finger food. The occupational therapy assistant notes that Rosetta would benefit from contrast between her food and serving dishes. In the computer lab, she is unfamiliar with operating a computer. Even with enlarged fonts, Rosetta's visual limitations interfere with her ability to locate the cursor on the screen. Since she does not have finger isolation on the involved side, she needs to learn one-handed keyboarding and would benefit from a one-handed keyboard. On the playground, Rosetta joins a dodgeball game but quickly gets tagged out. After consulting with the occupational therapist, the occupational therapy assistant meets with the teacher and classroom teacher to demonstrate how to modify playground games to include Rosetta.

The occupational therapist meets with the vision specialist, who determines that Rosetta requires hand held magnification in order to access the written materials in the classroom, and will require adaptations throughout her environment to increase the contrast and lighting. They collaborate on adaptations needed in the computer lab.

After team members complete their evaluations, they meet with Rosetta's grandmother to share the results. Though Rosetta has had limited exposure to English and formal education, she does not have cognitive limitations according to IDEA guidelines. Rosetta qualifies, however, for an Individualized Education Program (IEP) based on her visual limitations. Occupational therapy is included as a **related service** to address environmental adaptations and provide training in low vision aids. In consultation with the vision specialist, the occupational therapist and occupational therapy assistant adapt the classroom to accommodate her low vision needs. They install high intensity desk lighting and adjust classroom blinds to eliminate the glare on the chalkboard. They instruct Rosetta and the classroom staff in the use of a freestanding mounted magnifier that can slide across the surface of printed materials. They modify Rosetta's computer workstation, installing a one-handed keyboard and utilizing the computer's accessibility options to adjust the screen contrast, font size, and mouse tracking system. After making these modifications, they monitor Rosetta's needs, making adjustments as needed as the year continues. ■

Jamelle

Jamelle, a 16-year-old student in a large, urban high school has moderate to severe spastic quadriplegic cerebral palsy. He enjoys watching and talking about the high school football team with his friends. He lives with his grandmother and has a personal care attendant to help with his morning and evening care. Jamelle currently is exploring career options for when he turns 21 and transitions from high school. He wants to obtain employment where he is talking and interacting with people. Since he has breath control issues, the speech and language pathologist recommends tasks such as answering questions at an information desk or reception duties at a medium size office rather than telemarketing work. Gainful employment could be obtained at area universities, museums, and hospitals.

Jamelle relies upon extensive technology to complete his daily tasks. Although he is dependent in self-care, he is able to operate his customized electric wheelchair. A motion sensor controlled by slight head movements allows him to maneuver the chair within his environment, operate his electric feeder, and access a computer. Jamella's reading and vocabulary is at a tenth grade level; however, he has a math-related learning disability but is able to complete math computations.

His current transition plan includes goals that address his ability to use public transportation, make choices for personal care, refine interpersonal skills, establish work habits, and identify personal leisure activities. Occupational therapy services are included on his transition plan.

As part of the transition team, the occupational therapist and occupational therapy assistant meet with Jamelle, his grandmother, high school teachers, a speech and language pathologist, and the high school administrator. After discussing the identified transition goals, the team decides that Jamelle would benefit from being involved in the student work program with placement consideration in the school office or library. These placements allow Jamelle to establish work habits and interpersonal skills necessary for successful job placement outside the high school environment. The team determines that the occupational therapist and the occupational therapy assistant should focus on two of the transition goals: identifying personal leisure activities and accessing public transportation. Other team members will focus on the other goals.

After discussing the intervention plan with the occupational therapist, the occupational therapy assistant helps Jamelle identify ways to expand his leisure activities. After describing his interest in the high school football team, the occupational therapy assistant suggests that Jamelle explore ways that he could get involved in the football program in hopes that this will lead to further community recreation opportunities. By adapting the motion sensing system of his customized wheelchair to access environmental controls, he is able to turn switches on and off with slight head movements. He volunteers to join the technical crew and begins to learn to operate the controls for the electric score board. He arranges to attend their after school training sessions, sits with the crew during the game, and observes the scoreboard operation. The occupational therapy assistant meets with Jamelle and the crew and helps determine how he can be part of the crew. They decide that Jamelle first would learn to control the ball possession indicator. The occupational therapy assistant demonstrates to the crew how to interface the scoreboard and the environmental control unit of Jamelle's wheelchair. During practice scrimmages, Jamelle practices operating the switch, getting ready for his first regular game.

Jamelle begins to develop friendships with the crew members and they encourage him to join them working the theater sound and lighting system. The technology crew's high school advisor supports Jamelle's involvement and helps the crew to identify specific tasks that Jamelle can accomplish. The occupational therapy assistant and Jamelle explore opportunities where Jamelle can become involved in this type of volunteer work within the community setting. She also helps Jamelle to explore Internet-based games that involve knowledge of football strategies. The occupational therapy assistant also works with Jamelle on accessing the public transportation system. Since Jamelle only knows how to use school buses or private vans, the occupational therapy assistant and special education teacher organize a field trip for Jamelle and other students in wheelchairs to travel by city bus. While on this trip, the occupational therapy assistant observes Jamelle and identifies specific skills needed to successfully use public transportation. The occupational therapy assistant consults with the special education teacher to include information about the transportation system into his classes. Janelle learns to read the route maps and becomes familiar with the tokens used for fares. She provides multiple opportunities for Jamelle to practice using his wheelchair outdoors crossing streets, locating curb cuts, and maneuvering in crowds. The occupational therapy assistant works with the classroom teachers to increase Jamelle's independence and to recognize when he needs to request assistance. ■

SUMMARY

Cerebral palsy is a heterogeneous group of disorders that develops as a result of damage to the brain before, during, or after birth. Children and adolescents with cerebral palsy demonstrate difficulties with movement and posture, resulting from abnormalities in muscle tone. Cerebral palsy can be mild, moderate, or severe, depending on the extent of the brain damage. There are three main types: spastic, athetoid, and ataxic.

Some children have characteristics of more than one type. Cerebral palsy not only is described by type, but by the predominant body parts involved. The suffix plegia is used to describe muscle paralysis; the suffix paresis is used to describe muscle weakness. Although the brain damage that causes cerebral palsy is nonprogressive, some children may appear to get worse as they age, as atypical movement patterns, tone, and gravity, combined with the child's growth may lead to the development of contractures (Nelson, 2001). In addition to the motor difficulties that define cerebral palsy, children and adolescents with this condition may have other problems such as mental retardation, seizures, vision deficits, and hearing problems.

There are many causes of cerebral palsy; the incidents associated with some of these causes, such as prematurity, are increasing. The incidents associated with other causes, such as asphyxia and jaundice, appear to be on the decline with medical advances. However, the overall incidence of cerebral palsy has remained relatively constant.

Managing cerebral palsy requires attending to the child's speech, social and emotional, and cognitive development. For this reason, a team of doctors, nurses, educators, and therapists are involved. Physicians provide a variety of medical and surgical interventions. Physical therapists focus on posture and ambulation while speech and language pathologists focus on swallowing, breath control, and language expression and understanding. At school, educators may adapt the curriculum to adjust to the specific needs of children and adolescents with cerebral palsy.

Occupational therapy practitioners collaborate with a variety of healthcare professionals to maximize the performance of children and adolescents with cerebral palsy. Occupational therapy practitioners pay close attention to person, environment, and occupation factors in designing interventions for children and adolescents with cerebral palsy, and may use biomechanical, neurodevelopmental, and compensatory approaches. The needs of children and adolescents change as they grow and develop. With intervention, most children and adolescents significantly improve their ability to participate in their home, school, and community life.

REVIEWING KEY POINTS

1. Explain the common characteristics and symptoms of cerebral palsy.
2. Explain the three types of cerebral palsy: spastic, athetoid, and ataxic.
3. Define the terms diplegia, hemiplegia, and quadriplegia.
4. Explain the difference between the suffixes paresis and plegia.
5. Describe the most common causes of cerebral palsy.
6. Describe medical and surgical interventions for cerebral palsy.
7. Describe professionals who provide services to children and adolescents with cerebral palsy.
8. Explain what is meant when occupational therapy services are described as itinerant or related.

APPLYING KEY CONCEPTS

1. Further investigate one or more of the intervention approaches that occupational therapy practitioners use when working with youngsters with cerebral palsy: NDT, biomechanical, or compensatory. Visit an occupational therapy department that uses at least one of these approaches.

2. Explain one or more ways in which occupational therapy practitioners collaborate with other educational and health professionals in working with children and adolescents with cerebral palsy.
3. With a partner, demonstrate the positioning and handling suggestions for Michael (Figure 20.4). What other suggestions can you add to this list?
4. Refer to Minnie's case study. What modifications do you anticipate she will need when she enters later grades?
5. Explore the topic of low vision aids. Based on the information in Rosetta's case study, what aids may be helpful for her?
6. Explore the topic of English as a second language (ESL). What safeguards are in effect that assure that children and adolescents with ESL are not misidentified as having mental retardation?
7. Refer to Jamelle's case study. Identify what additional skills he will need to access public transportation. Design a series of intervention sessions that address those skills.
8. After reviewing the case studies, consider the follow topics:
   a. How important is interdisciplinary collaboration between occupational therapy practitioners and other disciplines?
   b. How do the needs of children and adolescents with cerebral palsy change as they get older?

REFERENCES

American Academy of Pediatrics (2000). Changing concepts of sudden infant death syndrome: Implications for infant sleeping environment and sleep position. *Pediatrics, 105,* 650–656.

Beery, K. Buktenic, N., & Beery, N. (2005). The Beery-Buktenic Developmental Test of Visual-Motor Integration (Beery™ VMI) manual. Minneapolis, MN: NCS. Person, Inc.

Bonnier, B. (2006). Effects of constraint-induced movement therapy in adolescents with hemiplegic cerebral palsy: A day camp model. *Scandinavian Journal of Occupational Therapy, 13,* 13–22.

Bly, L. (1983). *The components of normal movement during the first year of life and abnormal motor development.* Oak Park, IL: Neurodevelopmental Treatment Association.

Charles, J. (2001). Effects of constraint-induced therapy on hand function in children with hemiplegic cerebral palsy. *Pediatric Physical Therapy, 13,* 68–76.

Charles, J., & Gordon, A. M. (2005). A critical review of constraint-induced movement therapy and forced use in children with hemiplegia. *Neural Plasticity, 12,* 245–261.

Christiansen, C., Baum, C. M., & Bass-Haugen, J. (Eds.). (2005). *Occupational therapy: Performance, participation, and well-being.* (3rd ed.). Thorofare, NJ: SLACK.

Colangelo, C. (1999). Biomechanical frame of reference. In P. Kramer & J. Hinojosa (Eds.), *Frames of reference for pediatric occupational therapy* (pp. 233–305). Baltimore: Williams & Wilkins.

Crocker, M. D., Mackay-Lyons, M., & McDonnell, E. (1997). Forced use of the upper extremity in cerebral palsy: A single-case design. *American Journal of Occupational Therapy, 51,* 824–833.

Doster, S., & Politano, P. (1996). Augmentative and alternative communication. In J. Hammel (Ed.), *AOTA self-paced clinical course: Technology and occupational therapy—A link to function.* Rockville, MD: AOTA.

Dunn, W., Brown, C., & McGuigan, A. (1994). The ecology of human performance: A framework for considering the effect of context. *American Journal of Occupational Therapy, 48,* 595–607.

Dunn, W. (2000). *Best practice occupational therapy in community service with children and families.* Thoroughfare, NJ: SLACK.

Fetters, L., Figueiredo, E. M., Keane-Miller, D., et al. (2004). Critically appraised topics: Is constraint induced movement therapy an effective intervention for the treatment of upper extremity dysfunction in children with spastic hemiplegic cerebral palsy (CP)? *Pediatric Physical Therapy, 16,* 77.

Folio, M. R., & Fewell, R. R. (2002). *Peabody Developmental Motor Scales (PDMS-2)* (2nd ed.). Denver: Pro Ed.

Glover, J. E., Mateer, C. A., Yoell, C., & Speed, S. (2002). The effectiveness of constraint induced movement therapy in two young children with hemiplegia. *Pediatric Rehabilitation, 5,* 125–131.

Gordon, A. M., Charles, J., & Wolf, S. L. (2005). Methods of constraint-induced movement therapy for children with hemiplegic cerebral palsy: Development of a child-friendly intervention for improving upper-extremity function. *Archives of Physical Medicine & Rehabilitation, 86,* 837–844.

Hart, H. (2005). Can constraint therapy be developmentally appropriate and child-friendly? *Developmental Medicine & Child Neurology, 47,* 363.

Hoare, B. (2004). There is weak evidence that forced-use therapy provided for 1 month without additional therapy improved the fine motor function of children with hemiparesis. *Australian Occupational Therapy Journal, 51,* 110–111.

Howle, J. (2002). *Neuro-developmental treatment approach: Theoretical foundations and principles of clinical practice.* Laguna Beach, CA: The North American Neuro-Developmental Treatment Association.

Kielhofner, G., Tham, K., Baz, T., & Hutson, J. (2002). Performance capacity and the lived body. In G. Kielhofner (Ed.), *Model of human occupation: Theory and application* (3rd ed.). Baltimore: Lippincott, Williams & Wilkins.

Law, M., Baptiste, S., Carswell, A., McColl, M., Polatajko, H., & Pollock, N. (1998). *Canadian Occupational Performance Measure* (3rd ed.). Ottawa: CAOT Publication.

Law, M., Cooper, B., Strong, S., Stewart, D., Rigby, P., & Letts, L. (1996). The Person-Environment-Occupation model: A transactive approach to occupational performance. *Canadian Journal of Occupational Therapy, 63 (1),* 9–23.

Law, M., Missiuna, C., Pollack, N., & Stewart, D.(2005). Foundations for occupational therapy practice with children. In J. Case-Smith, *Occupational therapy for children* (5th ed.), pp. 53–87. St. Louis: Mosby.

March of Dimes (2004). *Cerebral palsy.* Retrieved June 10, 2006 from http://www.marchofdimes.com/printableArticles/681.

Menkes, J. H. (2001). *Textbook of child neurology.* Baltimore: Williams & Wilkins.

Morris, S. E., & Klein, M.D. (2000). *Pre-feeding skills: A comprehensive resource for mealtime development* (2nd ed.). San Antonio: Therapy Skill Builders.

Nelson, C. A. (2001). Cerebral palsy. In D. Umphed (Ed.), *Neurological rehabilitation* (4th ed.), pp. 259–286. St. Louis: Mosby.

Park, T. S., & Owen, J. H. (1992). Surgical management in spastic diplegia in cerebral palsy. *New England Journal of Medicine, 326,* 745–749.

Pellegrino, L. (2002). Cerebral palsy. In M.L. Batshaw (Ed), *Children with disabilities,* pp. 443–666. Baltimore: Brookes.

Rogers, S. (2005). Common conditions that influence children's participation. In J. Case-Smith *Occupational therapy for children* (5th ed.), pp. 160–215. St. Louis: Mosby.

Schoen, S., & Anderson, J. (1999). Neurodevelopmental treatment frame of reference. In P. Kramer and J. Hinojosa (Eds.), *Frames of reference for pediatric occupational therapy* (2nd ed.). Philadelphia: Lippincott Williams & Wilkins.

Schkade, J. K., & Schultz, S. (1992). Occupational adaptation: Toward a holistic approach to contemporary practice, part 1. *American Journal of Occupational Therapy, 46,* 829–837.

Shumway-Cook, A., & Woollacott, M. (2006). *Motor control: Translating research into clinical practice* (3rd ed.). Philadelphia: Lippincott Williams & Wilkins.

Stamer, M. (2000). *Posture and movement of the child with cerebral palsy.* San Antonio: Therapy Skill Builders.

Stanley, F. J., Blair, E., & Alberman, E. (2000). *Cerebral palsies: Epidemiology and causal pathways* (Vol. 151). New York: Cambridge University Press.

Taub, E., Miller, N. E., Novack, T. A., Cook, E. W., Fleming, W. C., Nepomuceno, C. S., Connell, J. S., & Crago, J. E. (1993). Technique to improve chronic motor deficit after stroke. *Archives of Physical Medicine & Rehabilitation, 74,* 347–354.

Taub, E., Ramey, S. L., DeLuca, S., & Echols, K. (2004). Efficacy of constraint-induced movement therapy for children with cerebral palsy with asymmetric motor impairment. *Pediatrics, 113,* 305–312.

Willis, J. K., Morello, A., Davie, A., et. al. (2002). Forced use treatment of childhood hemiparesis. *Pediatrics, 110,* 94–96.

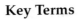

Chapter 21

Children and Adolescents with Autism Spectrum Disorder

Janet V. DeLany and David Kresse

Key Terms

Applied Behavior Analysis
Asperger syndrome
Autistic disorder
Autistism spectrum disorder
Childhood disintegrative disorder
DIR/Floortime
Discreet trial
Echolalia
Engagement
Epidemiologists

Pervasive developmental disorder
Rett syndrome
Shared attention
Social modeling
Social stories
TEACCH
Two way purposeful interactions
Two way problem solving

Objectives

- Explain autism spectrum disorders (ASD).
- Examine how ASD impacts the daily occupations of children and adolescents within the context of their family and environment.
- Describe occupational therapy interventions to support the capacity of children and adolescents with ASD to participate in their daily occupations.
- Examine how occupational therapists and occupational therapy assistants problem solve together during the intervention process.
- Describe how occupational therapists and occupational therapy assistants work with families and other professionals to provide services to children and adolescents with ASD.

INTRODUCTION

According to the *Diagnostic and Statistical Manual of Mental Disorders* (4th ed., rev) (DSM-IV TR), which is used to diagnose mental disorders, **pervasive developmental disorders (PDD)** are a group of early neurobiological disorders that include the following subtypes:

- Autistic disorder
- Asperger disorder
- Pervasive developmental disorder, not otherwise specified (NOS)
- Childhood disintegrative disorder
- Rett syndrome (APA, 2000)

Other terms are used interchangeably to describe these same conditions. Although listed as Asperger disorder in DSM-IV, in most of the literature it is referred to as **Asperger syndrome**. Though inconsistent with DSM-IV classification, the term **autism spectrum disorder (ASD)** is used synonymously with the term PDD to include all of the subtypes (Janzen, 2003). Sometimes, people use the word autism also to refer generically to all of the subtypes of ASD; other times they use the term autism to refer specifically to Autistic disorder.

Children and adolescents with ASD exhibit varying degrees of impaired social skills, communication disorders, and restricted, stereotyped patterns of behavior (AOTA, 2005). They may be delayed in some or all areas of their development, including physical, cognitive, and social-emotional. In addition they may have some difficulty

- Controlling motor and verbal responses
- Modulating and integrating sensory stimulation
- Scanning the environment to identify and focus on essential information
- Processing auditory information efficiently and reliably
- Understanding the meaning of visual information
- Accurately perceiving time concepts
- Understanding the varying meanings of words and concepts
- Organizing and retrieving information in its correct sequence
- Organizing and analyzing information to elicit meaning and determine relationship of new information to past experience
- Finding new or alternative solutions to problems
- Modulating and controlling emotional responses
- Coping with and adapting to change (Janzen, 2003).

In contrast to these areas of difficulty, children and adolescents with ASD may

- Learn and consistently follow routines appropriate to the situation
- Use applicable visual information effectively
- Understand and follow established rules and procedures
- Remember information for a long period of time
- Focus on a specific topic of an extended period of time
- Communicate in a straightforward manner (Janzen, 2003).

Though clustered together under the same diagnostic category, each child and adolescent with ASD has a unique set of capacities and needs. What look like non-compliant behaviors may be an inability to filter or process information. What appear to be belligerent behaviors or withdrawal may be the way the child has to defend himself or communicate feelings in the absence of adequate language (Notbohm, 2005).

ASD can occur alone or in combination with other conditions such as mental retardation, Down syndrome, fragile X syndrome, cerebral palsy, fetal alcohol syndrome, deafness, and blindness. There is widespread concern that the prevalence of ASD is increasing. **Epidemiologists**, scientists who study changes in patterns of health across populations, currently attribute a large portion of this increase to better understanding and reporting of this disorder, a broadening of the classification of ASD, and increasing public attention to ASD. Within school districts, the number of children receiving services for ASD is on the rise (Blaxill, 2004; Gurney, et al., 2003; Newschaffer et al., 2005; Palmer et al., 2005). The Center for Disease Control (CDC) reports rates as high as 20 to 60 per 10,000 for ASD (CDC, 2006).

Mutations on several different genes and chromosomes are suspected to be the major cause of ASD (APA, 2000; Barrett et al., 1999; Lauritsen et al., 2005; Miller-Kuhaneck, 2004). Abnormalities in the structure, chemistry, and physiology of the brain occur, though it is not clear if autism causes or is caused by these changes. Multiple areas of the brain may be affected, including the cortex, limbic system, cerebellum, and brain stem (Miller-Kuhaneck, 2004; Pelphrey et al., 2005; Reed, 2001). Research by Courchesne, Carper, and Akshoomoff (2003) suggested the "clinical onset of autism appears to be preceded by 2 phases of brain growth abnormality: a reduced head size at birth and a sudden and excessive increase in head size between 1 to 2 months and 6 to 14 months. . . . [and that] abnormally accelerated rate of growth may serve as an early warning signal of risk for autism" (p. 337).

Research also has shown an increased family prevalence of ASD, especially in studies of identical twins who share much of the same genetic material. A child has a 60 to 90 percent chance of having autism if his identical twin has autism. Siblings of children with autism have a 10 percent chance of having autism (Muhle, Trentacoste, & Rapin, 2004). Also, research describing sensory arousal is promising. In two separate studies, Miller et al., (2001) and Schaaf and Miller (2005) noted that children with autism demonstrated hypo responsive sympathetic and parasympathetic nervous systems functions to various types of auditory and visual stimuli. Typically, sympathetic nervous system functions predominate during periods of stress. The heart rate increases, bronchioli dilate, and sweat glands become more active, while digestive functions become less active. Typically, parasympathetic functions dominate during periods of nonstress. The heart rate decreases, bronchioli constrict to normal size, and peristolic and gastrointesinal secretions increase.

While alternative theories have been posed about factors contributing to the rise in the number of cases of ASD, additional research is needed to substantiate them. A study by Herbert (2005) found correlations between the increase in the incidence of autism and toxic sites in Texas. However, other studies examining the possible influence of environmental factors such as toxins to autism remain inconclusive (Edelson & Cantor, 1998; Miller et al., 2005; Miller-Kuhaneck, 2004; Vojdani et al., 2003). Suggestions that childhood immunizations are related to increased incidence of ASD have not been validated (Honda H, 2005; Madsen et al., 2002; Smeeth, et al., 2004). Though children and adolescents with ASD appear to have increased gastrointestinal problems and food allergies (Murch, 2005; Niehus, & Lord, 2006; Valicenti-McDermott et al., 2006), effective approaches to treat these difficulties remain unclear.

Currently, no effective biological test exists to determine whether a child or adolescent has ASD at birth. Determination is based on interviews with family members and teachers, family history, medical examination, clinical observations of behaviors, and psychological, communication, educational, and occupational assessments (National Dissemination Center for Children with Disabilities [NICHCY], 2003). However, current research about early detection of ASD is promising. Zwaigenbaum et al. (2005) found that children at 12 months of age, who were diagnosed later with ASD, demonstrated numerous abnormal behaviors. They had difficulty with visual tracking, visual attending, orienting to name, reacting to and imitating the actions of others, socially smiling, displaying social interest and affect, and engaging in sensory-oriented behaviors. The infants exhibited "marked passivity and decreased activity level at 6 months, followed by extreme distress reactions, a tendency to fixate on particular objects in the environment, and decreased expression of positive affect by 12 months [and] delayed expressive and receptive language" (Zwaigenbaum et al., 2005, p. 143). Mitchell et al. (2006) also found that children with ASD showed delays in early language and communication compared with non-ASD siblings and controls. At 12 months, the children with ASD understood significantly fewer phrases and produced fewer gestures than did non-ASD children. At 18 months, the children with ASD continued to exhibit delays in their understanding of phrases, their comprehension and articulation of single words, and their utilization of body and hand gestures. In a multiple year study, Landa and Garrett-Mayer (2006) found detectable fine motor, gross motor, and receptive and expressive language delays using standardized tests as early as 24 months. Landa (2006) also found signs of language and motor complications in 6-month-old infants who were later diagnosed as having autism. It is hoped that this improved ability to diagnose autism when the children are very young will enable interventions to be initiated earlier.

The prognosis for children and adolescents with ASD varies considerably. There is a continuum of functioning from severely impaired to mildly impaired. Children and adolescents with higher language and cognitive skills have a better prognosis (APA, 2000). Approximately one-third of children and adolescents with ASD achieve some level of independent living (APA, 2000; Howlin et al., 2004). Howlin reported that in a study of 68 children with ASD who were followed into adulthood, a few lived alone, had close friends, and sustained permanent employment. Some of the adults lived in group homes and participated in supported work. Their communication difficulties and stereotyped behaviors persisted. Those with more severe forms of ASD needed lifelong support for performing activities of daily living and instrumental activities of daily living.

Autistic Disorder

Children and adolescents with autistic disorder have qualitative impairment in social interactions and communication, and restricted, repetitive, and stereotyped patterns of behaviors, interests, and activities (APA, 2000). Seventy percent of these children and adolescents have mild to severe mental retardation. Often, they are over or under sensitive to sensory input, such as light, textures, smells, movement, and sounds. Behavioral complications include hyperactivity, short attention span, impulsivity, aggressiveness, temper tantrums, and self-injurious behaviors such as biting, scratching, and head banging. Because change frequently exacerbates these negative behaviors, families often try to develop functional and predictable routines to enable their children and adolescents to participate in some of the daily home activities and rituals (Larson, 2006).

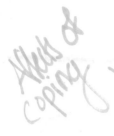

New interpretations are emerging about the reason for the behaviors that children with autism frequently display. Previously viewed as physiologically predetermined, behaviors such as spinning, repeatedly uttering particular phrases, and head banging now are viewed as coping mechanisms. Emotional inexpressiveness and mental retardation may be the result of communication difficulties rather than emotional or cognitive limitations.

To be diagnosed with autistic disorder, children must display the symptoms by age 3 (APA, 2000). Usually, the features associated with autism can be observed during infancy and early toddlerhood, though the signs can be subtle and dismissed initially as being a part of the range of normal development. Autistic disorder occurs in males four to five times more frequently than in females (APA, 2000).

Asperger Syndrome

Similar to those with autistic disorder, children and adolescents with Asperger syndrome demonstrate qualitative impairments in social interactions and exhibit repetitive and stereotyped patterns of behaviors, and restricted areas of interests, though to a lesser degree than those with autistic disorder. They may struggle with feelings of anxiety and depression that arise from social interaction challenges, particularly as they enter adolescence. Those who are anxious tend to be hypersensitive to sensory stimuli; those who are coping with depression tend to be hyposensitive to sensory stimuli (Pfeiffer, Kinnealey, Reed, & Hersberg, 2005). However, unlike those with Autistic Disorder, children and adolescents with Asperger syndrome do not have significant deficits in language skills, nor do they have clinically significant delays in cognitive development (APA, 2000). While children and adolescents with Asperger syndrome may struggle socially, have a limited number of friends, and adhere to highly established routines and interests, they typically have the language and cognitive skills that allow them to live and function independently in society. As adults, they are more likely than those with autistic disorder to hold jobs and form intimate relationships with others (APA, 2000).

Pervasive Developmental Disorder Not Otherwise Specified

Children and adolescents with pervasive developmental disorder NOS (PDD NOS) exhibit some but not all of the symptoms associated with autistic disorder (APA, 2000; Janzen, 2003). Frequently, they have difficulty with reciprocal social interactions, and verbal and nonverbal communication skills. As infants they may avoid eye contact, and demonstrate little interest in human voices and affection. They do not tend to exhibit separation anxiety or interest in playing with other children. By middle childhood, these children may show more affection toward and involvement with family members, but still have difficulty responding to other people's interests, emotions, or humor. Able to show joy, fear, or anger, they tend to show the extreme rather than the subtle forms of emotions. Thus, they still may have problems with group interactions and forming peer relationships (NICHCY, 2003).

Some of the children with PDD NOS experience significant cognitive delays; others have age appropriate cognitive skills. Generally, they do best on tasks requiring manipulative or visual skills or immediate memory, but struggle with tasks requiring symbolic thought and sequential logic. A few children and adolescents have excellent rote memories and special skills in music, mechanics, and mathematics (NICHCY, 2003).

Those who have significant cognitive limitations develop only a limited understanding of speech. Similar to children with autistic disorder, those with PDD NOS may communicate using **echolalic** speech, that is, repetitive use of particular words or phrases. Those with less severe impairments may follow simple verbal instructions and gestures. They may speak in a monotone, flat voice with little variation in pitch or emotional expression, or use a sing-song like cadence. Pronoun reversals, such as substituting "you" for "me" can occur. Others may struggle only with comprehending subtle or abstract meaning and with the turn taking during verbal exchanges.

Children and adolescents with PDD NOS also may display ritualistic or compulsive behaviors, develop strong attachments to inanimate objects, resist change in routines, and develop a pervasive interest in a few select activities. They may be over or under responsive to visual and auditory sensory input, and may dislike gentle touch but crave rough-and-tumble play. Some eat only a limited range of foods while others do not seem know when they are full.

However, in spite of these potential areas of difficulty, the extent of the developmental delay is less severe for children with PDD NOS than for those with classical autism. As a result, they may not be diagnosed until 3 to 4 years of age. Also, because of the possibility that PDD NOS and autistic disorder are on a continuum, the precise distinction between them is not always clear. A child's diagnosis may switch from autistic disorder to PPD NOS or from PPD NOS to autistic disorder as he or she develops and exhibits more definable behaviors (NICHCY, 2003).

Childhood Disintegrative Disorder

Childhood disintegrative disorder, or Heller syndrome, is a disintegrative disorder that primarily affects boys. The boys appear to develop normally for the first one or two years of life, but then lose previously acquired social, language, play, and motor skills over a period of weeks or months. Similar to those with autistic disorder, children with childhood disintegrative disorder have difficulties in at least two of the following three areas: impaired social interactions; impaired communication; and restricted, repetitive, and stereotyped patterns of behaviors, interests, and activities (APA, 2000). They also may lose their ability to control bowel and bladder functions. A history of the child's early development is necessary to make such a diagnosis (Yale Developmental Disability Clinic, 2006).

Rett Syndrome

Rett syndrome, a neurodevelopmental disorder, primarily affects girls. It tends to appear following a period of apparent normal development during the first 6 to 18 months of life. Though currently clustered with other ASD diagnoses, Rett syndrome is different than autism and may be removed from that categorization in future editions of *DSM*. Rett syndrome is a progressive disorder caused by a mutation in the MECP2 gene on the X chromosome. It results in the failure of the neurons in the brain to continue to synapse near the end of pregnancy or within the first few months after birth. As a result, cells responsible for sensory, emotional, motor, and autonomic function do not develop normally. The girls start to stagnate in development as their head growth slows. Over time they lose communication skills and purposeful use of their hands, and exhibit stereotypical hand wringing and handwashing movements. They also may have difficulty with walking, breathing, eye gaze, and motor control. Often misdiagnosed as autism, Rett occurs in 1 : 10,000 to 1 : 23,000 live female births (IRSA, 2007). The level of severity ranges from mild to severe. Initially, some of the girls are able to accomplish their daily life tasks independently. As the disease progresses, their life expectancy decreases. Most need assistance for such basic tasks's bathing, dressing, and feeding, and use an augmentative device to communicate (IRSA, 2007).

INTERVENTIONS

Considering the severity and breadth of challenges that children and adolescents with ASD and their families face, it is important for professionals to work collaboratively to provide needed services. Some of these professionals include: the primary care physician, teacher, psychologist, social worker, developmental pediatrician, occupational therapist, occupational therapy assistant, speech and language pathologist, audiologist, and physical therapist (AOTA, 2005). Early interventions for children with ASD focus on goals identified by the family. They might include strategies for providing positive parenting to the child, promoting expressive and receptive communication; facilitating physical, sensory, and perceptual skills; developing self-care, social, and play skills, designing safe home environments, managing disruptive behaviors and sleep patterns, and establishing respite services. As the child becomes school age, the focus of these interventions expands to emphasize the curricular and cocurricular educational needs of the child. The ability of the child to participate in family and community activities remains a central concern. By the time the child turns 16 years of age, interventions also need to address postsecondary transition to employment opportunities, additional education, community participation, and community living.

Learning Based Interventions

Professionals use various learning models to guide the interventions they provide to children and adolescents with ASD. The model they select may reflect their professions' philosophical perspectives. Three of the more common learning interventions are Applied Behavior Analysis, DIR/Floortime model, and TEACCH.

Applied Behavior Analysis

Based on the initial research of Ferster, Lovaas, Wolf, and Risley in the 1960s, **Applied Behavior Analysis** (ABA) utilizes positive reinforcers and other methods, such as incidental teaching and peer support, to teach and to shape the behaviors of children and adolescents with ASD. Initially, the child or adolescent may learn to perform a skill through **discreet** trial (DT) teaching. Discreet trial teaching is a process whereby a task is subdivided into smaller, measurable steps that are taught through repeated drilling. The instructor uses reinforcers that the child likes, such as bits of food, tickles, books, or a favorite toy, to build upon the child's initiation of an action and to reward the child for closer and closer approximations of the targeted behavior (Lovaas, 1987; McEachin, Smith, & Lovaas, 1993; Sheinkopf, & Siegel, 1998). The following illustrates the use of discreet trial training.

FOUAD

The classroom teacher wants to increase Fouad's ability to sit in the classroom. Her first goal is to have Fouad sit for 10 seconds when given the directive "Sit in the chair." The teacher uses a form to record Fouad's response each time she gives the directive. If Fouad does not do the desired behavior, the teacher physically cues him to sit. If Fouad sits for 10 seconds the teacher rewards him with his favorite toy. The teacher repeats this procedure for 2 minutes, and then switches to another goal. For a number of additional times throughout the day, the teacher repeats the discreet trial training for sitting until Fouad follows the directive 90 percent of the time for three or more days. Once Fouad masters the goal, the teacher modifies it to include greater demands, such as sitting for longer periods of time or in the presence of other children.

Initially, the child or adolescent may learn the skill in a contrived environment, that is, a learning environment specifically created to help the child learn. Emphasis is placed on acquiring the appropriate behavior. Redirection is used to replace repetitive or self-injurious behaviors with socially accepted ones. After the child masters the skill in the contrived environment, learning shifts to the natural environment, such as the classroom or the cafeteria, to enable generalization of the skill to other situations. Natural and social rewards, such as hugs and praise, gradually replace food based awards.

Those schools and home based programs that implement an intensive ABA approach provide one on one instruction for each child and adolescent for 35 to 40 hours per week. The curriculum is individualized, based on the child's or adolescent's capacities and needs, and systematically leads them through stages of learning. Early programming may focus on developing motor and verbal imitation skills, following basic directions, and making simple requests. Programming then may emphasize asking and responding to simple questions, talking in sentences, completing several step tasks, and playing with others. Goals for older children may address self-help skills, functional communication, school and community involvement, participation in family life, and peer interactions (Lovaas Institute, 2006).

Debate exists about the effectiveness of the ABA approach. Those who criticize it feel that the approach is too regimented and does not foster generalization of learning to new situations. Those who endorse ABA cite a large body of documented evidence regarding its effectiveness and believe that, when used correctly, it promotes generalization of learning.

DIR/Floortime Model

Greenspan and Wieder developed **DIR/Floortime** (Greenspan, 1992a; Greenspan 1992b; Greenspan & Wieder, 1998). DIR stands for *developmental, individual-difference, relationship-based.* Teachers, therapists, other professionals, and parents can use this approach. Based on developmental and humanistic principles, intervention begins by building on the limited routines the child exhibits. The adult interacts with the child first by allowing the child to select activities or actions that interest him. The adult looks to increase communication opportunities by slowly and deliberately building two-way interactions with the child (ICDL, 2000). Adhering to a developmental sequence, the adult tries to guide the child through the six stages of interaction: **shared attention, engagement, two-way purposeful interactions, two-way purposeful problem solving** interactions, elaborating ideas, and connecting ideas for thinking (ICDL).

- *Shared attention:* Initially, the adult encourages the child to briefly attend to the same object as the adult. The adult draws the child's attention to the object by tapping into the sensory system that the child prefers. This may be squeezing a toy to make a sound, or rubbing a toy across the child's hand. The adult also may use "playful obstruction" to facilitate the child's shared attention. To do so, the adult may put her hand over a specific object that the child wants. By forcing the child to move the adult's hand to get the desired object, shared attention takes place.

- *Engagement:* In the second stage, the adult tries to connect with the child by establishing a warm, trusting, and personal relationship. The adult follows the child's lead, rather than directs the child's behavior. The adult sets up the environment with various types of sensory and motor based play opportunities. Once the child selects the play materials, the adult joins the play, and builds on the child's interests to create more elaborate and functional play routines.

- *Two way purposeful interactions:* During the third stage, the adult engages with the child by responding to and building upon the child's nonverbal gestures and facial expressions. For example, the adult may help a child reach a toy in response to the child grasping the adult's hand and walking the adult to the toy shelf. The adult also notes and builds upon the child's facial expressions to model feelings such as pleasure, satisfaction, or curiosity.

- *Two way purposeful problem-solving interactions:* During the fourth stage, the adult fosters complex, preverbal problem solving. For example, the adult may feign an inability to open a door to prompt the child to observe and to problem solve how to respond to the situation.

- *Elaborating ideas:* During the fifth stage, the adult prompts the child to expand upon ideas to engage in imaginary play and to communicate with others. For example, using props, the adult models behaviors and encourages the child to hug and feed a doll or drive a riding toy through a pretend town.

- *Connecting ideas for thinking:* During this stage the adult encourages the child to use language to logically and functionally play and interact with the world. Through these interactions the adult focuses on increasing the child's range of emotional expression (ICDL, 2000).

While debate exists about the effectiveness of the DIR/Floortime approach, Greenspan and Weider (1997) reported that of the 200 cases using this approach, 58 percent had good to outstanding outcomes, 25 percent achieved moderate outcomes, and 17 percent had ongoing difficulties. Critics challenge that what determines good outcomes versus moderate outcomes versus ongoing difficulties needs to be more precisely defined. The following illustrates the use of the DIR/Floortime approach to increase shared attention and engagement with a 4-year-old child with autistic disorder.

GABRIELLA

Gabriella is a 4-year-old who has autistic disorder. The occupational therapy assistant allows Gabriella to pick her favorite activity, which is playing with and repetitively pouring sand over her hands. Initially, the occupational therapy assistant simply stands next to Gabriella and watches the routine. Then the occupational therapy assistant moves closer to Gabriella, pours sand over his hands, and then rubs his hands in the sand. The occupational therapy assistant repeats these actions as Gabriella makes brief eye contact for moments of shared attention. When Gabriella becomes comfortable with this level of interaction, the occupational therapy assistant orchestrates additional opportunities for engagement. He places other scooping toys in the sand box, and sets up other similar sensory tables such as a water table or rice table. Responding to Gabriella's gestures and facial expressions, the occupational therapy assistant pours sand and rice onto Gabriella's and his hands simultaneously. Over a period of sessions, the occupational therapy assistant slowly moves to more advanced levels of play and communication. Next, the occupational therapy assistant pretends to have difficulty with the scooping toys, and asks or waits for Gabriella's help. Next, the occupational therapy assistant encourages Gabriella to elaborate upon her play skills by playing with other sand and water toys, by scooping the sand into buckets, and by hunting for treasures buried in the sand and rice. During the last stage, the occupational therapy assistant models for Gabriella how to use language to describe what she is doing and how she is feeling.

TEACCH

Another education approach used with children and adolescents with ASD is the Treatment and Education of Autistic and Related Communication handicap Children (TEACCH) program. The goal of **TEACCH** is to manage the behaviors and increase the independent functioning of children and adolescents with ASD (Mesibov & Howly, 2003). Rather than trying to cure ASD, TEACCH outlines a method for teaching that incorporates the physical structure, the daily schedule, the work system, and the visual structure and information system (Mesibov et al., 1994; Mesibov & Howly, 2003; Miller-Kuhanek, 2004).

Physical Structure.   Those teachers who use this method arrange their classrooms in a consistent and highly structured manner. They divide the classroom into smaller learning areas to block out distracting stimuli and help the students focus their attention. The teachers may use furniture, tape, or other visual means to designate areas for whole class teaching, group work, play, and relaxation, and to provide clues as to acceptable behaviors for each of those areas. For example, to create a task area, the teacher might block off a corner of the room by putting up a screen, and removing distracting posters and other materials from the wall. To further minimize distractions, the teacher prepares all of the supplies needed for the learning task in advance. She then puts only those materials needed for the first step of the task on top of the desk, within the child's range of vision. She places the materials needed for the subsequent steps into covered bins, underneath or beside the desk. (See Figure 21.1■.)

Daily schedule.   The teacher also prepares a visual display of the classroom schedule to help the students see and understand what will happen during the day. The teacher lists each activity on a separate card using one or two words and a simple picture or photo of the activity. Because the cards are removable, the teacher can prepare the students in advance for changes in the schedule, as needed (see Figure 21.2■). Sometimes, rather than using one classroom schedule for all children, the teacher constructs individual schedules for each child, especially when several of them have a different sequence of tasks to follow.

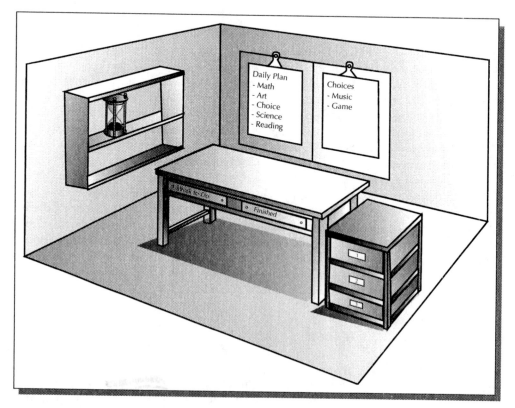

■ **Figure 21.1**
Task area.

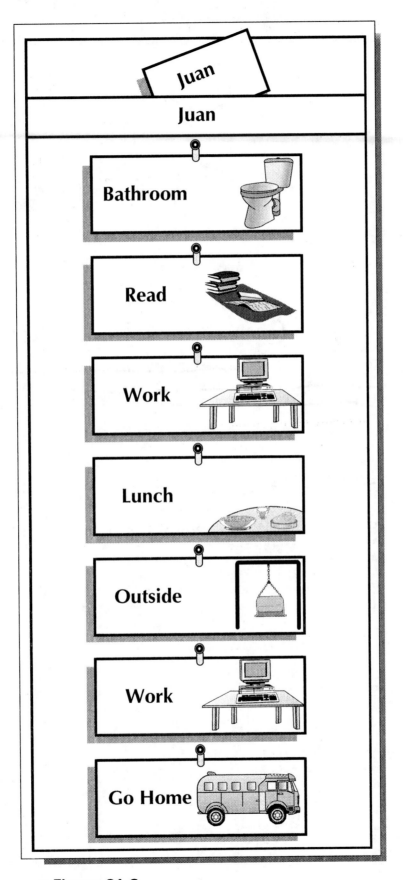

■ Figure 21.2
Daily schedule.

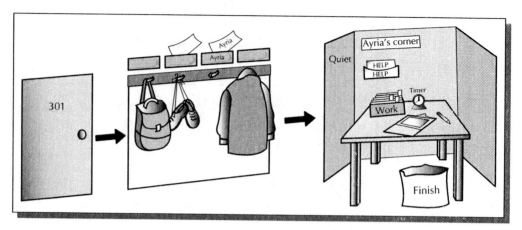

■ Figure 21.3
Work system.

Work Systems. Similarly, the teacher uses visual cues to help children and adolescents with ASD develop work habits to complete tasks as independently as possible. The teacher prepares a series of visual directions that show the students what task they are to perform; how they are to perform the task; how they are to know when they have finished the task; and what they are to do when they complete the task (see Figure 21.3■). Sensitive to the variances in learning abilities, the teacher adapts the number and complexity of the visual directions to match the capacities of the students.

Visual Structure and Information. When using the TEACCH method, teachers also focus on how they provide visual structure and information instruction. For example, for visual clarity, they may place carpet squares on the floor to indicate where each child is to sit during circle time, and use markers to highlight important details on a worksheet. To provide visual structure, they organize the classroom supplies and equipment into clearly defined groupings, using storage containers and pictorial labels. These groupings provide organization and filter out irrelevant sensory stimuli.

When wanting the child or adolescent with ASD to complete a specific task, the classroom instructor combines a number of the TEACCH methods. The following story illustrates the use of TEACCH in the classroom.

TERRELL

The classroom teacher wants Terrell to develop color matching skills. To promote this learning, the teacher directs Terrell to pick up the color sorting card from his daily schedule, and then escorts him to the individual task corner. She uses room dividers to mute the noises and activities of the other children in the room. She instructs Terrell to take different colored plastic fish out of a bin and place them into small boxes that match the color of the fish. The teacher provides visual instruction for this task using pictures that show a child:

- Picking up a fish from the bin
- Placing the fish in matching colored box
- Stopping the task after removing all of the fish from the bin
- Transitioning to the next activity.

The teacher draws a separate picture for each of these tasks, and places them in a top to bottom sequence so that Terrell knows in what order to perform each step.

Various studies have demonstrated increase in intelligence scores for preschoolers (Lord & Schopler, 1994), and greater academic achievement for children using

TEACCH than would otherwise be expected (Venter, Lord, & Schopler, 1992). In addition, studies have found correlations between those older children and adolescents who have been instructed using the TEACCH method and reduced rates of institutionalization (Handleman & Harris, 2001; Ozonoff & Cathcart, 1998; Panerai (et al., 2002;).

Health Care–Based Interventions

Often the primary health care physician or the pediatrician is the first professional to screen for and seek additional services for a child suspected of having ASD. As part of well baby and childhood healthcare screenings, the physician conducts a developmental assessment and may initiate referrals for audiological, speech and language, genetic, occupational therapy, and other neurological and other neurodevelopmental evaluations. The physician may provide medical interventions to address dietary and gastrointestinal concerns such as food refusal, nutrition deficiency, diarrhea and constipation, cyclical vomiting, and reflux that occur more frequently in children and adolescents with ASD. The physician also may recommend medical interventions to address the sleep disturbances, anxiety, aggressive and explosive behaviors, repetitive behaviors, obsessive-compulsive behaviors, self-injurious behaviors, and hyperactivity that children and adolescents with ASD may demonstrate. Medications such as melatonin, antipsychotic drugs, anticonvulsant mood stabilizers, antidepressants, and antianxiety medications help to manage these behaviors. Prior to prescribing such medications, the physician obtains a baseline of the frequency, duration, and intensity of such behaviors, and triggers that exacerbate such behaviors. In addition the physician screens for other contributing factors, such as physical pain, infections, and seizures. Once a baseline of behaviors is established, the physician monitors for changes in behavior and adjusts the dosages accordingly. Often the physician begins to carefully withdraw the medication after 6 to 12 months to assess if it is no longer needed (Myers, 2006).

As the adolescent reaches 18 years of age, the physician may need to help the family petition the courts for guardianship protection, if there is concern about the adolescent's capacity to make responsible decisions. At 18 years of age, adolescents become their own legal guardian unless the court assigns this responsibility to another person. Guardianship may be sought for some or all areas of decision making, including the procurement of medical services, insurance, a driver's license, community living, finances, and voting.

Occupational Therapy Interventions

Occupational therapy interventions focus on enabling children and adolescents with ASD to participate in their ADL, IADL, education, work, leisure, play, and social occupations. Interventions may focus on the occupations, the performance skills, performance patterns, or the performance context. The intervention strategies may include learning approaches such as TEACCH, ABA, and DIR/Floortime, neurodevelopmental approaches such as sensory integration and sensory modulation, and developmental approaches such as social skills training, and skill acquisition. In addition, interventions strategies may focus on modifying the environment and the task to support the children's or adolescents' participation in their occupations. The occupational therapist is responsible for determining which intervention approaches are most appropriate to help children and adolescents with autism participate in their daily life occupations, based on their performance capacities and occupational needs. The following stories about Juan, Tom, and Ayton illustrate three occupational therapy interventions.

Juan

Juan is a 5-year-old child who is severely autistic. He was diagnosed by the school psychologist as functioning in the moderate to severe range for mental retardation. He requires extensive support, that is, regular or daily support from an adult at home and at school (Heward, 2006). Juan recently started receiving special education services in a self-contained classroom for children with developmental delays. Because Juan struggles with a number of classroom tasks and routines, his teacher and parents request an occupational therapy evaluation. To obtain an occupational profile of Juan, the occupational therapist interviews Juan's teacher and parents. The teacher explains that Juan can sit for few minutes to attend to circle time and structured learning activities. He may look at a single object for several minutes, though he looks at people for only a few seconds. He enjoys touching and feeling objects, but struggles with prewriting and manipulative tasks, such as cutting, drawing, and pasting, that require fine motor and visual perceptual coordination. Juan eats a very limited range of foods served at school, primarily plain pasta, dry cereal, French fries, and soft cheese. He uses his fingers rather than a fork or spoon to feed himself and drinks from a sippy cup, preferring room temperature water or apple juice. He assists with pushing down and pulling up his pants, but requires others to put on and take off his coat and manipulate clothing fasteners.

Juan's parents report similar details. When given physical cues, he attempts to perform a simple physical activity that his parents request him to complete, such as placing an object in a container. He picks up and looks at toys, but usually does not play with them in a variety of ways. His prefers to watch the same video repeatedly and becomes angry if his parents try to turn it off before the story is over. They calm him by hugging him firmly and rubbing his back. Occasionally he interacts with his younger sister by rolling a ball back and forth to her. To make sure Juan is safe and does not wander away, one parent needs to continually supervise him. They are able to take him to the local playground where he can roam, but do not venture to take him to a restaurant or community event that requires him to sit. They avoid going to shopping centers, because he becomes overwhelmed with the noises and begins to bite his hand and to scream.

Based on this preliminary information, the occupational therapist asks the occupational therapy assistant to collect samples of how Juan engages in his school occupations in the classroom, at lunch, and on the playground, and to take notes about each of these environments. To organize her thinking about the assessment results, the occupational therapist selects the Person-Environment-Occupational Performance model. She chooses this model because it helps her design interventions that address Juan's personal capacities and needs; his current occupational performance levels; and the environment that affects these capacities, needs, and performance levels.

Evaluation Process

Using a site-specific form, the occupational therapy assistant completes the school based observations and prepares a written report for the occupational therapist. See Table 21.1■ for a summary of these observations.

Based on the conversation with the parents and classroom teacher and the report from the occupational therapy assistant, the occupational therapist decides to administer the Pediatric Evaluation of Disability Inventory [PEDI]

(Haley et al., 1992) and the Sensory Profile (Dunn, 1997). These are standardized assessments that can provide a baseline of Juan's occupational performance using information gathered through interviews with the parents and classroom teacher and additional observations of Juan in his natural environment. Because Juan has difficulty consistently following verbal directions, the occupational therapist does not administer standardized assessments that require him to complete series of prescribed tasks. The PEDI provides information about self-care, mobility, and social participation; the Sensory Profile assesses sensitivity and responsive to sensory input. In addition, the occupational therapist uses a developmental checklist to compare Juan's performance levels with those of other children his chronological age.

As measured by the PEDI, Juan needs moderate physical assistance from a caregiver to feed himself, brush his hair and teeth, and cleanse and dress his body. Though ambulatory, he is unaware of safety precautions, and wanders rather than purposefully moves from one location to another. Able to speak a few words, he communicates with others primarily through physical actions. He enjoys some rough and tumble play, though he has a limited repertoire of

■ **Table 21.1**
Sample of Juan's School-Based Performance Skill and Performance Patterns

Occupations Observed	Performance Skills and Performance Patterns Observed	Performance Context
Walking from bus to classroom Placing belongings in cubby Selecting and experimenting with materials at activity stations	Walked calmly as classroom aide placed her arm across his shoulder and escorted him to the classroom. With physical cuing from the aide, hung jacket and school bag on peg in cubby. Stopped for 10 seconds to 2 minutes at the stations to touch and pick up some of the toys. Ran fingers over wheels of truck for 2 minutes. Momentarily glanced at classmates but did not speak with them. Took a toy from another child; did not respond to or look at the child when she started to cry. Did not respond when verbally prompted by the teacher to return the toy to the child. Attempted to hit the child when physically cued by teacher to return the toy. Initially squirmed then quickly quieted when hugged firmly by the teacher to block the hits. Moved the teacher's hands and squeezed them firmly against his face and arms; smiling briefly.	School hallway Classroom with five activity stations that contain toys and prewriting materials Classroom filled with visual, auditory, olfactory stimuli from the objects, and the actions of the children and teachers in it
Singing songs and responding to teacher directed questions during circle time	Sat for two minutes independently, then stood up and began to wander around the room. Allowed classroom aide to physically direct him back to the circle. Sat with the group for five minutes when she placed her hands firmly on his shoulder and thighs. Sang same five words of song several times while currently clapping his hands; did not respond to questions.	Sitting on carpet squares in semicircle in the center of the classroom Background ambient noise from clock and street traffic
Completing manipulative matching, and prewriting tasks	Given verbal and physical cues, stacked six blocks. Held blocks against the palm of his hand rather than distally at his fingertips when he stacked them. Applied too much force and knocked over the tower. Matched colored blocks correctly 50 percent of time; matched one out of four objects to picture of object. With physical cues, placed fingers in scissor holes. Held arm in prone position and made jagged snips when attempting to cut along a solid line.	One on one session with classroom aide at a child size desk; aide used ABA approach to structure learning

■ **Table 21.1**

Sample of Juan's School-Based Performance Skill and Performance Patterns (cont.)

Occupations Observed	Performance Skills and Performance Patterns Observed	Performance Context
	Imitated scribbling vertical, but not horizontal, strokes with colored marker on paper, using an immature palmar grasp. Frequently tried to chew marker.	
	Repeatedly chewed and sucked on shirt during these activities, even though cued by classroom aide to stop.	
Eating lunch in the school cafeteria	Initially pushed children near him, then covered ears.	Noisy, brightly lit room with 20 tables
	Fed himself French fries using fingers. Ate applesauce from spoon, fed to him by classroom assistant. Pushed the spoon away when the aide encouraged him to feed himself.	Sat at a small table with the aide, separated from other children because of his frequent attempts to push and hit them
Playing outdoors after lunch recess	Repeatedly walked around the perimeter of the playground, dragging his fingers along the wire fence. Did not explore or use the playground equipment, except to push the swing. Briefly looked at but did not talk to or play with the other children.	Fenced playground area with swings, climbing gym, and grassy areas

exploratory play skills, performing the same few actions repeatedly. He completes some home and school tasks by imitating a series of one-two step familiar actions. As measured by the Sensory Profile, Juan has a high threshold for tactile stimuli, and a low threshold for auditory stimuli and oral sensory sensitivity. Based on a developmental checklist, Juan performs fine and gross motor skills in the 20 to 26 month range. He can walk forward and backward, run, jump down, and climb steps; he can scribble, insert shapes into form boards, turn pages, snip with scissors, and open containers.

During a supervisory meeting to discuss Juan, the occupational therapist and the occupational therapy assistant note similarities among the data gathered from the preliminary meeting with the parents and teacher, the classroom observations, and standardized assessments. First, Juan demonstrates developmental delays in a variety of daily living, education, and play occupations. These capacities are consistent with his moderate to severe range for mental retardation. Second, he likes touching objects, receiving firm, deep touch, and chewing resistive materials. He has a narrow tolerance for foods and noise levels. Third, he copes by biting, hitting, screaming, or covering his ears when his routine is changed, he is in noisy environments, or he cannot communicate his wants. These behaviors interfere with his ability to participate in school related activities. The occupational therapist and occupational therapy assistant also suspect that Juan's limited exploration and use of toys, school materials, and playground equipment may reflect dyspraxia, that is, difficulty knowing how to plan the movements of his body. In summary, cognitive delays, compounded by sensory modulation issues and dyspraxia, may negatively impact Juan's occupational performance.

Intervention Plan

In collaboration with his parents, the classroom teacher, and the other members of the team, the occupational therapist added the following goals to Juan's annual IEP:

Goal 1: Juan will demonstrate improved sensory modulation to participate with his peers in the school environment including the classroom, lunchroom, and playground.

Objective 1a: Juan will remain seated for 10 minutes to participate with his peers in classroom, lunchroom and other assembly functions, given periodic tactile cuing 4/5 times.

Objective 1b: Juan will seek and use materials and supplies in the classroom, such as headphones, fidget toys, beanbag chairs, and to modulate sensory input, 4/5 times.

Goal 2. Juan will complete self-care activities.

Objective 2a. Juan will put on and take off his clothes given physical assistance for fasteners, 4/5 times.

Objective 2b. Juan will eat at least one item from each food group daily, 4/5 days.

Objective 2c. Juan will feed himself using a fork and spoon, 4/5 times.

Objective 2d. Juan will wash and dry face and hands, and brush teeth, given minimum physical prompts, 4/5 times.

Goal 3: Juan will demonstrate an improved ability to explore and play with materials and equipment in the school environment.

Objective 3a: Juan will explore and play with a variety of classroom media and toys for 10 minutes, given modeling and verbal praise, 4/5 times.

Objective 3b: Juan will explore and play on several different pieces of playground equipment for at least 10 minutes, given physical and verbal cues, 4/5 times.

The occupational therapist and the occupational therapy assistant meet with the classroom teacher to devise a biweekly schedule to provide consultation and to work directly in the classroom with Juan. They contact the speech and language pathologist to help develop Juan's communication abilities. In collaboration with the parents, they determine how to observe and systematically respond to Juan's nonverbal gestures and spoken words. Appreciating that Juan communicates feelings of frustration and emotional distress by crying, biting, and hitting, they decide to provide deep tactile pressure and a calm, soothing voice to comfort him (Notbohm, 2005). When directing Juan to perform, they agree to cue him physically as to how to initiate the action. They also agree to design and teach Juan how to use a simple communication board that has photos of Juan performing specific actions. The occupational therapy assistant collects baseline data on how frequently Juan communicates with nonverbal gestures or pictures, follows simple directions, and behaves aggressively before starting the intervention, then once weekly for a four-week period after initiating the program, to document the effectiveness of the interventions.

Because Juan actively seeks and enjoys tactile input, the occupational therapy assistant helps the teacher design tactile based learning stations in the classroom. The stations include sand and soapy water tables, finger paints made from food items such as pudding and colored whipped cream, a ballpit, and weighted shoebox sized cardboard blocks covered with various fabrics. The occupational therapy assistant plays with Juan at these stations, modeling and providing physical cues regarding various ways to play with the materials. As Juan begins to initiate play with the materials, the occupational therapy assistant invites other children to join them. The occupational therapy assistant documents the length of time Juan plays with the materials and other children, the way he plays with the materials and other children, and the types of materials and play opportunities he explores.

The occupational therapist also suggests that Juan sit in a beanbag chair and hold tactile toys during circle time such as squeeze toy, stress ball, or a small textured beanbag. These fidget toys may satisfy some of Juan's tactile needs and allow him to sit for longer periods during this structured time. The occupational therapy assistant shows the classroom aide how to provide Juan with compression in a beanbag chair and how to provide deep tactile input while rolled up firmly in blanket if he becomes restless during circle time activities. To determine the effectiveness of these strategies, the occupational therapy assistant measures Juan's attention to tasks on three different activities before implementing the strategy and then once a week when implementing the strategy.

The occupational therapist also recommends a number of intervention strategies for lunchtime. To help with the cafeteria noise, the occupational therapist recommends that Juan try wearing headphones. Initially, she recommends that he wear them for only short intervals until he gets used to them. The occupational therapist also recommends that the parents try the headphones when they are in noisy locales in the community. To help with oral sensitivity, the occupational therapist initiates an oral desensitization program and encourages Juan to chew on various edible and nonedible objects. In collaboration with his parents, she gradually introduces Juan to new types of foods, slowly introducing slightly different textures, tastes, and temperatures. To help Juan learn to feed himself, she requests the occupational therapy assistant initially guide his movements by providing support to his elbow and wrist. As Juan initiates more of the movement to scoop the food from the dish and bring it to his mouth, she requests that the occupational therapy assistant fade out the level of assistance.

To address self-care skills, the occupational therapist, the occupational therapy assistant, the classroom teacher, and the parents agree to use a backward chaining teaching method. Using this method, Juan first learns to complete the last step of the task independently, then the second to last step, then the third to last step. He follows this sequence until he learns all of the steps. For example, when toileting, Juan first learns to push his pants down to his ankles, after the adult lowers them to his knees. He then learns to push the pants from his hips to his knees. Finally, he learns to un-fasten his pants, and push them over his hips and knees, to his ankles. This approach enables Juan to focus most of his attention on the completion of the task. The occupational therapist advises using a firm touch when providing physical assistance because Juan best tolerates this type of guidance.

The occupational therapy assistant also spends a num-ber of sessions on the playground with Juan. Initially, the occupational therapy assistant walks with Juan as he paces around the playground fence. Working with the adaptive physical education teacher, the occupational therapy assis-tant next guides Juan to the playground equipment, and en-courages him to follow the other children as they crawl into the tunnel because of its confining space. Once Juan masters the tunnel, the occupational therapy assistant encourages Juan to sit on and slide down the lower section of the slide. To help Juan feel more secure, initially the occupational ther-apy assistant sits with Juan as he goes down the slide. Over the course of five sessions the occupational therapy assis-tant and the physical education teacher introduce Juan to the jungle gym, encouraging him to watch and imitate the actions of his peers. With intervention aimed at Juan, his school and home environment, and the tasks that he is ex-pected to complete, Juan starts to make gradual improve-ment on a number of his goals. ■

Tom

Tom is an 8-year-old boy with autistic disorder who func-tions in the mildly mentally retarded range of cognitive abilities. He is in a third grade inclusion program. He re-ceives occupational therapy services in his school to ad-dress academic challenges resulting from sensory processing, fine motor, perceptual, and social skills difficulties. Tom's grandparents, who are his legal guardians, feel that while their grandson has made steady progress in many of these areas, they continue to have concerns about his participation in home and com-munity social activities. Because of social skill difficul-ties, he rarely is included to play with the neighborhood children, and is socially isolated when playing on com-munity sports teams. As a result, Tom's grandparents decide to take him to a pediatric center in their commu-nity that specializes in providing occupational therapy services for children and adolescents with ASD.

At the center, Tom's grandparents provide the occupa-tional therapist with a copy of a recent school occupational therapy evaluation. The grandparents explain that while they are aware of Tom's numerous needs, they are specifi-cally looking to address his at-home and community partic-ipation needs.

Evaluation Process

The occupational therapist interviews the grandparents, and asks permission to observe Tom interacting with neighbor-hood peers. The occupational therapist also asks Tom's grandparents to complete the Social Responsiveness Scale (Constantino, 2002).

Tom's grandparents explain that he has difficulty fol-lowing through on chores, occupying himself during leisure times, waiting to eat at restaurants, tolerating the noise and crowds at the mall, and changing routines (Larson, 2006). Unless they physically cue him to interact with children, he plays by himself. While the children in the neighborhood are generally polite to Tom, they are reluctant to play with him. He often invades their personal space, repeatedly asks unrelated questions, has difficulty staying focused, and oc-casionally hits other children—possibly as a way to try to interact with them. The results of the SRS questionnaire indicate that Tom has difficulty with social awareness, social information processing, and reciprocal social communication.

To augment this information, the occupational thera-pist directs the occupational therapy assistant to collect sam-ples of Tom's behavior while playing in the neighborhood. The occupational therapy assistant completes the summary shown in Table 21.2 ■

■ **Table 21.2**
Observations of Tom

OCCUPATIONS OBSERVED	PERFORMANCE SKILLS AND PATTERNS DEMONSTRATED	CONTEXT FOR PERFORMANCE
A large group of 12 children from the neighborhood play kickball; 20 minute observation. The children utilize motor skills such as coordination, mobility, and energy to run and kick, catch, and throw the ball. They understand the rules of the game and adapt to the various situations and conflicts that happen within the course of the game. They exchange information about how to play and win the game.	Tom sits on the curb and watches until his grandmother walks him over to where the group is playing and asks one of the older children if Tom can play. The child agrees and Tom is assigned to a team. Tom immediately goes to the plate to kick even though another child is already standing there. He does not respond to verbal cues to wait his turn. He finally moves to the back of the line when the child faces Tom, gestures to the back of the line, and touches his arm as a cue to move. Tom does not visually focus on the game as he waits his turn. When it is his turn he misses the ball repeatedly. After three "strikes" he does not leave the plate as expected under the rules of the game. The other team continues to give Tom a chance until he does kick the ball. After Tom kicks the ball he does not run toward first base until the girl behind him pushes him. He finally runs slowly towards the base. Though he is "put out" by the other team he stands on the base and refuses to leave. The other team allows him to stay. While on the base Tom talks to the first baseman, repeatedly asking questions about the sound of a fire alarm that can be heard in the distance. Tom stands very close to the other child as he is talking, though he does not make eye contact. When Tom's team is in the field he is put on third base. He stands directly on the base and rarely looks at the child kicking. When a foul ball is kicked near him he picks up the ball and examines it for almost 15 seconds before throwing it toward one of his teammates. Tom plays for two innings and then leaves the game and returns to his grandmother. The other children continue to play without him.	Quiet neighborhood street Group of children from neighborhood who know each other. The ages of the children appear to range from 6 to 10 years of age. Cultural expectation of competition and desire to win

Intervention Plan

Based on the results of the evaluation, the occupational therapist recommends that the grandparents try the following strategies to help Tom participate in his home tasks:

- Go to low sensory versus high sensory places when shopping.
- Minimize waiting time at restaurants.
- Divide large chores into several component parts, with a checklist for accomplishing each step.
- Describe alterations in the daily routine to prepare Tom for changes.
- Sandwich a difficult chore between two easy chores.
- Give Tom a choice between two options, and a choice of reward for completing required tasks.
- Build in slight variations into the routines; when possible, give Tom the choice of how to change the routine.
- Prioritize which chores are necessary for smooth functioning of the home and which routines are not necessary (Larson, 2006).

In addition, the occupational therapist describes two groups held at the center that might be appropriate for Tom, *Friends Club* and the *Explorers*. Friends Club, the first group, runs for eight weeks. It is a small group of four to six children with ASD, with similar levels of functioning. The focus of this group is to teach and use basic social skills.

The occupational therapist and the occupational therapy assistant begin the Friends Club with a brief introduction describing the activity for the day. Using the **social stories** approach (Gray 2000), they then use simple words to tell a story that depicts a problem a child has with a social situation. The stories address topics such as personal space, sharing, helping others, and making eye contact while talking to someone. Usually the story focuses only on one of these topics. Next, the occupational therapist and occupational therapy assistant lead a discussion about solutions, including suggestions specific for each group member (Gray, 2000). The discussion explores the feeling and actions of all of the people in the story as well as alternative actions that they might try. The occupational therapist and the occupational therapy assistant then encourage the group members to try these solutions while playing a game. The session ends with a summary of what has happened in the group and what they might have learned.

The second group, the Explorers, has eight children, four who have ASD and four who are siblings of children with ASD. The purpose of the Explorers group is to integrate the children with ASD with typically developing peers, and to learn and practice social skills in actual context. Having the typically developing peers in the group allows the children with ASD to learn social skills and develop social competencies through **social modeling**. Social modeling involves presenting an adaptive model of social behavior that allows the children with ASD to learn through example. Over an eight-week period, the group members play a variety of indoor and outdoor group games and plan a final field trip and party at the local bowling alley. Through these activities, group members learn how to take turns, share, make requests, and listen to and respond to the feedback of others (Gray, 2000). Initially, the occupational therapist and occupational therapy assistant provide cues for working together, or model appropriate dialogue to resolve conflict, but decrease this cuing and modeling as the sessions continue. The occupational therapist and occupational therapy assistant gradually introduce new activities involving more complex social skills. These more advanced skills focus on respecting the personal space and considering the perspective of others, attending and reacting appropriately to the actions of others, and generalizing and adapting the rules of one game to other games. The occupational therapist and occupational therapy assistant conclude each session of the Explorers with a discussion of the behaviors and feelings of the group members during the activities.

To measure the success of these interventions, the occupational therapist readministers the Social Responsive Scale at the end of the Explorer group. She interviews the parents about their perceptions of the change in Tom's social competences and requests the occupational therapy assistant to complete observations of the type, complexity, and length of Tom's interactions with the neighborhood children. ∎

Ayton

Ayton is 13 years old. He attends middle school and is in the seventh grade. Because the seventh graders are divided into teams, Ayton has several teachers and rotates through their classes during the day. One teacher serves as the lead teacher.

Ayton has Asperger syndrome. He is highly intelligent and is near the top of his class in academic performance. However, his lead teacher explains that he has difficulty organizing his belongings. His writing is messy, particularly when he rushes to complete the work. He also tends to look unkempt. Often his hair is uncombed, his pants are twisted on his waist, and his shirt is buttoned incorrectly. Ayton has difficulty in large group situations; he complains when there is a lot of noise, too many distractions, or other children in his personal space.

Ayton is a serious boy with intense likes and dislikes. He enjoys bugs, something he has enjoyed since he was young. He often launches into a long talk about bugs and rarely allows the other adolescents to ask questions or give their opinions. If another adolescent disagrees with Ayton, he becomes very upset and argumentative. Though he has one friend who shares an interest in bugs, most of his other peers have learned to avoid him. In addition, they laugh at him when he misunderstands school directions.

Ayton's teachers are concerned about his difficulty interacting with peers in the stimulating middle school environment. After consulting with Ayton's family members, the lead teacher requests that the occupational therapist evaluate Ayton for self-care, handwriting, organizational, and social interaction skills.

Evaluation Process

To begin the evaluation process, the occupational therapist asks the occupational therapy assistant to collect samples of Ayton's performance while he eats lunch, participates in team sports during his physical education class, and works on group projects in the classroom. In collaboration with the teacher, the occupational therapist chooses these activities because they are the most socially challenging for Ayton. The occupational therapy assistant prepares the summary of Ayton's occupational performance shown in Table 21.3■ for the occupational therapist to analyze.

Based upon a review of the sample behaviors the occupational therapy assistant recorded and the comments shared by the lead teacher, the occupational therapist decides to administer several standardized assessments to gather additional information. The occupational therapist first asks Ayton to complete the Child Occupational Self Assessment (COSA) (Keller et al., 2005; Keller & Kielhofner, 2005). The COSA is a self-rating form that allows Ayton to share his perceptions about his competence to participate in various ADL, IADL, school, and social participation, and the importance of those occupations to him. On the form, Ayton indicates that he is very knowledgeable about bugs, and can draw detailed pictures of them. He can easily navigate through the Internet to find information, and can concentrate for long periods of time. He wants to but does not know how to talk to and make friends. He states that he gets upset easily and has a hard time calming down, particularly when he doesn't understand what others are saying, can't find his belongings, or when there are too many people. He gets embarrassed when corrected or teased about the way he is dressed.

The occupational therapist then asks Ayton to complete the Developmental Test of Visual Perception Adolescent and Adult (DTVP-A) and the Sentence Completion Test (Hedderly, 1995) to assess his visual motor and handwriting skills. The Sentence Completion Test is a timed writing test and is scored according to the average words per minute that Ayton produces. In addition, the occupational therapist asks Ayton to complete a nontimed writing sample. The results indicate that Ayton's visual motor skills are age appropriate, except for visual motor writing tasks. When Ayton writes slowly, his writing is legible. However, he tends to write quickly, compromising his ability to accurately write within the designated lines, leave space between words, and size letters correctly.

Finally the occupational therapist asks Ayton to complete the Adolescent/Adult Sensory Profile (Brown & Dunn, 2002) because of Ayton's apparent difficulty tolerating touch and noises. Consistent with the behaviors the occupational therapy assistant observed, Ayton indicates that he has a low threshold of tolerance for tactile stimuli, especially unexpected touch, messy materials, and certain fabrics. He also has a low threshold for auditory stimuli, particularly loud noises, and background noises when he needs to concentrate. In preparation for the meeting with the classroom teachers, Ayton's family members, and the rest of the IEP team, the occupational therapist prepares a summary of the challenges that interfere with Ayton's ability to participate fully in his education (Table 21.4■).

Intervention Plan

To address these challenges, the occupational therapist, in collaboration with the rest of the IEP team, identifies the following goals:

Goal 1. Ayton will notice and attend to his physical appearance throughout the school day.

> **Objective 1a.** Ayton will check and correct his physical appearance at the beginning and end of each class day 4/5 days per week.
>
> **Objective 1b.** Ayton will check and correct his hair and clothing before and after participating in physical education class, and using the bathroom facilities 4/5 times.

■ **Table 21.3**

Observation of Ayton's Performance Skills and Performance Patterns at School

Occupational Expectations	Occupational Performance Skills and Performance Patterns	Context
Work with a group of five other students to answer teacher-prepared questions about a movie they just saw—15 minutes Rearrange desks into clusters to form tables Communicate, and exchange information with peers to produce a group answer to each question Take turns recording the group's answers	Ayton had difficulty finding his pencil and paper in his disorganized schoolbag. He pounded his fist on the desktop four times. After a third reminder from the teacher, Ayton turned his desk to join the writing group. He made eyes contact with his peers four times. Twice he gave suggestions in a loud voice, abruptly talking over fellow students. He moved his chair away from group as the discussion became louder and more animated. He got up out of his chair and started toward the door when the teacher said "Oh. Look what time it is! We need to hurry up with our work and get out of here." Ayton jerked his shoulder away when another student gently touched his shoulder to get his attention. Soon afterward, Ayton walked to the classroom windows and remained there until group finished its work.	Classroom had 24 students. It contained desks and chairs for each student. The classroom was well lit and filled with conversation as students talked with one another in their respective groups.
Enter cafeteria and select seat Eat lunch and engage in unstructured social conversation with peers	Ayton placed his hands over his ears and started to rock as he entered the cafeteria and found his seat. After he finished eating, he covered his ears and read a book about bugs that he had brought to the cafeteria. He made two comments about the book he was reading, but did not wait for a response from the other students before returning to the book. He briefly looked, but did not laugh, when a peer told a joke.	School cafeteria was filled with 100 students; it was well lit and noisy with multiple conversations Students self-selected seats and tables
Change clothes to prepare for physical education class Follow verbal directions of physical education teacher regarding game rules Participate in a volleyball game	Ayton squirmed and yelled when bumped by another student, then moved to a corner of the bleachers to change into his gym shoes. He left his belongings scattered on the bench. He tied his sneakers and tucked his shirttail into his pants after the teacher reminded him to do so.	Gym bleachers Outdoor fields

■ **Table 21.3**
Observations of Ayton's Performance Skills and Performance Patterns at School (cont.)

Occupational Expectations	Occupational Performance Skills and Performance Patterns	Context
	He noticed and started talking about bugs while waiting his turn to begin playing volleyball. He did not respond to or elicit questions from peers about the bugs.	
	He argued with his teammates about the direction to rotate positions and about the way to keep score.	
	He attempted but reacted too slowly to make contact with the volleyball. In the process, he knocked over another player who was closer to the ball.	

■ **Table 21.4**
Summary Observations of Ayton

Challenges	Source of Information	Samples of Gathered Information
Attending to self-care dressing tasks	Teacher report Classroom observation Ayton's self-perception on the COSA	Displayed an unkempt physical appearance and twisted clothing in the classroom Needed verbal cuing and felt embarrassed when reminded to correct his physical appearance
Managing school organizational tasks	Teacher report Classroom observation Ayton's self-perception on the COSA	Had difficulty organizing and finding his classroom supplies Had difficulty organizing clothing at the locker Had difficulty pacing himself to write legibly Became upset when he could not find his belongings
Tolerating tactile and auditory stimuli	Ayton's report on the Sensory Profile Classroom observation	Disliked touching messy materials and certain fabrics Reacted negatively to touch, particularly unexpected touch from another person Disliked being in close physical proximity to others Reacted negatively to loud noises in the cafeteria by holding his hands over his ears Needed verbal cue to refocus on task when the classroom was noisy

■ **Table 21.4**
Summary Observations of Ayton (cont.)

CHALLENGES	SOURCE OF INFORMATION	SAMPLES OF GATHERED INFORMATION
Participating in social interactions with peers	Teacher report Classroom observation Ayton's self-perception on the COSA	Had difficulty concentrating when TV or radio was on at home Reacted angrily to sudden noises such as the sound from the fire alarm during an emergency drill Withdrew from classroom group as noise level increased Talked about a singular topic of interest, and interrupted the conversation of others Became upset and argumentative when others tried to share their opinions, give directions, or question him Did not understand jokes or figurative use of language Maintained only minimal eye contact with peers when talking with them Focused on the task rather than concurrently on the person and the task

Goal 2. Ayton will organize his materials, supplies, and tasks to complete school assignments.

Objective 2a. Using visual cues and space dividers, Ayton will keep his school materials organized 4/5 times.

Objective 2b. Using time management strategies, Ayton will pace himself to write legibly when completing class work and homework assignments 4/5 times.

Goal 3: Ayton will demonstrate improved ability to modulate sensory stimuli to participate in school activities 90 percent of the time

Objective 3a: Ayton will remain in a small group activity for 30 minutes 90 percent of the time.

Objective 3b. Ayton will follow safety procedures in response to emergency signals 90 percent of the time.

Objective 3c. Ayton quietly will create a small physical distance between himself and another person when accidentally bumped or touched 4/5 times.

Goal 4: Ayton will demonstrate improved social and communication skills to participate in peer interactions at school.

Objective 4a: Ayton will participate in give-and-take conversations and activities with another peer for five minutes 4/5 times a week.

Objective 4b: Ayton will respond to peers who disagree with his opinion without raising his voice or arguing 4/5 times.

Objective 4c. Ayton will wait his turn and speak in a modulated tone to express his opinion during a small group activity 4/5 times.

Intervention Implementation

To achieve these goals, the IEP team decides to use an interdisciplinary approach that provides interventions within the natural setting of the classroom and other school functions. In collaboration with the occupational therapist and occupational therapy assistant, the classroom teachers agree to consider adaptations to their classroom environments and some of the learning assignments to support Ayton's participation in the classroom. They:

• Use portable room dividers and carpeted areas to create quiet zones
• Supply Ayton with a set of headphones to muffle sounds
• Position Ayton's desk near a corner of the room and move his locker to the end of the row to minimize the number of times he is bumped accidentally

- Group Ayton with students who are quieter and less verbal for team projects
- Close the door to reduce hallway noise, and close the windows to decrease outside sounds
- Establish a system whereby Ayton can request to go to the library to complete his work if the classroom becomes too noisy for him
- Train peer buddies to provide visual and verbal directions about classroom assignments when he does not appear to understand the directions
- Train peer buddies to coach Ayton regarding game rules prior to beginning of gym class, using verbal and visual cues

In addition, the occupational therapy assistant

- Installs a nonbreakable mirror in Ayton's locker and instructs a peer to serve as "peer buddy" to cue Ayton to check his physical appearance before class, and before and after physical education
- Establishes and monitors a visual system for Ayton to organize his school bag, locker, and notebooks
- Works with Ayton to use visual aids to pace himself when writing and a self-check system to judge the legibility of his writing
- Meets with the classroom teachers weekly for two months to monitor and modify the changes as needed

Following the recommendations of the speech-language pathologist, all of those who work with Ayton agree to use clear language and avoid words with multiple meanings when communicating with him. The occupational therapy assistant works with the speech-language pathologist to conduct an eight-week social skills and competency group during the school's weekly activity period. Using Animal Exploration as the name of their group, they include peer buddies. Through the use of table games, collaborative projects, and role playing scenarios that focus on animals, they emphasize language usage, conversational timing, personal space and body language, and ways to include others in conversation. They also guide Ayton to broaden his interest to include more types of animals and habitats.

In addition, the occupational therapist develops strategies to address Ayton's sensory modulation difficulties. The occupational therapist meets with Ayton weekly for one month to teach him how to be more aware of his hypersensitivities, how to notice their effect on his performance in group situations, and how to use specific techniques to function more adaptively in these settings. For example, the occupational therapist teaches Ayton how to modify his physical environment to adjust the amount of extraneous sensory input. She encourages Ayton to wear form fitting undershirts and teaches him how to apply deep pressure to himself to decrease tactile defensiveness and modulate his sensory responses (Lane, 2002). At the end of the two-month period, the IEP team agrees to meet again to term the effectiveness of the plan. ■

SUMMARY

Pervasive developmental disorders are a challenging set of early neurobiological disorders that include autistic disorder, Asperger syndrome, Rett syndrome, childhood disintegrative disorder, and pervasive developmental disorder NOS. Pervasive developmental disorders also are known as autism spectrum disorders (ASD). Children and adolescents with ASD exhibit varying degrees of impaired social skills, communication disorders, and restricted, stereotyped patterns of behavior (AOTA, 2005). They may be delayed in some or all areas of their development, including physical, cognitive, and social-emotional development. Many cases of ASD probably have a genetic basis. They also may have environmental causes. ASD can occur alone or in combination with other conditions such as mental retardation, Down syndrome, fragile X syndrome, cerebral palsy, fetal alcohol syndrome, deafness, and blindness. There is widespread concern about the increase in number of children needing services for ASD. It is not clear if this increase is related to actual increase in the number of children and adolescents affected with ASD or to better diagnosis of ASD.

Currently, a diagnosis of ASD is based on interviews with family members and teachers, family history, medical examination, clinical observations of behaviors, and psychological, communication, educational, and occupational assessments.

Emerging research suggests that early indicators of autism can be observed in some infants as young as 6 months of age.

The prognosis for children and adolescents with ASD varies considerably. There is a continuum of functioning from severely impaired to mildly impaired. Children and adolescents with higher language and cognitive skills have a better prognosis. As adults, some will live independently in the community, have friends, and maintain permanent employment. Some will live in group homes and participate in supported work. Those with more severe forms of ASD need lifelong support for performing ADLs and IADLs.

It is important for professionals to work collaboratively to provide needed services. Some of these professionals include: the primary care physician, teacher, psychologist, social worker, developmental pediatrician, occupational therapist, occupational therapy assistant, speech and language pathologist, audiologist, and physical therapist. The family and the individual with ASD are the central members of the team. Common approaches used in educational settings include Applied Behavior Analysis, TEACCH, and DIR/Floortime. Medical interventions focus on managing the physical and behavioral health complications associated with ASD.

Occupational therapists and occupational therapy assistants provide interventions to address the occupational challenges confronting children and adolescents with autism spectrum disorder. As part of this intervention, occupational therapy practitioners consider how autism spectrum disorder impacts on the ability of the children and adolescents to participate in their ADL, IADL, work, education, play, leisure, and social participation occupations. They assess the children's and adolescents' performance skills, performance patterns, and performance context. As members of a healthcare and educational team of professionals, occupational therapists and occupational therapy assistants often pay particular attention to the social participation, daily living, sensory modulation, motor, and processing challenges confronting children and adolescents with autism spectrum disorder. As the number of cases of ASD continues to increase, the opportunity for occupational therapists and occupational therapy assistants to work with children and adolescents with this disorder also increases.

REVIEWING KEY POINTS

1. Explain the common characteristics associated with ASD.
2. Explain the main characteristics of autistic disorder, Asperger syndrome, pervasive developmental disorder NOS, childhood disintegrative disorder, and Rett syndrome.
3. Chart the key differences among autistic disorder, Asperger syndrome, and pervasive developmental disorder NOS.
4. List other conditions that a child or adolescent may have concurrently with ASD.
5. List professionals who provide services to children and adolescents with ASD.
6. Explain how to use ABA, DIR/Floortime, and TEACCH to work with children and adolescents with ASD.
7. Explain the focus of occupational therapy intervention for children and adolescents with ASD.
8. List occupational therapy evaluation procedures used to gather information about children and adolescents with ASD.
9. Describe areas of intervention occupational therapy practitioners consider when working with children and adolescents with ASD.

10. Describe the roles and responsibilities of the occupational therapist and the occupational therapy assistant during these evaluation and intervention processes.

APPLYING KEY CONCEPTS

1. Search the Internet for support programs for children, adolescents, and families that address:
   a. Asperger syndrome
   b. Autistic disorder
   c. Rett syndrome
   d. Pervasive developmental disorder NOS
   e. Childhood disintegrative disorder
2. Interview a sibling of a child or adolescent with ASD. Ask the sibling to explain how the daily life of the family is affected by ASD.
3. Further investigate one or more of the learning approaches used with children and adolescents with ASD: ABA, DIR/Floortime, or TEACCH.
   a. Give examples of how to incorporate each of these approaches in occupational therapy.
   b. Visit a school that utilizes one of these approaches.
   c. Search the Internet for a further explanation of these approaches.
4. Review the case study of Juan. Based upon the information in the story:
   a. Provide the preschool teacher with a developmentally appropriate play, educational, and ADL activities that would address Juan's current capacities and needs. (Hint: Consider his developmental and chronological ages.)
   b. Design a series of activities to address each of his goals.
   c. Create a visual schedule for Juan.
5. Review Tom's case study. Design a series of three therapy sessions that would help to facilitate his social competency. Focus on his participation in occupations at home and in the community. Consider his capacities and needs, the environment, and the demands of the activity.
6. Review Ayton's case study. Design a series of activities to address each of his goals. Focus on relating those goals to his participation in home and school occupations.
7. Read *Ten Things Every Child with Autism Wishes You Knew* (Notbohm, 2005). Write down 20 key statements that are important to remember when working with children with autism. Write a poem or create a piece of visual art that reflects the perspective of a person with autism as outlined by the author of the book.

REFERENCES

American Psychiatric Association (2000). *Diagnostic and Statistical Manual of Mental Disorders* (4th ed., rev.). Washington, DC: Author.

American Occupational Therapy Association (2005). The scope of occupational therapy services for individuals with autism spectrum disorders across the lifespan. *American Journal of Occupational Therapy, 59*(6), 680–693.

Barrett, S., Beck, J. C., Bernier, R., Bisson, E., Braun, T. A., Casavant, T. L., Childress, D., Folstein, S. E., Garcia, M., Gardiner, M. B., Gilman, S., Haines, J. L., Hopkins, K., Landa, R., Meyer, N. H., Mullane, J. A., Nishimura, D. Y., Palmer, P., Piven, J., Purdy, J., Santangelo, S. L., Searby, C., Sheffield, V., Singleton, J., & Slager, S. (1999). An autosomal genomic screen for autism. *American Journal of Medical Genetics/Neuropsychiatric Genetics, 88,* 609–615.

Blaxill, M. F. (2004). What's going on? The question of time trends in autism. *Public Health Report, 119*(6), 536–551.

Brown, C., & Dunn, W. (2002). Adolescent/Adult Sensory Profile. San Antonio, TX: Harcourt Assessment.

Cambridge Center for Behavioral Studies. (2006). *ABA and autism.* Retrieved July 17, 2006 from http://www.behavior.org/autism.

Center for Disease Control. (2006). *Autism Spectrum Disorder.* Retrieved June 1, 2006 from http://www.cdc.gov/ncbddd/autism/asd_common.htm.

Constantino, J. N. (2002). *The social responsiveness scale.* Los Angeles, CA: Western Psychological Services.

Courchesne, E., Carper, R., & Akshoomoff, N. (2003). Evidence of brain overgrowth in the first year of life in autism. *Journal of the American Medical Association, 16*(3), 337–344.

Dunn, W. (1997). *The Sensory Profile.* San Antonio, TX: Psychological Corporation, Therapy Skill Builders.

Edelson, S. B., & Cantor, D. S. (1998). Autism: Xenobiotic influences. *Toxicology and Industrial Health, 14*(4), 553–63.

Gray, C. (2000). *The new social storybook: Illustrated edition.* Arlington, TX: Future Horizons.

Greenspan, S. I. (1992a). Reconsidering the diagnosis and treatment of very young children with autistic spectrum of pervasive developmental disorder. *Zero to Three 13*(2), 1–9.

Greenspan, S. I. (1992b). *Infancy and early childhood: The practice of clinical assessment and intervention with emotional and developmental challenges.* Madison, CT: International Universities Press.

Greenspan, S. I., & Wieder, S. (1997). Developmental patterns and outcomes in infants and children with disorders in relating and communicating: A chart review of 200 cases of children with autistic spectrum diagnoses. *Journal of Developmental and Learning Disorders, 1,* 87–141.

Greenspan, S. I., & Wieder, S. (1998). *The child with special needs: Intellectual and emotional growth.* Reading, MA: Addison Wesley Longman.

Gurney, J. G., Fritz, M.S., Ness, K.K., Sievers, P., Newschaffer, C. J., & Shapiro, E.G. (2003). Analysis of prevalence trends of autism spectrum disorder in Minnesota. *Archives of Pediatrics and Adolescent Medicine, 157*(7), 619–621.

Haley, S. M., Coster, W. J., Ludlow, L. H., Haltiwanger, J. T., & Andrellos, P. J. (1992). *Pediatric evaluation of disability inventory: Development, standardization, and administration manual, version 1.0.* Boston: Trustees of Boston University, Health and Disability Research Institute.

Handleman, J., & Harris, S. (Eds.) (2001). *Preschool education programs for children with autism* (2nd ed.). Austin, TX: Pro-Ed.

Hedderly, R. (1995). Sentence completion test. *Dyslexia Review, 7*(2).

Herbert, M. (2005). Autism: A brain disorder or a disorder of the brain? *Clinical Neuropsychiatry, 2*(6) 354–379.

Heward, W. (2006). *Exceptional children: An introduction to special education* (8th ed.). Upper Saddle River, NJ: Pearson Prentice Hall.

Honda H., Shimizu Y., & Ratter, M. (2005). No effect of MMR withdrawal on the incidence of autism: A total population study. *Journal of Child Psychology and Psychiatry, 46*(6), 572–579.

Howlin P., Goode, S., Hutton, J., & Rutter, M. (2004). Adult outcome for children with autism. *Journal of Child Psychology and Psychiatry, 45*(2), 212–229.

Interdisciplinary Council on Developmental and Learning Disorders Clinical Practice Guidelines Workgroup, S.I.G.C. (2000). *Interdisciplinary Council on Developmental and Learning Disorders' clinical practice guidelines: Redefining the standards of care for infants, children, and families with special needs.* Bethesda, MD: Interdisciplinary Council on Developmental and Learning Disorders.

International Rett Syndrome Association (2007). Facts and questions. Retrieved July 8, 2007, from http://www.rettsyndrome.org/context

Janzen, J. (2003). *Understanding the nature of autism. A guide to the autism spectrum disorders* (2nd ed.). San Antonio, TX: Therapy Skill Builders.

Keller, J., Kafkes, A., & Kielhofner, G. (2005). Psychometric characteristics of the Child Occupational Self Assessment (COSA). Part One: An initial examination of psychometric properties. *Scandinavian Journal of Occupational Therapy, 12*(3), 118–127.

Keller, J., & Kielhofner, G. (2005). Psychometric characteristics of the Child Occupational Self Assessment (COSA). Part Two: Refining the psychometric properties. *Scandinavian Journal of Occupational Therapy, 12*(4), 147–158.

Landa, R. (2006). Infant markers for lasting deficits in reciprocal social interactions and communication deficits. Paper presented at The Spectrum of Developmental Disabilities XXVIII: Autism from Kanner to Current. Baltimore, MD: Johns Hopkins University School of Medicine.

Landa, R., & Garrett-Mayer, E. (2006). Development in infants with autism spectrum disorders: A prospective study. *Journal of Child Psychology and Psychiatry, 47*(6), 629–638.

Lane, S. (2002). Sensory modulation. In A. Bundy, S. Lane, & E. Murray, *Sensory integration theory and practice* (2nd ed.). Philadelphia F. A. Davis.

Larson, E. (2006). Caregiving and autism: How does children's propensity for routinization influence participation in family activities? *Occupation, Participation, and Health: An Occupational Therapy Journal of Research, 26*(2), 69–79.

Lauritsen, M. B., Pedersen, C. B., & Mortensen, P. B. (2005). Effects of familial risk factors and place of birth on the risk of autism: A nationwide register-based study. *Journal of Child Psychology and Psychiatry, 46*(9), 963–971.

Lord, C., & Schopler, E. (1994). TEACCH services for preschool children. In S. Harris & J. Handelman (Eds.), *Preschool education programs for children with autism,* pp. 87–106. Austin, TX: Pro-Ed.

Lovaas Institute (2006). The Lovaas Model for Applied Behavior Analysis. Retrieved July 17, 2006 from http://www.lovaas.com.

Lovaas, O. I. (1987). Behavioral treatment and normal educational and intellectual functioning in young autistic children. *Journal of Consulting and Clinical Psychology, 55,* 3–9.

Madsen, K. M., Hviid, A., Vestergaard, M., Schendel, D., Wohlfahrt, J., Thorsen, P., Olsen, J., & Melbye, M. (2002). A population-based study of measles, mumps, and rubella vaccination and autism. *New England Journal of Medicine, 347*(19) 1477–1482.

McEachin, J. J., Smith, T., & Lovaas, O. I. (1993). Long-term outcome for children with autism who received early intensive behavioral treatment. *American Journal of Mental Retardation, 97,* 359–372.

Mesibov, G. & Howley, M. (2003). *Accessing the curriculum for pupils with Autistic Spectrum Disorders: Using the TEACCH programme to help inclusion.* London: David Fulton Publishers Ltd.

Mesibov, G. B., Schopler, E., & Hearsey, K. A. (1994). Structured teaching. In E. Schopler & G. B. Mesibov (Eds.), *Behavioral issues in autism,* pp. 195–207. New York: Plenum.

Miller, L. J., Reisman, J., McIntosh, D. N., & Simon, J. (2001). The ecological model of sensory modulations. Performance of children with fragile X syndrome, autism, ADHD, and SMD. In S. Roley, R. Schaaf, & E. Blanche (Eds.), *Sensory integration and developmental disabilities.* San Antonio, TX: Therapy Skill Builders.

Miller, M. T., Strömland, K., Ventura, L., Johansson, M., Bandim, J. M., & Gillberg, C. (2005). Autism associated with conditions characterized by developmental errors in early embryogenesis: A mini review. *International Journal of Developmental Neuroscience, 23*(2–3), 201–219.

Miller-Kuhaneck, H. (Ed.) (2004). *Autism: A comprehensive occupational therapy approach* (2nd ed.). Bethesda, MD: AOTA.

Mitchell, S., Brian, J., Zwaigenbaum, L., Roberts, W., Szatmari, P., Smith, I., & Bryson, S. (2006). Early language and communication development of infants later diagnosed with autism spectrum disorder. *Journal of Developmental and Behavioral Pediatrics, 27*(Suppl 2), S69–S78.

Muhle, R., Trentacoste, S. V., & Rapin, I. (2004). The genetics of autism. *Pediatrics, 113*(5), 472–486.

Murch, S. (2005). Editorial: Diet, immunity, and autistic spectrum disorders. *The Journal of Pediatrics, 146*(5), 582–584.

Myers, S. (2006). Psychopharmacology. Paper presented at The Spectrum of Developmental Disabilities XXVIII: Autism from Kanner to Current. Baltimore, MD: Johns Hopkins University School of Medicine.

National Dissemination Center for Children with Disabilities [NICHY] (2003). Pervasive developmental disorder. Retrieved June 19, 2006 from http://www.nichcy.org/pubs/factshe/fs20txt.htm.

Newschaffer, C. J., Falb, M. D., & Gurney, J. G. (2005). National autism prevalence trends from United States special education data. *Pediatrics, 115*(3) 277–282.

Niehus, R., & Lord, C. (2006). Early medical history of children with autism spectrum disorders. *Journal of Developmental and Behavioral Pediatrics, 27*(Suppl 2), S120–127.

Notbohm, E. (2005). *Ten things every child with autism wishes you knew.* Arlington, TX: Future Horizons.

Ozonoff, S., & Cathcart, K. (1998). Effectiveness of a home program intervention for young children with autism. *Journal of Autism and Developmental Disorders, 28*(1), 25–32.

Palmer, R. F., Blanchard, S., Jean, C. R., & Mandell, D. S. (2005). School district resources and identification of children with autistic disorder. *American Journal of Public Health, 95*(1) 125–130.

Panerai, S., Ferrante, L., & Zingale, M. (2002). Benefits of the Treatment and Education of Autistic and Communication Handicapped Children (TEACCH) programme as compared with a nonspecific approach. *Journal of Intellectual Disability Research, 46*(Pt 4), 318–327.

Pelphrey, K. A., Morris, J. P., & McCarthy, G. (2005). Neural basis of eye gaze processing deficits in autism. *Brain, 128,* 1038–1048.

Pfeiffer, B., Kinnealey, M., Reed, C., & Herzberg, G. (2005). Sensory modulation and affective disorders in children and adolescents with Asperger Syndrome. *American Journal of Occupational Therapy, 59*(3), 335–345.

Reed, K. L. (2001). *Quick reference to occupational therapy* (2nd ed.). Austin, TX: Pro-Ed.

Schaaf, R., & Miller, L. (2005). Novel therapies for developmental disabilities: Occupational therapy using a sensory integrative approach. *Journal of Mental Retardation and Developmental Disabilities Research Reviews 11,* 143–148.

Sheinkopf, S., & Siegel, B. (1998). Home based behavioral treatment for young autistic children. *Journal of Autism and Developmental Disorders, 28,* 15–23.

Smeeth, L., Cook, C., Fombonne, E., Heavey, L., Rodrigues, L. C., Smith, P. G., & Hall, A. J. (2004). MMR vaccination and pervasive developmental disorders: A case-control study. *Lancet, 364*(9438), 963–969.

Smith, T., Groen, A. D., & Wynn, J. W. (2000). Randomized trial of intensive early intervention for children with pervasive developmental disorder. *American Journal of Mental Retardation, 105,* 269–285.

Valicenti-McDermott, M., McVicar, K., Rapin, I., Wershil, B. K., Cohen, H., & Shinnar, S. (2006). Frequency of gastrointestinal symptoms in children with autistic spectrum disorders and association with family history of autoimmune disease. *Journal of Developmental and Behavioral Pediatrics, 27*(2 Suppl 2), S128–S136.

Venter, A., Lord, C., & Schopler, E. (1992). A follow-up study of high functioning autistic children. *Journal of Child Psychology and Psychiatry, 33,* 489–507.

Vojdani, A., Pangborn, J. B., Vojdani, E., & Cooper, E. L. (2003). Infections, toxic chemicals and dietary peptides binding to lymphocyte receptors and tissue enzymes are major instigators of autoimmunity in autism.

International Journal of Immunopathology and Pharmacology, 16(3), 189–99.

Wagner, S. (2001). *Inclusive programming for middle school students with autism/Asperger syndrome.* Arlington, TX: Future Horizons.

Wilbarger, P. (1984). Planning an adequate "sensory diet": Application of sensory processing theory during the first year of life. *Zero to Three, 5*(1), 7–12.

Yale Developmental Disability Clinic. (2006). *Information about pervasive developmental disabilities.* Retrieved June 19, 2006 from http://info.med.yale.edu/chldstdy/autism/pddinfo.html

Zwaigenbaum, L., Bryson, S., Rogers, T., Roberts, W., Brian, J., & Szatmari, P. (2005). Behavioral manifestations of autism in the first year of life. *International Journal of Developmental Neuroscience, 23*(2–3),143–152.

Chapter

22

Children and Adolescents with Attention Deficit Hyperactivity Disorder and Learning Disabilities

Margaret J. Pendzick

Key Terms

Acquisitional approach
ADHD combined type
ADHD primarily hyperimpulsive
  type
ADHD primarily inattentive type

Alert Program
Developmental delay
Learning disability (LD)
Sensory diet

Objectives

- Explain attention-deficit/hyperactivity disorder (ADHD) and learning disabilities (LD) conditions.
- Examine how ADHD and LD impact the daily occupations of children and adolescents within the context of their family and environment.
- Describe occupational therapy interventions to support the capacity of children and adolescents with ADHD and LD conditions to participate in their daily occupations.
- Examine how occupational therapists and occupational therapy assistants problem solve together during the intervention process.
- Describe how occupational therapists and occupational therapy assistants work with families and other professionals to provide services to children and adolescents with ADHD and LD.

INTRODUCTION

This chapter contains an overview of attention-deficit/hyperactivity disorder (ADHD) and learning disabilities (LD), and occupational therapy interventions to support children and adolescents coping with such challenges. While some children and adolescents experience either ADHD or LD, others have both ADHD and LD. Vignettes throughout the chapter highlight occupational therapy services for children and adolescents who have ADHD and LD at various points in their occupational development.

ADHD

ADHD is the most commonly diagnosed childhood and psychiatric condition; 3 percent to 5 percent of American school aged children are diagnosed with these conditions (Scanlon, 2006). Central to ADHD is the child's or the adolescent's frequent difficulty with sustaining focus on a task and increased activity level compared to other children or adolescents of the same age. Although these behaviors are present at a young age, they often are not recognized until school age, when a child is required to sit and attend for longer periods of time to age appropriate tasks.

There are currently three subclassifications of ADHD. **ADHD primarily inattentive type** refers to the inability to maintain focus on a task. A child or adolescent with ADHD inattentive type often daydreams, and responds to information slowly. **ADHD primarily hyperimpulsive type** describes inattentive behaviors due to hyperactivity or impulsive actions. A child or adolescent with this type of ADHD has difficulty sitting at a desk to complete schoolwork and staying on topic when engaging in conversations. The child or adolescent with **ADHD combined type** has difficulty due to increased activity and impulsive and inattentive behaviors. The combination often results in safety concerns for the child or adolescent, and others (APA, 2000; Izenberg, 2000; Mosier, 1998).

Although no definitive cause of ADHD has been discovered, current research suggests that the inattention or hyperactivity may be due to reduced activity in the site of the brain that controls inhibition, attention, and executive reasoning. These centers are located in the right hemisphere of the frontal lobes (Scalon, 2006). Since the siblings and parents of children and adolescents with ADHD are more likely than those within the general population to have ADHD, genetic involvement is suspected (Stubbe, 2000). Popular concerns that a diet that includes refined sugars and preservatives contributes to the cause of ADHD have not been supported by current research (Mosier, 1998).

The inattentive and hyperactivity characteristics of ADHD interfere with a child's or an adolescent's ability to perform age appropriate motor, social, cognitive, and processing skills. Often the child or adolescent does not attend to a task long enough to develop useful habits and skills. Delays in social skills may occur because of difficulty attending to and interpreting social cues may result in exclusion from age appropriate groups. Cognitive skills may be delayed due to gaps in knowledge as a result of inattentive behaviors. Difficulties in refined motor skills, particularly those associated with balance and coordination, may develop because of inattentiveness to sensory feedback and lack of skill practice.

Interventions for ADHD involve a variety of different team members and strategies. Physicians often prescribe medications that stimulate different brain centers to help the child or adolescent to focus on a task. Common medications include Ritalin, Adderall, Dexedrine, and Cylert (Scalon, 2006). Psychologists, counselors, or social workers may provide behavioral modification techniques to positively reinforce on task behaviors and offer practical suggestions to parents and teachers regarding living with and teaching children and adolescents with ADHD. Classroom teachers may decrease distraction within the classroom environment, restructure class assignments into smaller steps, or place a child or adolescent closer to the teacher during whole class instruction (Heward, 2006; Mulligan, 2001).

Occupational therapy intervention addresses deficits in sensory modulation, social skills, behavioral regulation, and organizational skills that often interfere with the child's or adolescent's ability to perform age appropriate occupations. Practical application of these intervention strategies are illustrated through case studies later in this chapter.

LEARNING DISABILITY

The National Joint Committee on Learning Disabilities (NJCLD) defines a learning disability as a general term that refers to considerable difficulties that a person has in learning and using skills to speak, listen, read, write, comprehend, or reason. This disability is not the result of other conditions and can occur throughout the lifespan (Scanlon, 2006). In most situations, the cause of learning disabilities is unknown.

A learning disability also is defined by IDEA, as it relates to the educational process. In this context, the term learning disability refers to a group of disorders that interferes with a student's ability to learn within a typical classroom. There is usually a discrepancy between the student's cognitive ability and school performance; the student's academic achievement is below expected levels. The learning difficulty is not the result of a sensory loss, inadequate instruction, or lack of exposure to the learning materials. Because students with learning disabilities often have difficulties in academic subjects such as reading, written language, or math, they may require special instruction to achieve academic goals. Without educational intervention, students with learning disabilities struggle academically and achieve below their peers. Since they can compare their achievement with others, students with learning disabilities are at high risk for poor self-esteem and often are delayed in social skills (Heward, 2006).

Students with a learning disability also have difficulties completing tasks that require coordination and organization such as shoe tying, handwriting, riding a bicycle, and shopping for groceries. Although learning disabilities are life long, children or adolescents may compensate for a deficit or choose to avoid situations that are challenging. For instance, an adolescent may choose to keyboard or use a voice activated word processing program to prepare written homework if handwriting is illegible. A middle school child may realize that his ball skills are not developed enough to be chosen for the school soccer team and decide to avoid the competitive sport. Instead he may join a local choral group that does not require a tryout.

When identified as having a learning disability, the child or adolescent may receive intervention from a variety of different team members. In the school setting, a student may receive specific instruction by a special education teacher within the regular education room or pullout sessions in a resource room. Instruction may address academic areas such as reading problems, written language deficits, or math difficulties. In outpatient clinics or school settings, psychologists and social workers may address behavioral problems or issues of self-worth and self-esteem. If the child or adolescent also displays ADHD, a physician may prescribe medication.

Occupational therapists and occupational therapy assistants provide occupation based intervention directed at the specific needs of the child or adolescent with a learning disability. Although handwriting may be the initial reason for referral, occupational therapists and occupational therapy assistants often address the child's or adolescent's difficulty with organizational tasks, sensory modulation, behavioral regulation, ADL, IADL, and social skills. For example, an occupational therapy assistant might work with an adolescent with a learning disability on job skills. If the adolescent has difficulty loading the dishwasher or clearing tables within the job's allotted time at the restaurant where he works, the occupational therapy assistant might focus on establishing organized routines to speed up his work performance. That same occupational therapy assistant might work with a child with a learning disability who does not play with other children because of coordination problems. If the child experiences delays in the development of her group social skills because of these coordination problems, the occupational therapy assistant may involve the child in a small group to develop coordination, play, and social skills. By modeling and providing timely feedback, the child may develop the skills necessary to participate in age related groups. Regardless of the reason for intervention, however, it is important for the occupational therapist and occupational therapy assistant to carefully grade interventions so that the child or adolescent builds self-worth and self-esteem. This includes grading of the environment, the task, the expectations on the child or adolescent to perform the task, and the therapeutic interactions by the occupational therapist and the occupational therapy assistant.

Occupational Therapy Intervention

Ricky

Ricky, a 5-year-old who has ADHD, attends a developmental kindergarten where the classroom schedule includes a daily 15-minute group circle time followed by individual center time. Even though Ricky is on medication, he continues to have difficulty participating in the classroom routine; he often cries or refuses to attempt an activity. Ricky's parents and classroom teacher refer him for an occupational therapy evaluation because of his difficulty participating within the kindergarten classroom. Since Ricky does not have an IEP, he may receive occupational therapy services on a 504 plan.

Following a meeting with the parents, classroom teacher, and school administrator, the occupational therapist reviews the referral and considers what areas of occupational performance need to be assessed. Based on the information, the occupational therapist makes an initial assumption that Ricky is having difficulty processing sensory information. To determine if this assumption is accurate, she chooses to administer the Sensory Profile (Dunn, 1997) and to conduct classroom observations. She also decides to administer the Peabody Developmental Motor Scales (PDMS-2) (Folio & Fewell, 2002) in order to determine if Ricky's outbursts may result from being asked to perform fine and gross motor tasks that are too difficult for him. To obtain detailed data about Ricky's capacities within the classroom environment, the occupational therapist requests the occupational therapy assistant to observe Ricky during multiple occasions during the school day. The occupational therapy assistant uses a site specific checklist to record her observations and prepares a written report for the occupational therapist (Figure 22.1■).

As directed by the occupational therapist, the occupational therapy assistant distributes a Sensory Profile to the classroom teacher and sends one home for the parents to complete. After completing the observations and testing, the occupational therapist and occupational therapy assistant discuss their findings. The occupational therapist then prepares the evaluation report for the team meeting. The results of the evaluation (Figure 22.2■) suggest that Ricky's

---

Classroom Observation

Student Name: Ricky
Grade: K
Teacher: Mrs. B
Start time: 9:45 A.M.   End time: 10:45 A.M.

<u>Classroom Environment:</u> The kindergarten classroom is a large room with windows on one side, computers lining one wall, and cloakroom to the rear. Children's artwork is displayed on wall bulletin boards.
Circle time area, located at the front of the room by teacher's desk, consists of a teacher chair, felt board, and weather/calendar map. The letter of the week is placed on felt board. Children sit on low pile multicolored rug. Places are not assigned but children are instructed to sit facing front with legs like a pretzel.
There are six different centers located throughout the room, with low room dividers to create space. The classroom teacher explains that she changes the center activities weekly and she encourages the children to rotate from station to station throughout the day/week. Children may choose a center but each center has a participation number.
Art Corner consists of five easels, finger paint, paper, and paint shirts.
Reading Corner has books on low shelves and two tape recorders/headsets with a specific book for the week.
Science Table has a large basin of gak.
Math Table has a balance scale with different types of small balls to weigh—cotton, clay, koosh, ping-pongs, tennis, and rubber.
Housekeeping Corner consists of child sized appliances, pots and pans, cooking utensils and dress up clothes.
Writing Table has tablemats imprinted with the letter of the week with clay and wikki sticks to make the letters.

<u>Class Activity:</u> Letter of the week—R
Circle time (15 minutes): After the children assemble on the carpet, the teacher hands each child a brightly colored streamer and leads them in singing the rainbow song. As they sing the chorus, the children are instructed to wave their streamers in the air. After the song is completed, two children collect the streamers while another two pass out rhino facemasks. Wearing their rhino masks, the children sit on the carpet while the teacher reads a short story. When the story is completed, the masks are collected and the teacher reviews instructions for the different center.
Center time (40 minutes): Unless assigned to the computers, each child chose four different centers. The teacher rings a small bell when it is time to change centers.

<u>Student's Participation</u>
Circle time: Ricky sat with the children on the rug but when they started to hand out the streamers, he moved slowly to the back of the group, walking in a low squat position. When the children stood and waved the streamers, Ricky turned his body so that only his right side was facing the group. Whenever a streamer

(continued)

■ **Figure 22.1**
Ricky's classroom observation.

touched his arm, he took one step away from the group. When asked to put on his facemask, he immediately asked to go to the bathroom. When he was told he had to wait until the end of circle time, he started to cry and refused to wear the mask. The teaching assistant separated Ricky from the group for the rest of the story (three minutes).

Center time
First choice, Reading Corner: Ricky chose two different books and looked at the pictures. He smiled at his classmates and parent volunteer.

Second choice, Math Table: Ricky worked with a classmate to compare weights. He only chose to pick up the ping-pong balls and rubber balls. He only held the clay with his fingertips when he attempted to pick it up, then quickly asked to go to the bathroom to wash his hands. He finished this activity quickly, never smiling, and stood away from the table waiting for the time to change centers.

Third choice, Housekeeping Corner: Ricky joined two classmates as they pretended to make lunch. He chose not to wear a costume but watched the other children dress. One child chose to wear a fur jacket, while the other child wore high heels and a fuzzy scarf. Ricky played cooperatively with the other children for four minutes. While Ricky was standing next to one child, the scarf came unraveled and had to be readjusted. When the child swung the scarf over her shoulder, Ricky backed away and for the remainder of the time played alone.

Fourth choice: When it was time to move to a new center, Ricky wandered around the classroom. When the teacher tried to direct him to a new center, he just shook his head and stood still. The teacher moved him to the open spot at the science center. He stood and stared at the gak on the table, keeping his hands to his side. When the teacher attempted to place his hands in the gak, Ricky began to cry and pull away. The teacher asked him what was wrong but Ricky just shook his head and continued to cry. The other children playing with the gak tried to convince Ricky to join the fun but he continued to cry. The teacher finally removed Ricky from the group and let him sit in a chair with a book.

End of observation.

■ Figure 22.1
Ricky's classroom observation. (cont.)

difficulties primarily are due to sensory modulation problems. He reacts negatively to different textures that often are included in classroom hands on activities. He displays discomfort when his legs or arms touch the carpet during circle time; he then fidgets and attempts to leave the circle. When given a choice, he chooses activities that have little texture variety, such as block building, looking at books, or coloring with crayons. When confronted with a messy activity such as finger painting, gluing, or glitter on art projects, he avoids the activity by indicating a need to use the restroom or by starting to cry. He plays in the housekeeping corner but avoids donning any costumes with feathers, fur, or corduroy. The results of the Sensory Profile that his parents complete indicate that he avoids these same situations at home.

The parents, classroom teacher, school administer, and occupational therapist meet to discuss the test results and

Ricky's difficulties processing tactile stimulation. The team decides that Ricky should receive occupational therapy services this school year under a Section 504 and develops the following goals and objectives.

Goal 1: Ricky will participate in all classroom activities, 4/5 days per week.
   Objective 1a: Ricky will participate in art activities, regardless of the medium, 3/5 days per week.
   Objective 1b: Ricky will sit quietly during entire circle time, 3/5 days per week.
Goal 2: Ricky will verbally express and inform others of his feelings, 4/5 times.
   Objective 2a: Rather than asking to go to the bathroom to avoid an uncomfortable situation, Ricky will verbally express his discomfort, 4/5 times.

Occupational Therapy Evaluation

Child's Name: Ricky
Grade/Age: 5 years, 6 months
Teacher: Mrs. Bentley
Date: 10/10/07

Ricky, a 5½-year-old kindergartener at Westside Elementary School, was referred for an occupational therapy evaluation by his classroom teacher, Mrs. Bentley. According to the classroom teacher, Ricky's cognitive skills are appropriate for a kindergarten program but he continues to have difficulty participating in classroom activities and dealing appropriately with stress. The parents and teacher are concerned that Ricky's lack of participation will interfere with learning. Since Ricky does not qualify for special education, occupational therapy intervention is being considered under a 504.

Evaluation results are based on classroom observations, standardized tests for fine motor skills and sensory processing, and clinical observations. As assessed by the Peabody Developmental Motor Scales (PDMS-2), Ricky's fine motor development is within the typical range for his age. He performs activities quickly and accurately, demonstrating right hand dominance with tripod grasp on writing utensils and superior pincer grasp of small objects. He spontaneously uses his nondominant hand to assist during cutting and block assembly.

Analysis of classroom observations and parent completed Sensory Profile suggest that Ricky is having difficulty modulating his response to tactile stimulation. In the classroom, his behavior deteriorates when he is confronted with activities that involve tactile input, often resulting in crying or being placed in time out. When given a choice of centers, he prefers to watch others or play with nontextured items such as blocks or books.

It is recommended that occupational therapy services under a 504 be considered for the remainder of the school year. Intervention strategies should include consultation to the teaching staff on ways to modify the classroom environment to best enhance Ricky's learning. Ricky would benefit from individual and small group occupational therapy intervention within the classroom setting to establish age appropriate coping strategies and to modulate his response to tactile stimulation.

■ **Figure 22.2**
Ricky's occupational therapy evaluation.

Objective 2b: Ricky will verbally express discomfort and refrain from crying during stressful situations, 3/5 times.

After the meeting, the occupational therapist and occupational therapy assistant meet to discuss how to best address Ricky's needs. They decide that a variety of different strategies will best help Ricky participate more fully in classroom experiences. Using the *Ecology of Human Performance* (Dunn, Brown, & McGuigan, 1994) to guide decisions, the occupational therapist decides to direct intervention toward Ricky, the environment, and the tasks. The occupational therapist and occupational therapy assistant help Ricky tolerate more tactile stimulation utilizing sensory modulation principles. For instance, before the occupational therapy assistant engages Ricky in a tactile experience, she applies deep pressure, which often decreases tactile defensiveness (Lane, 2002). The occupational therapy assistant also designs tactile experiences within enticing age appropriate games so that Ricky is encouraged to tolerate the sensation in order to play the game. At the same time, she adapts classroom tasks so that Ricky can experience immediate success and begin to abandon his avoidance behaviors and crying. For example, since Ricky reacts negatively when sitting on the carpet during circle time, the occupational therapy assistant suggests that the teacher offer the option that the children may sit either directly on the carpet or on a vinyl placement on top of the carpet. In the art center, the children may choose to paint with their fingers or use tongue depressors to spread the paint.

The occupational therapist works with the parents and the teacher to understand Ricky's difficulties and modify sensory experiences within his environment. The classroom teacher identifies a day and time that the occupational therapist can work individually with Ricky, grading sensory input so that he better tolerates the stimulation. The teacher also agrees to have the occupational therapy assistant set up a sensory center. The occupational therapy assistant designs hands on activities that incorporate a strong element of appropriately graded sensory stimulation. For example, if the letter of the week is B and the classroom theme is bears, the occupational therapy assistant hides pieces of a bear puzzle in a container filled with seeds. Shifting through the seeds in order to find the pieces, Ricky develops tolerance to increased sensory stimulation in order to complete the puzzle. If Ricky has difficulty tolerating the sensation, the occupational therapy assistant provides a small scoop so that Ricky only needs to tolerate the sensation on one hand at a time. If Ricky tolerates the sensation, the occupational therapy assistant increases the tactile experience by substituting sand for seeds or asking Ricky to close his eyes while searching through the seeds for the puzzle pieces. The occupational therapy assistant also might have Ricky stuff a corduroy bear with cotton batting, pieces of burlap, or mini-sponges at the sensory center. Because Ricky can complete the project over multi-days, he can switch to a different center if he needs a break.

As Ricky's tolerance for tactile sensation increases, the occupational therapist and the occupational therapy assistant engage Ricky in additional sensory activities with his peers that are consistent with sensory modulation principles. For instance, after discussing Ricky's progress in individual sessions, the occupational therapist and the occupational therapy assistant decide that Ricky should be able to tolerate some mild textures on his hands during play with his peers. Knowing that the classroom teacher is introducing the letter M that week, the occupational therapy assistant designs a center where the children squirt mustard on the paper, then use their fingers to draw pictures of objects that start with the M sound. The occupational therapy assistant engages Ricky in drawing pictures without emphasizing the media. The occupational therapy assistant models how to express feelings verbally by asking the children to talk about their likes and dislikes. If Ricky's body language suggests displeasure, she encourages him to express his feelings verbally, and to attempt the activity in a series of brief intervals, rather than to avoid the activity or cry. Sensing Ricky's reaction to the tactile experience, she attempts to end the session while he is finding the session pleasurable rather than distasteful.

The occupational therapist and occupational therapy assistant maintain written documentation of all interventions they provide (Jackson & Arbesman, 2005). They carefully record Ricky's reactions to sensory input and progress on his goals and keep copies of home and classroom suggestions. Though these records are separate from Ricky's 504 report, the occupational therapist and occupational therapy assistant use them when they prepare school progress reports. ■

Kendra

Kendra is a 13-year-old with ADHD whose condition has a different impact on her occupational performance than it does for Ricky. Kendra was never a behavioral concern at home or schools but she frequently seemed to be daydreaming. Due to frequent family moves, Kendra was enrolled in different schools each year; her inattentiveness was misattributed to being in new surroundings.

By seventh grade, Kendra's lack of attention interfered with her academic, social, and family life; the school psychologist diagnosed Kendra with ADHD primarily inattentive type. At school, Kendra has difficulty orienting to changing classes, using a locker, and following different classroom routines. She frequently is off task and needs instructions to be repeated. Even though Kendra struggles with these tasks, she still earns grades in the B/C range. She is a member of the cross country and track team, but she has difficulty making friends, often sitting alone during lunch, practice, or school assemblies. She would like to run in the 4X800 relay but the coach feels her inattentiveness would interfere with the handoff. Kendra's need to receive frequent reminders to complete her homework and family chores causes tension between Kendra and her parents.

Since Kendra is successfully passing all her subjects, she is not eligible for services under IDEA. Her parents discuss their concerns with the family physician who refers them to a community based wellness clinic that provides adolescent and adult occupational therapy services.

The occupational therapist and occupational therapy assistant discuss the referral and speculate that Kendra would be appropriate for an adolescent social skills group and the **Alert Program** (Williams & Shellenberger, 1996). The Alert Program would help Kendra to recognize when her attention is waning and what sensory stimulation helps her focus on a task.

In order to get an understanding as to how Kendra feels as she reacts to sensory input, the occupational therapist asks Kendra and her parents to complete the Adolescent Sensory Profile (Dunn, 1997), though independent of one another. The occupational therapy assistant arranges to observe Kendra during an after school track practice. The occupational therapy assistant uses a site specific checklist to record her observations and prepares a written report for the occupational therapist (Table 22.1■).

The occupational therapist reviews the results of the Adolescent Sensory Profile and the occupational therapy assistant's

■ **Table 22.1**
Kendra at Track Practice

Occupations Observed	Performance Skills Demonstrated	Performance Patterns Demonstrated	Context for Occupation
Arriving at and preparing for track practice; 10 minutes	Listened to but did not spontaneously join the conversation of the other girls. Giggled when asked direct questions by the other girls, and shrugged her shoulders. Dressed for practice; brought appropriate clothes to practice. Left the bleachers for the field at the sound of the whistle. Bumped her shin on one of the metal benches as she returned to the bleachers for her water bottle.	Sat to the side of the group. Took one sneaker out of her bag, started to put it on but stopped; began to brush hair, pulled out a second sneaker from her bag; searched her bag for socks; looked in the bag then around the bleachers for both of her sneakers; left her bag opened and her street shoes and jacket scattered on several bleachers.	Metal bleachers on side of track field
Attending track team meeting; 10 minutes	Responded on the second time the coach called her name for attendance, after being poked by another student. Told the coach that she did not have the parental permission slip necessary for her to ride the bus to the next day's track meet when he asked her for it. Accepted a cell phone from another student when directed by coach to call home for the permission slip, but did not make eye contact with or thank the student for the help.	Sat at the periphery of the circle. Twirled her hair and rubbed her legs in the grass while the coach talked.	Grassy knoll by side of the track field

■ **Table 22.1**
Kendra at Track Practice (cont.)

Occupations Observed	Performance Skills Demonstrated	Performance Patterns Demonstrated	Context for Occupation
	Attempted to dial phone number several times before pushing the correct sequence of numbers.		
Participating in practice drills and training program; 60 minutes	Followed the lead of her peers to complete warmup drills. Ran quickly, keeping pace with her peers during 100 and 200 meter practice races. Needed verbal and physical reminder from a peer to bring baton and to line up on the field for the relay practice run. Between the practice races, joined the other girls in a conversation about TV shows.	Smiled frequently and twirled herself during the drills. Continued to talk about her interest in cartoons geared for younger children, even after the other girls began to "roll their eyes" and attempt to change the subject.	
Preparing to depart for home; 10 minutes	Joined the other girls as they splashed one another with the water from the water cooler. Searched for her jacket and street shoes that she had left scattered on the bleachers before practice. Left her school bag on the bleachers as she began to exit the field.	Continued to splash the other girls when they had stopped, until one of the girls yelled "quit it."	Water cooler with paper cups by track field; bleachers

observation report prior to seeing Kendra and her parents. During the assessment, the occupational therapist interviews her parents and asks Kendra to complete the Canadian Occupational Performance Measure (COPM; Law, et al., 1998) and the Self-Awareness Assessment (Williamson & Dorman, 2002).

After analyzing the evaluation results, the occupational therapist prepares a report that indicates that Kendra is having difficulty modulating sensory information to be at her optimum state of arousal. This difficulty contributes to her inattentive behaviors. While completing the COPM, Kendra identifies and prioritizes her occupation based goals as having friends at school, being chosen to run on the track relay team, and having fewer arguments over homework with her parents. She rates herself at a level 2, indicating that she is dis-

satisfied with her level of performance in these occupations See Figure 22.3■, occupational therapy evaluation report.

Goal 1. Kendra will learn and integrate strategies to regulate her level of arousal to environmental cues to attend to tasks at home and school.
   Objective 1a. Kendra will identify what type of sensory input, sleep, and eating patterns are optimal for her to attend to activities (occupations) at home and school, and with her peers.
   Objective 2a. Kendra will develop a routine for integrating these optimal arousal strategies before beginning activities (occupations) at school and home, and with peers.

Child's Name: Kendra
Grade/Age: Seventh grade; 13 years old
Date: 3/12/07

Reason for Referral

Kendra is a 13-year-old female who is a seventh grader at Susquehannock Middle School. Kendra's primary care physician, Dr. Kov, referred her to the Community Wellness Center for an occupational therapy evaluation in response to concerns raised by her parents. The school psychologist recently diagnosed Kendra as having ADHD inattentive type. Her parents stated that Kendra's attention difficulties interfere with her academic, social, and family life. However, because she earns grades of Bs and Cs, her parents also stated that she is not eligible for school based occupational therapy services according to her school district's interpretation of IDEA guidelines.

Evaluation Results

Evaluation results are based on parental reports, standardized tests for sensory processing and occupational performance (i.e., the ability to perform daily life activities), a checklist of self-awareness, and observations of Kendra's occupational performance skills and pattern during an after school sports program. Kendra and her parents cooperated fully in the evaluation process, and stated they answered all questions to the best of their ability. Thus, it is assumed that the evaluation results accurately reflect Kendra's occupational performance capacities and challenges.

The results of the Adolescent Sensory Profile that Kendra and her parents completed separately indicate that Kendra has a low registration for sensory arousal. That is, compared to other adolescents, Kendra is less likely to notice and therefore respond as quickly to visual, auditory, tactile, sensory input that occurs within her everyday environment. In contrast, she is more likely to seek movement oriented sensory input.

This difficulty with noticing and responding to visual and auditory sensory input is consistent with how Kendra rated herself on the Self-Awareness Assessment. On that form, she indicated that she needs reminders from others to notice when things need to be done, or when other people need her help. As reflected in her words, "It is like I am in a fog sometimes." On that same form, Kendra indicated that she has difficulty making friends, knowing how to talk with peers to make decisions, or knowing how to ask for and successfully receive assistance.

Observations of Kendra during her after school track practice support these findings. Difficulties fully attending to visual and auditory details within her environment compromised her ability to efficiently organize herself to accomplish the required tasks. For example, several times while dressing for the track practice, she became distracted by other articles of clothing, thus did not follow through on putting on the original articles of clothing she retrieved from her bag. In the process, she left her belongings scattered on the bleachers and needed to spend additional time looking for them. In the course of practice, she forgot several items, including her water bottle, permission slip, baton, and school bag. While retrieving the water bottle she did not notice location of the metal bench and bumped her shin on it. In an attempt to dial home for a permission slip, she did not carefully attend to and thus pushed the wrong sequence of buttons several times. She needed additional verbal and tactile cues from the coach and her peers to attend to instructions during the team meeting, and to prepare herself for the practice runs. Concurrently, she appeared to seek

(continued)

■ **Figure 22.3**
Occupational therapy evaluation report.

and respond to movement oriented sensory input. She smiled while moving her body during practice drills, and kept pace with her peers during practice runs.

Kendra's attending difficulties also compromised her ability to effectively engage in social interactions with her peers. Though she enjoyed participating in movement oriented play with them, she did not notice when they were no longer interested in continuing the play. When conversing with them she did not notice the age level differences in interests or the visual cues to change topics. In addition, she did not verbally acknowledge assistance given to her by a peer.

On the Canadian Occupational Performance Measure (COPM), Kendra indicated that she has difficulties making friends, performing well on the track team, and getting along with her parents. She prioritized her occupation based goals as having friends at school, being chosen to run on the track relay team, and having fewer arguments over homework with her parents.

Summary Analysis

Kendra is having difficulty modulating sensory information, to be at her optimum state of arousal. This difficulty contributes to her inattentive behaviors and organizational challenges. In turn, these inattentive behaviors and organizational challenges compromise her ability to efficiently and effectively engage in her school, home, and social occupations (daily life activities). Strong movement oriented sensation appears to help increase her state of arousal.

Recommendations

It is recommended that Kendra participate in occupational therapy services biweekly for an eight week period to address her sensory modulation, inattention, organizational, and social skill challenges. Specifically, it is recommended that Kendra participate in the Alert and Social Competences programs biweekly to modulate her sensory responses, to learn attending strategies, and to develop social competencies.

■ Figure 22.3
Occupational therapy evaluation report. (cont.)

Goal 2. Kendra will learn and integrate attending and organizational strategies to complete tasks at home and school.

Objective 2a. Kendra will learn strategies such as using writing aids, time sensors, and visual charts to attend to and organize her daily routines, and home and school activities.

Objective 2b. Kendra will select which of these strategies are most useful and integrate them into her daily routine.

Goal 3. Kendra will learn and integrate social skills to participate in age appropriate interactions with her peers.

Objective 3a. Kendra will identify and learn how to respond to nonverbal cues of others during social exchanges.

Objective 3b. Kendra will learn how to ask questions to seek needed assistance from others.

Objective 3c. Kendra will learn strategies for initiating and continuing conversation with her peers.

Objective 3d. Kendra will learn how to adapt the topic of her conversation in response to the interest of the listener.

In order to meet Kendra's needs, the occupational therapist suggests a **sensory diet** that includes specific sensory stimulation activities to help Kendra modulate her sensory responses (Wilbarger & Wilbarger, 2002). She includes Kendra in a biweekly young adolescent Alert Program that also addresses social competency. While in the program, Kendra learns strategies to help her focus during her track meets, in the class, and at home, and during social conversations. In addition, Kendra also learns social, time management, and organizational skills. To supplement this program, the occupational therapist requests the occupational therapy assistant to draft a list of suggestions that Kendra can implement at home to help her complete her homework and family chores (Figure 22.4■). ■

Organizational and Time Management Strategies for Homework

- Establish a time immediately before or after supper every night to complete homework.
- Before beginning homework, do an "alerting task" for five–ten minutes, such as a brisk walk or stretching exercises.
- Do homework in a brightly lit, distraction reduced environment; wear headphones and consider playing background instrumental music to block out house noises.
- Before beginning homework, make a list and read aloud all homework assignments and steps for each assignment. Make the list using a chart, day planner, or personal data assistant. Arrange the list to correspond with the sequence of classes. Estimate time needed to complete each assignment. Set a timer to correspond with estimated start and stop times for each assignment.
- Arrange books and materials in the same order as the written homework assignments. Use a color code system to keep all materials and books for a class together.
- Check off each assignment as it is completed and put corresponding books and materials in the school bag in the order needed for classes.
- Place all forms and materials that need to be handed in to the teachers in a separate folder at the front of the school bag. Place a sticky note on the front of the folder as a reminder as to what materials each teacher needs to receive the next day.
- When finished with homework assignments, throw away unnecessary materials and store materials that need to be saved but not carried back to school in color coded files.
- Check gym and athletic bags. Remove soiled clothing. Using a checklist, place clean clothing and needed equipment in designated sections of the bag. Consider marking those sections with words or pictures of the clothing and equipment.

Organizational and Time Management Strategies for House Chores

- Establish a time when arriving home from school or on the weekend to complete family chores.
- Before beginning chores, make a list and read aloud all chores, supplies, and steps for each chore. Make the list using a chart, day planner or personal data assistant. Arrange chores to complete those that are most physical first. Estimate time needed to complete each chore. Set a timer to correspond with estimated start and stop times for each chore.
- Check off each chore as it is completed, put corresponding materials in locations where they belong, and throw away unnecessary materials.

■ **Figure 22.4**
Home program.

Nikki

The following two vignettes of Nikki illustrate how occupation based intervention changes as a child or adolescent with a learning disability develops and faces new challenges. Notice that as a preschooler, Nikki's condition is referred to as a **developmental delay** but later is changed to a learning disability. Developmental delay is often the generic term used to describe a young child who struggles with achieving developmental milestones but is too young for cognitive testing to be conclusive. As the child becomes older, additional testing can be conducted to determine a more precise diagnosis. Regardless of the identified condition, occupation based intervention addresses the child's or adolescent's challenges to participate in developmentally appropriate occupations and roles.

NIKKI AS A PRESCHOOLER

Nikki, a 4-year-old preschooler with a developmental delay, attends a noncategorical half-day developmental preschool within a large urban school district. She currently has an IEP and receives speech intervention. Nikki enjoys riding the school bus. Her special education preschool teacher reports that she is very friendly with the other children and teaching staff. Nikki's overall development resembles a 3-year-old's. She likes to look at picture books and listen to short stories. She can match but not name primary colors of red, blue, and yellow. She likes to recite familiar nursery rhymes and songs. She speaks in three word sentences and often talks to herself. She finger feeds herself and is toilet trained. Her current IEP includes goals for prewriting skills and independence in ADLs. Although Nikki is exposed to a variety of developmental activities throughout the day, she still has difficulty performing self-help skills in the classroom setting.

The special education preschool teacher and parents refer Nikki for an occupational therapy evaluation due to difficulty manipulating fasteners, eating with utensils, and building with blocks. She uses a full-fisted grasp to pick up and transfer objects. Since Nikki currently has an IEP for preschool special education and speech therapy, occupational therapy services are available under IDEA. The occupational therapist meets with the teacher and parents to discuss the referral, obtain information about Nikki's skills at home, and prioritize parent and teacher concerns.

After meeting with the parents and teacher, the occupational therapist considers possible reasons for Nikki's delayed skills. Since there is no evidence from the parents' or teachers' report that Nikki is experiencing sensory modulation problems, the occupational therapist concludes that delays in fine motor development are interfering with her participation in school related tasks. Since Nikki needs to develop and adjust her performance skills and patterns to meet a wide variety of different classroom tasks, the occupational therapist decides to use the Person-Environment-Occupation model (Law et al., 1996) to guide the evaluation and focus on Nikki's occupations as they relate to her student role. She assigns the occupational therapy assistant the task of observing Nikki multiple times in the classroom and recording how she completes school-related ADL tasks (Table 22.2■). Since the occupational therapy assistant often is in the vicinity of the preschool classroom, he arranges to observe Nikki when she naturally performs the ADL skills. After completing his observations, the occupational therapy assistant prepares a written report that he shares with the occupational therapist.

The occupational therapist also observes Nikki within the classroom routine to identify any difficulty with classroom tasks. She decides to use the Peabody Developmental Motor Scales (PDMS-2) and clinical observations to assess Nikki's performance skills and patterns. After analyzing the test results, observations, and conversations with parents and teacher, the occupational therapist prepares her report (Figure 22.5■). She considers the impact of Nikki's motor delays on all areas of occupation, but focuses the results on occupations related to Nikki's role as a student. The occupational therapist determines that Nikki would benefit from an **acquisitional approach** that provides Nikki with multiple opportunities to establish performance skills and patterns. Rather than recommending that Nikki receive occupational therapy services on a one to one basis, the occupational therapist proposes that she receive occupational therapy consultative services. The occupational therapist makes this decision because she believes that the classroom teacher and aide can provide multiple opportunities during the daily class routines for Nikki to acquire the skills given suggestions by the occupational therapist as to how to do so. Collaborative consultation initially involves assisting the teacher in creating an environment that encourages Nikki to establish her fine motor skills while directly demonstrating intervention techniques. The consultation time allotted can be adjusted to the needs of the preschool teacher and aide. Below is an example of a report that the occupational therapist might write to summarize these details.

After reconvening the IEP team, the occupational therapist shares the result of her evaluation and the team discusses how she will implement services. Because Nikki's IEP already includes goals to address self-care skills and fine motor skills, the team adds the occupational therapist to the list of service providers.

Before meeting with the preschool teacher, the occupational therapy assistant consults with the occupational

■ **Table 22.2**
Nikki's ADL Observations

Occupations Observed	Performance Skills Demonstrated	Performance Patterns Demonstrated	Context for Performance
Completing morning routine after arrival on school bus; 10 minute observation	Independently removed knit cap from head when she entered the classroom. Recognized her cubby and placed hat on shelf. Spontaneously pulled on zipper to open coat. Attempted to doff coat but initially was not successful. After receiving assistance, child completed the remaining steps to doff coat. Hung coat up on hook.	Attempted to remove coat by wiggling rather than using her hands to pull on the sleeves. Did not request assistance of classroom aide but stood quietly until the aide saw she needed assistance. Needed momentary assistance to initiate pulling on sleeves.	In a preschool classroom with 10 children, one special education preschool teacher and one aide Standing in a corner of the classroom where child height hooks are placed on wall for coats and cubby is above each hook. Cubby and hook are labeled with child's name and a unique symbol—Nikki, blue star. Children chatted with teacher and aides. Each child left area as they completed their morning routine.
Eating snack in preschool classroom; 20 minute observation	Recognized placemat with name and symbol and sat in chair. Attempted to open pudding and utensil containers but was unsuccessful. Held spoon with fisted grasp when scooping. Independently drank from child size cup. Placed napkin, bowl, and spoon in trash when finished.	Needed hand-over-hand assistance to open containers. Had difficulty scooping pudding with spoon. Did not spontaneously use her nondominant hand to steady the pudding cup while scooping. Successfully placed in mouth. No choking during snack.	Preschool classroom with two round tables and five children at each table. Teacher and aide provided supervision. Children and classroom personnel engage in quiet conversation.
Dressing and hygiene during toileting; 3 minute observation	Independently pulls down elastic waist pants prior to toileting. Initiated but unsuccessfully pulled up pants. Independently turned faucet on and off. Unable to pump liquid soap.	Needed hand-over-hand and verbal cues to pull up pants. Does not grasp waistband but rather tries to push up material without grasping waist band. Does not automatically use nondominant hand to steady pump, but attempts to complete with one hand.	Bathroom adjacent to preschool classroom. One to one assistance with aide during toileting. Liquid soap container sits on top of child size sink.
Preparing to depart for home; 10 minute observation	Locates her coat and cubby without assistance. Pulls coat off hook and hat off shelf.	Needs verbal directions and hand-over-hand assistance to don coat.	Two children at a time are in the coat area getting ready for dismissal.

■ **Table 22.2**
Nikki's ADL Observations (cont.)

Occupations Observed	Performance Skills Demonstrated	Performance Patterns Demonstrated	Context for Performance
	Needs maximum assistance to don coat. Needs assistance to zip coat closed. Child independently puts on hat.	Classroom aide engages front separated zipper. Child needs hand-over-hand assistance to hold bottom of coat while pulling up zipper.	

Occupational Therapy Evaluation

Nikki (CA = 4 years, 2 months) attends the developmental preschool at Lincoln Grade School. She was referred by her preschool teacher for an occupational therapy evaluation due to difficulty manipulating fasteners and eating utensils, and building with blocks. Mrs. Lawrence, the preschool teacher, indicates that Nikki's cognitive skills are at a 3–3 1/2-year-old level, but she has made significant gains in speech since her enrollment in the program four months prior. Her vocabulary is expanding and currently includes approximately 500 words. She speaks in three–four word sentences and likes to pretend that she is talking on the phone. She often plays parallel to other children, but occasionally joins others in the housekeeping corner or when a story is being read. She stays with an activity for about three minutes.

Nikki was cooperative and friendly during the evaluation. During the administration of the Peabody Developmental Motor Scales-2, she attempted all tasks presented, often humming to herself as she worked. Nikki had no adverse reactions to movement or sensory stimulation during classroom observations or individual testing sessions.

Nikki's ADL skills were observed within the context of the classroom routine. During the classroom snack time, Nikki was able to chew and swallow different textured foods and drink from a cup independently. She needed assistance unwrapping all food and utensils. She held the spoon with a tightly fisted gross grasp and had difficulty scooping food from container. During toileting she easily pulled down her elastic waist pants but did not attempt to grab the waistband to pull them up. She unzipped her jacket and attempted to wiggle it off her body. She required assistance to fully doff the jacket. She required maximum assistance to don her jacket or manipulate the separating zipper. Throughout the observations, Nikki performed most tasks unilaterally and did not use her nondominant hand spontaneously to provide assistance.

Nikki's upper extremity active range of motion, muscle tone, and strength were within functional limits. As measured by the Peabody Developmental Motor Scales-2, Nikki performed overall fine motor skills at the 2 1/2-year-level with subtests of hand grasp skills and visual-motor skills in the 18–24 month level. She has not yet developed consistent hand dominance but displayed a right hand preference and more developed right hand prehension skills. Although she preferred to use a full fisted grasp, when presented with smaller items, Nikki spontaneously used an inferior pincer grasp and static tripod grasp. She used a pronated grasp on scissors, which hindered her ability to snip successfully. Since she did not spontaneously adjust the pile with her nondominant hand, Nikki stacked only two–three blocks successfully. She spontaneously scribbled with the marker but did not attempt any specific strokes.

Summary: Nikki demonstrates difficulties completing self-help and classroom tasks that require fine motor skills and bilateral coordination. Nikki's skill level is

■ **Figure 22.5**
Nikki's occupational therapy evaluation.

delayed for her developmental age. It is recommended that occupational therapy consultative services be added to Nikki's current IEP to assist the teacher in creating opportunities for Nikki to establish these skills.

therapist and begins to prepare a list of possible classroom suggestions (Figure 22.6■). He must consider the following points to ensure that his suggestions are consistent with the occupational therapist's chosen models of practice and compatible with the classroom routine.

- *Occupation-based model:* Since the occupational therapist has chosen the P-E-O model, the occupational therapy assistant considers the person, occupation, and environment. In this situation, he realizes that the occupations are defined by the preschool setting, but that adaptations may be needed for Nikki's success. Interventions also need to be directed toward the person in establishing performance skills and patterns and toward the environment that creates opportunities for Nikki to learn and practice skills.
- *Non–occupation based frames of reference:* Recalling his knowledge of the acquisitional approach, the occupational therapy assistant realizes that he must choose interventions that allow Nikki to have multiple opportunities to practice skills and receive feedback. He considers activities that are self-correcting so that Nikki can monitor her success.

- *Occupation based goals and objectives:* He carefully analyzes and selects activities based on their potential impact on goals and objectives.
- *Developmentally and culturally appropriate:* He chooses activities compatible with Nikki's age and culture.
- *Practical considerations:* He considers how an idea will impact the classroom routine and is mindful of the preschool teacher's style and preferences. When possible, he chooses ideas that can be incorporated easily into current classroom activities and involve minimum preparation by the teaching staff.

Consultation to the preschool teacher and aides helps to create an enriching environment for Nikki to establish and refine developmentally appropriate performance skills and patterns. As the preschool teacher identifies new concerns, the occupational therapy assistant can make suggestions to the classroom environment, the specific classroom activity, or activity instructions. Since Nikki's skills are developing in a typical sequence though at a slower rate, the preschool teacher easily incorporates and generalizes these ideas into her current preschool curriculum. Eventually she finds that she no longer needs consultation from the occupational therapist or occupational therapy assistant.

Classroom Suggestions

Increase self-dressing opportunities
- Require Nikki and the other children to don/doff dressing vests prior to beginning their turn on indoor playground equipment and to taking turns in relay races.
- Replace over the head paint smocks with button down paint shirts.
- Provide dress up clothes in housekeeping area

Increase toys and activities that require bilateral hand use
- Provide rolling pins for play dough activities.
- Increase number of bilateral toys on free play shelf, such as plastic nuts and bolts, pop beads, and Duplos®.
- During circle time, introduce bilateral musical instruments such as cymbals, rhythm sticks, and sandpaper blocks.
- Incorporate cutting activities into daily job chart, such as cutting brown paper off the roll to use as placemats, and cutting paper ends off snack utensil packs.

Encourage refined pincer grasp
- During art activities, use small rather than large pieces of chalk or crayons to draw and color.
- When offering finger food such as fish crackers or raisins, instruct the children to pick them up one at a time using a tripod grasp.
- Encourage Nikki to pick up puzzle pieces using the small knobs.

■ Figure 22.6
Classroom suggestions.

NIKKI AS A SECOND GRADER

During her three year re-evaluation to requalify for special education services, the school psychologist determined that Nikki has a learning disability that interferes with her written language skills. As a second grader, Nikki now receives special education support within her regular education classroom. She is making slow but steady progress in her reading and math skills. Her teacher, Mr. Hazel, is concerned about Nikki's ability to complete written work. Although Nikki has had repeated instruction, she continues to have difficulty producing legible handwriting. Her letters are not in proportion to the grade level lines and spaces. Her papers often are torn or smudged due to erasing. After discussion with Nikki's grandparents, who are her guardians, the teacher requests an occupational therapy evaluation. Besides handwriting, the grandparents and teachers also are concerned that Nikki does not participate in nonacademic activities with her classmates. The playground staff reports that Nikki often stands by the fence watching her classmates as they jump rope, play hopscotch, or converse in small groups. The grandparents would like Nikki to be involved in the school social programs but Nikki always refuses, stating that she doesn't know anyone.

While reading the referral, the occupational therapist decides that besides conducting an evaluation of handwriting, she also needs to investigate Nikki's reluctance to participate in social groups. She interviews the physical education teacher, Mr. Crawford, and finds that Nikki's gross motor skills are average for her age and grade and she should have no difficulty participating in the playground activities. The occupational therapist asks the occupational therapy assistant to observe Nikki in a variety of different social contexts, with emphasis on how she is interacting with others. The occupational therapy assistant observes Nikki during art and music classes, during lunch and recess, and during a classroom group project. He prepares a written report (Table 22.3■) and discusses the information with the occupational therapist.

In order to assess Nikki's handwriting skills, the occupational therapist collects classroom handwriting samples, administers standardized and nonstandardized evaluations, and completes clinical observations. Based upon an analysis of her evaluation and the observations completed by the occupational therapy assistant, the occupational therapist prepares the evaluation report (Figure 22.7■) and presents it at the IEP team meeting.

After discussing the occupational therapy evaluation, the IEP team decides that occupational therapy services should be included on Nikki's current IEP to address difficulties in handwriting and social participation. The following goals are added to the current IEP:

Goal 1: Student will demonstrate legible printing on class assignments.

Objective 1a: Student will print upper and lowercase letters with correct formation, 9/10 attempts.

Objective 1b: Student will produce upper and lowercase letters in proportion to printed lines, 8/10 attempts.

Objective 1c: Student will erase mistakes without tearing paper, 5/7 attempts.

Goal 2: Student will demonstrate age appropriate social competency skills.

Objective 2a: When arriving at the playground, student will initiate participation in a group, 3/5 days per week.

Objective 2b: When conversing with others, student will use appropriate voice volume and maintain eye contact, 3/5 attempts.

Objective 2c: Student will participate in group decision making by expressing her opinion or contributing an idea, 2/5 attempts.

In order to meet Nikki's needs, the occupational therapist recommends that Nikki receive direct and consultative occupational therapy intervention services. The occupational therapist provides consultation to the teacher to recommend strategies that minimize the impact of Nikki's visual perceptual difficulties. The occupational therapy assistant collaborates with the occupational therapist to draft a list of possible immediate alterations to environment and tasks (Figure 22.8■). The occupational therapist shares these strategies with the teacher and discusses positive ways to encourage Nikki to increase participation with her peers.

The classroom teacher and occupational therapist arrange for Nikki to attend the social skills group and handwriting club that the occupational therapy assistant conducts in her school building. During the social skills group, Nikki engages in role playing and group tasks that allow her to develop her social competency skills. The occupational

■ **Table 22.3**
Observation of Nikki

Occupation Observed	Performance Skills and Patterns of Most of the Children	Performance Skills and Patterns of Nikki	Context for Occupation
Morning arrival at school; 15 minute observation	Children engage in quiet conversation as they enter the building. As children join the group, they greet each other.	Nikki does not participate in conversation. Walks with head down, dragging her backpack across the floor. Nikki does not acknowledge a new person to the group.	In the school hallways Small groups of children
School lunchroom procedure; 15 minute observation	Children carry trays through line. They engage in quiet conversation, answer questions from food servers, and give lunch ticket to cashier. As they leave the line, children take any available seat or sit together in small groups.	Nikki proceeds through line without talking with other children. When asked, she requests a hamburger, fries, and strawberry milk. Doesn't have her lunch ticket ready and searches through her pockets. Hands in the ticket looking down and mumbles, "here it is." When Nikki comes to the end of the line, she gazes across the room and then chooses a solitary seat.	In school cafeteria during lunch Children sit in small groups at tables.
Completing a group collage in art class; 25 minute observation	Children choose their assigned seat and listen to teacher directions. One student starts organizing the group and hands out materials. Group members discuss the project.	Nikki quickly takes her seat and listens attentively during directions. Nikki takes scissors and magazines that are next to her area and starts cutting out pictures and putting them in a pile. When asked by her peer why she is cutting out those pictures, she puts down the scissors and just looks down. Does not share ideas or contribute to the group discussion. When asked directly for her opinion, she shakes her head and gives no answer.	In the art room with high stools around a raised wooden tables. Children are assigned six to a table. All necessary materials are placed in the middle of table.

■ **Table 22.3**
Observation of Nikki (cont.)

Occupation Observed	Performance Skills and Patterns of Most of the Children	Performance Skills and Patterns of Nikki	Context for Occupation
Selection and participation in a lunchtime recess activity; 20 minute observation	As children enter the playground, they choose an activity to join. As new children arrive in the area, they approach the kickball game and ask which team they can join. Five girls walk around the playground chatting and talking to each other and other children. Three children walk directly over to Nikki and ask her to join them in a game of dodge ball.	As Nikki enters the playground, she watches the kickball game from the building steps. She walks past the game, but stands next to the fence. She doesn't ask to join the group. When the girls pass Nikki, she does not greet them spontaneously. When they wave to her, she vocalizes a quiet "hi" but does not leave the fence area. As the group approaches, Nikki does not look up until they greet her. Nikki responds "OK" and follows behind the group to the selected play area. She remains with the group for the remainder of the recess period.	Large school playground surrounded by a fence. There is a blacktop area where ball games occur and grassy area with benches. Children are walking around in small groups. A kickball game is being played on the blacktop.

Occupational Therapy Evaluation

Name: Nikki   Date: 10/10/07

Nikki (CA = 8 years) attends second grade at Kennedy Elementary School and receives special education support services for reading and math. Mr. Hazel, Nikki's classroom teacher, referred her for an occupational therapy evaluation due to illegible handwriting. The classroom teacher indicated that Nikki's writing is large, irregular, and often not within the second grade lined paper. Although she does remember to print her name on the paper, she often does not print it in the upper left hand corner of the paper, as instructed. She has difficulty using the eraser, often tearing the paper. Mr. Hazel and grandparents also are concerned about Nikki's social competencies. Nikki does not make friends easily and often stands alone during recess. Mr. Hazel has observed that Nikki does not participate fully in group activities and feels that this interferes with learning. The grandparents would like Nikki to participate in after school programs and other social groups.

Nikki was observed as she engaged in social interactions on the playground, in the cafeteria, during art class, and in the school hallways. During all of these settings, Nikki demonstrated difficulties participating in age appropriate social situations. Although she was physically capable of participating in playground activities, she did not initiate joining a group play and consistently waited until a group member requested her participation. When communicating with others,

■ **Figure 22.7**
Nikki's occupational therapy evaluation report.

she did not engage in conversation and only answered direct questions with a very soft voice. She usually kept her head down when speaking and walking, and rarely looked at others when listening or speaking. During small group discussions, she did not express an opinion or contribute to the conversation. When directly asked, however, she joined a play group and participated for an extended period of time.

Nikki's handwriting skills were assessed by examining typical work samples, observing Nikki during classroom written tasks, and administering standardized assessment tools. During classroom writing tasks, she consistently held the pencil with a right handed tripod grasp. No involuntary movement patterns interfered with her ability to control the pencil. Although she was observed performing bilateral skills throughout the day, she did not use the left hand spontaneously to stabilize the paper. As the paper moved across the desk, she often smudged her work or tore the paper while attempting to erase a mistake.

On the Developmental Test of Visual Perception, Nikki scored at the 12th percentile for visual-motor integration due to a low score in design copying and visual-motor speed. She scored at the 3rd percentile in motor-reduced visual perceptual skills, having the most difficulty with Figure–Ground and Position in Space subtests, which have a strong influence on her ability to produce legible handwriting.

Nikki's writing samples displayed illegible handwriting that consistently was worse when required to use paper with lines and spaces. She formed letters incorrectly, frequently starting at the bottom rather than top of letters and having difficulty producing counterclockwise circles. She inconsistently placed letters on the lines, often paused during printing and pondered where to place the next letter.

Summary: Nikki demonstrated delays in social competency skills that hinder her full participation in the school environment. She has difficulty participating in group activities and engaging in age appropriate social situations.

Nikki's ability to produce legible handwriting is hindered by her difficulties in visual perceptual skills of figure–ground and position in space. Incorrect letter formation and letter proportion, and bilateral skills difficulties, contribute to her poor production of written work.

It is recommended that occupational therapy services be added to the current IEP to address social competence and handwriting.

- Decrease visual distractions
  - Classroom environment
    - Decrease visual distractions from teaching aids and charts.
    - Minimize amount of information written on classroom board at a time.
  - Tasks
    - Eliminate unnecessary visual decorations on worksheets.
    - Decrease amount of information on a handout.
    - Allow Nikki to print answer on separate piece of paper that only includes writing baseline.
  - Provide positional cues
    - Highlight left corner of paper where name should be written.
    - Provide tactile feedback to writing lines
  - Increase social interaction opportunities
    - Assign Nikki a classroom task that requires her to approach each student directly.
    - Instruct all students to look directly at each other while speaking in groups.
    - When working in small groups, reassign Nikki a role that requires her to interact with others.

■ **Figure 22.8**
Classroom suggestions.

therapy assistant grades and alters situations and models social skills so that Nikki can learn through active experimentation and observation. During the weekly handwriting club meeting, Nikki receives instruction in correct letter formation and erasing methods. During this small group session, she has the opportunity to meet and interact with peers and practice social skills addressed in her other group.

At the IEP meeting, the grandparents ask for suggestions that they can incorporate into Nikki's home routine to address her goals. The occupational therapist suggests that they encourage Nikki to play various games and activities such as puzzles and picture searches that stimulate her visual perceptional skills. They also discuss after school activities and groups that Nikki can join. The classroom teacher gives the grandparents a list of programs that the school offers and indicates ones that her classmates regularly attend. The occupational therapist suggests that the grandparents visit different groups with Nikki and encourages them to notify her if they needed further assistance. The occupational therapist schedules a followup meeting with the teacher and grandparents to monitor Nikki's progress in social competency skills. ■

SUMMARY

Children and adolescents with learning disabilities and ADHD often have difficulty completing daily occupations. Occupational therapists and occupational therapy assistants can utilize occupation based interventions and therapeutic use to self to address deficit performance patterns and skills. Applying occupation based theories and therapeutic models of intervention, occupational therapists and occupational therapy assistants can make use of a variety of different strategies and techniques that may enhance a child or adolescent's motor, processing, and social skills. When working with children and adolescents with learning disabilities and ADHD, occupational therapists and occupational therapy assistants need to be mindful of underlying social and emotional issues that may impact self-esteem and self-worth.

REVIEWING KEY POINTS

1. Explain the differences among the three types of ADHD.
2. Explain the differences between the two definitions of learning disabilities.
3. Explain what is meant by social competence.
4. Explain how ADHD and LD impact the daily occupations of children and adolescents within the context of their family and environment.
5. Explain a method for recording observations of the child's or adolescent's occupational performance. Refer to Tables 22.1, 22.2, and 22.3 for examples.
6. Describe how occupational therapy interventions support the capacity of children and adolescents with ADHD and LD conditions to participate in their daily occupations.
7. Describe how occupational therapists and occupational therapy assistants work together to provide occupational therapy services to children and adolescents with ADHD.
8. Describe how occupational therapist and occupational therapy assistants work with families and other professionals to provide services to children and adolescents with ADHD and LD.

APPLYING KEY CONCEPTS

1. Review the case study of Ricky. Based upon the information provided, design another sensory experience for the kindergarten classroom.

2. Further investigate the Alert Program. If possible, visit a group session.
3. Review the case study of Nikki as a preschooler. Provide the preschool teacher with a developmentally appropriate activity that would address Nikki's current needs.
4. Review the case study of Nikki as a second grader. Consider the role of the occupational therapy assistant and design a session for the social skills group and the handwriting group. Critique your ideas with your peers. If possible, role play the session and make modifications to your initial ideas.

REFERENCES

American Occupational Therapy Association (2002). Occupational therapy practice framework: Domain and process. *American Journal of Occupational Therapy, 56*(6), 609–639.

American Psychiatric Association (2000). *Diagnostic and statistical manual of mental disorders: DSM-IV-TR.* Washington, DC: American Psychiatric Association, <http://alias.libriaries.psu.edu/eresources/STATREP>.

Dunn, W. (1997). *The Sensory Profile.* San Antonio, TX: Psychological Corporation, Therapy Skill Builders.

Dunn, W., Brown, C., & McGuigan, A. (1994). The ecology of human performance: A framework for considering the effect of context. *American Journal of Occupational Therapy, 48,* 595–607.

Folio, M. R., & Fewell, R. R. (2002). *Peabody Developmental Motor Scales (PDMS-2)* (2nd ed.). Denver, CO: Pro Ed.

Heward, W. (2006). Exceptional children: An introduction to special education (8th ed.). Upper Saddle River, NJ: Pearson Prentice Hall.

Izenberg, N. (Ed.) (2000). *Human diseases and conditions.* New York: Charles Scribner's Sons.

Jackson, L., & Arbesman, M. (Eds.) (2005). *Occupational therapy practice guidelines for children with behavioral and psychosocial needs.* Bethesda, MD: AOTA Press.

Lane, S. (2002). Sensory modulation. In A. Bundy, S. Lane, & E. Murray. *Sensory integration theory and practice* (2nd ed.). Philadelphia: F. A. Davis Company.

Law, M., Baptiste, S., Carswell, A., McColl, M., Polatajko, H., & Pollock, N. (1998). *Canadian Occupational Performance Measure* (3rd ed.). Ottawa: CAOT Publications.

Law, M., Cooper, B., Strong, S., Steward, D., Rigby, R., & Letts, L. (1996). The person-environment-occupational model: A transactive approach to occupational performance. *Canadian Journal of Occupational Therapy, 63,* 9–23.

Mosier, W. (1998). Toward a psychology of understanding attention-deficit/hyperactivity disorder. *Journal of the American Academy of Physician Assistants,* http://jaapa.com/issues/j19980200/articles/j2w056.html. Retrieved 07/05/07.

Mulligan, S. (2001). Classroom strategies used by teachers of students with attention deficit hyperactivity disorder. *Physical & Occupational Therapy in Pediatrics, 20*(4), 25–44.

Scanlon, D. (2006). Learning disabilities and attention deficits. In K. Thies & J. Travers (Eds.), *Handbook of human development for health care professionals.* Sudbury, NJ: Jones and Bartlett Publishers.

Stubbe, D. (2000). Attention-deficit/hyperactivity disorder overview: Historical perspective, current controversies. *Child & Adolescent Psychiatric Clinics of North America, 9,* 469–479.

Wilbarger, P., & Wilbarger, J. (2002). The Wilbarger approach to treating sensory defensiveness. In A. Bundy, S. Lane & E. Murray (Eds.), *Sensory integration: Theory and practice* (2nd ed.). Philadelphia: F. A. Davis.

Williams, M. S., & Shellenberger, S. (1996). *How fast does your engine run? A leader's guide to the alert program for self-regulation.* Albuquerque, NM: Therapy Works.

Williamson, G., & Dorman, W. (2002). *Promoting social competence:* San Antonio, TX: Therapy Skill Builders.

Appendix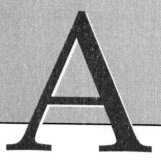

Development Charts

Age	Motor Milestones
Birth to 1 month	Holds hand in a fist; turns head from side to side when placed in a prone position; attempts to follow objects that are out of direct line of vision
1 to 4 months	Holds head up when help upright; lifts up on arms when lying on stomach; grasps with entire hand; raises head and upper body on arms when in a prone position; reaches for and grasps objects; sits when supported; begins to roll from side to side by turning head to one side and allowing trunk to follow
5 to 8 months	Rolls over; sits up; begins to crawl; holds bottle; transfers objects from one hand to the other; uses finger and thumb to pick up objects; sits alone without support
9 to 12 months	Stands alone; climbs, removes lids from containers; begins to prefer one hand over the other
12 to 18 months	Stands alone and is able to sit in a chair; carries small objects while walking; waves bye-bye and claps hands; walks without help
18 to 24 months	Walks well; rolls a large ball; picks up toys without falling over
2 years	Turns pages while reading; walks backwards; likes to push, pull, fill, and dump; builds block towers; holds pencil or crayon; throws large balls; climbs upstairs; walks down stairs (both feet on each step)
3 years	Stands on one foot for up to 5 seconds; uses riding toys; throws balls overhand; kicks large balls; feeds self with spoon; uses scissors; holds writing instrument in hand between thumb and fingers; draws vertical, horizontal, and circular lines
4 years	Walks a straight line; hops on one foot; pedals and steers a tricycle skillfully; jumps over objects five to six inches in height; uses fork and spoon; threads beads on a string; makes identifiable objects out of clay
5 years	Learns to skip; throws balls overhead; cuts on a line with scissors; establishes hand dominance; goes up stairs with alternating feet; walks backwards; manipulates most buttons and zippers without assistance
6 years	Enjoys physical activity—running, jumping, climbing, and throwing; moves constantly; has increased dexterity and eye–hand coordination; makes movements that are more deliberate and precise; ties own shoes
7 years	Maintains control over gross and fine motor skills; balances on either foot; uses alternating feet when running up and down stairs; throws and catches small objects (balls)
8 years	Exhibits improvements in agility, balance, speed, and strength; enjoys vigorous activities; seeks out opportunities to participate in team/group sports
9 and 10 years	Throws ball with accuracy; performs fine motor skills with improved coordination; likes to run, climb, ride bicycles; uses hands for different projects—arts and crafts, cooking, and/or building or taking apart objects

AGE	MOTOR MILESTONES
11 and 12 years	Exhibits increased strength in completing gross motor activities; continues to improve fine motor skills; displays coordinated and smooth movements; however, may be clumsy during growth spurts

Allen, K. E., & Marotz, L. (2007). *Developmental profiles: Pre-birth through twelve* (5th ed.). Clifton Park, NY: Delmar Learning.
Berk, L. (2000). *Child development* (5th ed.). Needham Heights, MA: Allyn & Bacon.
Oliver, S. J. *Playing for keeps.* Retrieved April 24, 2006 from http://sites.target.com/site/en/kids.

AGE	COGNITIVE PERCEPTUAL MILESTONES
Birth to 1 month	Blinks eyes in response to fast approaching objects; begins to study own hand; follows objects that are moved vertically in front of face or are moved in a slow moving arc pattern; synchronizes body movements with speech patterns of parent or caregiver; develops sense of smell present at birth, turning away from unpleasant odors
1 to 4 months	Explores objects with mouth; distinguishes familiar faces; distinguishes between colors across the spectrum; prefers complex visual and sound patterns; looks in the direction of a sound source; continues to gaze in direction of moving objects that have disappeared; watches hand intently; moves eyes from one subject to another, focuses on and reaches for small objects; attempts to keep objects in hand in motion
5 to 8 months	Understands simple cause and effect actions; focuses on and reaches for small objects; imitates actions that child has seen many times; anticipates an expected action; experiments with simple physical relationships (objects hitting one another, retrieval of objects thrown); uses hand, mouth, and eyes in coordination to explore own body, toys, and other items; picks up objects to explore, may pick them up in an inverted position.
9 to 12 months	Groups objects that are alike; explores small switches and openings that turn; recognizes the names of some objects; solves problems through trial and error; imitates actions seen at another time or in another place; reaches for toys, objects that are visible but out of reach; recognizes reversal of an object; begins to demonstrate understanding of functional relationships
12 to 18 months	Enjoys object hiding activities; demonstrates understanding of functional relationships; takes things apart; identifies objects in a book; enjoys playing peek-a-boo; begins to understand and follow simple directions
18 to 24 months	Shows preference between toys; manages multiple toys at once; listens to short stories; offers toys or objects to others; names everyday objects; begins to understand spatial and form discrimination; puts objects into containers and empties container of objects
2 years	Enjoys stories, songs, and rhymes; wants to learn how to use things; likes to look at books and name objects; puts objects together and takes them apart; sorts objects according to type
3 years	Matches objects and picture; identifies common colors; puts on shoes; recognizes everyday sounds; draws a circle and square; listens attentively; plays realistically; understands and recognizes basic shapes (circle, square, triangle) by pointing to them
4 years	Places objects in a line from largest to smallest; recognizes some letters if taught and may be able to print name; recognizes familiar words in simple book or signs (i.e., STOP sign); counts to 20 or more; identifies missing puzzle parts when looking at picture
5 years	Understands sequential orders of objects based on size; understands that stories have a beginning, middle, and end; understands that books are read from left to right, top to bottom; draws pictures that represent animals, people, and objects; sorts objects based on two dimensions or common feature

Age	Cognitive Perceptual Milestones
6 years	Displays knowledge of time (today, tomorrow, yesterday) and simple concepts of motion; utilizes increased attention span; enjoys "thinking" activities and games (puzzles, mazes, matching games)
7 years	Exhibits better understanding of cause and effect; enjoys reading; tells time using a clock; understands concept of time and space
8 years	Likes to read and work independently; organizes and collects items according to classifications; begins to understand concepts of conservation; uses logic in understanding everyday events; shows interest in what others are doing around them
9 and 10 years	Learns through "hands-on" learning; demonstrates improved understanding of cause and effect; recalls events from memory; reads and writes for leisure
11 and 12 years	Thinks in abstract terms; demonstrates longer attention span; enjoys problem solving; creates plans and lists to reach goals; performs tasks without thinking; demonstrates increased memory; demonstrates increased understanding of more complex cause and effect

Berk, L. (2000). *Child development* (5th ed.). Needham Heights, MA: Allyn & Bacon.
Allen, K. E., & Marotz, L. (2007). *Developmental profiles: Pre-birth through twelve* (5th ed.). Clifton Park, NY: Delmar Learning.

Age	Speech and Language Milestones
Birth to 1 month	Reacts to loud noises by blinking, moving, stopping a movement, shifting eyes, or making a startle response; turns head in an effort to locate voices and other sounds; makes occasional sounds other than crying.
1 to 4 months	Smiles when talked to; makes cooing sounds; turns the head in response to the human voice; communicates needs primarily through crying; imitates facial expressions
5 to 8 months	Makes vowel and consonant sounds while cooing; begins to babble, which contains all the sounds of the human speech
9 to 12 months	Uses gestures, eye contact, and verbal sounds to communicate; repeats certain syllables (e. g., "ma-ma"); understands some words, may say a few; experiments with word sounds
12 to 18 months	Says hi or bye if encouraged; points or uses single words; looks at person talking to him/her; talks by pointing or gesturing toward things
18 to 24 months	Utilizes a vocabulary of more than 50 words; uses some two word phrases; says please and thank you when prompted
2 years	Speaks using several hundred words; uses two to three word sentences; repeats words others say; says names of items when asked
3 years	Talks in complete sentences of three to five words; uses a vocabulary of about 1,000 words; listens attentively to short stories; likes familiar stories told without any changes in words
4 years	Speaks fairly complex sentences; learns name, address, and phone number, if taught; follows two unrelated directions
5 years	Enjoys telling his or her own stories; enjoys riddles and jokes; identifies some letters of the alphabet and few numbers
6 years	Enjoys talking; asks questions; learns up to 5 to 10 new words daily; uses vocabulary of approximately 10,000 to 14,000 words; uses correct verb tenses and sentence structure; enjoys fictitious stories and being read to; talks self through problem solving situations

Age	Speech and Language Milestones
7 years	Uses gestures to illustrate conversations; enjoys storytelling; uses more precise use of language with descriptive adjectives and adverbs; describes personal experiences in detail; demonstrates understanding and carry through of multiple step instructions
8 years	Uses language to compliment and/or criticize others; repeats slang and/or curse words; demonstrates understanding of grammar rules in conversation and writing
9 and 10 years	Enjoys talking at great lengths; expresses feelings and emotions through words; uses slang expressions common among peers in conversation; understands double meanings of words; demonstrates continued understanding of grammatical sequences
11 and 12 years	Incorporates longer and complex sentences into writing, conversation; understands concepts of sarcasm, irony, and implied meaning; demonstrates ability to shift language style from formal to informal.

Berk, L. (2000). *Child development* (5th ed.). Needham Heights, MA: Allyn & Bacon.
Allen, K. E., & Marotz, L. (2007). *Developmental profiles: Pre-birth through twelve* (5th ed.). Clifton Park, NY: Delmar Learning.

Age	Social Emotional Milestones
Birth to 1 month	Experiences a short period of alertness immediately following birth; likes to be held close and cuddled when awake; begins to establish emotional attachment with parents and/or caregiver; begins to develop sense of security or trust with parents and caregivers
1 to 4 months	Imitates, avoids, and ends social interactions; enjoys being cuddled; coos, smiles, and squeals in response to friendly faces; frowns or becomes anxious to loud or unfamiliar voices
5 to 8 months	Establishes attachment to primary caregiver; differentiates between people; likes rhythmic activities; seeks attention by verbalizing and moving body; becomes upset if familiar objects are removed; remains friendly toward strangers; imitates and responds differently to various facial expressions, sounds, and actions of others
9 to 12 months	Demonstrates stranger anxiety; wants caregiver in visual field; communicates needs for caregiver by extending arms or clinging; becomes attached to a favorite object; repeats behaviors to get attention of others; enjoys being a part of family activities; begins to assert will by resisting caregiver's directions
12 to 18 months	Shares toys with and responds to facial expression of others
18 to 24 months	Shows a wide range of emotions including fear, angry, frustration, joy, and empathy; laughs at silly actions
2 years	Demonstrates willingness to separate from parents; displays basic understanding and expression of range of emotions; shows empathy toward others; observes other adults and children; uses "no" frequently in an effort to exert control; becomes shy around strangers; enjoys companions and shows interest in peers
3 years	Enjoys being with other children; demonstrates increased interest in self-help skills; shows empathetic behavior to others who are hurt; participates in simple games and group activities; attempts challenging activities; demonstrates awareness of turn taking and social aspects of conversation
4 years	Understands rules and begins to actively follow them; demonstrates mood changes; enjoys group activities and time with friends; likes silly activities
5 years	Exhibits affection, empathy, and care toward others; demonstrates increased capability to boost self-esteem; maintains friendships with those who share mutual interest vs. those who are available to play; demonstrates an understanding of the feelings of others; plays in groups of two to four

AGE	SOCIAL EMOTIONAL MILESTONES
6 years	Experiences sudden swings in moods; begins to shift dependence from parents to developing friendships; becomes easily disappointed and frustrated; has difficulty calming and soothing self when frustrated; may become increasingly fearful of external situations that have an element of risk; views situations from a self-centered perspective; seeks adult approval and reassurance
7 years	Sees humor in situations; becomes more cooperative with and likes to help adults; worries about being liked; blames others for mistakes; feels situations acutely; takes responsibility seriously
8 years	Seeks acceptance from but becomes argumentative with peers about being right; imitates dress and language of others; desires attention and recognition from adults; enjoys talking on the phone with friends; begins forming opinions about right and wrong; enjoys playing with several best friends; becomes easily upset when a task does not meet expectations
9 and 10 years	Seeks out friends based on common interests and proximity; has several good friends and some enemies; defends self by name calling and teasing; has difficulty dealing with failure or frustration; takes criticism as a personal attack
11 and 12 years	Likes and cares for animals; views image of self as important; becomes more self-conscious and self-focused; recognizes loyalty, honesty, dependability, and trustworthiness; uses words and gestures to handle frustrations; spends more time with peers than with parents

Allen, K. E., & Marotz, L. (2007). *Developmental profiles: Pre-birth through twelve* (5th ed.). Clifton Park, NY: Delmar Learning.
Case-Smith, J. (2005). *Occupational therapy for children* (5th ed.). St. Louis: Elsevier Mosby.

AGE	PLAY MILESTONES
Birth to 1 month	Enjoys light, brightness, and face-to-face positioning; stares at faces
1 to 4 months	Plays briefly with fingers, hands, and toes; likes to be tickled and jiggled; reaches out to familiar people and objects; enjoys physical activity such as kicking, turning head, and clasping hands
5 to 8 months	Plays with small toys that cause a reaction such as a noise or movement; bangs objects together; enjoys throwing and mouthing objects; talks to self; experiments with own voice
9 to 12 months	Enjoys large motor activities involving creeping, cruising, and walking; engages in sensorimotor and exploratory play; puts objects into and out of containers; likes opening and closing cupboards and drawers
12 to 18 months	Engages in functional and relational play; enjoys gross motor play; participates in parallel level play
18 to 24 months	Begins to demonstrate pretend and symbolic play; enjoys solitary play
2 years	Links multiple schemes together to create a sequence to pretend play; uses objects to represent people and objects; imitates adults and animals; likes rough and tumble play; engages in drawing and assembling simple puzzles; rides riding toys; engages in cooperative play
3 years	Creates imaginary stories that combine real and imaginary sequences; engages in constructive play; enjoys circle time, singing, and dancing; participates in associative play with others
4 years	Likes to role play adult actions, make up stories, and play dress-up; builds complex structures with construction toys; plays group games with simple rules; participates in simple organized games
5 years	Plays board games and computer games with rules; participates in competitive and cooperative games; creates elaborative imaginary games that reconstruct the real world; participates in sports teams and organized group activities
6 years	Has a clear sense of likes and dislikes; becomes possessive about own toys and belonging; forms friendships with a few friends; participates in cooperative play

Age	Play Milestones
7 years	Prefers same gender playmates; likes to play in groups; likes competitive board and card games but will bend rules to suit self; wants to be part of social situation and to keep up with friends
8 years	Enjoys competitive activities; reinterprets rules to improve chances of winning; eager to join sports teams but will quit if competition is too intense
9 and 10 years	Fluctuates activity level between high and low intensity; develops new hobbies and special interests; likes to form and join secret clubs
11 and 12 years	Prefers goal directed activities, making money, and being part of a team; enjoys outdoor skill activities; prefers organized activities and sports

Allen, K. E., & Marotz, L. (2007). *Developmental profiles: Pre-birth through twelve* (5th ed.). Clifton Park, NY: Delmar Learning.
Case-Smith, J. (2005). *Occupational therapy for children* (5th ed.). St. Louis: Elsevier Mosby.

Appendix B

Reflexes, Righting, and Equilibrium Reactions

PRIMITIVE REFLEXES

These are automatic and specific motor responses that typically are present during the first year of life. They occur in response to a particular sensory stimulus and facilitate early sensory-motor experiences for the infant. As the nervous system matures, these limited automatic motor responses develop into a variety of different voluntary and complex movement patterns. Environmental stimulation and skill repetition contribute to the development. If nervous system damage occurs, these primitive reflexes can persist, resulting in stereotyped movements (Cronin & Mandich, 2005).

Asymmetrical Tonic Neck Reflex (ATNR) As the head turns to the side, the extremities on the skull side flex while the extremities on the chin side extend. This reflex is present at birth and usually integrates by 6 months (Cronin & Mandich, 2005). If this reflex is obligatory and allows no alternative movements, it interferes with the development of bilateral hand skills and hand to mouth movements.

Symmetrical Tonic Neck Reflex (STNR) As the neck flexes, both upper extremities (BUE) flex while both lower extremities (BLE) extend. When the neck extends, BUE extend while BLE flex. This reflex assists the infant in learning to prop sit by extending the UE to take weight when the head bobs forward (Cronin & Mandich, 2005). If the reflex becomes a compulsory movement, it interferes with independent arm and neck movement patterns.

Rooting Reflex When the check is stroked, the infant turns the head toward the stimulation. This reflex is present at birth and assists the infant in turning the head toward the breast to nurse (Kail, 2002). By 3 months, this reflex is no longer present. If the reflex continues to persist, it interferes with the head maintaining a midline position.

Sucking Reflex When the roof of the mouth is touched, the infant immediately begins to suck. This reflex is present in babies who are born full term (Kail, 2002) but often absent with premature infants, resulting in feeding difficulties. By 3 months, this reflex is no longer a prominent movement pattern, allowing a more mature feeding pattern.

Grasp Reflex When an object is placed in the palm of the hand with pressure over the metacarpals, the fingers flex automatically. The full term newborn baby's hands are in a full flexion pattern with thumb resting in the palm and all fingers flexed. The involuntary grasp response slowly diminishes as the central nervous system matures and the infant interacts with the environment. In prone, the infant takes weight through the hands, which begins to elongate the finger flexors. In supine and supported sitting, the infant begins to bat out at objects. Before 11 months of age, this reflex gradually decreases its dominance to allow the development of voluntary grasp and release of objects (Cronin & Mandich, 2005; Alexander, Boeme, & Cupps, 1993).

Moro Reflex (Startle Reflex) When the head falls or when a loud noise sounds, an infant quickly throws his arms out and then brings them inward (Kail, 2002). By 6 months, this reflex is no longer dominant. Since the automatic response can cause a loss of balance, this reflex must be diminished before an infant can sit independently.

Landau Reaction When an infant is supported under the waist and suspended in a horizontal position, the head, neck, and lower extremities extend while the upper extremities extend and abduct. This reaction appears at the 3–4 month stage and diminishes around 24 months. If this reaction is seen earlier, it may be an indication of increased tone (Alexander, Boehme, & Cupps, 1993). In older children, this total antigravity position is referred to as a *pivot prone position* (Cronin & Mandich, 2005).

RIGHTING REACTIONS

This group of automatic responses allows subtle body shifts to occur which allow the person to align the head in space and the other body parts in relation to the position of the head and ground. This process keeps the person in an upright position and allows stability during movement. Righting reactions begin to appear at 4 moths of age and become part of the person's posture (Shumway-Cook & Woollacott, 2001).

PROTECTIVE REACTIONS (PARACHUTE REACTIONS)

Protective reactions are automatic responses that trigger a person to extend the upper extremities to protect the proximal body parts when falling. They develop in the following directions and in the following sequence: downward, forward (anterior), lateral, and backward (posterior). Once developed, these reactions are present throughout life (Cronin & Mandich, 2005).

EQUILIBRIUM REACTIONS (TILTING REACTIONS)

Equilibrium reactions automatically occur when a person attempts to regain balance. Regardless of the position of the person, these automatic responses are the same. The trunk curves or bends against the direction of displacement. The extremities on one side of the body increase in tone and elongate while the opposite extremities abduct. These reactions develop sequentially: first prone, then supine, then sitting, then kneeling, and finally standing. They remain present throughout life (Cronin & Mandich, 2005).

ATYPICAL RESPONSES

Tonic Bite Reflex The tonic bite reflex is an atypical response, only seen in individuals with neurological condition. Following stimulation to the gums or teeth, there is a sustained jaw closure whereby the mandible forcefully clamps upward. Increased tone is present and it is difficult to relax the jaw (Cronin & Mandich, 2005).

Associated Reactions An associated reaction is an atypical response, only seen in individuals with neurological conditions. Often present in individuals with hemiplegic cerebral palsy, there is an involuntary increase of postural tone in the effected side as the result of voluntary effortful movement on the noninvolved side. The postural tone on the involved side remains increased even after the voluntary action ceases (Shumway-Cook & Woollacott, 2006).

REFERENCES

Alexander, R., Boehm, R., & Cupps, B. (1993). *Normal development of functional motor skills.* Tucson: Therapy Skill Builders.

Cronin, A., & Mandich, M. (2005). *Human development and performance.* Clifton Park, NJ: Thomas Delmar Learning.

Kail, R. (2002). *Children.* Upper Saddle River, NJ: Pearson Education.

Shumway-Cook, A., & Woollacott, M. (2006). *Motor control: Translating research into clinical practice* (3rd ed.). Philadelphia: Lippincott, Williams, & Wilkins.

Appendix C

Sequence of Grasp

Sequence of Hand Grasp Development

AGE	SKILL DEVELOPMENT
0–3 months	Can not voluntarily grasp objects Exhibits grasp reflex Opens and closes hands involuntarily in response to sensory stimuli
3–6 months	Contacts objects with palmar surface of hand Begins to demonstrate grasp in the following order: • Ulnar grasp • Palmar grasp
7 months	Uses crude raking action to pick up small objects
8–9 months	Refines grasp patterns Exhibits radial digital grasp pattern develops (thumb opposed to two or more fingers) Uses finger surface and thumb to make contact with small objects (finger surface contact)
9–12 months	Refines thumb and finger pad control with small objects (finger pad contact)
12–18 months	Further refines grasp patterns Increases control of intrinsic muscles
18–36 months	Develops power grasp: disc grasp, cylindrical grasp and spherical grasp Begins to demonstrate lateral pinch

Sequence of Voluntary Release Patterns

AGE	SKILL DEVELOPMENT
0–6 months	Cannot release objects voluntarily
6–9 months	Begins to bring objects to mouth and to midline
	Transfers objects from one hand to the other, using the receiving hand for stability
9–12 months	Releases objects without using the other hand for stability
12 months	Releases objects using shoulder, elbow, and wrist stability present
	Exhibits instability of MCP joints
12–18 months	Demonstrates stability of MCP joints
	Begins to demonstrate control to release objects into small containers and stack blocks
18–36 months	Refines release patterns
	Improves graded movements of the fingers and intrinsic muscles for greater control of release

Sequence of In-Hand Manipulation Skills

AGE	SKILL DEVELOPMENT
1–2 years	Demonstrates beginning of hand manipulation skills
	Moves objects from fingers to palm (finger to palm translation)
2–3 years	Further develops hand manipulation
	Moves objects from palm into fingers without help from other hand (palm to finger translation)
	Turns objects over with fingers acting as one unit (simple rotation)
3 years	Demonstrates increase in in hand manipulation skills
	Turns objects over using isolated finger and thumb movements (complex rotation)
	Make slight adjustments of objects by finger pads (shift)

REFERENCES

Exner, C. E. (1996). Development of hand skills. In J. Case-Smith, A. S. Allen, & P. N. Pratt (Eds.), *Occupational therapy for children* (3rd ed.), pp. 268–306. Baltimore: Mosby.

Exner, C. E. (2006). In-hand manipulation skills. In A. Henderson & C. Pehoski (Eds.), *Hand function in the child: Foundations for remediation*, pp. 239–266. St. Louis: Mosby.

Mulligan, S. (2003). *Occupational therapy evaluation for children: A pocket guide*. Philadelphia: Lippincott Williams & Wilkins.

Appendix D

Legislation

LEGISLATIVE ACTS RELATING TO EARLY INTERVENTION AND SCHOOL BASED PRACTICE

1958 PL 85-926   EDUCATION TO MENTAL RETARDATION CHILDREN ACT
- Funds colleges and universities to train persons assuming leadership roles in educating children with mental retardation
- In 1963, expanded to include additional disability groups

1968 PL 90-538   THE HANDICAPPED CHILDREN'S EARLY EDUCATION ASSISTACE ACT
- Funds experimental program for children less than 8 years old with disabilities

1973 PL 93-112   THE REHABILITATION ACT, SECTION 504
- Any agency receiving federal funding not allowed to deny services based on disability
- No funding or monitoring of the act; therefore, often ignored

1975 PL 94-142   THE EDUCATION OF ALL HANDICAPPED CHILDREN ACT OF 1975
- Free appropriate public education for 6- to 21-year-old individuals
- Least restrictive environment
- Individual Education Plan (IEP)
- Occupational therapy as related service
- Part B: incentive grants for preschool programs

1986 PL 99-457   EDUCATION OF THE HANDICAPPED ACT AMENDMENTS
- Part B: services for 3–21-year-old individuals

  Mandated special education services

  Occupational therapy as a related service

- Part H: services children from birth to 2 years

  Established incentives for states to develop systems of coordinated care for infants and families

  Individual Family Service Plan (IFSP)

1990 PL 101-476   INDIVIDUALS WITH DISABILITIES EDUCATION ACT (IDEA)

- Part B: 3- to 5-year-old individuals and 6- to 21-year-old individuals

  Mandates service

  Occupational Therapy as related service

  Individualized Educational Program (IEP)

  Added Transition Services

- Part H: children birth to two years

  Entitlement

  Occupational therapy as primary service

  Individualized Family Service Plan (IFSP)

1997 PL 105-17   IDEA-R (IDEA revised)

- Part H renamed Part C
- Changes to discipline section, emphasizing positive behavioral intervention

2001 PL 107-110   NO CHILD LEFT BEHIND ACT OF 2001

- Requires public schools to raise achievement of all students

2004 PL 108-446   INDIVIDUALS WITH DISABILITIES EDUCATION IMPROVEMENT ACT OF 2004

- Aligns with NCLB Act
- High expectations ensuring access to general education curriculum in a regular classroom, to the maximum extent
- Maintains all provisions of previous IDEA

From *The future of children*, a publication of the Woodrow Wilson School of Public and International Affairs at Princeton University and the Brookings Institution.
FULL JOURNAL ISSUE: *Special education for students with disabilities*
ARTICLE: Legislative and litigation history of special education
Edwin W. Martin, Reed Martin, and Donna L. Terman.

Appendix E

Web Resources

Organization Name	Contact Information	Web Address
Alliance for Technology Access	1304 Southpoint Blvd., Suite 240, Petaluma, CA 94954, 707-778-3011	www.ataccess.org
Attention Deficit Disorder Association	P.O. Box 543, Pottstown, PA 19464, 484-945-2101	www.add.org
Autism Society of America	7910 Woodmont Avenue, Suite 300, Bethesda, MD 20814, 301-657-0881 or 800-3AUTISM	www.autism-society.org
Beach Center on Disability	University of Kansas, Haworth Hall, 1200 Sunnyside Avenue, Room 3136, Lawrence, KS 66045, 785-864-7600	www.beachcenter.org
Children and Adults with Attention-Deficit/ Hyperactivity Disorder (CHADD)	8181 Professional Place, Suite 150, Landover, MD 20785, 800-233-4050	www.chadd.org
Interdisciplinary Council for Developmental and Learning Disorders	4938 Hampden Lane, Suite 800, Bethesda, MD 20814, 301-656-2667	www.icdl.com
International Rett Syndrome Association	9121 Piscataway Road, Clinton, MD 20735, 800-818-RETT	www.rettsyndrome.org
Learning Disabilities Association of America	4156 Library Road, Pittsburgh, PA 15234	www.ldaamerica.org
Muscular Dystrophy Association (MDA)	3300 E. Sunrise Drive, Tucson, AZ 85718, 800-FIGHT-MD 800-344-4863	www.mdaa.org
National Association for Down Syndrome (NADS)	Post Office Box 206, Wilamette, IL 60091, 630-325-9112	www.nads.org
National Center for Learning Disabilities	381 Park Avenue South, Suite 1401, New York, NY 10016, 212-545-7510	www.ncld.org
National Dissemination Center for Children with Disabilities	P.O. Box 1492, Washington, DC 20013, 800-695-0285	www.nichcy.org
National Down Syndrome Society	666 Broadway, New York, NY 10012, 800-221-4602	www.ndss.org

Organization Name	Contact Information	Web Address
National Institute of Child Health and Human Information Resource Center	P.O. Box 3006, Rockville, MD 20847, 800-370-2943	www.nichd.nih.gov
National Institute of Mental Health (NIMH)	National Institutes of Health, DHHS, 6001 Executive Blvd., Rm. 8184, MSC 9663, Bethesda, MD 20892-9663, 301-443-4513	www.nimh.nih.gov
National Organization on Fetal Alcohol Syndrome	900 17th Street, NW, Suite 910, Washington, DC 20006, 202-785-4585	www.nofas.org
The United Brachial Plexus Network	1610 Kent St., Kent, OH 44240, 866-877-7004	www.ubpn.com
United Cerebral Palsy	1660 L Street, NW, Suite 700, Washington, DC 20036, 800-872-5827	www.ucp.org
U.S. Department of Health and Human Services Administration for Children and Families Administration on Developmental Disabilities	HHH 405-D 370, L'Enfant Promenade, SW, Washington, D.C. 20201, 202-690-6590	www.acf.hhs.gov

Appendix F

Equipment Resources

Organization Name	Contact Information	Web Address
AbleLink Technologies	528 N. Tejon Street, Suite 100, Colorado Springs, CO 80903, 719-592-0347	www.aslelinktech.com
AbleNet, Inc.	1081 Tenth Avenue, Minneapolis, MN 55414-1312, 800-322-0956	www.ablenetinc.com
Abilitations, Inc.	One Sportime Way, Atlanta, GA 30340-1402, 800-850-8602	www.abilitations.com
Achievement Products for Children	P.O. Box 9033, Canton, OH 44701, 800-373-4699	www.specialkidszone.com
Action Products, Inc.	22 N. Mulberry St., Hagerstown, MD 21740, 800-228-7763	www.actionproducts.com
Adaptive Mobility Services, Inc.	1000 Delaney Ave., Orlando, FL 32806, 407-426-8020	www.adaptivemobility.com
Advanced Keyboard Technologies	P.O. Box 186, Paso Robles, CA 93446	www.keyboardinstructor.com
Advanced Therapy Products, Inc.	P.O. Box 3420, Glen Allen, VA 23058-3420, 804-747-8574	www.atpwork.com
AlphaSmart, Inc.	973 University Ave., Los Gatos, CA 95032, 888-274-0680	info@alphasmart.com www.alphasmart.com
Apex-Carex Healthcare Products	1808 Aston Ave., Suite 190, Carlsbad, CA 92008, 760-602-3150	www.apex-carex.com
Attainment Company, Inc.	P.O. Box 930160, Verona, WI 53593-0160, 800-327-4269	info@attainment-inc.com www.attainment-inc.com
Beacon-Ridge	20951 Baker Rd., Gays Mills, WI 54631, 800-737-8029	info@beacon-ridge.com www.beacon-ridge.com
Beyond Play—Early Intervention Products	1442-A Walnut St. #52, Berkeley, CA 94709, 877-428-1244	www.beyondplay.com
CAST Universal Design for Learning	40 Harvard Mills Square, Suite 3, Wakefield, MA 01880-3233, 781-245-2212	cast@cast.org www.cast.org

ORGANIZATION NAME	CONTACT INFORMATION	WEB ADDRESS
Chewy Tubes	P.O. Box 2289, South Portland, ME 04116, 207-741-2443	www.chewytubes.com
Computer Resources for People with Disabilities: A Guide to Assistive Technologies, Tools, and Resources for People of All Ages (4th ed.)	AOTA Products, P.O. Box 0151, Annapolis Junction, MD 20701-0151, 877-404-AOTA	www.aota.org
Creative Communicating, Inc.	P.O. Box 84060, Park City, UT 84060, 435-645-7737	www.creative-comm.com
Don Johnston Inc.	26799 West Commerce Drive, Volo, IL 60073, 800-999-4660	info@donjohnston.com www.donjohnson.com
Dycem	83 Gilbane Street, Warwick, RI 02886, 401-738-4420	www.dycem.com
Easy Access Clothing/Finnease Adaptive Fashions	P.O. Box 6521, San Rafael, CA 94903, 800-775-5536	www.easyaccessclothing.com
Envision Technology	4905 Del Ray Ave., Suite 220, Bethesda, MD 20814, 800-582-5051	www.envisiontechnology.org
Franklin Learning Resources	122 Burrs Road, Mt. Holly, NY 08060, 800-266-5626	www.franklin.com
Freedom Scientific	11800 31st Court North St., Petersburg, FL 33716-1805, 800-444-4443	www.freedomscientific.com
Georgia Project for Assistive Technology	1870 Twin Towers East, Atlanta, GA 30334, 404-463-3597	www.gpat.org
Inspiration Software, Inc.	7412 SW Beaverton Hillsdale Highway, Suite 102 Portland, OR 97225, 503-297-3004	www.inspiration.com
IntelliTools, Inc.	1720 Corporate Circle, Petaluma, CA 94954, 800-899-6687	info@intellitools.com www.intellitools.com
Johns Hopkins University Center for Technology in Education; Adapted Pencils to Computers	6740 Alexander Bell Drive, Suite 302, Columbia, MD 21046 410-312-3800	http://cte.jhu.edu/index.html
Kidzplay/Theragifts	1 F Commons Drive, Suite 38, Londonderry, NH 03053, 603-437-3330	www.theragifts.com
Low-Tech Assistive Devices: A Handbook for the School Setting	AOTA Products, P. O. Box 0151, Annapolis Junction, MD 20701-0151, 877-404-AOTA	www.aota.org
Maryland Assistive Technology COOP	One Oakwood Center, 7050 Oakland Mills Road, Suite 160, Columbia, MD 21046	info@matcoop.org
Mealtime Notions LLC	P.O. Box 35432, Tucson, AZ 85740, 520-323-3348	www.mealtimenotions.com
North Coast Medical, Inc.	18305 Sutter Boulevard, Morgan Hill, CA 95037, 408-776-5000, ext. 155	www.ncmedical.com

ORGANIZATION NAME	CONTACT INFORMATION	WEB ADDRESS
Onion Mountain Technology	74 Sexton Hollow Road, Canton, CT 06019-2102, 860-693-2683	www.onionmountaintech.com
OT Ideas, Inc.	P.O. Box 124, Morris Turnpike, Randolf, NJ 07869, 201-895-3622	
Otto Bock Health Care	Two Carlson Parkway, N., Suite 100, Minneapolis, MN 55447, 763-489-5110	www.ottobockus.com
Pediatric Prosthetics, Inc.	12926 Willowchase Drive, Houston, TX 77070, 281-897-1108	www.kidscanplay.com
Pocket Full of Therapy	P.O. Box 174, Morganville, NJ 07751, 732-441-0404	www.pfot.com
Really Good Stuff	448 Pepper Street, Monroe, CT 06468, 877-867-1920	www.reallygoodstuff.com
Sammons Preston Rolyan	P.O. Box 5071, Boilingbrook, IL 60440-5071, 800-323-5547	www.sammonspreston.com
S & S Worldwide	75 Mill Street, Colchester, CT 06415, 800-642-7354	www.ssww.com
See It Right! Corporation	P.O. Box 1117, Rancho Cucamonga, CA 91729, 951-272-6700	www.seeitright.com
Sensory Tools	P.O. Box 44219, Madison, WI 53719, 608-819-0540	www.sensorytools.net
Southpaw Enterprises, Inc.	617 N. Irwin Street, Dayton, OH 45403, 937-258-4373	www.southpawenterprises.com
Space Tables, Inc.	11511-95 Avenue, N., Maple Grove, MN 55369, 800-328-2580	www.spacetables.com
The Pencil Grip	P.O. Box 67096, Los Angeles, CA 90067, 310-315-3545	www.thepencilgrip.com
Therapro, Inc.	225 Arlington Street, Framingham, MA 01702-8723, 800-257-5376	www.theraproducts.com
Therapy Skill Builders	555 Academic Court, San Antonio, TX 78204-9498, 800-228-0752	www.harcourtassessment.com
Vision Technology, Inc.	8501 Delport Drive, St. Louis, MO 63114, 314-890-8300	www.visiontechnology.com

Appendix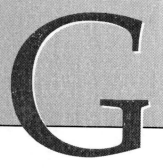

Abbreviations

A
AAMR: American Association of Mental Retardation
ABA: Applied Behavior Analysis
ADA: Americans with Disabilities Act
ADL: Activities of daily living
AFO: Ankle-foot orthosis
AFP: Alpha-fetoprotein
AIMS: Academic Intervention Monitoring System™
AIMS: Alberta Infant Motor Scales™
AMPS: Assessment of Motor and Process Skills™
ASD: Autism spectrum disorders

C
CAPE: Children's Assessment of Participation and Enjoyment™
CIMT: Constraint induced movement therapy
CNS: Central nervous system
COPM: Canadian Occupational Performance Measure™
COSA: Child Occupational Self Assessment™
CP: Cerebral palsy

D
DSM-IV: Diagnostic and Statistical Manual of Mental Disorders (4th ed.)
DT: Discreet trial
DTVP: Developmental Test of Visual Perception™

E
EBD: Emotional and behavioral disorders
EHP: Ecological Model of Human Performance
ESL: English as second language
ETCH: Evaluation Tool of Children's Handwriting™

F
FAS: Fetal alcohol syndrome

H
HELP: Hawaii Early Learning Profile Preschool Checklist™

I
IADL: Instrumental activities of daily living
ICF: International Classification of Functioning, Disability, and Health
IDEA: Individuals with Disabilities Education Act
IEP: Individualized education program
IFSP: Individualized family service plan
ILEP: Intermittent, limited, extensive pervasive supports system
IQ: Intelligence quotient

J
JRA: Juvenile rheumatoid arthritis

L
LD: Learning disability
LRE: Least restrictive environment

M
MAP: Miller Assessment for Preschoolers™
MOHO: Model of Human Occupation
MR: Mental retardation
MVPT: Motor-Free Visual Perceptual Test™

N
NCLB: No Child Left Behind Act
NDT: Neurodevelopmental treatment
NJCLD: National Joint Committee on Learning Disabilities
NSAIDSs: Nonsteroidal anti-inflammatory drugs

O
OA: Occupational Adaptation Model
OTPF: Occupational Therapy Practice Framework: Domain and Process

P
PEO: Person-Environment-Occupation Model
PEOP: Person-Environment-Occupational Performance Model
PAC: Preferences of Activities of Children™
PACS: Pediatric Activity Card Sort™
PBS: Positive behavioral interventions and supports system
PDD: Pervasive developmental disorders
PEC: Picture Exchange Communication™
PEDI: Pediatric Evaluation of Disability Inventory™

S
SFA: School Function Assessment™
SI: Sensory integration frame of reference
SIPT: Sensory Integration and Praxis Test™
SOAP: Subjective, Objective, Assessment, Plan
SRS: Social Responsiveness Scale™

T

TBI: Traumatic brain injury

TBPA: Transdisciplinary Play-Based Assessment™

TDD: Telecommunication devices for the deaf

TEACCH: Treatment and Education of Autistic and Related Communication Handicap Children program™

TIME: Toddler and Infant Motor Evaluation™

TSFI: Test of Sensory Functions in Infants™

W

WS: Williams syndrome

Glossary

A

Academic preparation—Formal academic subjects such as math, science, reading

Accessibility options—Program within most computer control panels that allows adjustments or configurations for vision, hearing, and mobility needs

Accommodation—Modification of existing schema to incorporate and make sense of new information and achieve a new state of equilibrium

Acquisitional frame of reference—Principles and assumptions from a combination of learning theories, including behavioral theory and social learning theory; behavior occurs in response to environmental cues

Active participant observation—Approach that allows a person to facilitate and respond to specific behaviors of the child or adolescent, and to adjust the task and the environment to encourage various adaptive responses

Activities of daily living (ADL)—Activities that people perform to take care of their bodies: bathing, bowel and bladder management, dressing, eating, feeding, functional mobility, personal device care, sexual activity, sleep and rest, toilet hygiene, grooming and hygiene

Activity—Actions or tasks people do to achieve a goal

Activity demands—Inherent parts of an activity, including the use of specific objects and tools, space, body parts, sequence and timing demands, and adherence to social rules which are required in order to perform various activities

Adaptation—Modifying and grading activity demands

Affordance—Visual clue to the function of an object

ALERT program—Intervention approach which focuses on increasing a child's or adolescent's self-regulation of behavior

Alpha-fetoprotein—A type of antigen or protein present in the developing fetus

Alternative and augmentative communication (AAC)—Communication that supplements or does not require speech and that can be individualized to the needs of the person

American Association of Mental Retardation (AAMR)—International association that promotes policies, research, effective practices, and universal human rights for people with intellectual disabilities

Analysis of occupational performance—Use of clinical reasoning to gather, synthesize, and interpret observable performance skills and performance patterns the client uses to engage in activities and occupations

Anencephaly—Type of neural tube defect in which the majority of the brain, skull, and skin fail to form during fetal developing, exposing the brain stem

Ankle-foot orthosis (AFO)—Splint often used to correct foot drop

Anorexia—An eating disorder during which a person severally restricts intake of necessary nutrition

Anxiety disorder—A group of mental health challenges categorized by excessive anxiety and worry about life situations

Applied behavior analysis (ABA)—Learning based intervention that utilizes positive reinforcers and other methods, such as incidental teaching, to teach and to shape the behaviors of children and adolescents with autistic spectrum disorders

Areas of occupation—Activities of daily living (ADL), instrumental activities of daily living (IADL), education, work, play, leisure, and social participation

Arms first method—Dressing technique in which the person inserts his arms into a jacket first before inserting other body parts

Arnold Chiari malformation—Associated condition present in almost all children and adolescents with spina bifida that involves a downward displacement of a portion of the brain into the neck through the foramen magnum, an opening in the base of the skull through which the spinal cord passes

Asperger Syndrome—Type of pervasive developmental disorder characterized by qualitative impairments in social interactions, repetitive patterns of behaviors, and restricted areas of interest, though to a lesser degree than those with Autistic Disorder.

Asphyxia—Deprivation of oxygen

Assessment—Specific observations, chart reviews, interviews, and measurement tools that are used to gather information

Assimilation—Process of taking in new information and interpreting it in a manner that conforms to an existing view or schema of the world

Associative group interactions—Level of interaction that involves sharing of some materials from those who are physically near and are separately engaging in similar activities

Associative play—Type of play that typically develops during preschool years; children engage in a similar activity, sharing and borrowing materials, but no common goal

Asymmetrical bilateral movements—Arms and hands on one side of the body perform coordinated but different movements of the arms and hands on the opposite side of the body

Asymmetrical pattern—Irregular configuration

Asymmetrical tonic neck reflex (ATNR)—Reflex typically seen in infants up to the age of 4 to 5 months that occurs when the baby turns the head and neck to the side, resulting in extension of the arm on the face side, and flexion of the arm on the skull side

Atlanto-axial joint—Joint between the first and second vertebrae

Attachment—An enduring emotional bond that often develops between the child and the parent or primary caregiver, through social interactions

Augmentative communication devices—Piece of equipment used by a person often with limited or absent verbal abilities to interact with and share information and ideas with others

B

Backward chaining—A technique in which the person learns how to complete the last step of the task first, then the second to last step, then third to last step, until all of the steps are learned

Behavioral disorders—Cluster of behaviors categorized by negative actions that reflect disrespect for or violations of major rules regarding expected conduct

Behavioral theory—A learning theory developed by Skinner to explain facilitators or inhibitors of behavior

Biomechanical model—Schema for using theories of physics and physiology to explain how gravity affects the body physically, mechanically, and physiologically as it moves

Biomechanical techniques—Methods consistent with the biomechanical approach such as strengthening, stretching, positioning, and joint alignment

Bite reflex—An exaggerated, uncontrolled clamping down with the jaws when an object is inserted into the mouth

Body-powered prosthesis—Manmade limb with five components: socket, harness, stainless-steel cable, wrist unit, and terminal device

Body schema—Internalized sense of how one's body is configured and occupies space

Bridging—Procedure a person uses to lift up his buttocks when lying supine on a flat surface by bending his knees and pushing down on the surface with his feet

Bulimia—Eating disorder involving binge eating and purging

C

Cable—Part of an upper limb prosthesis which attaches to the harness on one end and to the functional component of the prosthesis on the other end

Calibrate—Ability to modulate amount of grip strength required to hold an object

Capacity—Level of ability a person possesses to perform an action or a task without any assistance or adaptations

Ceiling effect—Upper limit of the test where there is no room to detect further improvements

Central nervous system lesion—Damage to pathways and structures within the brain

Centration—The focusing on one feature of a situation, while ignoring other features

Cephalocaudal—Principle explaining that motor development occurs first in the upper parts of the body then the lower parts of the body

Checklist—Compensatory learning strategy for multi-step tasks

Childhood Disintegrative Disorder, or Heller Syndrome—A disintegrative disorder that primarily affects boys; the boys appear to develop normally for the first one or two years of life, but then lose previously acquired social, language, play, and motor skills over a period of weeks or months

Classification—Arrangement items into categories based on certain characteristics

Client—Children and adolescents, their parents, caregivers, and extended families, organizations, and populations who receive services

Client factors—Body functions and body structures of the person

Client-centered—Process by which the children, adolescents, and their family members or caregivers are actively involved in the decision about the need for services, the goal of those services, and the types of services received

Clinical reasoning—Use of conceptual models to guide and make judgments about service delivery

Close-ended questions—Questions that elicit a single word or short phrase response

Cock-up splint—Rigid forearm and wrist support that positions wrist into slight extension allowing free movement of fingers

Code of ethics—Set of principles regarding adherence to a high standard of professional behaviors

Cognitive maps—Mental images of how to align various spaces and tasks in relation to one another

Cognitive theory—Developed by Piaget, who examined cognitive development of children, including how they think, gain knowledge, become self-aware, and understand their environment

Coincidence-anticipation timing—Individual's ability to predict the speed of a moving object and coordinate a motor action in response to that prediction

Communication device use—IADL involving the use of equipment to convey written or spoken language

Community mobility—Various means individuals use to move around their communities, including the use of personal and public transportation and assistive mobility devices

Compensation—Intervention approach that focuses on modifying the context or the demands of the task

Competitive play—Level of play that includes elements of succeeding better than others or of winning, either individually or as part of a team

Concept—Abstract or intangible idea built from a number of concrete or tangible examples

Conceptual model—Set of constructs and assumptions, organized in a systematic manner to represent their interrelatedness

Concrete operations—Piaget's third stage of development during which children develop their ability to use inductive logic

Conservation—An understanding that the quantity of an object remains unchanged even when it is reshaped or rearranged

Constraint-induced movement therapy (CIMT)—Intervention approach that increases voluntary usage of the involved side of the body by restraining the non-involved side

Construct—Interconnected concepts

Consultation Process—The process of providing information to the client to help identify problems and create and propose solutions

Constructive play—Form of play that involves manipulating objects to create something

Context—Variety of interrelated conditions that are part of and external to the person, and influence what the person does

Contracture—Tightness of the muscles, ligaments, and tendons that hinders joint movement

Conventional—Process by which individuals make decisions based on the norms and rules of the group

Cooperative play—Type of play that involves members working toward achieving a common goal

Cooperative groups—Group in which the members are able to establish and abide by group rules, divide the workload, and assume roles to accomplish a common task

Cosmetic hand—Part of an upper limb prosthesis; terminal device which looks more natural and can function to push, pull, and stabilize objects

Criterion referenced—Assessments which use criteria to compare the performance of an individual to an established standard or level of expectation of performance

Cultural context—Context comprised of the beliefs, attitudes, values, and expectations of a society

Cyclothymic disorder—Mental health problem characterized by numerous depressive and hypomanic episodes over a period of a year or longer

Cylindrical grip—Type of grasp used to hold relatively large objects by flattening the transverse arch of the palm, slightly abducting the fingers, and flexing the IP and MCP joints to accommodate to the size of the objects

Cytomeglovirus (CMV)—Mild infection that often causes birth defects

D

Decentering—Perceptual process by which the person focuses on multiple features of a situation

Deductive reasoning—Way of thinking that leads from first considering the gestalt and then the particulars (or from the effect to the cause)

Delusion—False belief that is inconsistent with a person's knowledge and with evidence in the environment

Depth perception—Judgment of the distance between two objects, or two points on an object

Developmental delay—Diagnosis given to young children who demonstrate deficits in adaptive behaviors and delays in achieving developmental milestones

Developmental, Individual-Difference, Relationship-Based (DIR)/Floortime model—Learning-based intervention that utilizes developmental and humanistic principles to elicit interaction skills in children

Developmental norms—Guidelines for explaining and measuring the progression of skill acquisition

Diagnostic and Statistical Manual of Mental Disorders (4th ed.) (DSM-IV)—Manual used to define and identify behavioral and mental health challenges

Diplegia—Muscle paralysis primarily in lower extremities

Directed play—Type of play organized by adults such as sports, motor programs

Discrete trial (DT)—Teaching process whereby a task is subdivided into smaller, measurable steps that are taught through repeated drilling

Distant observation—Approach that allows for minimal influence by the observer on the behaviors of the person being observed, and on the surrounding environment

Dominating habits and routines—Habits and routines that restrict adaptation by requiring rigid adherence to a specific way to perform the behavior

Downgrade—The steps to make an activity easier or simpler to perform

Dynamic balance—Ability to maintain one's center of gravity while shifting weight from one direction to the other

Dynamic systems—A system which is affected by stimuli or information coming into it and which affects stimuli and information leaving it; it also is affected by and affects the context that surrounds it

Dyspraxia—Difficulty developing the idea of how to move one's body, planning and sequencing the course of actions to move the body, and using feedforward and feedback input to fluidly execute and modify movements in response to environmental clues

E

Eating—Series of coordinated tasks including opening containers, manipulating eating utensils, bringing the liquid and food to the mouth, and managing the liquid and food within the mouth

Eating disorders—Cluster of maladaptive eating patterns that are harmful, including anorexia, bulimia, and obesity

Echolalic speech—Repetitive use of particular words or phrases

Education—Knowledge acquired by learning and instruction

Education occupation—Formal, informal, and exploration learning activities

Egocentric—Perspective of seeing and interpreting situations from one's own vantage point, rather than from that of another person

Egocentric cooperative groups—Groups in which the members cooperate with one another because they realize that, through this cooperation their individual needs are met

Emergent literacy—Beginning of understanding that written words are meaningful

Energy conservation techniques—Strategies utilized to help pace the effort needed to perform a task and avoid excessive fatigue

Engagement—Second stage in the DIR/Floortime program during which the adult tries to connect with the child by establishing a warm, trusting, and personal relationship; the adult follows the child's lead, rather than directs the child's behavior

Environment—Characteristics of natural and human made space, the objects in it, the services, policies, and systems in it, and the supports, attitudes, and relationships of people in it

Environmental adaptations—Modifications made within the home, community, or workplace to enable people to navigate, and to perform daily occupations

Environmental factors—Aspects extrinsic to the individual that include societal factors, social interactions, social and economic systems, culture environments, built environments and technology, and natural environments

Epidemiologist—Scientist who studies changes in patterns of health across populations

Epigenetic principle—Assumption that each part of the personality has a particular time for development to occur until all the parts develop to form the whole of the individual

Equilibrium—Stable, balanced, or unchanging system

Establish—The learning of a skill for the first time

Ethnic identity—Self-identification with and acceptance of the values, attitudes, and occupational roles of a specific group of people

Evaluation—The process of gathering and interpreting relevant data to make judgments about the need for, scope of, and types of services

Evaluation report—Written summary and analysis of standardized and nonstandardized assessments, the intervention plan, and the proposed outcomes of services

Exacerbation—Flareup of the symptoms of the disease

Exercise bulimia—An eating disorder involving overexercising to burn calories

Exploratory play—Type of sensorimotor play, emerging around 1 year of age, in which children investigate their surroundings and begin to develop cause/effect relationships

Expressive language—Ability to speak words and sentences

Extensive support—Regular or daily support provided to children and adolescents in at least some environments, such as work or home

Extensor position—A body position in which the extensor muscles dominate

Externally powered prosthesis—Prosthesis activated by a power source other than the person's muscles

Extinction—Process used to systematically reduce or eliminate a behavior

Extrinsic feedback—Sensory information that comes from the environment or another person

F

Family focused—Early intervention services that are delivered in a way that compliment the strengths and wishes of the individual and the family

Fantasy play—Type of play in which imagination and makebelieve dominate

Far transfer—Process of generalizing learning to a novel or different situation; specific to the multicontext treatment approach, the activity is physically different but conceptually the same as the initial skill

Feeding—Process of providing liquid and food that is nutritional and adequate for self or another person

Feedback—Information provided about the accuracy of a movement, behavior, or thought once it is executed

Feedforward—The co-contraction of muscles in preparation for a goal-directed movement

Figure-ground—Identification of an object from the background surrounding it

Finger-to-palm translation—Movement of an object from the fingers to palm of the hand

Flaccid paralysis—Loss of sensation or movement accompanied by low or floppy muscle tone

Flexor position—Body position in which the flexor muscles dominate

Floor effect—Lower limit of the test where there is not room to detect further deterioration

Flow—Smooth, controlled movement

Foreclosure—Acceptance by an individual of familial or culturally defined occupations or belief systems without reassessing the choices

Form constancy—Recognition that a shape is the same regardless of size, position, or background

Form perception—Ability to recognize and identify the shape of an object

Formal education participation—Involvement in academic participation, nonacademic participation, and vocational preparation

Formal operations—Ability to use the formal logic

Forward chaining—Technique whereby the steps of a task are taught in the order in which they occur

Frame of reference—Model, applied to a specific area of practice that guides evaluation, intervention, and outcome procedures

Full physical assistance—Comprehensive physical support provided by another individual to complete most or all activities of daily life

Functional play—Type of play in which toys and objects are used for their intended purpose

Functional prosthesis—Prosthesis that has the capability of grasping and holding objects

G

Games with rules—Type of play that involves identifying, accepting, and abiding by a set of directions for actions and interactions

Gender cleavage—Child's natural gravitation toward same gender when engaging in play and other activities

Gender identity—Individual's internal sense of being male or female

Generalization—Individual's ability to appropriately and spontaneously apply skills learned on one task to a variety of other tasks

Gesture—Motion to emphasize or alert one to a specific step of a task

Goals—Reflects outcomes which are global in scope and usually take an extended period of time to accomplish

Grammar—Organized system of word structures and word arrangement

Gross motor play—Use of large body muscles to move through space and to explore objects

H

Habits—Automatic behaviors that allow a person to respond in a consistent way in familiar environments

Habituation—Routines and patterns embedded within the behaviors used to perform occupations; provides routine and familiarity to people's daily lives

Hallucination—Visual, auditory, olfactory, gustatory, or tactile perception of a sensory experience that does not exist

Hand held walker—Adjustable mobility aid designed to be pushed in front of individual (anterior walker) or pulled behind the individual (posterior walker)

Hand-over-hand assistance—Physical prompt; directly guiding one through a motion

Hand-to-mouth movements—Action of moving an object that is in the hand to the mouth

Harness—Part of a prosthesis that is worn across the back and shoulders or around the chest, and fastens to the socket to secure the prosthesis

Hemiparesis—Muscle weakness involving extremities on one side of the body

Hemiplegia—Muscle paralysis involving extremities on one side of the body

Home-schooling—Program whereby children participate in their formal education at home

Hook—Part of an upper limb prosthesis that has greater grip and tension than the prosthetic hand

Hook grasp—Type of grasp pattern typically used to carry objects by a handle

Human agency—Motivation that enables individuals to effectively use the social, material, and personal resources available within their environments to learn, problem solve, and achieve goals that contribute to life satisfaction

Hydrocephalus—Condition in which cerebrospinal fluid accumulates in the ventricles of the brain, causing an increase in brain size, potentially resulting in damage of the brain tissue

Hyperbilirubinemia—Yellowing of the skin due to the build up of a pigment called bilirubin in the blood

Hypertonicity—Increased muscle tone that often restricts full range of motion within the joints

Hypothetico-deductive reasoning—Reasoning that involves if-then logic to generate plausible hypothesis and systematic problem solving to change and measure the effect of one variable at a time to solve abstract problems

Hypotonicity—Decreased muscle tone that often results in an inability to stabilize against gravity; floppiness

I

Identity—Individual's behavioral characteristics that define a person's values and interests

Identity achievement—Stage in personal turmoil that results in a resolution about belief systems and occupational roles

Identity diffusion—Absence of experiencing a personal turmoil and coming to a resolution about belief systems and occupational roles

Identity status—Internal beliefs about oneself based on own experiences and those learned through social relationships

Imaginary audience—Individual's belief that everyone in the environment is attending to and making judgments about the individual's behavior and appearance

Imitate—Mimic an action or task

Impoverished habits and routines—Habits and routines which do not provide enough structure to enable one to effectively organize time and activities

Inclusion—Setting whereby students with disabilities are educated within a regular classroom

Incontinent—Inability to control bowel and bladder functions, often because of muscular or neurological damage

Individualized education program (IEP)—Legal document developed for each child or adolescent who qualifies for special education services; it outlines required related services, intervention goals, and objectives, when appropriate

Individualized family service plan (IFSP)—Legal document developed in collaboration with the family to address the developmental needs of infants or toddlers who display delays in development or are at risk to develop delays

Industry—Development of a sense of mastery which arises from opportunities to experiment with materials in a safe environment that allows for mistakes and fosters success

Industry versus inferiority—Erikson's fourth stage of psychosocial development during which children ages 6 through 12 are interested in how things work and are constructed, and through exploration, develop a sense of mastery and competency

Inferior pincer grasp—Type of grasp pattern in which the thumb is placed against the volar surface of the index finger and the first and second digits are used as unit

In-hand manipulation—Process of repositioning an object within the hand by that hand

Initiation—Individuals' ability to begin an activity or task

Initiative versus guilt stage—Erikson's third stage of psychosocial development during which children between the ages of 4 and 5 years develop a sense of the ability and guilt about initiating actions

Instrumental activities of daily living (IADL)—Occupations which involve a sequence of tasks that require decision making and responsibility to and for other people or objects

Interdisciplinary team—Group of individuals from different disciplines who collaborate with one another and the family to share and interpret their findings and design integrated interventions

Interests—What individuals find pleasurable and satisfying to do

Intermediate transfer—Process of generalizing learning to a novel or different situation

Intermittent support—Support provided to children/adolescents on an as needed basis; typically short term and needed during life span transitions at home and school

Intermittent, limited, extensive pervasive supports system (ILEP system)—Organizational system that defines four levels or intensities of support needed for the child/adolescent

International Classification of Functioning, Disability, and Health (ICF)—Document created and published by the World Health Organization (WHO) to provide a structure for discussing, researching, and documenting the health and health related states of all individuals, not just those with disabilities

Intervention—Design and implementation of skilled services or solutions in order to facilitate improvement in a client's function

Intervention plan—The determination of services for the client that incorporate the client's beliefs, values, and goals for therapy; the client's performance skills and performance patterns; the physical, social, and cultural environments; the demands of the activity; the functioning capacity of the client's body structure; and the setting for or circumstances of intervention

Intrinsic feedback—Sensory information that comes from the body such as feeling the movement or seeing the results

Intrinsic reinforcement—Sense of internal satisfaction that comes from accomplishment of a behavior independent of any external feedback

Itinerant—Staffing pattern whereby therapists move from one location to another

J

Joint protection techniques—Strategies utilized to protect joints and to prevent excessive force on joints during engagement in occupations

K

Knowledge of performance (KP)—External feedback that comments on the quality of the movement pattern of an individual

Knowledge of results (KR)—Feedback which alerts the individual to the results or outcomes of the performance

Kyphosis—Excessive forward curvature of the thoracic vertebrae that results in a "hunchback" appearance and rounding of the shoulders

L

Lateral prehension—Use of the first two digits to grasp a small item; characterized by partial thumb adduction, MCP flexion, and slight IP flexion

Lateral tripod grasp—Functional, alternative tripod grasp which involves stabilizing an object with the distal phalanges of the index and middle finger, and the IP joint of the thumb

Least restrictive environment (LRE)—Provision mandated by federal law in which students with disabilities are educated whenever possible in learning environments with their nondisabled peers

Leisure—Exploratory and participatory activities which are nonobligatory and are done during discretionary time; may satisfy an area of curiosity or interest, may be done alone or with others, and may provide pleasure or opportunities to learn and create

Level of lesion—Term used to indicate the point of spinal cord damage associated with neural tube defects

Limited support—Support provided to children and adolescents, typically more intensive than intermittent support; it is time bound and directed to the accomplishments of a specific objective

Longitudinal anomaly—Congenital anomalies where only the pre- or postaxial portion of the limb is affected

Lordosis—Excessive forward curvature of the lumbar vertebrae that results in a sway-back or hollow back appearance and often is accompanied by anterior pelvic tilt and hip joint flexion

M

Mainstream—Type of educational system in which students with disabilities are included with their nondisabled peers for nonacademic instruction such as music, physical education, or art

Maintain—Process of preserving an individual's capacity to perform occupations without loss of functional skills

Manic—Symptom of a mental health disorder characterized by a flight of ideas, unstable mood swings, aggressive behaviors, excessive activity, and irritability

Meal preparation and clean-up—IADL involving meal planning, preparing, serving, and necessary clean-up

Measurement tool—Instruments for systematically gathering and recording information about an individual

Memory notebook—Compensatory strategies (e.g., daily planners, PDA) to recall information

Menarche—First menstrual period, usually occurring during puberty

Meningocele—Type of neural tube defect in which the meninges or covering around the spinal cord are pushed out through the opening in the spine and through an opening in the skin

Metacognition—Ability to think about one's thinking capacities, including how one looks for and attends to information and how one organizes and memorizes details

Metamemory—Knowledge gained through memorizing and recalling multiple details

Micrognathia—Unusually small jaw

Middle childhood—Children between the ages of 6 and 12 years

Mild level of mental retardation—Represents an IQ range of 55–70 and the ability to perform academic tasks at the third- through seventh-grade level

Mirror image—Reverse view; may cause directionality confusion

Mobility—Movement against gravity

Modeling—Demonstration; teaching technique often used in social skills training

Moderate level of mental retardation—Represents an IQ range of 40–55 and the ability to perform academic tasks at the second-grade level

Moratorium—Stage of personal turmoil in which a person has not yet arrived at a resolution

Moral development—Stages of development, based on questions related to justice

Motion hypothesis—Hypothesis that self-initiated, active movements likely contribute to development of depth and spatial perception

Multicontext treatment approach—Type of intervention approach that considers the complexity of context and how multiple contexts influence the ability to generalize a skill

Multidisciplinary team—Group of individuals from different disciplines who inform one another of their evaluation results and their interventions, but operate individually

Muscle tone—Resistance of the muscle to passive elongation or stretch

Myoelectric hand—Externally powered prosthetic hand

N

Narrative note—Type of documentation used in healthcare practice that contains all pertinent information, written in a concise paragraph

Natural environments—Geographic terrain, weather, temperature, amount of sunlight, noise level, and air quality within nature

Near transfer—Process of generalizing learning to a novel or different situation; specific to the multicontext treatment approach, the new activity is very similar to the initially learned skill

Negative reinforcement—Process used to increase the likelihood that a desired behavior will occur so that something unpleasant will stop

Neural tube defect—Group of birth defects that occur during the first thirty days of embryonic development because the layer of cells that become the central nervous system fail to completely fold onto itself and become a closed tube

Neurodevelopmental (NDT) model—Sensorimotor technique to address movement related difficulties, developed by Bobath and Bobath

Nonacademic participation—Involvement in activities and occupations that are not centered around education or school

Nonstandardized assessments—Assessments which do not have a specified content, administration, or scoring procedure to follow

Nonsteroidal anti-inflammatory drugs (NSAIDs)—Regime of drugs used treat JRA and other forms of arthritis

Norm-referenced assessments—Assessments that compare the performance of an individual to that which is typically expected within the normal population

O

Obesity—Eating disorder involving caloric intake that results in an excessive body mass

Object permanence—Ability to realize that objects exist independent of a person's ability to see and hear them

Objectives—Subsets of long term goals that direct the focus of the intervention sessions and serve as benchmarks to measure progress toward achieving those goals

Occupation—Activities people do that hold a central meaning and purpose in their life and contribute to a sense of identity and competency

Occupational competence—Ability to capably perform various occupations, enabling the person to lead a satisfying and meaningful life

Occupational form—Sequence of rule-bound activities that are recognized, named, and understood by the members of the society and that are available for individuals to do within a particular social and physical environment

Occupational profile—Information gathered about the client's occupational histories or life experiences, daily living routines, interests, values, the problems with performing daily life tasks, and priorities

Occupational Therapy Practice Framework: Domain and Process—Document first published by the American Occupational Therapy Association (AOTA) in 2002 that outlines the domain and process of occupational therapy

Occupation based activity—Engage in the occupation that matches the client's determined outcome (e.g., manipulate locker combination during change of classes, make a sandwich, play a card game with peers)

Onlooker play—Stage in the development of play skills during which a child becomes aware of and watches how others play

Open-ended questions—Questions that allow respondents to talk about the topic in their own words, adding important and meaningful details

Oppositional defiant disorder—Mental health disorder categorized by a persistent pattern of negativistic, hostile, and defiant behaviors that lasts at least 6 months; is inconsistent with the child's developmental age, and interferes with social, academic, and occupational tasks

Orthosis—Device worn on a human body part that functions to control or enhance joint movement, to support the body part, or to prevent bone movement or deformity

Osteoporosis—Decreased bone density that may develop due to disuse and lack of weight bearing on joints, or result from changes in body chemistry

Outcome—Measurement of the degree to which the interventions addressed the issues identified during the evaluation

Outcome studies—Research conducted to determine the benefits of the intervention plan and the intervention

P

Palm-to-finger translation—Movement of an item from the palm of the hand back to the fingers

Parallel image—Teaching strategy in which the activity is demonstrated, step by step, and completed within the learner's view, and without visual reversals

Parallel play—Type of play that typically develops between 2 and 3 years in which the children are physically near but do not directly interact with one another

Paresis—Muscle weakness

Partial physical assistance—Physical prompts with minimal physical contact (e.g., lightly guide hand, brief touch or tap to body part)

Participation—Involvement in a life situation (WHO, 2001)

Passive prosthesis—Prosthesis which has no moveable parts and often is used to provide postural balance or to assist the functional limb

Performance capacity—Level and types of skill needed to perform the occupations; it involves the objective physical and mental components necessary and the subjective experiences associated with doing the activity

Performance patterns—Habits, routines, and rituals that individuals use when engaging in daily life activities

Performance range—Scope of a person's ability to select and complete a task

Performance skills—Observable behaviors that a person demonstrates when selecting and engaging in a task

Person factors—Neurobiological, physiological, cognitive, psychological, emotional, and spiritual factors that are intrinsic to the individual

Person permanence—Ability to realize that people exist independent of the ability of an individual to see and hear them

Person variables—Personal values, interests, experiences, and skills relative to a task

Personal causation—Individual's belief about his or her capabilities

Personal context—Nonhealth features of a person such as age, gender, educational level, and economic status

Personal fable—Romantic and heroic images and stories an individual creates about one's self, believing that no one else can understand that experience

Personal safety—IADL that involves recognition and avoidance of hazards and following established safety standards

Pet care—IADL that provides for the well-being of a personal pet or service animal

Pervasive developmental disorders—Group of early neurobiological disorders that include the following subtypes: autistic disorder, Asperger's disorder, pervasive developmental disorder NOS (not otherwise specified), childhood disintegrative disorder, and Rett syndrome

Pervasive support—Constant, high intensity support provided to individuals with severe cognitive and physical challenges that impact all aspects of life and have a potential life sustaining nature

Phocomelia—Congenital anomaly where distal portion of the extremity attaches directly to a proximal part; e.g., arm attaching to upper humerus

Physical context—Nonhuman objects, terrains, buildings, plants, and animal aspects of an environment

Physical environment—Natural or manmade settings or objects

Physical prompts—Type of touch cue given to an individual to encourage problem solving or completion of the next step of a task

Pincer grasp—Type of grasp pattern characterized by thumb in opposition to the first digit with pad-to-pad contact

Play—Exploratory and participatory activities that provide pleasure or amusement, stimulate curiosity and creativity, or offer diversion and entertainment

Playfulness—Individual's attitude toward play

Plegia—Muscle paralysis

Position in space—Ability to recognize the direction that an object is turned and aligned within the physical environment

Positive Behavioral Interventions and Supports system (PBS)—System designed to promote socially appropriate behaviors within the school or community program using positive instead of punitive approaches

Positive reinforcement—Process used to increase the likelihood that the desired behavior will occur again

Postconventional—Decisions based on principles that address the needs of the larger society and transcend the needs of any particular individual, such as issues of justice, equality, and compassion across groups of people

Posttraumatic stress disorder—The experience of a significant trauma resulting in sustained and significant anxiety; the anxiety lasts for a minimum of one month, during which the person re-experiences the trauma, remains hypervigilant, and may avoid stimuli related to the trauma

Postural control—Ability to use proprioceptive input to respond to gravity and maintain the alignment of the body

Posture—Position or alignment of the body

Power grasp—Type of grasp pattern that utilizes the full strength of the hand

Pragmatics—Element of communication that involves the production and comprehension of communicative acts or speech

Praxis—Ability to plan how to execute nonhabitual motor acts and to adapt body movements to complete coordinated, complex movements

Precision grasp—Type of grasp pattern that involves opposition of the thumb and fingers

Preconventional—Moral decisions based on an external source of authority that is powerful and near to the individual

Preoperational stage—Piaget's second stage of cognitive development that typically occurs between 2 and 7 years of age, during which children learn to use symbols such as pictures, language, and pretend objects to represent real objects and events in the world

Preparatory methods—Activities such as stretching, nonresistive exercises, and visual imaging to prepare individuals for participation in purposeful activities and occupations

Press—Expectation to perform in a particular manner

Prevent—Intervention approach that focuses on stopping the development of barriers that may limit occupational participation

Profound level of mental retardation—Represents an IQ below 25 and requires extensive supports to live in the community

Progress note—Form of written documentation used to record the progress of the intervention process; contains information about the individual's current status on projected outcomes and interventions

Promote—Intervention approach that focuses on creating opportunities for occupational participation

Prosocial behaviors—Acts or deeds intended to benefit others

Prosthesis—Artificial device fabricated to substitute for a missing body part

Psychometric properties—Validity, reliability, utility, and responsiveness of a measurement or assessment tool

Psychotic symptoms—Characteristics associated with severe mental health disorder and include delusions, hallucinations, disorganized speech and behaviors, or disturbances in affect and thought

Pulmonary hypoplasia—Underdeveloped or atrophied lungs

Punishment—Process used to cause an unwanted behavior to cease that involves discomfort or negative stimuli

Purposeful activity—Tasks that develop skills a person needs to engage in daily life occupations

Q

Quadriparesis—Muscle weakness involvement in all four extremities

Quadriplegia—Muscle paralysis involvement in all four extremities

R

Radioulnar synatosis—Fusion of the lower radius and ulna causing limitations in forearm supination

Rapport-talk—Conversations marked by turn taking and sharing of feelings

Reactive attachment disorder—Affects young children who received grossly inadequate or harmful care from their primary caregivers; the children have severe difficulty with personal relationships in most social and interpersonal contexts

Receptive language—Ability to comprehend what is said or conveyed by another person

Re-evaluation—Stage in the intervention process to determine progress and the need to continue, modify, or discontinue services

Referral—Written request for another discipline to evaluate or consult with a client

Reflex—Involuntary response to a stimulus

Rehabilitation Act of 1974 (Section 504)—Legislation which allows students with disabilities to receive support services within their educational environment; if a student with disabilities does not qualify for special education

Reinforcement—Process used to increase the likelihood that a desired behavior will increase

Related service—Scope of transportation, developmental, corrective, and other supportive services that may be required to support the educational participation of a child with a disability

Relational aggression—Verbal form of bullying used more frequently by girls than by boys to hurt one another; it involves the use of name-calling, rumors, gossip, printed and verbal insults, and shunning rather than physical violence to cause emotional and social pain

Relational play—Type of play that involves combining a sequence of related actions to expand upon the complexity of the play

Reliability—Psychometric property, based on statistical procedures, used to determine how consistently an assessment measures a particular factor over multiple administrations

Remediation—Type of intervention approach which attempts to reduce or diminish dysfunction

Report-talk—Type of communication exchange that involves providing information and giving directives to one another

Resting pan splint—Rigid, static support of the forearm, wrist, and hand providing rest for joints in functional position

Restore—Intervention approach that focuses on helping a person regain lost skills

Rett syndrome—Progressive disorder caused by a mutation in the MECP2 gene on the X chromosome, primarily affecting girls; it results in the failure of the neurons in the brain to continue to synapse near the end of pregnancy or within the first few months after birth

Reversibility—Process by which objects that have been changed may be returned to their original state

Rheumatologist—Physician specializing in non-surgical treatment for patients with arthritis

Ritual—a type of routine that holds special meaning and purpose to the person, and that can be socially, culturally, and spiritually influenced

Role confusion—Sense of task futility, role inhibition, self-doubt, and isolation

Role experimentations—Actions taken by individuals to stretch the boundaries of the roles they currently have

Role fixation—Actions that a person takes to maintain existing roles and avoid role experimentation

Roles—Scripts of expected behaviors placed on people within their social systems that provide a way to identify who they are and what they do within the social system

Rough and tumble play—Type of play that involves gross motor rolling actions and physical contact with another person

Routines—Sequences of behaviors that an individual clusters to accomplish a task and organize time efficiently, without careful attention to each step

S

Schema—Mental frameworks individuals use to cope with and respond to environmental information

Schizophrenia—Mental health disorder characterized by psychotic symptoms including delusions, hallucinations, disorganized speech and behaviors, or disturbances in affect and thought

Scoliosis—Spine curved in an S shape and can cause uneven pressure on the ischium; the internal organs may become compressed and pushed out of their proper position as the body collapses upon itself

Scope of impact—Amount of influence a specific performance skill, pattern, or habit has on successful participation within various contexts

Screening—Initial step in the evaluation process to determine whether more intensive assessments need to be conducted

Secondary circular reactions—Nonreflex based response to a stimulus in the environment resulting in a continuation of the response pattern

Selective dorsal rhizotomy—Neurological surgical procedure used to reduce lower extremity muscle spasticity

Self-awareness—Ability to recognize when a task is completed satisfactorily

Sensation seeking—Behaviors which involve an individual consciously or subconsciously looking for various types of sensory input

Sensitivity—Psychometric property that indicates how much change in behavior a person needs to demonstrate before the assessment registers that change

Sensorimotor—Piaget's stage of development that lasts from birth to approximately 2 years of age and involves learning about the world through integrating sensory and motor experiences

Sensory diet—Specific sensory stimulation activities designed to meet an individual's sensory needs

Sensory hypersensitivity—Overreactive sensory systems when exposed to certain stimuli

Sensory integration (SI)—Frame of reference that (1) addresses how the brain receives, processes, interprets, and responds physically and emotionally to sensory information; and (2) focuses intervention on facilitating effective integrating, processing, and responding to sensory information

Sensory modulation—Individual's ability to regulate responses to tactile, auditory, visual, oral, gravitational, rotary, or other movements

Separation anxiety disorder—Excessive anxiety about separating from the primary caregiver or other person and place with whom the person is emotionally attached

Severe level of mental retardation—Represents an IQ range of 25–40 and the ability to learn to communicate basic ideas and perform self-care tasks

Service competency—Ability to (1) understand the purpose, scope, and bounds of various aspects of a service; (2) know the language to use and the procedures to follow when delivering the services; and (3) obtain the same information and outcomes as would a person when providing the same services

Shaping—Process to reinforce progressively closer approximations of a desired behavior

Shared attention—First stage of the DIR/Floortime program during which the adult encourages the child to briefly attend to the same object as the adult

Shift—When related to prehension, applies to the ability to use the pads of the thumb and fingers to separate two items (e.g., pages of a magazine)

Shopping—IADL encompassing the total shopping experience, including list preparation, item selection, purchase method, monetary transaction

Shunt—a thin, flexible tube with a one-way valve and reservoir that is inserted into a ventricle and then threaded under the skin and inserted into the abdominal cavity or the atrium of the heart to drain excess fluid in the brain

Simple rotation—When related to prehension, applies to the ability to roll an item between pads of the thumb and fingers

SOAP Note—Type of documentation that is divided into four sections and includes subjective information, objective information, assessment information, and a plan

Social competency—Ability of an individual to discriminate demands of a social setting, determine verbal and nonverbal skills necessary for the situation, execute those skills in a fluid manner appropriate to social norms, effectively perceive the reactions of others, and adjust to this feedback

Social context—Relationships of people with one another in groups, organizations, and societal systems

Social environment—Social groups and the occupational form that surround an individual's participation in activities and occupations

Social modeling—Involves presenting an adaptive model of social behavior that allows a person to learn through example

Social participation—Interactions with family, friends, peers, and community members in organized patterns that are recognized by society

Social play—Type of play which involves interaction with others; depending on the stage of development, it can involve attachment, bonding, imitation, and turn taking

Social referencing—Ability to attend to the emotional reactions of others to determine how to respond to ambiguous situations

Social skills training—Intervention technique that teaches individuals how to effectively listen to and communicate with others, manage behaviors, take turns, compromise, problem solve, and resolve conflicts

Social stories—Technique that uses simple words to tell a story depicting a problem a child has with a social situation

Socket—Part of a prosthesis which fits snugly over the residual limb and is the fundamental component to which the others are attached

Solitary play—Type of play in which the person centers on own activities

Spasticity—Type of cerebral palsy characterized by increased muscle tone and difficulty isolating individual muscle activity

Spatial perception—Ability to recognize spatial relationships between objects, including size, distance, and position

Spina bifida—Term commonly used to describe the myelomeningocele level of neural tube defect

Spiritual context—Sense, purpose, and meaning that individuals associate with their lives; may incorporate religious beliefs

Splint—External device that is applied to a body part for support, to provide immobilization, to correct or prevent deformity, or to provide assistance with movement of the body part

Spontaneous play—Type of play which involves engaging in play occupations without the elicitation of others

Stability—When related to posture, reflects the ability of an individual to hold one's position

Standardized assessments—Assessments based on established norms or criteria that allow comparison of performance across individuals and that follow specified administration, data recording, and scoring protocols

State of arousal—Internal state of readiness

Static balance—Ability to keep one's head, shoulders, hips, and feet aligned against gravity without moving

Structured environment—Contrived or simulated settings set up in a particular manner to elicit certain behaviors

Substance abuse—Maladaptive behaviors resulting from abuse of a legal or illegal substance, but does not involve a history of tolerance and withdrawal reactions

Substance dependence—Maladaptive behaviors resulting from abuse of a legal or illegal substance that involve tolerance and withdrawal reactions or patterns of compulsive usage

Superior pincer grasp—Type of grasp pattern characterized by the thumb tip in opposition to the first digit tip

Supervision—Cooperative process in which the supervisor and the supervisee are mutually responsible for the content, format, quality, and frequency of the feedback regarding performance

Support walker—Mobility aid designed for individuals who have some use of the legs, but require support at the pelvis and chest, and possibly the upper extremities and/or head

Swallowing—Act of bringing the saliva, liquid, and food from the mouth, through the esophagus, and to the stomach

Symbolic play—Type of play which develops between the ages of 2 to 3 years in which the child uses objects to represent something else and takes on imaginary roles

Symbolic representation—The understanding that an object, gesture, or word has meaning; children demonstrate this ability during pretend play

Symmetrical bilateral movements—Use of both hands and arms, or both legs to perform the same movement

Syntax—Arrangement of words in sentences

T

Tasks—Series of objective behaviors sequenced to achieve a specific goal

Telecommunication devices for the deaf (TDD)—Apparatus which allows individuals to send typed messages to one another through the telephone network that results in a visual and paper copy of the typed message

Temperaments—Manner of thinking, behaving, or reacting characteristic of a specific person

Temporal context—Point in time in the day, year, activity cycle, or life stage in which one engages in occupation; measurement is personally and culturally determined

Temporal factors—Person's chronological age, developmental stage, life cycle, and/or health status

Temporal organization—Initiation, continuation, sequencing and termination of a task or activity

Tendon release—Orthopedic procedure which involves lengthening of a muscle

Tendon transfer—Orthopedic procedure which moves the point of attachment of a tendon on a bone

Teratogens—Toxic substances or agents which cause malformations in a developing fetus

Terminal device—Part of an upper limb prosthesis which functions to grasp and hold objects; user can choose between two styles of terminal devices, a hook or a cosmetic hand

Tethered cord—Abnormality in which the spinal cord becomes trapped within the spinal column, which may result in changes in sensation, movement, or bowel and bladder function

Theory—Set of constructs organized in a particular manner to provide a systematic understanding of, and predictions about, the relationship between events or phenomena

Therapeutic use of self—Use of one's personality, insights, and judgments in a planned way within the intervention process

Thumb loop splint—Usually made from Neoprene™, assists in positioning thumb into abduction and opposition

Tongue thrust—Exaggerated, uncontrolled pushing of the food or fluid forward out of the mouth with the tongue

Topographical orientation—Understanding of the route to a location

Toxoplasmosis—Mild parasitic infection often causing birth defects

Transdisciplinary team—Group of individuals from different disciplines who work together collaboratively throughout the evaluation, intervention, and outcome processes, blending their expertise

Transformation—The understanding of how an object can change in size, shape, consistency, and color

Transition plan—Document included in a student's Individualized Education Program (IEP) which includes specific goals related to employment and/or any additional postsecondary education and outlines services required to meet these goals; should also include domestic, leisure, and community goals

Transition process—Procedure including formation of a transition team, development of a transition plan, and implementation of the transition plan goals and objectives

Transition services—Coordinated set of activities for a student with a disability that is designed to promote movement from school to postschool activities and is based on the individual student's needs, strengths, and interests; involves the development of a transition plan

Transition team—Committee consisting of the high school student, parent, school and community personal chosen to design and implement a transition plan to prepare the student to leave school and enter the community

Transverse—Congenital anomalies where the defect extends across the entire limb

Transverse complete forearm deficiency—Congenital below-elbow amputation

Transverse complete humeral deficiency—Unilateral above-elbow amputation

Treatment and Education of Autistic and Related Communication Handicap Children (TEACCH) program—Learning based intervention designed to manage behaviors and increase independent functioning of children and adolescents with special needs

Tripod grasp—Type of grasp pattern which involves opposition of the thumb to the index and middle fingers to provide increased stability when holding an object

Trust versus mistrust—Stage of development when infants learn to form basic trusting relationships as a result of positive and secure interactions with their caregivers

Two-way purposeful interactions—Third stage of the DIR/Floortime program during which the adult engages with the child by responding to and building upon the child's nonverbal gestures and facial expressions

Two-way purposeful problem-solving interactions—Fourth stage of the DIR/Floortime program during which the adult fosters complex, pre-verbal problem solving

U

Ulnar deviation—A drift of the metacarpalphalangeal joints toward the small finger

Ulnar deviation splint—Support fashioned around the metacarpophalangeal joints to maintain a neutral position or counter the drift of the joints toward the small finger

Universal design—Development of products, services, and environments which are created to be used by as many people as possible regardless of age, ability, or situation

Unoccupied play—Play which occurs when an infant is not interacting with others; the infant may momentarily watch an activity that occurs in their environment or engage in body play and gross motor activities

Upgrade—Slight changes made to increase the difficulty of an activity so that an individual is successful and correctly challenged for his/her present abilities

Useful habits and routines—Habits and routines that provide enough structure to enable a person to perform daily life tasks efficiently, yet allow enough flexibility to enable to adapt to various situations

V

Validity—Psychometric property, based on statistical procedures, used to determine how accurately the assessment tool measures what it purports to measure

Values—Feelings and thoughts individuals have about what is important to them

Vascular stenosis—Constriction of blood vessels

Verbal prompts—Words/phrases (verbal cues) or questions (verbal hints) to help refresh an individual's memory to encourage problem solving or initiation of the next step of a task

Verbal rehearsal—Memory technique of verbally reciting the steps of a task before initiating the skill

Very far transfer—Process of generalizing learning to a novel or different situation; specific to the multicontext treatment approach, to transfer skills learned during intervention to everyday situations

Violence prevention programs—Community- and school-based interventions to reduce or eliminate violence at the systems level by helping the students to master five core competences: self-awareness, social awareness, self-management, relationship skills, and responsible decision making

Virtual context—Electronic and other nonphysical context across time and distance

Visual attention—Alertness during visual task; ability to divide visual focus between two tasks

Visual closure—Ability to visualize a complete figure, even though it is partially drawn

Visual discrimination—Ability to detect differences and spatial relationships; includes the visual perceptual skills of form constancy, visual closure, figure-ground, and position in space

Visual imagery—Ability to visualize objects, actions, and ideas without seeing them

Visual memory—Ability to recall immediate (short-term memory) and distant (long-term memory) visual information

Vocational preparation—Knowledge and skill training necessary to gain employment

Volition—Motivational aspects of occupations

Voluntary release—Ability to intentionally let go of a handheld object; typically develops around 7 months of age

W

Work—Occupations that include paid and volunteer activities

Wrist unit—Part of an upper limb prosthesis that pronates, supinates, and rotates the terminal device to position it for various functional needs

Written directions—Clear and concise printed instruction

Index